A SHORT TEXTB

UNIVERSITY MEDICAL TEXTS

General Editor

SELWYN TAYLOR
D.M., M.Ch. (Oxon.), F.R.C.S.
Surgeon, Hammersmith Hospital,
Dean of the Royal Postgraduate Medical School

A Short Textbook of Surgery
(Second Edition)

SELWYN TAYLOR
D.M., M.Ch. (Oxon.), F.R.C.S.
Surgeon, Hammersmith Hospital,
Dean of the Royal Postgraduate Medical School

L. T. COTTON
M.Ch. (Oxon.), F.R.C.S.
Surgeon, King's College Hospital, London

A Short Textbook of Gynaecology and Obstetrics

G. D. PINKER
M.B., F.R.C.S., F.R.C.O.G.
Consultant Gynaecological Surgeon and Obstetrician, St. Mary's Hospital

D. W. T. ROBERTS
M.Ch., F.R.C.S., F.R.C.O.G.
Consultant Obstetrician and Gynaecologist, St. George's Hospital, London

A Short Textbook of Chemical Pathology
(Second Edition)

D. N. BARON
M.D., D.Sc., M.R.C.P., F.C.Path.
Professor of Chemical Pathology, Royal Free Hospital School of Medicine, London

A Short Textbook of Medical Microbiology
(Second Edition)

D. C. TURK
D.M., M.R.C.P., M.C.Path.
Senior Lecturer in Bacteriology, University of Newcastle upon Tyne

and

I. A. PORTER
M.D., M.C.Path.
Consultant Bacteriologist to the Ayrshire Area Laboratory Service,
Formerly Senior Lecturer in Bacteriology, University of Newcastle upon Tyne

A Short Textbook of Orthopaedics and Traumatology

J. N. ASTON
F.R.C.S.
Orthopaedic Surgeon, St. Bartholomew's Hospital, London

A Short Textbook of Psychiatry

W. L. LINFORD REES
B.Sc., M.D., F.R.C.P., D.P.M.
Professor of Psychiatry, St. Bartholomew's Hospital Medical School

A SHORT TEXTBOOK
OF
MEDICINE

J. C. HOUSTON
M.D., F.R.C.P.
Physician and Dean of the Medical and Dental Schools, Guy's Hospital, London

C. L. JOINER
M.D., F.R.C.P.
Physician, Guy's Hospital, London

J. R. TROUNCE
M.D., F.R.C.P.
Professor of Clinical Pharmacology and Sub-Dean of the Medical and Dental Schools, Guy's Hospital, London

THE ENGLISH UNIVERSITIES PRESS LTD

ISBN 0 340 08375 1 boards edition
ISBN 0 340 07518 X paper edition

First Edition 1962.   Reprinted 1964
Second Edition 1966.   Reprinted 1967
Third Edition 1968.   Reprinted 1970, 1971 (with revisions)
Fourth Edition 1972.

The English Universities Press Ltd
St Paul's House Warwick Lane London EC4P 4AH

Printed and bound in Great Britain
by Hazell Watson and Viney Ltd, Aylesbury

EDITOR'S FOREWORD

"Books must follow sciences, and not sciences books"

FRANCIS BACON

Textbooks of medicine are all too often so vast that the student could not possibly read them through but only use them as works of reference. Alternatively they are so brief and synoptic as merely to provide aides-mémoires in those crowded revision weeks before the final examination.

This entirely new text is intended for the medical student during his clinical apprenticeship. It is a concise account of the subject with more than enough material to satisfy the examiners for the final medical degree. It is intended to be read and reread until, with tattered covers, it is discarded, having served its purpose well.

Medicine is developing so rapidly at the present time that any textbook is out of date almost before it is published, therefore the days of great and comprehensive textbooks, like those of William Osler and Clifford Allbutt, are departed. What are required today are expendable texts based on the sure foundations of physiology and anatomy and giving due stress to the more recent advances in the subject.

This book is not designed for future reference, but rather for present instruction. It will be found that there is a freshness about its style which bespeaks the authors' active participation in the subject presented.

The demand for a new edition is very gratifying and a fitting tribute to such an excellent textbook. By dint of revising the text skilfully every three years, the authors have kept their book extremely up to date.

Royal Postgraduate Medical School,   SELWYN TAYLOR
Hammersmith Hospital,
London, W.12.

AUTHORS' PREFACE

The need for an inexpensive short textbook of medicine has been long felt and frequently expressed. Both the theory and practice of medicine are changing so quickly at the present time that any textbook is out of date within a very few years; what the clinical student requires, therefore, is a convenient and expendable manual of current medical practice rather than a large and comprehensive work "which he can use all his life". For wider reading he should be encouraged into the habit of consulting original sources in his medical school library, and to this end we have appended a few key references to the principal chapters. The practitioner anxious to keep abreast of the times may also welcome a book of this size, for we have deliberately given rather fuller treatment to the more rapidly developing branches of medicine.

Apart from four special chapters, the whole book has been written jointly by the three authors, the original draft of each section, written by one of us, being subjected to very free criticism and discussion by the other two before its final form was agreed. Our aim has been to write of medicine as we have seen it and practised it and to avoid wherever possible second-hand information and traditional statements. The book has not been produced with any examination in mind, but in spite of its small size we believe it provides a sound basis of reading for the Membership and more than enough to satisfy the Finals' examiners. There is no section on diseases of children, but all the other specialities which come from time to time within the province of the general physician have been included.

We are particularly grateful to Dr. A. G. Bearn for the chapter on human genetics; to Professor W. J. H. Butterfield for the chapter on medical aspects of radiation; to Dr. I. C. K. Mackenzie for the chapter on the nervous system; and to Dr. D. Stafford-Clark for the chapter on psychiatry.

Our thanks are due also to Dr. G. W. Scott, who revised the chapter on the respiratory system and contributed the section on respiratory function tests; to Mrs. C. Dawbarn and Mrs. K. Hasler of the Department of Medical Illustrations, Guy's Hospital; to Mr. W. H. G. Hill, who prepared the index; to Mr. J. Fennel, who reviewed the names of the drugs and the doses quoted throughout the book; and to the publishers, for their help and forbearance during the book's long gestational period.

J. C. HOUSTON
C. L. JOINER
J. R. TROUNCE

Guy's Hospital
London

PREFACE TO SECOND EDITION

The whole text has been very thoroughly revised and although many additions have been made, judicious pruning has enabled us to keep the increase in size to 10 pages.

We extend a welcome to Dr. G. W. Scott, who has now become responsible for the whole of the respiratory section. We are very grateful to the many friends and colleagues from all over the world, too numerous to mention, who have sent us helpful comments and suggestions. Particular thanks are due to Dr. M. J. Langman for help in revising the alimentary section, to Dr. W. L. Gent for invaluable assistance with the new chapter on acid-base regulation and to Mr. W. H. G. Hill who has again been responsible for the index. Our thanks are due also to the *Lancet* for permission to reproduce in modified form the figure on p. 108, and to the publishers for their continued excellent work on the production of the book.

PREFACE TO THIRD EDITION

The whole text has again been revised and major changes have been made in the chapter on the cardiovascular system. Disorders of water and mineral metabolism are now discussed with those of acid/base balance in a single chapter.

We are grateful to Professor S. Cohen for help with the chapter on auto-immune phenomena, to Miss Cynthia Lynes for the diagrams illustrating disorders of adrenal function, and to Dr. J. S. Cameron and the *Nursing Mirror* for permission to reproduce the figure on p. 373.

PREFACE TO FOURTH EDITION

The major change in this edition has been the complete revision of the chapter on disorders of immunity, with a new section by Professor S. Cohen on immunological reactions in clinical medicine. The chapter on medical aspects of radiation has been omitted.

The whole text has again been revised to keep it in line with modern medical practice but as a result of judicious pruning there has been very little increase in the total length of the book.

CONTRIBUTORS

A. G. BEARN, M.D.

Professor and Chairman, Dept. of Medicine,
Cornell University Medical College,
Physician-in-Chief, The New York Hospital, New York.

W. J. H. BUTTERFIELD, O.B.E., M.D., F.R.C.P.

Vice-Chancellor, University of Nottingham,
formerly Professor of Medicine, Guy's Hospital Medical School, London.

S. COHEN, M.D.

Professor of Chemical Pathology, Guy's Hospital Medical School, London.

I. C. K. MACKENZIE, M.D., F.R.C.P.

Physician for Nervous Diseases, Guy's Hospital, London.

G. W. SCOTT, M.D., F.R.C.P.

Physician, Guy's Hospital, London.
Physician to the Chest Clinic, Guy's Hospital, London.

D. STAFFORD-CLARK, M.D., F.R.C.P., D.P.M.

Physician for Psychological Medicine, Guy's Hospital, London.

CONTENTS

CHAPTER ONE

HUMAN GENETICS

Man is the product of his hereditary endowment interacting with his external environment. The bulk of this book is devoted to describing the ways in which alteration of man's environment causes disease, whereas this section will consist of a brief discussion of some of the hereditary aspects of disease. A hereditary component of variable importance exists in the aetiology of all disease. In infectious diseases, for instance, the hereditary component is usually relatively unimportant; in hypertension, it appears to be a contributory factor but not decisive, whereas in diseases such as haemophilia the genetic component is critical and the environmental influences unimportant. The subsequent discussion will be restricted to conditions in which the hereditary component is crucial. A few elementary facts should be recalled.

Chromosomes, the bearers of the hereditary material, are present in the cell nucleus of all tissues. In man, all somatic (diploid) cells have forty-six chromosomes; forty-four of these chromosomes are the same in both males and females and are called the autosomes. Females have in addition to the forty-four autosomes two X chromosomes; males have in addition to the autosomes one X and one Y chromosome. The bearers of the hereditary elements arranged linearly along the chromosomes are called genes and are composed of deoxyribonucleic acid (DNA). The specificity of non-genic molecules such as proteins is determined by the arrangement of purine and pyrimidine bases within the DNA molecule, and therefore the sequence of base pairs is referred to as the genetic code.

Mitosis

During mitosis, each chromosome duplicates and when cell division takes place one of the identical daughter chromosomes passes to each daughter cell. In this way, each daughter cell preserves the identical chromosomal constitution that occurred in the parental cell.

Meiosis

If the chromosome complement is to be retained at forty-six, a halving of the number of chromosomes must take place during the development of ovum and sperm for the normal complement to be restored in the fertilised ovum (zygote). This process of halving the number of chromosomes is called meiosis and results in a gamete with a haploid number of chromosomes (twenty-three). The essential feature of meiosis is that the cells divide twice while the chromosomes divide once.

CHROMOSOMAL ABNORMALITIES

Chromosomal abnormalities are found in approximately 20 per cent of spontaneous abortions and 0·7 per cent of births.

Disturbances in the normal mechanism of meiosis or mitosis may result in the formation of cells with an abnormal number of chromosomes. Until recently it had been assumed that variation in the total number of chromosomes would be lethal. Abnormal segregation of the chromosomes during meiosis or mitosis results in cells with an abnormal number of chromosomes. The most frequent abnormality is non-disjunction in which two chromosomes, members of the same pair, are incorporated in one daughter nucleus. Meiotic non-disjunction occurs more frequently with increasing maternal age.

Transfer of a chromosomal segment to a non-homologous chromosome is called a translocation. In this way chromosomal aberrations may occur despite a normal number of chromosomes. When the translocation results in an excess of chromosomal material, a specific error of development occurs in the zygote; no such effect is seen when there is deficiency of chromatin. Errors in somatic cell division may give rise to individuals with populations of cells with different chromosome numbers (chromosomal mosaics).

Mongolism (Down's Syndrome) (1 in 650 live births)

This disease, which accounts for 5 per cent of institutionalised patients with mental deficiency, is usually associated with forty-seven chromosomes. Rarely the additional chromosomal material is rearranged so that 46 chromosomes are seen but one chromosome appears larger than its normal partner (translocation). The mean age of the mother at the birth of a mongol child is thirty-seven compared with a mean of twenty-nine for all births. If the mother is age 25, the risk is 1/2,000, but at age 45 it is increased to 1/50. If the parents have had one mongol child the recurrence risk is about 2 per cent independent of maternal age. Exceptionally familial mongolism may occur.

Although the majority of mongols have three free 21 chromosomes (trisomy 21), a number of different chromosome complements have been described. Mitotic non-disjunction may lead to mongols who are chromosomal mosaics in which some of the patient's cells are trisomic 21 and some are normal. Some of these mosaics are so mildly affected as to be almost indistinguishable from normals, but they have a considerable risk of having mongol offspring, as cells in the gonadal tissue may be trisomic 21.

An important type of mongolism is due to translocation, often between chromosomes of the 13–15 group and a 21. As a consequence of receiving the 13–15/21 translocation, these mongols have only 46 chromosomes. The normal mothers of such mongols often carry the translocation chromosome and have 45 chromosomes (balanced translocation carriers). Familial mongolism, particularly in young mothers, is commonly due to translocation.

Klinefelter's Syndrome and Turner's Syndrome (1 in 400 male and 1 in 2,000 (XO) female live births respectively)

These diseases, which are described in detail elsewhere, are examples of non-disjunction of the X chromosome. Individuals with Klinefelter's syndrome have forty-seven chromosomes with an XXY constitution, whereas in Turner's syndrome the chromosome constitution is XO and the total complement only forty-five chromosomes. Mosaicism in sex anomalies is not infrequent.

XYY Syndrome (1 in 1,000 male births)

This recently described syndrome is characterized by a chromosomal complement of 47 with an extra Y chromosome. Individuals with this syndrome are often unusually tall and are particularly liable to exhibit aggressive criminal behaviour. In many instances, however, such individuals are physically and mentally normal.

GENETIC VARIATION

The position on the chromosome occupied by a gene is called a locus. At each locus there may be alternative genes (alleles). When both chromosomes carry the same gene at a particular locus individuals are said to be homozygous at that locus; if the genes are different they are said to be heterozygous. At some loci there may be multiple alleles (e.g. ABO blood groups). Five main types of inheritance can be recognised, autosomal dominant, autosomal recessive, autosomal co-dominant, sex-linked (X-linked) dominant and sex-linked (X-linked) recessive. Certain diseases may be inherited in more than one way. For example, there are two types of Hurler's syndrome (gargoylism), one of which is inherited as an autosomal recessive and one as an X-linked recessive.

Autosomal Dominant Traits

Dominant traits are those which are determined by a gene in the heterozygous state. Except for mutation, each affected individual will have one parent affected. On the average, affected individuals will have normal and abnormal offspring in equal proportions; the usual 1:1 ratio of a dominant gene. Normal offspring have all normal children, whereas abnormal children have normal and abnormal offspring in equal proportions. Sometimes the gene may be incompletely manifest, so that the descendants of the apparently unaffected person may be affected. This is called skipping of generations. Examples of autosomal dominant inheritance include lobster claw deformity, achondroplasia, neurofibromatosis and Huntington's chorea.

Autosomal Recessive Traits

A disease or trait which is only recognizable when a gene is present in the homozygous state is called recessive. Both parents of an affected individual are usually heterozygous for the gene in question, but are clinically normal. Although parents and all immediate ancestors are normal, sibs are likely to be affected. On the average, one quarter of the offspring of parents heterozygous for the same gene will be affected, one quarter will be normal and one half will be unaffected heterozygous carriers, like their parents. All children of affected individuals will be heterozygous for the abnormal gene. Due to the bias in locating families through an affected individual, the proportion of affected members in small sibships will usually exceed one-quarter. The incidence of consanguinity in the parents of individuals suffering from a *rare* recessive disease will be much greater than in the normal population. In some instances, the incidence of first-cousin marriage in the parents of affected individuals may be as high as 35 per cent instead of the normal incidence of 0·1–0·4 per cent in the United Kingdom. Most of the classical inborn errors of metabolism are inherited in an autosomal recessive fashion. Such conditions include phenylketonuria, albinism, alkaptonuria, Wilson's disease, galactosaemia and fibrocystic disease of the pancreas. Detection of heterozygous carriers of recessively determined disease is becoming increasingly important. A partial deficiency of the enzyme galactose-1-phosphate-uridyl transferase exists in the red cells of individuals heterozygous for galactosaemia, and a diminution of the enzyme phenylalanine hydroxylase is present in the liver of those carrying the gene for phenylketonuria.

Autosomal Co-dominant Traits

The abnormal haemoglobins illustrate this variety of inheritance. If an individual is homozygous (AA) for the gene which directs the synthesis of normal haemoglobin, only normal haemoglobin is synthesised. If he is homozygous for sickle haemoglobin (SS), only sickle haemoglobin is formed. The heterozygote (AS), in whom there is a gene for normal haemoglobin and a gene for sickle haemoglobin, will produce approximately equal amounts of normal and sickle haemoglobin.

Dominant X-linked Traits

Affected males will transmit the trait to their daughters but not to their sons. Heterozygous affected females will transmit the trait to half their sons and half their daughters. Vitamin D resistant rickets due to renal phosphaturia and glucose-6-phosphate dehydrogenase deficiency are transmitted as dominant X-linked traits.

Recessive X-linked Traits

Haemophilia is the classical example of an X-linked recessive disease. The pedigree is highly characteristic. The disease is restricted to males but transmitted by females. Affected individuals frequently have affected maternal uncles. An affected man who marries a normal woman will have normal sons and normal daughters. All his daughters, however, will be carriers. When such a carrier marries a normal man, on the average half the sons will be affected and half the daughters will be carriers. These facts can be verified by the construction of a chromosome diagram.

Biochemical Genetics

Understanding of classical Mendelian genetics is a necessary prerequisite to the interpretation of pedigrees of disease, but human genetics extends beyond these narrow bounds. Biochemical genetics, as a result of the early work of Archibald Garrod, has progressed so far that it is now possible, in a few instances, to pin-point the precise function of a gene. The only detectable difference between normal and sickle haemoglobin is that in the molecule of sickle haemoglobin valine has been substituted for glutamic acid in one peptide; this is a remarkable example of how the substitution of a single amino acid in a protein molecule can determine the difference between health and disease.

Genetic Counselling and Amniocentesis

The need for genetic counselling in inherited disease is increasing rapidly and includes two facets: the estimate of the genetic risk and the humane presentation of the risk to the patient. In clear cut inherited disease the risks follow Mendelian laws as outlined above; in many congenital abnormalities or diseases in which the magnitude of the genetic component is unclear, such as congenital heart disease, precise information on the risk of recurrence is not available and counselling must rely on 'empiric risk figures'. Recently, genetic counselling has been greatly advanced by the introduction of the technique of amniocentesis. Withdrawal of amniotic fluid can be safely performed between the 14th and 16th week of pregnancy. Culture of the fetal cells contained in the amniotic fluid enables the detection of a variety of chromosomal abnormalities including mongolism. In addition, using appropriate biochemical techniques an increasing number of inborn errors of metabolism such as Gaucher's disease and Tay Sachs disease can be detected. As a result of such studies, abortion of the affected fetus may be indicated.

FURTHER READING

Fraser Roberts, J. A. *An Introduction to Medical Genetics*. 5th edition. Oxford, 1970.

Clarke, C. A., *Genetics and the Clinician*. 2nd edition. Blackwell, Oxford, 1964.

Stanbury, J. B., Wyngaarden, J. B. and Frederickson, D. S., *The Metabolic Basis of Inherited Disease*. 3rd edition. McGraw-Hill, New York, 1971.

CHAPTER TWO

PSYCHIATRY

THE NATURE OF THE SUBJECT

Psychiatry is that part of medicine which is primarily concerned with disorders of thought, feeling, and behaviour. In one sense all illness or injury, and indeed all suffering of any kind, involves disorder of feeling; and this is one of the reasons why the basic principles of psychiatry are vital to a proper understanding of medicine and surgery as a whole. But the special province of psychiatry is the understanding of those disorders of subjective experience or objective behaviour which are themselves a cause of disability.

They may be primary, or secondary to some other illness or structural damage. The disturbance of experience or behaviour to which they give rise may be apparent to the sufferer, in which case he is said to have insight for the nature of his illness; or he may be entirely unaware that he is ill or disabled in this way, and may attribute his experience or predicament to changes in the world around him. All this every doctor must be able to acknowledge, to understand, to diagnose, and, at least in some degree, to treat. Psychiatry in fact includes in its concern that most human aspect of human beings, their awareness of themselves, and their capacity to communicate with each other.

THE CLINICAL APPROACH

As in general medicine and surgery, this consists in the discovery of the presenting complaint—or reason for the consultation, if the patient is not personally complaining of anything—followed by history and examination.

The first necessity is to permit the patient to tell his troubles in his own words. A few minutes' patient listening will often elicit a tale of woe whose degree of involvement of thought, feeling, and general experience may point clearly to the nature of the underlying diagnosis. The next step is an adequate history whose foundation rests upon the following aetiological considerations:

(1) Heredity and constitution.
(2) Environmental factors; including past physiological and psychological stresses, and present life situation.
(3) The cumulative effect of these two in producing disturbance of normal psychophysiological equilibrium.

Family History

Family history is important for the light it throws upon the start which the patient had in life, as well as the stock from which he sprang. It should extend back as far as the grandparents on both sides of the family, and should include available information about first cousins, uncles, and aunts, as well as parents and siblings. Specific enquiries should be made about the incidence of serious illness or 'nervous breakdown' in the family. More intensive investigation need be undertaken in this field only if there is evidence of a strong genetic factor in the illness.

In general, constitutional factors are of greatest importance in mental deficiency, certain disturbances of instinctual development and behaviour such as homosexuality or addiction, profound instability of mood, and schizophrenia; and considerably less important in acute emotional re-actions to severe environmental stress, and acquired patterns of behaviour arising from them.

Personal History

Personal history carries the story from infancy up to the present per-sonal, marital, or occupational difficulties, tracing these and the develop-ment of personality which preceded them, through childhood and re-lationships with parents and siblings, school days and relationships with fellow pupils and teachers, adolescence, with awakening of psycho-sexual needs and relationships with members of the same and opposite sex, adult life, and the achievement of present relationships with fellow human beings and the rest of the world. Against the background of this life-story must be sought the readjustments, ambitions, daydreams, and disappointments which have contributed to shaping the character and behaviour of the patient.

History of Previous Illnesses

Must cover all serious illnesses to which the patient has been subject, both structural and functional. Particular attention should be paid to unexplained absence from school or work, or vague periods of ill health. It is always worth while enquiring whether the patient has ever had any kind of nervous breakdown, or suffered from a similar illness to the one which afflicts him now.

Personality before Illness

This should be an assessment of the kind of person the patient was, in the estimation of a reliable relative, friend, or other informant.

> Examples: ? Energetic, bright, cheerful . . .
> ? Always a worrier . . .
> ? Bold or timid; boisterous or a quiet sort of per-son . . .
> ? Conscientious or lackadaisical . . .

The general level of mood, and capacity for relationship with other people, should be included.

History of Present Complaint

Establish when the patient was last quite well. Establish the circumstances of onset of the condition and the symptoms at that time. Try to find out as much detail as possible about the situation in which the patient was placed when the illness began; his home environment, social situation, work situation, etc. Then trace the development of the illness from this onwards, noting the factors which influenced its course.

A complete history along these lines may take between half and three-quarters of an hour. The time will be well spent. Such a history will achieve two invaluable goals; not only will a complete picture of the patient as well as his complaint steadily emerge, but the rapport, gratitude, and confidence felt by a patient for the doctor who thus displays so careful and penetrating an interest in his case will itself prove of therapeutic importance.

Physical Examination

This is important whether or not there is any evidence of structural abnormality, and whether or not the patient complains of physical symptoms. Physical examination, gently but purposefully and professionally undertaken, creates a bond of sympathy and acceptance. Anything the doctor may subsequently have to say to the patient will have gained strength and authority from this essential preliminary, even when physical findings indicative of structural disease have neither been anticipated nor obtained.

Examination of Mental State

This is as definite and invaluable a technique as the physical examination, and is as indispensable a part of the equipment of the clinician.

Observations should be assessed and recorded under the following headings:

(1) General appearance and behaviour.
(2) Talk: manner and content.
(3) Subjective state: mood and attitude to consultation.
(4) Content of thought.
(5) Contact with reality.
(6) Sensorium and formal intelligence.
(7) Insight and judgement.

Observations under the first three headings will already have been made during the course of the general history and physical examination. Patient's situation may include subjective distress as well as disturbance of thought, feeling, or behaviour of which he may not be wholly aware.

Such distress will presumably have been mentioned in the statement of initial complaint when this has been made, and may have been described as pain, exhaustion, uneasiness, apprehension, fear, or a vague and general sense of malaise.

In recording observations about the patient's manner and content of talk, attention should be paid to any special characteristics such as slowing, flight of ideas, incoherence, or evasiveness. Similarly, his attitude to the consultation should have become apparent by the time formal examination of mental state has been reached.

Disorder of mood requires assessment in the light of the patient's life situation. *Anxiety* is the commonest of all unpleasant human emotional experiences. It has been described as fear spread out thin. *Depression* of mood, with sadness or foreboding which exceed the patient's own capacity to justify or explain, or which may be related to a general and intolerable deterioration in himself and the world, may also be directly conveyed. Less often *unreasonable exaltation* may be encountered; and the patient may show an elevation of mood which may shade off into *frank excitement*, clearly abnormal and inappropriate to his circumstances.

Content of thought will include:

    (1) Disorders of thinking.
    (2) Obsessive compulsive symptoms.
    (3) Ideas of reference.

Disorders of thinking include *thought block*, whereby the patient's capacity to maintain a train of thought is constantly interrupted; *retardation* when thinking is perceptibly slowed, or *acceleration*, when it is speeded up to produce an effect of incoherence with ideas tumbling over each other as the patient attempts to express them. *Flight of ideas*, with multiple associations, may have been revealed in talk by an incoherent jumble of senseless rhymes or puns.

Obsessive compulsive ideas emerge as preoccupations, which are recognised as unreasonable, but from which the patient cannot free himself. Such obsessive ideas, and actions dictated by them, form a particular group of distressing symptoms which patients may be prepared to discuss only when they feel that the doctor is at least familiar with the possibility of their occurrence, and sympathetic to their description.

Ideas of reference involve a disturbance of judgement and interpretation of external reality whereby the patient tends to relate external circumstances to himself, and so comes to believe that almost everything that happens has some special meaning directed towards him. This kind of thought disorder leads naturally to *delusions*, in explanation of the otherwise incomprehensible picture of the world which the patient obtains.

Contact with reality may be disturbed by *delusions, hallucinations*, and *illusions*. A *delusion* is a false or mistaken belief, which has for the patient the force of conviction, and is firmly held despite all evidence to the contrary. A *hallucination* is perception through one of the senses, which does not correspond to any stimulus in the outside world; whereas an *illusion* is a similar perception, which, although produced by an external stimulus, is misinterpreted by the patient in purely subjective terms.

Examples will make these three descriptive terms clear. If someone believes that he is being kept under constant observation by unknown enemies through radar or television, is having his food poisoned, or the air in his room contaminated by gas pumped through the ceiling, and cannot be induced to modify these beliefs, although they remain demonstrably untrue, then he is suffering from delusions. If he hears voices or sees visions, which no one else can hear or see, or smells, for example, the gas which he believes to be entering the room, and if these experiences are in fact projections of his own fantasy, released by illness, then he is hallucinated. If, on the other hand, he mistakes his doctor or nurse for his father or mother, or for the devil come to take him away, then he is suffering from illusions, which are being grafted on to the normal experience of seeing people, whose identity he misconstrues.

Delusions may be primary or secondary. Primary delusions are ideas which arise spontaneously in the patient's mind, and which, although manifestly false, possess for the patient a degree of subjective certainty and conviction which nothing can alter. Secondary delusions are equally mistaken ideas of similar intensity and conviction, but which represent the patient's attempt to find a reasonable explanation for hallucinations, ideas of reference, or primary delusions, otherwise naturally inexplicable.

A more diffuse disturbance of contact with reality is provided by a loss of that subjective conviction of the actual identity between one's self and one's body, or of the actuality of the rest of the world, normally taken for granted. Impairment in these fields is called depersonalisation, or derealisation, respectively.

Sensorium and Formal Intelligence

Particular attention should be directed to recent and remote memory, to attention, concentration, grasp, and judgement. The patient's ability to understand what is said to him, and to make appropriate response, although naturally subject to interference by hallucinations or delusions, ideas of reference, or occasionally by obsessive preoccupation with painful, unpleasant or frightening ideas, will also come under this heading. Direct testing will elicit:

Orientation. For place, date and persons.

Memory. (a) Remote past (this will have been tested in taking the preliminary history).

(b) Recent past—some account of the last few days.

(c) Immediate retention. Telephone number, name, address; name of a flower, objects shown, repetition of a series of digits forwards and backwards (normally six digits should be retained forwards and at least four reversed). A simple anecdote, taking not more than one or two minutes to tell, can be repeated by the patient in his own words; and a formal sentence, such as the Babcock sentence, given to the patient for immediate repetition.

'One thing a Nation must have to become rich and great is a good secure supply of wood.'

Attention. Steady or fluctuating; distractability.

Grasp of general information (current news in press or on radio).

Ability to perform simple calculations. Change for small sums of money; serial subtraction of 7 from 100 (note errors: time in seconds).

Judgement. Ability to make reasonable plans.

Insight into illness. Does the patient realise that he is ill? If he does, is he able to accept his illness as responsible for the symptoms of which he complains, or does he consider, for example, that the persecution to which he is being subjected is the cause of his illness, and not the outcome of it?

EVALUATION OF FINDINGS

Examination of the mental state provides the raw material for the clinical study of personality in health and sickness, in terms of thought, feeling, and behaviour. Their respective contribution to the total personality of an individual can conveniently be assessed in terms of three abstractions:

(1) Intelligence.
(2) Emotional integration.
(3) Instinctual drive.

The purpose of abstractions of this kind is to provide a framework for clear description and understanding; just as the concepts of dimensions, length, breadth, and thickness and mass are useful abstractions in the description of solid objects.

Intelligence may be defined as the capacity to interpret experience, to learn from it, and to modify behaviour in the light of it. It can be measured with reasonable objectivity and accuracy, and is distributed throughout the population in a predictable way.

Formal tests of intelligence are not based upon the subject's knowledge, but upon his ability to learn, and particularly to recognise and abstract logical patterns from experience, and to apply these patterns to the solution of problems. Tests of intelligence can be adjusted to the overall capacity of the subject under examination. The natural development of intelligence, like physical growth, is normally completed by about the age of sixteen. Wisdom, judgement, and experience continue; but the innate capacity which has been achieved by the late teens or early twenties may not thereafter increase.

Emotion may be defined as a combination of subjective feeling and objective physiological change. It provides the drive underlying behaviour, as well as the subjective response and accompaniment to experience.

Emotional integration is not necessarily related to intelligence. This is exemplified in everyday experience by the fact that childishness in adults is not confined to the stupid. Emotional integration can be regarded as the capacity of an individual to preserve a balance and consistency both in the way he feels about people and things, and what he does about them.

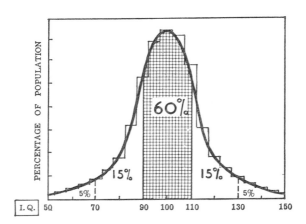

This figure indicates the characteristic graph obtained when the numbers of any large random sample of a population are plotted against the I.Q. levels of the individual members. It will be seen to be a symmetrical normal curve of distribution. Taking the Intelligence Quotient of 100 as the standard mean average level for the population, significant features are

(1) 60 per cent of the population have an I.Q. between 90 and 110.
(2) A further 30 per cent are distributed symmetrically on either side of this (15 per cent 70–90; 15 per cent 110–130).
(3) The remaining 10 per cent show an equally symmetrical distribution between subnormality (5 per cent below I.Q. 70) and outstanding intellectual endowment (5 per cent 130 upwards).

As general guiding indications, successful completion of a professional training demands an I.Q. of not less than 120: 4 'O' levels in G.C.E., not less than 110; and a strictly average I.Q. of 100 equips its owner for no more than artisan occupation under supervision.

It provides an index of the resilience and stability of a personality; and, like intelligence, it normally matures with age.

Instincts are innate combinations of emotion and behaviour, directed towards goals unrelated to previous experience, which emerge spontaneously during the lifetime of an individual, and develop without having to be learned or acquired from outside. Strength of instinctual drive, like intelligence and capacity for emotional integration, varies from one individual to another; it is the principal determinant of that individual's basic level of persistence, flexibility, explosiveness, or stability of conduct.

CLASSIFICATION

A convenient and practical classification arises naturally from the developmental approach:

A. Disorders primarily due to failure of normal development

(1) *Amentias.* Under the new Mental Health Act, the official designation of patients with this disability is subnormal, or severely subnormal. The intellectual failure is the most evident component, but emotional maturation is inevitably involved.

(2) *Immaturities of Personality.* These are essentially emotional in origin, and do not necessarily involve any kind of intellectual impairment.

(3) *Anomalies of Instinct.*

B. Disorders primarily due to abnormal development, or reaction to internal or external stress (including infection, exhaustion, structural and physiological change, as well as emotional experience)

(4) *Functional Neurosis:*
   Hysterical Reactions.
   Obsessive Compulsive Reactions.

(5) *Affective Disorders:*
   Anxiety States.
   Depressive Illnesses.
   Mania.
   Hypomania.

(6) *Schizophrenic psychoses.*

(7) *Acute confusional states* and other psychiatric emergencies.

(8) *Puerperal psychoses.*

(9) *Psychosomatic reactions*, and special syndromes.

(10) *Dementias.*

The distinction between neuroses and psychoses implicit in the immediately preceding section is arbitrary and purely clinical, but of considerable practical value. Under its terms, a *neurosis* is a disorder of mental function whereby patients are abnormally emotionally vulnerable or upset but retain touch with external reality, whereas a *psychosis* is a form of mental illness, whether acute or chronic, which actually interferes with the patient's understanding and appreciation of what is going on in the world about him. As has already been indicated, this distortion of contact with reality, and interpretation of experience, is characteristically produced by ideas of reference, primary delusions, or hallucinations, thereafter supported by delusions, with a total disruption of normal judgement and appreciation of normal reality.

This classification, considered in detail under separate headings, will be found to cover the whole range of clinical psychiatry, with the exception of that special branch of the subject dealing with children.

THE COMMON AND IMPORTANT CLINICAL CONDITIONS

AMENTIAS

This term can be used to cover all conditions characterised by subnormal mental development, present at birth or early childhood, and presenting essentially as a limitation of intelligence. The intelligence quotient, expressed as a percentage of the average level of intelligence of the community as a whole, is below 70–75 in patients suffering from amentia.

Before the Mental Health Act, 1959, three categories were officially recognised for administrative and practical convenience: feeble-minded, or high-grade defectives, with intelligence quotients of 50–75; imbeciles from 20–50, and idiots below 20. The practical value of this classification is that high-grade defectives can learn to perform simple tasks and to this degree can become self-supporting; imbeciles, while requiring care and protection throughout their lives, can at least feed themselves and develop human relationships; while idiots are considerably less intelligent than domestic animals, and have to be guarded against common physical dangers. The official legal term for high-grade defectives is now SUBNORMAL, and for imbeciles and idiots, SEVERELY SUBNORMAL.

Incidence. It is probable that some degree of amentia is present in 5 per cent of all live births. However, the mortality of idiots is high in infancy, and the number of individuals surviving the age of two with amentia probably represents about 2 per cent of the population.

Aetiology. Amentia is primarily a constitutional disorder, although environmental factors are believed to play a significant part in some cases. The genetic component is probably multiple and recessive; in the majority of individuals it is not pathological. The genetic difference between a high-grade defective and someone who is simply dull and rather stupid is one of degree rather than of intrinsic quality. But in the lower ranges of amentia there are certain specific genetic factors which make it impossible for normal development to take place.

Environmental contributions include damage in utero from virus infections, for example rubella during the second month of pregnancy; birth injury; hypoxia during intra-uterine life, or in the course of delivery; and major disasters in the form of injury or infection involving the brain in infancy or early life.

Clinical Features. Generally speaking the lower the scale the patient is placed mentally, the greater the extent to which anatomical and physiological congenital abnormalities will be combined with defect. Deformed or misshapen skull structure, variations in size of the head, limbs or body, and in development of the cardiovascular system, are common anomalies. At the upper end of the scale, normal physical development is the rule.

Idiots are wholly dependent. They cannot be taught to feed themselves, to keep themselves clean, nor can they recognise other people or communicate with them except in the crudest and most primitive way. Their emotional responses reflect this general crudity: when frustrated they may bite or scratch themselves. They tend to pull out their hair and eat it. Unlike imbeciles, whose emotional state is usually readily apparent, they appear to be neither happy nor unhappy in the accepted sense of these descriptions.

Imbeciles, while being by definition unable to learn in the ordinary sense of the word, may acquire certain striking accomplishments on an essentially automatic basis. For example, they may be able to memorise railway timetables, and produce answers to questions put purely along these lines with startling rapidity and accuracy. However, they are unable to apply these feats, which are a form of 'party piece', to any general purpose, and their capacity for dealing with abstract thought is negligible. They tend to be happily dependent creatures who appreciate affection and respond frequently with docility and obedience to kind and sympathetic handling. However, the immaturity and instability of their emotional and intellectual balance may be brought out disastrously by their response to sexual or aggressive impulses. Allowed to roam about without care or supervision they may commit murder, rape, or arson with as little concern or appreciation of the nature of their actions as they show towards some minor delinquency. A high proportion of the ranks of prostitutes, vagrants, and petty recidivists are found on examination to suffer from a degree of mental defect.

The personality of people with amentia, like that of everybody else, varies widely from one individual to another. Some are gentle and kindly, others rough, deceitful and vindictive. Like everybody else, they display in this not only a constitutional but also a reactive and environmental aspect. With the best available type of upbringing, less than 10 per cent of all defectives show anti-social or troublesome behaviour. But the capacity of even the highest patients with amentia, those who can be taught a simple trade, depends as much upon their character and personalities as upon the level of their intelligence.

Diagnosis. This is based essentially upon examination of the features immediately described, together with formal intellectual testing. The special clinical types of amentia such as cretinism, mongolism, and those due to specific biochemical anomalies such as phenylketonuria, are essentially parts of the domain of child psychiatry and as such are excluded from consideration in this textbook.

Other forms of specific mental defect with a clear-cut genetic pattern, such as tuberose sclerosis (epiloia) and familial amaurotic idiocy (Tay-Sachs's disease), due respectively to a simple dominant and to a simple recessive gene, are of interest purely as curiosities, and will not be further described.

Treatment. Apart from cretinism and biochemical anomalies such as phenylketonuria, treatment for mental defect is essentially the provision of adequate care, management, and training suited to the innate capacities of the individual. The prognosis for all cases is limited by the innate constitutional and structural nature of the underlying disorder, which is a failure in the complexity and development of the brain and nervous system. Nevertheless, high-grade aments can lead useful and productive lives, often performing with encouragement tasks which give them satisfaction, but which would be too repetitive and boring for more fortunately endowed members of the community to tolerate.

PERSONALITY IMMATURITY
      (1) Psychopathic personality.
      (2) Hysterical personality.
      (3) Marginal immaturity.

Psychopathic Personality
Definition. Psychopathic personality represents a failure of maturation of personality whose impact is evident not so much in the mind or feelings of the patient, as in his conduct, and particularly in his failure to make an effective adjustment with the rest of society. This is the fundamental abnormality of the psychopath, and although characteristically independent of any degree of intellectual impairment or mental defect, it corresponds in terms of personality development to a failure to emerge from the explosive period of early infantile development. The psychopath has not matured emotionally beyond the age of four or five.

This failure is evident in a number of related fields: the E.E.G. record tends to be dominated by wave forms of frequency and distribution normally seen only in children below the age of five. Capillary structure, directly visible through the skin of the nail-bed, displays a corresponding preponderance of infantile forms. The psychological attitudes, no less than the personal history and day-to-day behaviour of the psychopath, remain understandable on a basis of explosive childishness rather than by postulating any other kind of abnormality of adult function.

Incidence. The incidence of psychopathic personality in the population as a whole is almost impossible to estimate. It is probably not higher than 0·25 per cent. One objective estimate of incidence which has been made, concerns that proportion of psychopaths to be found among the prison population. Research studies suggest that 5 per cent of the prison population are of psychopathic personality.

Aetiology. Hereditary, constitutional, and environmental factors have all been invoked. The hereditary component is difficult to assess, but where present is probably related to multi-factorial recessive genes. The constitutional element is undoubted, and will often account for the emergence of psychopathic personality in one member of the family, when parental relationships and siblings are apparently normal in every respect. Further supporting evidence for a constitutional component is to be found in the E.E.G., capillary, and other psychophysiological findings. The striking lack of correlation with intellectual development remains unexplained.

Clinical Features and Diagnosis. The psychopath can be regarded as falling between the insane and the criminal personality. He is recognisable as 'the black sheep of the family', the 'bad hat', or the 'bad penny who is always turning up'. At one time he was sent abroad to become a remittance man, nowadays he may attempt to solve his problems by crime or sponging on family or friends, and frequently ends up in prison. Psychopaths are essentially people who seem completely unable to live on ordered terms with society: their inadequacy or badness is part of a true disability for which we have no wholly satisfactory treatment.

They tend to be explosive personalities with a very low tolerance for stress, who either cannot or will not conform to existing standards of behaviour. They may display tantrums, sulks or running away as patterns surviving from childhood, when they cannot cope with the situation. An example was a young man who landed himself in a military prison on the eve of being commissioned because he masqueraded as an officer two days before he actually would have become one, simply to impress a casual acquaintance. Psychopaths want what they want immediately, whatever the consequences. They seem unable to postpone gratification for the sake of future stability or success. They may be intelligent or dull; but are especially inadequate in social relationships; and they tend to work out their problems on their environment, rejecting medical or psychological help except as an emergency measure in extreme crises. Even then they will exploit such help rather than co-operate with it if they can. They appear to have strong inner demands, and are emotionally intractable. They act on impulse, attempt to live out their fantasies, and very rarely display foresight or wisdom. They attempt instead to distort and misinterpret reality to make it fit their own self-centred concepts.

The environmental factor, particularly the relationship existing between child and parents in the first ten years of life, is clearly important. In practice the diagnosis is reserved for adults, since apparently psychopathic behaviour in childhood and adolescence may subside without lifelong disturbance following.

The diagnosis is reached by means of the life history and the evidence of physiological and psychological immaturity already indicated. Of particular importance is the work record, in which a large number of jobs whose average duration does not exceed six months over several years is characteristic.

Treatment. In this, as in all subsequent clinical sections, treatment will be referred to simply in terms indicating its general nature. There is a special section on treatment in general on p. 46.

Patients with psychopathic personality rarely complain of their personality disorder as such: they are likely to seek treatment either for the immediate predicament in which they have become involved or for the reaction which it has evoked: for example, a state of anxiety or depression.

Basically the object of treatment must be to reinforce whatever latent tendency may exist towards maturation of personality. This can sometimes be achieved by group psychotherapy, preferably under residential conditions; very occasionally by skilled intensive individual psychotherapy. Such work is particularly liable to involve the doctor in disappointment and frustration because often the psychopath will attempt to exploit the medical relationship in exactly the same way as he has attempted to exploit all other relationships throughout his life. But this is not a reason for refusing to try to help psychopaths, since, in their variety, pathos, and sporadically savage or helpless lovelessness, these people constitute a formidable challenge, not simply to medicine but to mankind.

Hysterical Personality

Definition. Hysterical personality is the outcome of a failure of maturation less profound than that of psychopathic personality but, nevertheless, sufficiently marked and definite to constitute a basic psychological syndrome. Whereas the psychopath's emotional development has remained infantile, the patient with hysterical personality has reached the stage of childhood but has failed to emerge from adolescence. Once again, this failure of emancipation from a childhood relationship with parents and the rest of the world is quite unrelated to intelligence.

Incidence. This can be estimated only on clinical impression; but it is probable that between 5 and 10 per cent of the population display emotional immaturity of this degree of severity.

Aetiology. As with psychopathic personality, constitutional and environmental factors are both important. In the environmental contribution, the key factor appears to be an incomplete and very often deeply divided emotional relationship to one or both parents, characteristically the parent of the opposite sex. It is as though the patient had failed to complete that part of the growing-up process whereby the child's dependence upon the parent is replaced by adult respect and regard.

Clinical Features. The person with an hysterical personality tends to be characterised on the psychological side by an outgoing extroverted attitude, a relatively good capacity to make superficial contact with other people, a histrionic type of behaviour with a strong tendency to dramatisation, and a measurably high degree of suggestibility. On the physical side there is evidence of anatomical and physiological immaturity comparable to that of the psychopath, but correspondingly less pronounced.

People of this kind tend, therefore, to be both over-demanding and yet shallow in their relationships to others, to display something of the irresponsibility of children towards adult decisions, and a good deal of the child's helplessness in dealing with the complications with which such irresponsibility inevitably confronts them. This is apt to be the more striking, and socially unacceptable, because of the articulateness and obvious intelligence often possessed by this type of individual. In the light of this it is understandable that such patients frequently develop neurotic reactions to the inevitably painful and infinitely complicated processes of adult emotional adjustment, for which they are not fully equipped.

Diagnosis. This is essentially a matter of clinical assessment, and is not difficult once the existence of this type of personality disorder is recognised. The decisive feature is the apparently incorrigible, manipulative childishness displayed throughout the patient's entire attitude to life. The manipulative quality is particularly characteristic. Just as an insecure child plays off one parent against the other in his unconsciously desperate attempt to gain some kind of relative security, so the adult with hysterical personality contrives the same kind of manipulation between doctors, family, and friends, helplessly, almost always to his own ultimate detriment, and yet with an uncannily perceptive intuitive skill which creates its own tensions and exploits the vulnerability of all who come into contact with the patient.

Treatment. This is usually required for symptoms of overt hysterical illness, anxiety, or depression, arising out of the general circumstances created by such patients in their ineffectual attempts to deal with the problems of adult life. The initial impression is that here, above all, is a most suitable subject for individual psychotherapy. The combination of intelligence, rapport, apparent insight, and a sincerely appealing and convincing desire for help is apt to prove irresistible. Unfortunately, experience is a bitter guide, since the innate and constitutional element of immaturity tends ruthlessly to limit both the degree of co-operation and therefore the amount of progress of which such patients are capable. Supportive psychotherapy is often in the long run the best that can be offered, together with appropriate symptomatic treatment for the particular syndrome which they present on the occasion of consultation.

Marginal Emotional Maturity, not amounting to psychopathic or hysterical personality, probably underlies a good deal of the aetiology of all neurotic illnesses. It will be further mentioned in descriptions of the specific syndromes to which it contributes.

INSTINCTUAL ANOMALIES

    (1) Homosexuality.
    (2) Sexual perversions.
    (3) Addiction to drugs or alcohol.

Homosexuality

Homosexuality occurs as a normal phase in sexual development, during adolescence. It may persist into adult life as a specific failure of emotional maturation, or reappear under conditions of stress or deprivation—for example, in prison. Twin studies suggest that constitutional factors are more important than environmental contributions to its aetiology, but there is no discoverable structural or endocrinological basis for the disorder. It has been estimated that about 4 per cent of the adult population of both sexes are confirmed homosexuals—having never experienced either sexual desire or orgasm except with their own sex—while up to 25 per cent of men and about 15 per cent of women enter upon frankly homosexual adult relationships at one time or another.

This latter group may respond to individual psychotherapy by completing instinctual development to established heterosexuality; but the most that can be offered the 4 per cent of confirmed homosexuals is mitigation of their sense of social isolation, ostracism, guilt, and shame. This is not made easier, in the case of men, by the existent criminal law.

Sexual Perversions

Bestiality is the name given to intercourse with animals. It is virtually confined to grossly emotionally and intellectually immature men in close contact with beasts—for example, shepherds, cowmen, and ostlers.

Fetishism is the substitution of a symbolic object for the normal goal of union with a member of the opposite sex, as fulfilment of the sexual instinct. The object may be a particular part or aspect of the normal goal, such as the hair or the feet or buttocks; or it may be more remote—for example, an article of clothing. This in turn may have to be worn by the intended partner for orgasm to be possible; or in some cases orgasm may be prompted by the sight or touch of the object alone.

Fetishism is almost exclusively a male perversion, probably because projections and symbolic associations to sexual excitement normally contribute much more to male than to female instinctual patterns.

Successful treatment by appropriate individual psychotherapy is possible in about half the cases.

Transvestism means literally the wearing of clothes characteristic of the opposite sex, and in some cases may represent a special form of fetishism, in which subject and object are combined. Often, however, transvestites identify themselves completely with the opposite sex, and may even develop delusional convictions along these lines. These may lead them to press for 'Change of Sex operations', for which there can never be psychiatric justification. A proportion of such patients do, however, respond to psychotherapy.

Sadism and *Masochism* are pathological exaggerations respectively of the normal aggressive and submissive components of sexuality. Wherever they violate self-respect or consideration for others they constitute an indication for psychotherapy. Contrary to lay expectation, sexual relationships based upon complementary characteristics of this kind are not satisfactory: rather indeed do they tend to be disastrous because their mutual repercussions can prove exacerbatory to a suicidal or even murderous degree.

Addiction to Drugs or Alcohol

Some degree of dependence upon sedatives and particularly upon alcohol is the price paid by many people for participation in competitive, complex society. Addiction, however, can be defined as a dependence upon drugs or alcohol which exceeds the subject's capacity to moderate or control, and destroys both his physical health, his psychological equilibrium, and ultimately his social and personal relationships.

Incidence. Alcoholism and drug addiction are currently increasing in the United Kingdom. Together they represent probably not more than 5 per cent of all mental illness sufficiently serious to require admission to hospital, although it must be remembered that patients suffering from addictions are normally extremely resistant to in-patient treatment, and the amount of social and personal misery caused by alcoholism, although impossible adequately to assess, is very much greater than any figures for hospital admission can possibly indicate.

Aetiology. Constitutional and environmental factors are, as always, of complementary importance. The hereditary element may be both specific, in terms of a hypothetical biological component, and more general in terms of an immaturity of personality, leading to increasing dependence upon immediate relief of tension. The symptomatic use of alcohol or drugs to tide an individual over a period of intense anxiety or depression must be distinguished from chronic or sporadic but specific addiction as the principal cause of disability.

Clinical Features. Drunkenness itself is socially recognisable and will not be further described. It can be arbitrarily regarded as appearing when the concentration of alcohol in the blood reaches 0·2 per cent by volume. There are, of course, individual variations. Sedatives and tranquillisers of all kinds reinforce alcohol, producing retardation, slurred speech, and often clumsiness of movement amounting in some cases to ataxia. Nystagmus is an important sign, frequently present, and often overlooked.

In the wider sense, the characteristic features of addiction are that the individual turns to the bottle, the tablets, or the injection, at first as an alternative to personal stress, particularly to difficulties in human relationships, and, later, to mitigate the suffering which existence without drugs or alcohol has begun to impose. Withdrawal symptoms in the form of pains in the limbs or body, unbearable physical and psychological tension, tremulousness, exhaustion, anorexia, and sleeplessness are all secondary symptoms. Deterioration in personality follows, with evasiveness, suspicion, paranoid and pathological jealousy or guilt and resentful attitudes towards those most closely related to the patient, culminating finally in a humiliating collapse of personal integrity and reliability. Secondary physical effects include vitamin depletion and acute delirium, when a combination of intercurrent illness or injury, combined with withdrawal, produce far-reaching changes in metabolism. (See toxic confusional states, p. 36.)

Diagnosis. The characteristic symptoms and signs, together with the possibility of a resort to alcohol and drugs, can often be clinched by the discovery of ways in which these are being obtained. The patient frequently denies the situation up to and beyond the point at which it has become all too evident to everybody else.

Treatment

(1) Individual psychotherapy.
(2) Vitamin saturation.
(3) Specific biochemical measures.
(4) Social readjustment.

Individual psychotherapy is a fundamental aspect of psychiatric treatment and receives necessarily brief but general exposition in the special section on treatment. (See p. 46.)

Vitamin saturation with ascorbic acid and the entire B complex is a sound traditional procedure whenever the effects of alcohol upon metabolism have impaired the function of brain or central nervous system.

Specific Biochemical Measures. These are of two kinds: the administration of drugs incompatible with the metabolism of alcohol, so that the patient cannot drink while taking the medicine without suffering immediate and violent repercussions on autonomic equilibrium; and drugs designed to link the taking of alcohol with aversion or nausea, so that the desire for alcohol is diminished or destroyed. Examples of the former are tetraethylthiuram disulphide (antabuse), and citrated calcium carbimide (abstem); and of the latter apomorphine by mouth or by injection. Treatment along these lines may be initiated in hospital, and the appropriate regime and dosage stabilised before discharge. Regular supervision and maintenance remains essential for at least two years.

Social Readjustment. This can frequently be improved by the specific co-operation of the organisation 'Alcoholics Anonymous', whose contribution to the problem of alcoholism has probably been at least as great as that of any other single approach.

FUNCTIONAL NEUROSES

(1) Hysterical reactions.
(2) Obsessive compulsive reactions.

Hysterical Reactions

Definition. Hysterical reactions represent the attempt, never fully conscious and frequently unconscious on the part of the patient, to obtain relief from otherwise intolerable stress, by the exhibition and experience of symptoms of illness.

Aetiology. The constitutional component of hysterical personality is often important. Environmental contribution may come from the life situation of the patient, or from structural disease affecting the brain, or any other part of the body.

The mechanism of symptoms production rests upon the normal capacity of human beings to form concepts with an emotional significance and imaginative elaboration and to react to these concepts and their related associations as if they were real.

An example is the marked difference in the capacity of an average person to walk along a plank 6 inches wide when it is 1 foot from the ground, and when it is 200 feet in the air, despite the identical physical conditions of the subject's body and the plank's stability in both instances. The crucial factor is, of course, the suggestive power of the concept of the danger of falling, which affects both subjective well-being and motor control.

Hysterical symptoms appear to be produced by a *dissociation of normal mental processes*, whereby certain concepts, patterns of activity, and related associations affecting the patient's total well-being are separated from conscious awareness and relegated to the unconscious area of mental life. Here the effects of suggestion cannot be counteracted by insight or criticism, and the patient's capacity to comprehend or modify the experience is correspondingly limited.

In practice the relief afforded may be totally illusory, and the symptoms both painful and crippling; but the principle underlying the illness remains the same. In the most superficial types of hysterical illness the advantage tends to be comparatively obvious to the dispassionate observer, while the symptoms directed towards it may be equally transparent. It may indeed be difficult to draw a hard-and-fast line between deliberate and conscious malingering on the one hand and the more superficial type of hysterical illness on the other. Nevertheless, true malingering is exceedingly rare, if only because of the capacity inherent in every human being to believe what seems to be necessary or desirable to him; this in itself is an effect of suggestion and may explain why hysteria, in contrast to malingering, is comparatively common.

Clinical Features. The simplest forms of hysterical reaction involve the loss or distortion of normal motor or sensory function. Blindness, deafness, anaesthesia or paraesthesia, paralysis, or disturbance of reflex motor activity, for example in vomiting, may occur. Symptoms may be psychological rather than primarily physical: loss or disturbance of consciousness, hysterical hallucinations, or disturbance of behaviour may also occur. Often the symptoms will take part of their colouring from the stress which has precipitated them; for example, prolongation of structural disability following injury, long after the wound has healed or fractured bone has united.

Further contributory factors to the presenting clinical picture will be:

(1) The patient's own concept of the illness as it emerges.

(2) The capacity of the symptoms:

    (a) to produce some sort of solution to the patient's difficulties with relief of subjective anguish, and

    (b) to symbolise the sort of solution which would be emotionally acceptable to the patient, though in practice it may not be possible.

Hysterical symptoms are never unimportant; often because of their crudity or transparency to everyone but the patient, they provoke contempt and hostility, but always they are a warning that a human being in distress has found no better solution than a partial surrender. To unmask them is easy. To restore to true health the patient displaying them is often exacting and difficult, but there can be no doubt about which way the doctor's duty lies.

Treatment

(1) Attention to the underlying and provocative stress, whether in the patient's life situation, history of recent illness or injury, or current structural disorder.
(2) Supportive and interpretative individual psychotherapy.
(3) Following elucidation of the situation by (1) and (2) above, specific reversal of symptoms by hypnosis or other methods involving controlled suggestion may be employed. (See page 46.)

Obsessive Compulsive Reactions

Definition. These are mental experiences, ideas, images, impulses, or patterns of behaviour, in which a subjective sense of compulsion is opposed by an equally subjective, conscious, and deliberate resistance. They are usually repetitive, often unpleasant, always unwelcome, and accompanied by emotional tension.

Aetiology. The capacity to develop an obsessional preoccupation, for example with a tune in the head, or a senseless idea which recurs repeatedly, is perfectly normal. The tendency is often increased by fatigue or anxiety. A specific vulnerability to the development of this pattern of mental activity, to the extent that it becomes recognisable as an illness, has a strong constitutional basis; and this is to some extent hereditary. As in so many other forms of mental illness, the hereditary factor can also produce an environmental contribution. The parent from whom the patient acquires the genetic background will also probably have influenced the patient's early life by example.

Obsessive compulsive patterns of thought and behaviour are also apt to be released by damage to the brain: and so are seen in some cases following head injury, and also following encephalitis. For example, post-encephalitic parkinsonism is frequently accompanied by obsessive compulsive symptoms, as well as by oculogyric crises.

Clinical Picture. The symptoms may be general and diffuse, or, more frequently, related to one of a limited number of specific preoccupations. When general and diffuse they represent a pathological meticulousness which affects every aspect of the individual's life. They are particularly associated with the difficulty in finally completing any activity. For example, the patient cannot turn off a tap without returning several times to turn it on again and then off to make sure that it is properly turned off. Letters cannot be posted without the envelope having been opened and resealed a number of times, sometimes a specific number such as 3, 7, 9, 11, and so on. The day-to-day business of getting up, getting dressed, going to work, completing routine tasks, and returning home may become quite impossible, because the time taken to check and recheck each stage of each procedure, often complicated by having to do things in a certain prescribed and extremely complicated way, may delay completion even of the morning dressing and toilet until it is time to start going to bed. One patient of this kind took $2\frac{1}{2}$ hours to shave; much of this time being taken up in checking the exact setting of the razor, in making sure that all the adjustable parts were screwed to a particular degree of perfect balance and tension. Similarly, when punching a card either to clock in or to clock out at work, the card had to be taken back six to a dozen times to make quite sure that it had been properly punched, and that the time and date upon it corresponded accurately with the actual hour and day on which the operation had been undertaken.

Specific preoccupations which become the centre of obsessive compulsive rituals are usually:

> *Sexual:* connected with a fear of impregnating women, if the patient is a man, or of becoming pregnant, if the patient is a woman, or

> *Aggressive:* connected with a fear of causing injury, or doing harm, or

> *Contaminatory:* connected with a fear of conveying or acquiring infection or contamination by handling material from which dirt or germs may be picked up, either to harm the patient, or more frequently to be passed on by the patient to other people who will then be harmed by them.

These preoccupations lead to extremely complicated and vexatious rituals, expressly designed to avoid the contingencies expressed by the fears. For example, an obsessional man may be compelled to wash the bath out with disinfectant three or four times before taking a bath, then again after taking a bath; to avert contamination or insemination of the bath or bath-water which then might infect or impregnate the next woman to take a bath in the same tub. Such fears are in no way mitigated by their recognition as senseless and irrational.

The wearing of gloves, the repeated washing of the hands or the body, up to as many as twenty times before and after performing the simplest task, the inability to touch articles which may have been contaminated, however indirectly, by contact with other people, and at the same time the fear that other people will be themselves contaminated by contact with the patient, lead inevitably to an ultimately crippling complication of day-to-day life.

Treatment

(1) *Psychotherapy.* This is most likely to be successful in a proportion of cases seen early in the development of the disorder, and particularly in children. But in its widest sense it is necessary for the acceptance, effective aid, and comfort of all patients, who are already more than half-way towards expecting and dreading ridicule and contempt when they venture to communicate their symptoms.

(2) *Symptomatic medicinal treatment* in the form of tranquillising medicines (q.v.) has an important place. Specific treatment with certain hallucinogens, notably lysergic acid and cannabis indica, undertaken in hospital, can sometimes loosen and dissolve the rigid and automatic pattern of obsessive compulsive thought.

(3) If either of the two measures above have succeeded in releasing emotion, this will nearly always be predominantly depressive. Symptomatic treatment with *E.C.T.* can be salutary in such cases.

(4) Intractable anguish, unrelieved in any other way, may call for bi-medial *leucotomy* under certain circumstances.

AFFECTIVE DISORDERS

Anxiety State

Definition. A state of continual irrational anxiety and apprehension, sometimes flaring up into acute fear amounting to panic, accompanied by symptoms of autonomic and endocrine disturbance; with secondary effects on other mental functions such as concentration, attention, memory, and judgement.

Aetiology. Anxiety states are the commonest of all psychiatric disorders, and make up a considerable proportion of the complaints which bring patients to their general practitioner or to the general out-patient departments of hospitals. Constitutional and personality factors are important in some instances, but chiefly in the extent to which they render the patient vulnerable to states of anxiety in response to otherwise apparently trivial stress. All human beings are capable of developing this reaction if the threat to their confidence and well-being is sufficiently severe.

Clinical Picture. Anxiety itself may dominate the patient's subjective mental state; or, alternatively, the patient may complain of physical symptoms which are the outcome of the normal adrenergic component of anxiety, such as tachycardia, restlessness, loss of appetite, insomnia, sweating, tremulousness, and loss of weight. Periodic episodes of acute fear amounting to panic are common.

Some patients may experience either their basic anxiety, or these crises of blind and overwhelming fear, accompanied by physical sensations of choking or suffocation, tremulousness, sweating, and a sense of impending collapse, mainly or exclusively in response to certain specific stimuli. For example, they may be unable to face travelling on an underground train or going in a lift, or they may be acutely afraid of venturing out alone on the one hand, or meeting people or going into a crowded place on the other. Specific fears of this nature are described as *phobias*, and so-called phobic states can be regarded as a variety of anxiety states in general.

In practice it is most rare for any phobia to be so restricted to a specific type of experience that the patient remains free of anxiety in all other circumstances. What usually happens is that the underlying and persistent anxiety is heightened to an unbearable degree by the activation of the particular phobia concerned.

Physical symptoms include the autonomic accompaniments of anxiety already mentioned, which in turn lead to the vegetative disturbances, weight loss, exhaustion, and insomnia. *Sleep disturbance* takes a characteristic form, the patient being unable to get to sleep for hours, tossing and turning restlessly, and finally falling into a broken slumber often disturbed by vivid and terrifying dreams from which he may awake tense, sweating, and trembling. It is common for patients to claim that they have had less than an hour of unbroken sleep at night for many weeks or months.

As well as the fear and the accompanying malaise, hypochondriacal preoccupations are common and may be related either to the physiological symptoms of anxiety on the one hand, or to the unbearable apprehension and sense of impending disaster experienced by the patient on the other.

Treatment

(1) *Psychotherapy.* This is the treatment of choice in every case, whatever additional measures are adopted.

(2) *Symptomatic Medicinal Treatment.* Tranquillisers, sedatives and vitamin B.

(3) Occasionally acute tension may require some *interviews under intravenous barbiturates*; more rarely, a period of *continuous sleep*.

(4) *Hypnosis* can be employed after the essential exploration, elucidation, and interpretation of the causal mechanisms have been satisfactorily completed. It should not be employed to suppress anxiety whose basis has not been investigated.

Depressive Illnesses

Definition. Depressive illness is a combination of misery and malaise, which occurs either spontaneously, or exceeds in duration and intensity the normal reaction to any provocative disaster or misfortune. The misery tends to be compounded of guilt, anguish, and despair; and the malaise of exhaustion, insomnia, anorexia, constipation, headache, and multiple bodily discomfort.

Aetiology. Heredity and constitutional factors are of some importance. The incidence of depressive illness in the population as a whole is about 0·4 per cent; the increase in incidence with a family history of depressive illness is shown in the following table:

Relationship					*Approximate Incidence*
Parents, children, siblings	..	..	..	..	10%
Aunts and uncles ..	..	..	..	..	5%
Cousins, nephews, etc.	..	..	..	..	2·5%

However, certain investigators have questioned these findings, which are none the less widely quoted in textbooks. Tomassen in Iceland carried out a very careful investigation in which he personally traced and interviewed all the descendants, collaterals, and surviving grandparents of twenty-five patients with a classical manic depressive illness. These totalled some 2,463 people, yet Tomassen was unable to satisfy himself that there was any greater incidence of depression among his special group than among the population as a whole.

Reactive factors will be elicited in the patient's history. Bereavement, or other overwhelming personal disaster, material loss, intense disappointment of long cherished hopes, or the threat or certainty of abandonment or betrayal by others in whom the patient has trusted, are examples. But it is only when the depression exceeds both in severity and duration what can normally be regarded as appropriate to the total life situation, that it can be regarded as a form of mental illness.

Depression may also occur in association with other serious intercurrent illness; for example, it may complicate anaemia, myxoedema, carcinoma, or any chronic debilitating disorder.

Clinical Picture. The condition commonly reveals itself in three areas: in mood; in the response of the patient to physical and intellectual stimulation; and in the functioning of the autonomic nervous system.

The patient's mood is characterised by dejection and unhappiness, with some blunting and withdrawal of interest from the outside world, general retardation of mental and physical activity, indecision, and often subjective difficulty in thinking. Feelings of guilt may be intense and occasionally provide the basis for delusions. Such delusions may be self-punitive, including convictions of impoverishment, or hypochondriacal. For example, the patient may believe that he is financially ruined, or is to suffer some dreadful persecution or disaster; and this belief may then be accompanied by hallucinations taking the form of accusatory voices, which simply din into the patient's ears the same melancholy and appalling ideas with which he is already assailed from the sources of his own introspection. Or he may be tormented by convictions that his bowels are blocked, his brains have rotted away or turned to water, or that his whole body is putrefying and a source of offence to others. The key to understanding these apparently diverse symptoms is the recognition that each is the product of an underlying state of mind characterised by a mood of consistent sadness and abject despair.

The response of the patient to stimulation in the intellectual or physical plane is explicable in terms of the retardation already mentioned. Response to questioning, to the necessity of making decisions, and even to the performance of normal everyday tasks may become quite unendurably difficult. The housewife may dread going out to do the shopping, partly because of the physical and intellectual effort which it costs her, and partly because her indecision in the face of various items of choice in the shops makes it almost impossible for her to complete this routine task. The pressure of necessity for examination may then lead to a final breakdown into tears which have hitherto been held back only by a tremendous effort. It is a characteristic of many cases of depression that this effort will have been made, and that a façade of apparent although exceedingly brittle cheerfulness may be the presenting feature of the patient's approach.

Sometimes there is a complicating element of agitation; not only is the patient slowed up but he is also restlessly preoccupied with distressing and painful ruminations. There is often a diminished awareness of external events, with increasingly painful introspection and narrowed range of thought.

In the sphere of autonomic function, the symptoms of outstanding importance are:

(1) Disturbance of sleep rhythm with early morning waking.
(2) Loss of appetite and weight.
(3) Constipation and dyspepsia.

The disturbance of bowel function corresponds to the retardation seen in the sphere of thought and action. The bowels are not moved regularly within the normal twenty-four-hour cycle, as though the passage of ingested food through the gastrointestinal tract has become increasingly retarded until eventually the patient is severely constipated. This constipation often bulks largely in the patient's mind, and may provide grounds for some of the hypochondriacal delusions already mentioned.

The pulse is usually slow, full and bounding, even in the more agitated patients. The skin is likely to be warm and dry, by contrast with the clammy sweating skin of the patient of acute anxiety. However, attacks of sweating occasionally occur, often in the early morning when the patient awakens drenched with sweat, wholly unrefreshed, restless and oppressed with morbid thoughts and fears.

During the daytime there is a constant sense of fatigue and listlessness. Everything is an effort and nothing seems worth while any more. To the patient, all this may seem essentially physical. It may be very hard for him to describe it in convincing terms, or to pin it down to physical symptoms which he can effectively recount. Unable to sleep, to eat, to work efficiently, to hope, or to enjoy any of the simple pleasures of life, it is not surprising that all too often he despairs of living; and if his doctor appears to have no understanding of his plight, to die may then seem to him to be all that is left.

Depression appearing spontaneously is often called *endogenous*: when it follows external events which are regarded as having precipitated it, it is called *reactive*. Such distinction is, however, rarely clear-cut. There are three main clinical types: *simple depression*, the depressive phase of *recurrent depression or manic depressive illness*, and *involutional melancholia*.

Simple depression is characterised by retardation rather than agitation, by apathy and inertia, but rarely by delusions or hallucinations. In quality it resembles a normal grief reaction; for example, the phase of mourning after bereavement.

The depressive phases of **manic depressive illness** or *recurrent depression* are characterised by a greater degree of loss of judgement, and of separation from reality; and are more likely to be accompanied by delusions and hallucinations.

Phases of normality, or of exaltation and elation, may alternate with phases of depression. The cycle may vary in duration from days and weeks to months or even years. There may be intervening periods during which the patient shows no symptoms of any kind. Sometimes depression and manic episodes may alternate gradually or violently without normal phases occurring at all.

Involutional melancholia occurs characteristically at the junction of the middle and latter thirds of life, and is apt to be particularly severe. Agitation is frequently a predominant feature of the illness and may be expressed by repeated importunate complaints of bodily or mental suffering, with wringing of the hands, restlessness, and lamentation. Hypochondriacal ideas and delusions of impoverishment are particularly common in this form of illness; moreover, the patient's suffering may be increased by a sense of intolerable guilt. Under such circumstances severe adverse moral judgements tend to be passed by patients upon themselves. They may say that they are unworthy to be saved, have committed the unpardonable sin, are damned, decadent, and degenerate, and will bring horror and disgrace upon all who are associated with them. Severance from reality is most acute in this form of the illness, and therefore, of course, the risk of suicide is correspondingly grave.

Suicide is a real danger in any case of depression which exceeds normal limits of a stable individual's response to personal unhappiness. In the absence of effective treatment, probably all seriously depressed patients have contemplated suicide, and at least 20 per cent of them attempt it, of whom about half are successful.

Studies of large series of suicides from all causes show that between a quarter and a half have suffered from depression to a degree which would have made them certifiable; but less than 10 per cent of all patients who commit suicide have been seen by a psychiatrist before they took their life. This suggests that the diagnosis is being made far too infrequently, and that a significant proportion of the patients who die undiagnosed could have been saved if prompt and effective treatment had been undertaken.

Pathology. The basic disorder in depression is probably a biochemical disturbance of neuro-endocrine origin. Its psychopathology is therefore secondary, in the sense that whatever in the patient's past recollection, or present situation, is capable of tragic interpretation will form a prominent part of his preoccupations. In this sense, depression has been compared to the thalamic syndrome, whereby all sensory experience is felt as pain. In depression, all emotional experience is felt as sorrow.

Treatment

(1) Supportive psychotherapy.
(2) Specific anti-depressant and symptomatic medicines. } See
(3) Electrical treatment. } p. 46.
(4) Indications for leucotomy in special cases. }

(1) and (2) can often be effectively administered on an out-patient basis, if the patient's general condition is compatible with out-patient supervision and care. The risk of suicide must never be forgotten under such circumstances, but need not overwhelm clinical judgement if the physician is prepared to accept the calculated risk in carrying a depressed patient on an out-patient basis, properly assessed, following frank enquiry, and the foundation of a sincere relationship of mutual trust between the patient and doctor.

Specific electrical treatment for depression should always be initiated in hospital, though it may subsequently prove possible to complete it at out-patients.

Mania and Hypomania

Definition. Just as depression is a combination of misery and malaise, so the opposite side of the coin is an equally pathological combination of elation and energy. This is equally pathological, because equally liable to progress to final exhaustion and disaster.

Aetiology. This is essentially a constitutional predisposition. The incidence is probably about one-fifth to one-quarter of depressive illness, at least in Western society.

Clinical Features. Hypomania is the milder form of the illness. By contrast with the depressed retarded inert apathetic patient, a person afflicted with hypomania shows elevation of mood, and an acceleration and extension of stream of thought, with flight of ideas, pressure of talk, and apparently inexhaustible energy.

Such patients are restless and excitable, cannot sleep, often will not be bothered with food and must always be busy, dashing purposelessly about, taking up one activity after another. They may plan or launch innumerable tasks, and then, constantly abandoning one to embark upon another, finish none, while seeming to thrive upon the mounting chaos of their own contrivance.

Like depression, elation is an aspect of the normal experience of human beings; and often only gradually and imperceptibly emerges into an abnormal degree of intensity. But when the sense of wellbeing and confidence not only exceeds all degree of appropriateness to the patient's life, but begins to colour and to cloud judgement and responsibility to a point at which the normal capacity to adjust to reality and manage affairs becomes impaired, then it constitutes a condition of illness, no matter how little the patient may complain of it.

In more severe cases, complete physical collapse from lack of sleep and nourishment may follow, unless treatment controls the situation. While gaiety and goodwill often form the superficial characteristics of the patient's mood, irritability and exasperation are apt to be provoked by the slightest attempt to control or restrain him. Great tact is therefore necessary in handling such patients. The severest form of the disorder is *mania*, wherein the patient is uncontrollably excited, while flight of ideas and pressure of thoughts may render him incoherent. Violence and exasperation may lead to homicidal assaults by such patients on those who endeavour to control them, and in these extreme conditions hallucinations and delusions are again apt to occur.

Treatment

(1) Establishment of rapport: this is a prime necessity if any further progress is to be made.

(2) Admission to hospital: it is impossible to treat any form of hypomania or mania effectively without admission.

(3) Symptomatic medicinal measures: sedation and tranquillisation.

(4) Specific medicinal measures, including, if necessary, continuous sleep and vitamin saturation.

(5) Electrical treatment. (See p. 53.)

SCHIZOPHRENIC PSYCHOSES

Definition. Schizophrenia is a generic name for a group of disorders characterised by a progressive disintegration of emotional stability, judgement, contact with and appreciation of reality; which produces considerable secondary impairment of personal relationships and intellectual function of the affected patient.

Aetiology. Schizophrenia can be regarded as a form of mental illness displayed by human beings subjected to various kinds of stress where response is governed by a specific constitutional handicap, not yet fully understood. It may be partly genetic (*vide infra*).

Incidence. Schizophrenia has an incidence of about 0·85 per cent of the general population. Surrounding the clinical concept of the disease itself is the wider social concept of the schizoid personality, estimated to occur in about 3 per cent of the general population. This concept rests upon manifestation of marked social and personal withdrawal, often in association with shyness, reticence, eccentricity and a tendency to suspicion and hypersensitivity. While it is certainly true that cold, potentially ruthless, dreamy eccentrics or lonely, diffident, sensitive and suspicious people may often be described as displaying schizoid traits, it is their inability to deal successfully with external reality which links them in practice. The essential importance of this type of personality in the aetiology of frank schizophrenia is indicated by the fact that from 35 to 50 per cent of all people who develop the illness have previously shown personality traits of this kind.

The following table, based on Kallmann's work in 1946, illustrates the general incidence of schizophrenia and schizoid personality among the relatives of the patient.

INCIDENCE OF SCHIZOPHRENIA
Kallmann 1946

In summary the weight of evidence suggests a probability that schizophrenia is a disturbance of physiological function, possibly with an hereditary component, whose psychological effects are reflected at the level of cortical integration—and thence, by interaction upon hypothalamus and anterior pituitary, produce the widespread autonomic and endocrine changes so often characteristic of the illness.

Clinical Features. The essential features of the illness can be summarised under four main headings:

(1) Disorder of thinking.
(2) Disorder of feeling and mood.
(3) Disorder of contact with reality: hallucinations.
(4) Disorder of conduct.

Thought disorders include *thought block; ideas of reference, passivity,* and *influence*; and *primary delusions,* including mysterious convictions of inexplicable changes in the universe, or within the body of the patient.

The potential impact of such disorder is exemplified by the case of a young man who, while listening to the radio, suddenly became aware that the entire programme was about him. This conviction was absolute, and he found himself waiting for evidence which would convince another person; he was himself already completely convinced. During the programme a song 'Don't laugh at me 'cos I'm a fool' was broadcast. The patient smashed the set.

Secondary delusions occur as part of the patient's understandable attempt to make some sort of sense of the ideas of reference and disturbance of thought and feeling from which he suffers. Such delusions in fact show that the patient's powers of reasoning and judgement are preserved at least to the extent that he tried to keep order and system in the world of his experience. But the more ill the patient, the more disintegrated his personality, the more disordered, unrelated, and chaotic are his delusions likely to be.

Emotional incongruity is often a most striking feature. Apart from a certain bewilderment and perplexity, the patient may show astonishingly little concern about the uncanny nightmarish life which he describes as his own. But the outcome of suspiciousness or persecutory delusions may sometimes be impulsive murderous attacks, just as the response to some mysterious vision or message may be a state of ecstasy striking and evident, but transcending the power of the observer to share or in any way experience.

Hallucinations themselves are common although by no means essential in the clinical picture. Most frequently they take the form of voices repeating the patient's thoughts, explaining, praising, criticising, abusing, or ridiculing his actions even before he acts, thereby often distracting him so much that no outward action follows; but visual hallucinations including quasi-mystical experiences are not particularly rare. Sensory hallucinations are probably responsible for the common delusions of electrical or radio-active stimulation, and may lead to belief that the patient is being erotically caressed by invisible admirers. Such experiences may at one and the same time form the subject of vigorous complaints and obvious satisfaction. This preoccupation with a vivid but unreal world, of course, releases the patient from the demands and limits of normal existence, and this withdrawal from reality underlies almost all the symptoms.

In the schizophrenic, love and hate, trust and suspicion, joy and sorrow, terror and confidence, may co-exist or alternate so rapidly as to be indistinguishable in the patient's mind. It is not hard to see how such a chaos of mental and emotional existence can lead to **impulsive action** or **eminently bizarre and incomprehensible behaviour.**

Clinical Varieties. The clinical varieties of schizophrenia are conveniently described under four headings:

    (1) Simple schizophrenia.
    (2) Hebephrenic schizophrenia.
    (3) Catatonic schizophrenia.
    (4) Paraphrenia or paranoid schizophrenia.

The first two can be largely summarised by saying that they differ from each other only in severity and chronicity, and are characterised by early onset, a chronic course, and all too often an eventual dementia which may persist for many years; these are the types which earned from Kraepelin the name of dementia praecox. The initial stages of both these forms may send the patient on a round of consultations through medical and surgical out-patients, with constant changes of general practitioner, complaining of a variety of symptoms which actually overlie a deepening conviction of profound ill health whose true basis is never recognised.

The third group, catatonic forms of schizophrenia, include the wild and bizarre postures and activities of the obvious madman, which may alternate with periods of complete stupor and withdrawal. They carry the most favourable outlook, and a single attack may be over in a matter of weeks or months and never recur. The fourth group comprises all those disorders which at one time were considered separately from schizophrenia and called paranoia. They are distinguished by the prominence of delusions of persecution which may be logical and systematic, and could often be accepted as reasonable were their premises true. Such delusions may remain fixed and apparently unalterable without subsequent deterioration or disintegration of the personality. But nearly always there is an eventual insidious and progressive disorder of thought and feeling, sometimes accompanied by hallucinations, with a splitting and crumbling of existing delusions into diverse and inconsistent fragments so that the final picture is unmistakably schizophrenic.

Treatment

(1) Individual psychotherapy.
(2) Specific medicinal measures: the greatest single contribution to treatment in this field has come from the development of the phenothiazine group of drugs. (See p. 52.)
(3) Electrical treatment. (See p. 53.)
(4) Consideration of indications for bi-medial leucotomy in chronic resistant cases, characterised by intractable anguish and suffering. (See p. 55.)

Deep insulin treatment is now essentially of historical interest only.

Prognosis. Manfred Bleuler's study of 500 cases in 1941 remains the most solid basis for the estimation of prognosis. He estimated that 25 per cent of all cases of schizophrenia make a complete recovery from their first attack, while a further 25 per cent show a very marked improvement with slight residual defect. The remaining 50 per cent can again be divided almost equally into 25 per cent who show some improvement, but in whom there is a severe residual degree of disability, and 25 per cent who do not recover at all. The effect of successful treatment is to move a proportion of cases from each group into the group above. A reduction in the 25 per cent of formerly irrecoverable cases, who may have remained ill for anything from 5 to 20 years, can only be hoped for in some instances from bi-medial leucotomy.

ACUTE CONFUSIONAL STATES AND OTHER PSYCHIATRIC EMERGENCIES

Psychiatric emergencies arising in the course of intercurrent medical or surgical illness, and presenting usually as a progressive loss of contact between the patient and his environment, with varying degrees of clouding of consciousness, and associated excitement, stupor, or panic, can be divided into two main groups:

(1) Toxic and confusional reactions.
(2) Acute reactive psychotic episodes.

Toxic Confusional States

These can all be regarded as varieties of acute dementia. Dementia is more commonly recognised as the chronic deteriorative outcome of progressive degeneration of brain structure or function. (See p. 43.) But when seen in its acute and reversible form, it retains the same clinical characteristics, although these are, of course, telescoped together so that their individual recognition tends to be obscured. The general clinical characteristics of such states include:

(1) Clouding of consciousness.
(2) Failure of recent memory.
(3) Failure of attention, concentration, and judgement.

All these three features tend to produce:

(4) Disorientation in space and time; to which are added—
(5) Emotional lability, and finally—
(6) Hallucinations and misinterpretations of external reality.

From these six spring all the rest: delusions, excitement, panic, disturbance of behaviour, and the entire phenomenon of the frightened and frightening patient who is temporarily out of touch and beyond control.

Aetiology

(a) *Direct Causes*

(1) Hypoxia, directly affecting the neurones of the cerebral cortex.
(2) Depletion of intracellular glucose.
(3) Accumulation of toxic metabolites.
(4) Cortical enzyme inhibition.
(5) Disturbance of fluid and electrolyte balance (particularly by steroids).
(6) Specific histotoxic effect upon cortical neurones (particularly by amphetamine and belladonna preparations).

From these factors it will be evident that the excessive loading of a patient with an acute toxic confusional state with barbiturates or atropine preparations, can complicate, rather than improve, the clinical picture. It is also worth remembering that large doses of amphetamine or alcohol may have been taken by the patient before the onset of the acute confusional syndrome.

(b) *Indirect Causes.* More remote, but equally important, factors leading to the direct causes above include:

(1) Infections producing toxic effects and dehydration.

(2) Cardio-vascular disturbance, *via* hypoxia.

(3) Respiratory disturbance, *via* hypoxia.

(4) Vitamin deficiencies (for example, in debilitating illness, or after prolonged alcoholism leading to delirium tremens).

(5) Post-operative conditions complicated by residual anaesthetic effects and shock, both leading to hypoxia.

(6) Metabolic disorders (for example, diabetes mellitus, hepatic failure, or uraemia).

(7) Endocrine disturbance (for example, immediate puerperal disorder or myxoedematous crisis).

(8) Unwise exhibition of drugs (particularly bromides, phenobarbitone, dexamphetamine, paraldehyde, and, of course, alcohol).

In warning against massive sedation in the attempted therapy of these conditions, it is perhaps important to stress that intramuscular paraldehyde can be the most disruptive of all attempts at sedation which misfire. Paraldehyde intramuscularly is painful, can cause local abscess formation, frequently produces an exacerbation of confusion, and may lead the confused and delirious patient to believe that he has suffered a further unpremeditated assault (as indeed he has).

Acute reactive psychotic episodes are really sudden explosions of the classical forms of mental illness, occurring in people constitutionally liable to such illness, and released in this instance by the stress of medical or surgical crisis. They comprise essentially:

(1) Acute schizophrenic episodes.

(2) Acute depressive episodes.

(3) Acute mania.

(4) Acute hysterical episodes.

Their differential diagnosis from toxic confusional states can usually be made relatively easily on three grounds:

(a) The history, both previous personal and medical history, and family history, in which evidence of the latent psychosis may be apparent.

(b) The absence of the toxic confusional physiological state, and particularly of the six factors listed as direct causes on p. 36.

(c) The clinical picture itself, which it may nevertheless take an expert eye to differentiate in a particular case.

In general, acute psychotic episodes tend to last longer than toxic confusional states, involving as they do a more profound disturbance of basic personality, and they tend to occur in a setting nearer the normal physiological equilibrium than that seen in the acute toxic deliria.

Treatment. The first essential to treatment is to remember that the patient is frightened, estranged and for this reason often inaccessible and perhaps frankly hostile to the normal somewhat detached clinical approach. No matter how disturbing the patient's conduct may be to others, it is he himself who suffers and is disturbed the most of all. And it is to him primarily that the doctor's and nurse's obligation to understand, accept, and relieve must be fulfilled. Bearing in mind these essential considerations, whose importance cannot be overemphasised, the following general principles then clearly emerge.

(1) Nurse the patient in a *side ward* or private room, preferably with regular and constant attendants who become recognised as friends and protectors, who sit with him when he is frightened, talk to him when he calls out, and soothe him by an understanding presence. Clearly the room must not be entirely dark, nor need it be brightly lit by night; but moving shadows and dark corners should be avoided.

(2) *Obviate cerebral hypoxia* by:

   (a) Review of existing treatment and state.
   (b) Administration of oxygen if necessary.
   (c) Secure adequate pulmonary ventilation (if inadequate, Rx. choline theophyllinate, aminophylline, etc.).

(3) *Hydration.* Bland glucose fluids by mouth.

(4) *Vitamins.* Vitamins B and C are essential, and should be given by intravenous route in the first instance. These injections cause no pain. Parentrovite is a suitable preparation, containing all the essential vitamins of the B group together with ascorbic acid. It is put up in twin ampoules which must be mixed for injection; high potency strength intravenously 3 times daily for the first 48 hours, then daily injections for the next 5 days. This can be followed by oral becosym, oral vitamins B and C in high concentration.

(5) *Sedation.*

   Avoid

      Bromide always.
      Intramuscular paraldehyde always.
      Short-acting barbiturates usually.

Give

Oral chloral 2–3 g.
Oral paraldehyde 8–12 ml.
Oral chlorpromazine 75 to 100 mg.
If intramuscular or intravenous therapy is necessary—
R. Chlorpromazine 100 to 150 mg. stat.
+ six hourly
Morphine 15–20 mg. in emergency (but this in fact is rarely necessary).
Haloperidol 5–10 mg. can now replace morphia for most acutely disturbed patients.

(6) *Minimal physical restraint,* and no hostility, remain golden rules.

Final General Principles

(1) Remember that this condition is not uncommon and often avoidable.

(2) Think ahead and think early (6 p.m. will often see a sick patient restless, who by 2 a.m. will, untreated, have become wildly disturbed and violently excited).

(3) Accept the management of these cases as part of every doctor's and every nurse's job: not as a disgraceful catastrophe for which responsibility can be shelved, or shoved elsewhere Remember that among other things doctors and nurses need to stand in patients' eyes as pillars of confidence, acceptance, charity in the true sense, and abiding care. No self-respecting doctor or nurse would shrink from a stinking wound or a sudden haematemesis; still less should they dissociate themselves from the proper care of the acutely disturbed and critically ill patient. As in so many therapeutic techniques, success or failure is ultimately determined by intelligent imaginative anticipation, and the fundamental attitude of mind in approaching the problem.

PUERPERAL PSYCHOSES

These do not differ in their essential nature from comparable psychoses seen apart from the puerperium. Their commonest forms are affective disorders, notably classical depression, sometimes with suicide and infanticide as dire complications; and severe persistent states of anxiety with considerable secondary depersonalisation and hysterical manifestations. Schizophrenic illnesses may also occur in the puerperium, and occasionally obsessive compulsive illnesses make their first appearance during this time.

Aetiology. Puerperal psychoses as a group are defined by their occurrence within one year of delivery. A great majority of them occur within three months, and are usually of relatively short duration and good prognosis. Specific aetiological factors in addition to those present in the basic disorder, whenever it is seen, are probably:

(1) The additional psychological stresses and challenges of pregnancy

and labour, with all the emotional significance attaching to the prospects of childbirth and motherhood, and

(2) The considerable and sudden biochemical changes secondary to the endocrinological crises following delivery.

Incidence. Puerperal mental illness is a relatively uncommon complication of pregnancy and delivery, having an incidence of not more than 0·5 per cent. By contrast, mild and relatively transient disturbances of mood and judgement (referred to immediately above) not amounting to frank illness, and rarely lasting more than 24 hours, are to be expected during the first 10 puerperal days, and may be accepted as normal.

Clinical Features. Apart from a tendency for all syndromes to be accompanied by a rather higher proportion of hysterical symptoms and frequently to be complicated by severe depersonalisation, the clinical picture does not differ essentially from that seen in comparable illness at other times.

Treatment. This again must be based essentially upon the appropriate measures for the illness itself. Special features requiring attention in puerperal illness are, by the nature of the additional aetiological factors:

(1) Elimination of any toxic exhaustive factor. (See p. 36.)

(2) When major psychiatric disturbance is encountered within the first ten days of delivery, a deliberate reduction in the gradient of decline of progesterone may be achieved by giving diminishing doses of progesterone by injection. The initial dose should be100 mg. diminishing by 25 mg. daily over the next three days.

Prognosis. Prognosis for all forms of mental illness appearing in and related to the puerperium is relatively better, with appropriate treatment, than for illnesses occurring spontaneously and without this additional aetiological component. Long-term prognosis need not be regarded with apprehension in terms of further pregnancies. Provided that the general health, constitution, and hereditary background of the mother are otherwise sound, a second pregnancy will often go through with adequate supervision without incident or puerperal disturbance, even though the first pregnancy has been attended by psychiatric illness. Except in the case of chronic schizophrenia with puerperal exacerbations, a history of puerperal illness is not in itself an indication for avoiding further pregnancies.

TERMINATION OF PREGNANCY ON PSYCHIATRIC GROUNDS

In this writer's view, termination of pregnancy on psychiatric grounds can only be justified when continuation of the pregnancy would certainly carry a risk to the mother's life, or permanent destruction of her health. It can never be justified on purely sociological or personal grounds. Severe depression, with the open threat of suicide if the pregnancy is not terminated, cannot in itself constitute an indication for termination. The indication which it does constitute is of course for appropriate treatment of the depression. Termination in itself (in fact) is often a dangerous treatment for depression (quite apart from being ethically unjustifiable). Intense exacerbation of depression with additional guilt, remorse, and occasionally severely paranoid ideas, can follow termination when the mother comes to realise that, even perhaps at her own insistence, her child has been killed.

PSYCHOSOMATIC REACTIONS

Definition. Psychosomatic reactions may be defined as structural changes significantly related to emotional factors.

Aetiology. In essence every form of illness to which human beings are subject has its psychosomatic aspects. In fact, the essential link between psychiatry, general medicine, surgery, and obstetrics lies in the ultimate impossibility of treating states of mind apart from states of body, or states of body apart from states of mind.

The anatomico-physiological basis for psychosomatic reaction is, on reflection, self-evident. The central nervous system, the autonomic nervous system, and the neuro-endocrine system, whose pivotal centre can be regarded as the pituitary gland, represent three inter-related systems of communication whereby the individual maintains equilibrium respectively between himself and his external environment, and within his own organism.

Although interaction between these systems is a constant and invariable aspect of human health and sickness, it tends all too often to be ignored in the practice of medicine.

Clinical Implications. These are simply that in taking a history and conducting an examination of the patient, attention must be paid to the entire life situation of the person concerned, to his background and personal history, as well as to his presenting complaint.

One valuable and illuminating way of arranging the data thus obtained, is by constructing a life chart for the patient. This consists of three vertically ruled columns, the first of which contains the date, and age of the patient throughout the life history, the second the circumstances of his life and development at the relevant times, and the third the symptoms from which he has suffered, including exacerbations, relapses, and remissions of existent illnesses, and fluctuations in general health. Correlations which become evident in this way will enable every doctor to become a more observant, careful, effective, and humane physician.

SPECIFIC CLINICAL SYNDROMES OF PARTICULAR PSYCHIATRIC IMPORTANCE IN GENERAL MEDICINE

(1) Anorexia nervosa.
(2) Hypochondriasis.
(3) Sexual disorders.

Anorexia Nervosa

This is a condition in which there is a profound aversion to food, often leading to severe self-starvation, accompanied at least initially by subjective well-being and protestations of energy. Emaciation, and even death from starvation or secondary infection, are significant risks in untreated cases.

Aetiology. The disorder is almost entirely confined to adolescent or young adult girls; although cases have been encountered occasionally in young men. In a recent survey of clinical material in Guy's Hospital, the underlying psychopathology was regarded as hysterical in 75 per cent of the cases, schizophrenic in 20 per cent, with depression and obsessive-compulsive disorder accounting for the remaining 5 per cent.

Clinical Features. The combination of emaciation, subjective well-being, and a determined, sometimes a desperate, refusal or inability to accept a normal diet, in the absence of other primary pathology, is characteristic.

Differential Diagnosis. This is essentially from endocrine disorders such as hypopituitarism on the one hand, and from severe latent infection such as chronic miliary tuberculosis on the other. The loss of secondary sexual characteristics such as pubic and axillary hair, and breast contour, are common in endocrine disorder and absent in anorexia nervosa.

Treatment must be divided into two stages. The first is the establishment of initial contact, sympathy, and rapport, together with the restoration of the patient to normal body weight and capacity for living, by a carefully maintained nursing, dietetic, and supportive therapeutic regime in bed in hospital. The second stage is the treatment of the underlying psychopathological disorder, whatever this may be.

Prognosis. Immediate prognosis in treated cases is good: long-term prognosis, unfortunately bad. Over 60 per cent of patients who have suffered from anorexia nervosa either experience further attacks in later life, or display relatively crippling disorders of personality, usually on a hysterical basis.

Hypochondriasis

Definition. Hypochondriasis may be defined as a morbid preoccupation with the maintenance of bodily health or the possibility of disease.

Incidence. Hypochondriasis is probably one of the commonest bugbears of general practice. In one form or another it is responsible for about 10 per cent of all regular attendances at doctor's surgeries or hospital outpatients. Subjectively it can be exhausting, humiliating, and disabling for the patients concerned.

Differential Diagnosis. It is the importance of recognising the underlying disorder of which hypochondriasis may be the most insistent syndrome, which merits its inclusion as a special item in this section. Hypochondriasis may in fact constitute the presenting feature of an anxiety state or depressive illness, may represent a hysterical or obsessive compulsive reaction, or may form part of the clinical syndrome of chronic or insidious schizophrenia or even of dementia.

Sexual Disorders

Male Impotence and Female Frigidity

These two general terms embrace a wide range of afflictions involving human sexual incapacity; and can in varying degrees be productive of untold personal misery and humiliation. Three simple but comparatively detailed communications out of many published, cover between them much essential information for the student and practitioner.[1] Without reproducing the detailed content of these already published papers here, it is important to remember the essentially simple and reflex aspects of human sexual performance, as well as their enormous psychological importance to the individual, to which these papers have drawn much needed attention.

Investigation and Treatment. The first essential is to make the patient feel that the doctor has time and is interested to listen to the problem, and to pay attention to the patient's feelings and way of describing them without interruption. The examiner should avoid premature questioning or jumping to conclusions, and above all guard against creating the impression that he is inclined to dismiss the complaint as trivial on the one hand, or on the other that he approaches it with an attitude of defeat and despair.

Much of this will be familiar to the general practitioner who already knows his patient. There remains this golden rule: generally speaking, *it is not so much what the doctor tells the patient, but what the patient tells the doctor*, which brings the initial relief and confidence. Naturally, when the patient has had his or her say there will often be simple explanation, reassurance, and advice which in good time the doctor will be able to impart. Relative failure or difficulty at any stage is less important than the patient's realisation that, given confidence, practice, and an acceptance of the situation on both sides, things will tend to come right. Occasions of intercourse should not be feared or avoided because the possibility of failure lurks for ever in the patient's mind as a perpetual source of misery and discouragement. It may therefore be helpful to offer to talk to the partner, so that their joint attitude towards what may well have seemed to each of them a particularly personal disaster, may become less catastrophic and less bound up with a deeper fear that they are either unloved, unlovable, or incapable of loving.

It is no exaggeration to say that at least a quarter to a third of all patients consulting doctors about this kind of difficulty can be relieved in this way in the course of perhaps six to a dozen interviews, within two or three months.

---

[1] Stafford-Clark, David, 1954, 'The Etiology and Treatment of Impotence', The Practitioner, 172, April 1954, p. 397; Malleson, Joan, 1954, 'Sex Problems in Marriage', The Practitioner, 172, April 1954, p. 389; Dawkins, Sylvia, and Taylor, Rosalie, 1961, 'Non-Consummation of Marriage', The Lancet, November 4, 1961, pp. 1028–33.

DEMENTIA

Definition. In essence, dementia represents the deterioration of previously normal mental function, secondary to brain damage or disease. Some physicians, however, reserve the term for conditions in which the deterioration is progressive and the underlying brain pathology irreversible. The wider usage will be employed here.

Incidence. Exceptionally, dementia can occur at any time in life; but its incidence is most important in the latter third, where it has been variously calculated as affecting from 0·25 up to 0·5 per cent of the population.

Aetiology. Dementia may be primary, or secondary to intercurrent damage or disease. The basis of *primary dementia* is largely unknown; its essential characteristic is the diffuse atrophy of neuronal tissue of the brain, remorselessly but sometimes unevenly progressive.

Genetic and constitutional factors appear to be of some importance in certain cases. Huntington's chorea provides a special but rare example of a progressive dementia accompanied by involuntary movements usually appearing between 35 and 50 and inherited as a Mendelian dominant.

Important causes of *Secondary Dementia* include:

(1) Damage from *injury*.

(2) Damage by *poisoning*: (a) by alcohol;
   (b) by lead and other heavy metals such as antimony or manganese.

(3) Damage from *anoxia*: particularly from carbon monoxide poisoning and asphyxia.

(4) Damage from *infection*: For example, following encephalitis or cerebro-vascular syphilis (general paralysis of the insane).

(5) Damage from *metabolic error*: For example, vitamin B deficiency (beri-beri) or as a further less direct complication of chronic alcoholism.
   Another example of metabolic error producing a reversible type of dementia is the disturbance of protein metabolism secondary to chronic liver damage which may produce a characteristic form of dementia long before the onset of hepatic coma.

(6) Damage by *neoplasm*: This may be intra- or extra-cerebral (meningioma); and in the case of intra-cerebral neoplasm may be primary or metastatic.

(7) *Degenerative conditions*: Hypertension and arteriosclerosis.

Pathology. The essential pathology of primary dementia is the replacement of destroyed neurones by neuroglia.

The pathology of secondary dementia is essentially that of the primary cause. In both instances the gross appearance of the brain shows a shrinking, with distortion of normal contour and outline, flattening of the gyri, widening sulci, and expansion of the ventricles often apparent upon air encephalography.

There is frequently some rise in protein (>40 mg per cent) in the cerebrospinal fluid in primary dementia, and, in secondary dementia, changes characteristic of the primary disorder.

Clinical Features. The impairment of mental function inevitably affects all three aspects of personality: intelligence, emotional integration, and behaviour. But in practice the relative degree of evident deterioration in each aspect may vary considerably, producing a variety of clinical pictures. Epileptic attacks may occur at an early stage.

Failure of recent memory is the most consistent disability. This may be so gross that the patient may be unable to remember the nature or the place of his last meal, where he is now living, and the whereabouts or even the death of his closest relatives or friends. The tendency to fill in what are in fact blank spaces in the subjective memory of recent events by entirely confabulatory accounts, for which the patient has no insight whatever, is a characteristic of dementia of this type.

By contrast, remote memory may be relatively unimpaired and may indeed remain for the patient the sole source of vivid interest and recall. Concurrent with the failure of recent memory there is correspondingly failure of attention, concentration, and judgement; and, with these, a total lack of interest in contemporary events, so that such patients neither read nor discuss items of contemporary news or interest, and are frequently grossly disorientated in time and space.

Before recognition has led to appropriate care being taken of such patients, they may have slithered into appalling confusion and disintegration in their personal life. Their rooms may be in the state of indescribable squalor and disorder, their underclothes filthy, their belongings jumbled and scattered, suitcases stuffed with rubbish, sweets and half-consumed meals hoarded in cupboards or littering the bed. Much of their day-to-day conduct may be explicable as a mixture of greed, apprehension, slothfulness, bewilderment, and sheer incapacity. In their relationship with others they may also display a capricious querulousness alternating with a shallow remorse. The more sordid and unappetising their predicament, the more necessary it is to remember the tragedy which it bespeaks. This is in essence an insightless atrophy and ultimate obliteration of normal mental life. Dementia is a remorseless enemy of the natural dignity of man.

Diagnosis. In the first instance this is made essentially on clinical grounds; these can then be supported by:

> (1) Formal psychological testing of intellectual function. Characteristic evidence of deterioration, in which vocabulary is least affected, and recent memory and capacity for calculation and logical thought most impaired, will be found.

(2) Lumbar puncture and air-encephalography may be justified where their outcome may confirm or exclude some treatable condition; but in view of the increase in disturbance which may follow air-encephalography, it is questionable whether this should be undertaken with patients in whom the diagnosis of primary dementia on clinical grounds appears to be beyond all reasonable doubt.

(3) Biopsy of cortical material may be used in certain cases; but the reservations expressed in (2) above should also apply here.

(4) Electro-encephalography and arteriography are of no help in diagnosis of primary dementia; but they may be indicated in investigating the cause of secondary dementia where appropriate.

In all cases of secondary dementia the diagnosis is naturally that of the underlying cause.

Treatment. The treatment of primary dementia is essentially only palliative. Its first essential is the acceptance of the patient's disability with kindness, understanding, and realism. But against this background the following measures may be taken:

(1) Establishment of whatever degree of rapport is possible with the patient.

(2) Frank explanation and discussion with the relatives of the implications of this condition, and their obligations to the sufferer.

(3) Saturation with vitamin B as a possible way of mitigating the rate of progress of the disorder by ensuring the maximum nutrition and metabolism of the surviving neurones, and the dilatation of the peripheral cerebral vascular tree.

(4) Symptomatic treatment of any intercurrent condition; for example, malnutrition, chronic infection, or reactive depression, if these are present.

(5) The measures outlined above will need to be combined with whatever social and administrative arrangements can be made to relieve the demented patient of personal burdens and responsibilities which he can no longer sustain, and to contrive circumstances in which his life is passed with as little personal unhappiness, embarrassment, or humiliation to others as is reasonably possible. On all these matters the sensible, detached, but humane advice of the doctor should be invaluable. (See page 60 for reference to legal implications.)

Prognosis. In the wide use of the term 'dementia', reversible cases of secondary dementia are included. The prognosis for these cases is the prognosis for the underlying condition, subject to treatment. But for primary dementia and for many cases of secondary dementia where the underlying cause itself is beyond effective treatment, the prognosis is necessarily hopeless. Recognition of this, and management of the case along lines dictated by the necessity for imagination, tolerance, and humanity, is the key to procedure.

TREATMENT

For as long as mental illness has been recognised, treatment has been divisible under two main broad headings: they can be called respectively, treatment by attempts at communication, and treatment by attempts at transformation.

Treatment by communication covers all forms of exchange of ideas, discussion, reasoning, and emotion; of the effort to reach out into the mind and world of a sick person and, by comprehending it, to make it comprehensible to him; even to enable him to see it in a different way, and to modify his behaviour along lines governed by a deeper and wider understanding and by an increased confidence. This is really the basis of psychotherapy. The term 'psychotherapy' means literally the treatment of the mind. It could therefore logically be applied to all methods of treatment for mental illness. Its use in practice is restricted to those methods which rely for their effect upon the exchange of ideas and understanding between patient and doctor, directed towards relief of the patient's symptoms and distress.

Treatment by transformation has a history as long as any form of medical treatment. Its underlying aim is to change the patient by some means which either does not depend at all, or depends only in the most concrete and limited sense, upon the patient's own co-operation, understanding, and interest. Under this heading come all the various forms of physical treatment which have been employed to relieve or cure mental illness.

Treatment by Communication: Psychotherapy

Psychotherapy can be of two main kinds, depending upon whether the object of communication between the patient and doctor is purely support to sustain the patient, or whether it is to effect some change in his personality or attitude towards his present difficulties, by interpretation of his feelings and predicament which may lead to a better understanding. Supportive psychotherapy and interpretive psychotherapy, which may also be called insight therapy, differ therefore considerably in technique. The former is usually simpler, less ambitious in aim, easier in execution and indicated primarily for patients for whom a more ambitious approach would be impracticable or unproductive.

Nevertheless supportive psychotherapy plays a great part in out-patient management of patients who might otherwise receive no help whatever from their doctor. It can include direct, simple and sympathetic advice, and sheer reassurance and encouragement; and may be combined with practical intervention in the social circumstances of the patient, whereby emotional complications of his family life or employment may be constructively modified through personal contact with the family or employer, usually by a trained psychiatric social worker attached to the out-patient clinic and under the supervision of the psychiatrist concerned.

Such advice or explanation as the doctor has to offer will be based not upon his own personal feelings about the desirability of any particular solution; still less upon a projection on his part of what he would do if he were in the patient's shoes: these being the two shortcomings from which so much well-intentioned lay advice so often suffers. By contrast, the doctor's advice and explanation will be based upon his objective assessment of the patient's individual needs and possibilities, gained from his knowledge of the patient acquired in the way described, and accepted without prejudice of any kind.

Psychotherapy of this limited but invaluable kind should be within the capacity of every practising doctor. The expenditure of a limited amount of time in this way is not only humane, but economical; for by the skilled use of a few hours spread out over weeks or months, the physician may not only avert the chronic invalidism and demoralisation of the neurotic patient, but may also spare himself the bitterness and frustration which inevitably assails a practitioner continually confronted with this aspect of human suffering, who has never acquired the interest or understanding necessary to deal with it effectively.

Interpretive Psychotherapy

All interpretive psychotherapy is based on three principles: they are—

(1) Behaviour is prompted chiefly by emotional considerations, but insight and understanding are necessary to modify and control such behaviour and the aims underlying it.

(2) A very significant proportion of human emotion, together with the action to which it leads, is not normally accessible to personal introspection, being rooted in areas of the mind which are beneath the surface of consciousness.

(3) It follows logically (and is supported empirically by experimental and clinical work) that *any process which makes available to individual consciousness the true significance of emotional conflicts and tensions hitherto repressed*, will thereby produce both heightened awareness, and increased stability and emotional control.

The application of these principles in practice can lead not simply to improved health in its widest sense, but also to a more mature and developed personality.

This in essence is the case for interpretive psychotherapy, but there is, alas, no space further to present it here. For information about the theoretical foundations and practical applications for the various analytic techniques of psychotherapy the reader is referred to the brief bibliography at the end of this section.

Ancillary and Special Psychotherapeutic Techniques

Hypnosis

Hypnosis can be used both in supportive and, in certain cases, in interpretive psychotherapy and in the special applications of deconditioning and learning theory in the treatment of phobic states. Its range of indications and techniques require direct instruction and experience and cannot be covered in a brief survey of this kind.

Abreaction, using physical methods

Abreaction is the term given to the explosively rapid release of emotion, in a psychotherapeutic setting. This can occur when previously repressed material is suddenly recalled, whether in normal psychotherapeutic interviews, under hypnosis, or in special circumstances, by the use of physical methods, such as partial anaesthesia with ether, or the intravenous injection of solutions of soluble barbiturate preparations, combined with methedrine. Abreactive techniques are apt to be particularly valuable when the buried material is comparatively recent and compact, as in the experiences of war, natural catastrophes such as fire, earthquake, avalanche, or other accidents in which the patient may have been involved. Often after such experiences, memory for the event which has been partly or completely lost can be restored in one or two periods of treatment in which much of the unbearable emotion returns, but is on this occasion accepted and integrated in consciousness.

Abreaction can be secured with ether, when an explosive emotional outburst is anticipated and can be controlled; less explosive or more protracted work of this kind can be done with the aid of intravenous barbiturate preparations. As well as states of amnesia, recent and severe attacks of acute anxiety will sometimes respond to treatment of this kind. It is obvious that the selection of cases suitable for this type of treatment must be made with great care, and must depend to a considerable extent upon the capacity of the patient to deal with the material released in this heroic fashion. The use of abreactive techniques in patients on the edge of schizophrenic illness, for example, can prove utterly disastrous.

TREATMENT BY TRANSFORMATION

(1) Symptomatic Treatment

(a) Sedation

Sedation by day has the aim of reducing the patient's subjective distress and objectively disturbed behaviour: by night it can combat the insomnia which in various forms is such a constant and distressing feature of many forms of psychiatric disorder.

(1) *Diurnal Sedation*

This can be achieved by soluble barbiturate preparations in small divided doses. Examples are amylobarbitone sodium, 50 mg. t.d.s., or b.d., or phenobarbitone 15 mg. t.d.s. It is most unwise to exceed the latter dose of phenobarbitone for diurnal sedation in psychiatry, since phenobarbitone is a relatively long-acting drug, can readily become cumulative in larger doses, and under such circumstances exerts a markedly depressant effect. *For this reason phenobarbitone should never be given to depressed patients.*

Methylpentynol (oblivon) is occasionally a useful substitute for barbiturates for sensitive patients, given in divided doses of 250–500 mg. three to four times a day.

(2) *Nocturnal Sedation*

Properly used, barbiturates are a standby: amylobarbitone sodium has already been mentioned and for nocturnal sedation, doses of 200–400 mg. are reasonable.

Other preparations of general use include:

> Quinalbarbitone sodium (seconal) 100–200 mg.
> Pentobarbitone sodium (nembutal) 100–200 mg.
> Butobarbitone (soneryl) 100–200 mg.

and various combinations of these put up by the proprietary firms.

As an alternative to barbiturates, chloral is both safe and reliable. Chloral hydrate, taken, for example, in fruit juice in doses of 1–3 g., is effective.

Methylpentynol (oblivon) in doses of 1–2 g. may also produce sleep.

Three general observations can be added on the subject of sedation:

(1) The day of bromides and of paraldehyde is past. Bromide preparations are cumulative, toxic, and readily lead to confusion and disturbance of sleep-rhythm rather than its consolidation. There is no longer any indication for the prescription of bromide as a sedative in psychiatry.

Paraldehyde, while less pernicious than bromide, is a malodorous and nauseating draught with no compensatory advantages: as an intramuscular injection it is crude, cruel, cumbersome, and carries a significant risk of abscess formation.

(2) Owing to the regularity with which overdoses of barbiturates are used for suicidal attempts, a number of proprietary firms have put out combinations of barbiturates with emetics or with antidotes such as megimide, incorporated in small doses. The effect of a large dose of such preparations is then either to produce vomiting or to prevent coma.

A wiser and more effective safeguard is to know and to control the dosage which each individual patient receives from the doctor. Very few patients in fact kill themselves with barbiturates prescribed by a single doctor on a single occasion. They either hoard them, which the doctor can at least bear in mind when repeating prescriptions; or they obtain a number of prescriptions from different doctors, or manage to take the same prescription to a number of different chemists. These activities are not always entirely beyond the imagination and control of the doctors and pharmacists concerned.

(3) Whenever barbiturates are prescribed regularly, an accompanying dose of vitamin B should be given (orovite or becosym forte, tabs 1 t.d.s.). This obviates the disturbance of carbohydrate metabolism which has been shown to follow prolonged barbiturate ingestion in the absence of additional vitamin B.

(b) Tranquillising Preparations

These may be given both as alternatives to diurnal sedation, and as adjuncts to nocturnal sedation. Their characteristic clinical action is to produce calmness and tranquillity without sedation as such. In general they are useful in conditions of chronic anxiety, and for the tension and agitation associated with some states of depression and obsessive compulsive disorder. They include:

(1) Meprobamate (Equanil: miltown) 400 mg. three or four times daily.
(2) Chlordiazepoxide (Librium) and diazepam (Valium): 5–10 mg. three or four times daily.
(3) The entire range of phenothiazine compounds (chlorpromazine, promazine, etc.). These will receive further mention in their more important roles as specific drugs in the treatment of schizophrenia; but in severe states of agitation and tension they have a useful symptomatic role as tranquillisers.

(2) Specific Medicinal Treatment

(a) Anti-depressant

Preparations which produce a specific reversal of the depressive syndrome in certain cases include:

(1) imipramine hydrochloride (tofranil)
(2) amitriptyline hydrochloride (tryptizol) and nortryptyline (aventyl)
(3) compounds having in common their function as amine-oxidase inhibitors.

The exact mode of action of these preparations is not yet fully understood, but it seems probable that they produce their effect by potentiating or prolonging the action of sympathin in the brain. Sympathin is largely compounded of adrenaline and nor-adrenaline, and is potentiated by serotonin. The first three of the compounds listed above may act directly by potentiating sympathin and may also potentiate serotonin itself.

The group of amine-oxidase inhibitors prolong the action of sympathin by interfering with its breakdown by amino-oxidase. They include:

> Nialamide (niamid),
> Isocarboxazid (marplan) and
> Phenelzine (nardil).

Dosage and technique of administration should be carefully supervised in accordance with the instructions of the manufacturers in every case.

Complications attendant upon some of these anti-depressant drugs have been jaundice and liver damage in some of the earlier preparations (not included among those mentioned above, and now largely abandoned); there is also the occasional risk that in the emergent phase from severe depression, some 2 to 3 weeks after the drug has begun to take effect, the patient may be sufficiently released from retardation to make a suicidal attempt, which previously only the severity of his psychomotor incapacity had held in check.

Side effects, including dizziness, dryness of the mouth, mistiness of vision, constipation, and a kind of irritable restless fatigue, are also to be expected within the first 10 days of starting a course of imipramine and some of the amine-oxidase inhibitors. Patients forewarned about this can usually tolerate it. Sometimes treatment for this reason has to be initiated in hospital. Treatment with (1), (2), or (3) (above) can be combined with E.C.T., but in many of the milder cases it may actually replace it. It is wiser not to combine E.C.T. with amine oxidase inhibitors.

(b) **Anti-excitement Preparations** (Anti-manic, anti-hallucinatory and particularly anti-schizophrenic drugs).

(1) Haloperidol, a butyrophenone derivative, has proved valuable in controlling hypomania.

(2) *Phenothiazine Derivatives*. This group of preparations has now reached enormous proportions. The parent drug is chlorpromazine (largactil); but a vast number of comparable preparations, each with allegedly specific indications, and differing doses, have been elaborated. They include:

> Promazine (sparine), 50–150 mg. t.d.s.
> Thioridazine (melleril), 25–75 mg. t.d.s.
> Trifluoperazine (stelazine), 5–15 mg. t.d.s.
> Perphenazine (fentazin), 2–6 mg. t.d.s.
> Prochlorperazine (compazine, stemetil), 10 mg. t.d.s.

They have in common the capacity to reduce the general level of excitement, disorientation, and confusion of a disturbed patient, and appear to have a specifically tranquillising and anti-hallucinatory effect in schizo-phrenia, where in large doses they make possible the establishment of rapport and contact with an otherwise inaccessible patient. Taking chlorpromazine as a standard, the normal dose is 25 to 75 mg. t.d.s., but doses as high as 400 mg t.d.s. can be given in hospital. Low regular doses can be used in chronic schizophrenics.

(3) *Reserpine and Related Alkaloids.* A number of alkaloids have been isolated from the plant rauwolfia serpentina. These substances liberate serotonin in the brain and have been used especially in the treatment of schizophrenia. They can be combined with phenothiazine derivatives in intensive in-patient therapy, and both preparations can be used in combina-tion with E.C.T., sometimes with extremely effective results.

Both phenothiazine and rauwolfia serpentina derivatives can produce a reversible syndrome either singly or in combination, involving parkin-sonism, and jaundice. The former is never serious, the latter must always be regarded as potentially so. Reduction of the dose will usually lead to a remission of symptoms, but liver function tests and extreme care in the exhibition of these preparations subsequently should always follow the reaction of jaundice in a sensitive patient.

(c) **Anti-delirium:** *Specific Medicinal Therapy*

The specific role of vitamin saturation in treatment of toxic confusion states has already been mentioned. The most effective immediate treat-ment is parenteral vitamin B and C in proprietary preparation (parentro-vite), the combination being mixed in a syringe from two small glass ampoules before injection. The other measures to be considered in the treatment of acute toxic confusional states have been outlined in detail, together with the contra-indications of certain traditional but disastrous specifics such as intramuscular paraldehyde, in the relevant section. (See p. 38.)

PHYSICAL METHODS OF TREATMENT

Special Techniques

Over the past forty years several careful but essentially empirical tech-niques have significantly improved the whole outlook for certain types of mental illness by providing methods of physical treatment which in many cases can relieve or cure conditions which were previously beyond the power of psychological medicine to control. Properly used they can produce changes in the function of the brain, autonomic nervous system, and neuro-endocrine system, through the use of electricity and neuro-surgery.

Electrical Treatment. Electroconvulsive Therapy (E.C.T.)

The modern version of this method of treatment consists in the pro-duction of an epileptiform convulsion modified by the specific muscle relaxant drugs, such as succinylcholine, under intravenous barbiturate anaesthesia, by the passage of a very small electrical current of the order of 250–500 milli-amps, for a duration of up to one second, at a voltage not exceeding 150 volts. The treatment is given with the patient in bed, the first stage being the production of anaesthesia, which is followed by the intravenous administration of a muscle relaxant, the establishment of artificial respiration with oxygen through a B.L.B. mask, and the passage of the current through electrodes placed on the scalp.

Apart from a temporary alteration in breathing, and a flickering in facial muscles and the peripheral muscles of the forearms, hands, and feet, which provides evidence of adequacy of the dose, there is no physical accompaniment to the patient's response. As soon as the response has been achieved, the sponge rubber gag, which is inserted to prevent damage to the teeth or jaws during the actual passage of the current, is removed, an airway inserted, and oxygen maintained until normal breathing is re-established within three or four minutes.

Within five to ten minutes the patient begins to recover consciousness, with no knowledge whatever of the details of the procedure and no memory of anything more unpleasant than the administration of the anaesthetic.

Treatment is usually given once or twice a week; the average number of treatments necessary completely to relieve a severe depressive illness is somewhere between six and twelve; however, since unilateral E.C.T. has proved to be the safest and most gentle form of treatment in most cases, up to twenty treatments may now be given. Treatment can, under special circumstances, be given on an out-patient basis, but it is generally preferable that it should be given in hospital, at least on the first occasion.

Its general effect is progressively to relieve depression until the patient is restored to full normal health and happiness. This effect is quite remarkable, and the nature of the relief accorded can be spectacular, when a tormented, agitated, weeping, suicidal patient is transformed into a calm, vigorous, active, and happy person. Needless to say, psychotherapy before, during, and after the course of electrical treatment is part of the whole process. In the early stages its most effective form is essentially that of encouragement and reassurance, based upon an appreciation of the patient's grief and fears. At a later stage, when improvement has begun, the degree to which personal problems may remain to be dealt with will vary among individual patients and will effect the nature of the psychotherapy required.

Pre-frontal Leucotomy

Pre-frontal Leucotomy. The principle underlying this operation is the partial isolation of the frontal lobes from connection with the rest of the brain, particularly the thalamus, hypothalamus, and temporo-parietal region. The fronto-thalamic relationship, which is deliberately impaired or sacrificed by this operation, appears to be essentially concerned with the emotional quality and elaboration of associations to incoming information.

In this sense it seems to play a fundamental part in colouring the whole of the patient's personal experience or, to put it in the simplest terms, the way he feels about things. The established patterns of activity and associated emotional experience mediated by this aspect of brain function appear to be stored largely in the tempo-parietal areas; certainly disturbances of the kind seen in temporal lobe epilepsy produce changes both in subjective emotion and observable behaviour of a consistent and characteristic kind.

Indications. The primary general indication for operation of this kind would seem to be otherwise intractable anguish or other severe and crippling distress, for example, persistent physical pain not accessible to surgery, in which tension and emotional suffering are paramount, while apathy and withdrawal are not. Such states of mental or physical extremity would normally need to have existed either continually or intermittently for at least one or two years, but ideally for not much more than two, and preferably for not more than five; and to have been treated by other appropriate physical methods either without success or with only temporary relief, before such operation is justified. There can be no doubt that this operation, whatever the particular form or technique adopted, is essentially a destructive procedure; moreover, its effects, in so far as they are under the control of the operator, are irreversible in most cases: so that while the undeniable and sometimes seemingly miraculous benefits which may accrue from it in suitable cases can never be excluded in weighing the indication for its use, the utmost care and deliberation is necessary before advising it, and the decision as to whether or not it is the right procedure is often one of the most anxious and difficult which the psychiatrist and neuro-surgeon in consultation may have to make.

GENERAL CONCLUSIONS

Although in this section physical and psychological methods of treatment have necessarily been described separately, in clinical practice they are essentially complementary; and, though in some cases it may be possible to bring relief and even to accelerate recovery by psychological methods alone, it is neither reasonable nor humane to rely upon physical intervention, without individual interest, compassion, and understanding, in the treatment of any patient for any disease.

FURTHER READING (PSYCHOTHERAPY)

Adler, A. (trans. P. Radin), (1924) *The Practice and Theory of Individual Psychology*, Kegan, Paul, Trench.

Freud, S. (trans. Sprott), *New Introductory Lectures on Psycho-analysis*. Hogarth Press, London (1933).

Jung, C. (1928), *Collected Papers on Analytical Psychology*. Baillière, Tindall and Cox.

Stafford Clark, D., *Modern Trends in Psychological Medicine*. Butterworths, London (1970).

PSYCHIATRY AND THE LAW

In all aspects of relationship between psychiatry and the law, it is the law which calls the tune. The law defines the basis of the relationship and by definition is the final arbiter in all interpretations of medico-legal problems. Four fundamental legal principles underlie the whole of forensic psychiatry, and from the standpoint of justice they are unexceptionable. They are:

(1) A sane man is assumed to be wholly responsible for his actions and to intend their consequences.

(2) Just as innocence must be presumed while guilt has to be proved, so equally must sanity be presumed and insanity proved to the satisfaction of a magistrate, judge or jury, before it can be legally accepted.

(3) No man may be indefinitely deprived of liberty, or of the privilege of managing his own affairs, on purely medical grounds: such deprivation, even if necessitated in a patient's own interests and entirely by his unsoundness of mind, may be recommended, and in emergency undertaken, by a doctor; but must always be ratified by the decision of the duly appointed and legally authorised representative body or individual—in the case of deprivation of liberty, by the appropriate mental health review tribunal of the local regional hospital board; and in the case of management of property, by the Court of Protection (see p. 60).

(4) Criminal responsibility is always and essentially an affair of mind as well as of body, of intention as well as of action. This is a principle which has been enshrined in English law for nearly 800 years: it is embodied in the famous legal tag, '*actus non facit reum nisi mens sit rea*' ('There cannot be a guilty act unless there is a guilty mind').

These principles form the foundation of all laws concerned with mental illness, now consolidated in the Mental Health Act 1959: they are held also throughout the whole body of common law, wherever this has to do with the assessment of a person's mental state.

In practice, the legal implications of psychiatry may be summarised under three headings:

(1) Civil responsibility.
(2) Criminal responsibility.
(3) Individual liberty.

Civil Responsibility

Medical opinion as to an individual's state of mind may be required in law to assist in deciding—

(a) whether he is competent to give evidence;

(b) whether he is competent to enter into a civil contract: this includes marriage as well as contracts of a more essentially commercial kind;

(c) whether he is competent to recognise and fulfil his normal legal obligations, independently of contract. An infringement or failure to respect the general rights of others, independently of contract, is known as a tort; the law of torts, and their relationship to unsoundness of mind, is one of the most complicated aspects of English jurisprudence;

(d) whether he is competent to make a valid will.

In every case the doctor must be guided by his knowledge of the patient, by his recognition of the nature of the disturbance of mental state which may exist, and by its probable effect upon the patient's capacity to undertake the various responsibilities above described. What is required is a lucid common sense and reasonable appreciation of the situation: no more, and no less.

Under the Matrimonial Causes Act of 1950*, and the Divorce (Insanity and Desertion) Act, 1958, a marriage may be declared null upon proof that either party to the marriage was at the time of the marriage suffering from unsoundness of mind, whether from mental defect or insanity: under certain circumstances supervening insanity is also a ground for the dissolution of a marriage. But before the Court can dissolve a marriage on these grounds it must be satisfied by medical evidence that the mental illness is effectively incurable, and that the patient has been continuously under care and treatment for at least five years immediately preceding the presentation of the petition. The Abortion Act of 1968 required psychiatric guidance for colleagues perplexed by unwanted pregnancies.

Criminal Responsibility

In law responsibility means liability to punishment. A plea of unsoundness of mind may be raised by way of defence to any criminal charge, but for all practical purposes such a plea is usually confined to charges of murder. The law as to responsibility of insane persons is still based upon the answers of the judges consulted by the House of Lords in 1843 after the murder of Mr. Edward Drummond, Private Secretary to Sir Robert Peel. Drummond was shot dead by a man called MacNaughton, who was suffering from delusions of persecution and who killed Drummond in mistake for Sir Robert Peel himself. MacNaughton was tried and, after evidence of his delusions had been heard, was acquitted on grounds of insanity on the judge's direction. The public reaction to this acquittal was most unfavourable, and eventually led to a debate in the House of Lords where a number of questions were put to those of its members who were judges. The answers have come to be known as the MacNaughton Rules, and are in essence as follows:

* The wording of the 1950 Act was amended by the 7th Schedule to the Mental Health Act, 1959.

In order to establish a defence on the grounds of insanity, it must be clearly proved *'that at the time of committing the act the accused was labouring under such a defect of reason from disease of the mind as not to know the nature and quality of the act he was doing; or if he knew what he was doing, that he did not know that it was wrong'*. The second important provision is that if the accused commits an act by reason of delusion, the degree of responsibility which must be attached to him, and therefore in law the degree of culpability which must be attributed, is based upon the justification which the delusion would provide, if it were true. The frank absurdity of evaluating insane delusions as if they were true, in assessing the sufferer's responsibility, while ignoring the underlying mental illness of which the delusions are themselves evidence, has been recognised for over eighty years; but this aspect of the rules is now rarely invoked.

The principal medical criticisms levelled against the rules are founded upon two points: the first, that the rules made no provision for the effect upon conduct of pathological disturbances of emotion as opposed to disturbances of reason or knowledge; the second, that the diagnosis of any kind of insanity is a complex medical task and cannot reasonably be finally entrusted to a panel of laymen, the jury.

In support of the first objection, there is the glaring inadequacy of the rules to take account of the nature of depression, one of the commonest forms of serious mental illness. A depressed patient may be driven by his illness to attempt to commit suicide; but if he has a dependent relative— for example, an aged mother—he may kill her first in his mood of utter despair and subsequently be apprehended before he can take his own life. In such a case it is clearly difficult for the honest expert medical witness to maintain either that the man did not know what he was doing, or that he did not know that it was wrong. But the balance of the patient's mind is no less overthrown, and his sanity therefore no less impaired, because the disturbance is primarily emotional rather than rational.

However, not all medical objections to the MacNaughton Rules are themselves free from confusion. Doctors have to remember that the law does not presume to define insanity. That is accepted as a medical question. What the law considers are the conditions which have to be satisfied in order that a person may be excused from criminal responsibility. Moreover the determination of such responsibility, like that of every other question of fact or opinion in the course of trial by jury, must finally be made by the jury themselves. The object of the MacNaughton Rules is to provide a clear, concise direction for the guidance of judges in advising juries as to the law with regard to criminal responsibility in particular circumstances. They have never pretended to define insanity from a medical point of view.

The measure of public support for them is based upon a salutarily jealous concern for the ultimate powers of the jury, reinforced by their apparent logic and common sense. But doctors are entitled to point out that this latter appearance is to some extent deceptive, since the rules are derived from an over-simplified and now obsolete concept of human mental processes. The Homicide Act (1957), by recognising that responsibility may be impaired by illness not amounting to legal insanity, has gone some way towards meeting this medical criticism.

Individual Liberty

This includes both physical liberty, and the normal freedom which an individual possesses to manage his own personal and financial affairs. Under the Mental Health Act of 1959, all previous Acts and Statutes are superseded. The underlying principles of this Act are that psychiatric patients should be able to seek treatment with no more formality than that required for any other type of illness; and that those patients who are incapable of appreciating their own need for in-patient treatment in hospital should be compulsorily admitted for observation or treatment only if it is urgently and immediately essential on medical grounds for their own safety and protection or for the safety and protection of others.

Compulsory admission, under such circumstances, can be arranged in any one of the following ways:

(a) Emergency admission for observation. This can be arranged by a doctor with the co-operation of the Mental Welfare Officer for the appropriate area, into any hospital with suitable facilities, for a period of 72 hours (Section 29).

(b) Admission for observation for 28 days. This normally follows emergency admission, and requires two independent medical recommendations (Section 25).

(c) Admission for treatment. This also requires two medical recommendations, and covers any period from 28 days up to a year (Section 26), but can be terminated at any stage either by the patient electing to remain voluntarily under medical care, or in any of the following ways (Sections 43–57):

(1) By discharge being requested by the nearest relative, who must then accept full responsibility.

(2) On the advice of the doctor in charge of treatment.

(3) As a result of the decision of the local authority, or

(4) Of the appropriate mental health tribunal. This tribunal is charged with the responsibility of reviewing every case independently at statutory intervals, or at the request of the patient himself (Sections 47 and 48).

(d) Special procedures for compulsory admission may follow a Court Order in an order by the Home Office, in the case of patients who have come into conflict with the law and subsequently have been discovered to be mentally ill (Sections 60–70). These provisions apply equally to patients with mental illness on the one hand and various degrees of mental deficiency on the other. The official legal terms for mental deficiency are subnormality and severe subnormality.

A fourth legal category exists under the Mental Health Act of 1959; that of psychopath. Psychopaths and subnormal patients can be compulsorily admitted for treatment upon a medical recommendation if they are under twenty-one years of age; the rationale underlying this procedure is that such patients have the greatest chance of benefiting from special treatment or training in the early years of life. Over the age of twenty-one they cannot compulsorily be admitted for treatment except by Court Order: nor can they be detained beyond the age of twenty-five years unless they have been proved to be dangerous to others. All patients under compulsory admission orders can appeal to the appropriate Mental Health Review Tribunal within six months of their admission.

In practice the Mental Health Act has gone some way towards recognising a change in public opinion and medical and legal practice which had been the direct outcome of enlightenment and advance in treatment and attitude for a number of years before the Royal Commission, which reported upon the desirability of changing the law, and the Act which implemented the changes. Over 80 per cent of all admissions to mental hospitals are in fact voluntary admissions, and over 80 per cent of all patients discharged from mental hospitals have been in-patients for less than six months.

Nevertheless it is important to remember that only a degree of unsoundness of mind amounting to insanity in law can be held to justify compulsory admission for treatment. It remains perfectly possible for a man or woman to refuse an operation or any other form of medical treatment, and to die from the consequences of this refusal, unless such refusal is based upon a degree of unsoundness of mind which would be recognised as insanity, in law. In practice here, as in every other aspect of medicine and surgery, and indeed in every other aspect of human affairs, the final determination of the issue rests upon the relationship of trust, acceptance, and humility between human beings, rather than upon purely legal provisions on the one hand or purely technical possibilities on the other.

Management of Property (M.H.A. Sections 101–121 and M. of H. Circular 23/60)

The Court of Protection exists to protect the property and interests of all people who are mentally incapable of managing their own affairs. An application to the Court (address 25 Store St, London, W.C.1) supported by an appropriate medical recommendation on the form of affidavit available therefrom is required in any case where the patient, whether in hospital or not, is 'incapable by mental disorder of managing or administering his property or affairs, (Section 101). The usual procedure is to appoint a receiver to act in the name of and on behalf of the patient. Such arrangements are not subject to time limit, but can always be terminated on recovery or discharge from hospital, such application requiring a supporting medical opinion.

CHAPTER THREE

THE ALIMENTARY SYSTEM

SYMPTOMS OF ALIMENTARY DISORDERS

1. Pain

There is still no general agreement either about the mechanism of abdominal pain or its classification. Following the observations of Kellgren, who showed that human volunteers could distinguish only two types of pain, a superficial variety elicited by stimulation of the skin and subcutaneous tissues and a deep variety felt when any structure deep to the subcutaneous tissues was stimulated, doubt has been cast on the validity of the traditional classification of abdominal pain into visceral and somatic types. Furthermore, the description of pain given by patients with visceral and somatic lesions, such as carcinoma of the stomach and retroperitoneal sarcoma, often fails to provide any distinguishing clue.

Nevertheless, certain types of pain are sufficiently characteristic to be of great value in diagnosis. *Colic*, originally pain arising in the colon, is a term now applied to painful spasm in any hollow muscular viscus, usually due to partial or complete obstruction of its lumen. Intestinal colic is a spasmodic pain, coming in a succession of waves which rise to a peak of intensity and then subside; renal and biliary colic, however, may persist at a steady and very severe level for an hour or more. The patient doubles up or writhes about when it is at its height and warmth applied to the abdomen helps to relieve it. There may be associated vomiting. Colic is usually poorly localised, but small intestine spasm is felt mainly in the centre of the abdomen, large intestine colic in the lower abdomen, renal colic in the loin radiating to the groin and testicle on the same side, biliary colic in the right upper quadrant or epigastrium sometimes radiating through to the back, and uterine colic in the lower abdomen.

Pain due to inflammation of the parietal peritoneum, on the other hand, is a sharp steady severe pain accurately localised over the site of the inflammation. Pressure on the area causes tenderness and reflex spasm in the overlying muscles (guarding or rigidity) and since the pain is aggravated by movement the patient usually lies quite still.

Patients with acute appendicitis provide a good illustration of these two types of pain. In the early stages when there is obstruction and consequent spasm in the appendix the patient has colicky pain vaguely referred to the area around the umbilicus, and he frequently vomits at the outset; but in a few hours, when inflammation has developed in the appendix and spread to involve the parietal peritoneum, the pain becomes sharper and shifts to the right iliac fossa directly over the site of the lesion.

Pain and tenderness occur in the liver only when its capsule is acutely stretched by sudden distension of the organ, as in congestive cardiac failure; and in the spleen when there is inflammation in its peritoneal covering, as by an infarct extending to the surface. The mechanism of pain in peptic ulcer is considered on p. 68.

2. Vomiting

Vomiting is produced by compression of the stomach between the muscles of the abdominal wall and the diaphragm, with simultaneous relaxation of the cardiac sphincter and reverse peristalsis in the stomach and oesophagus. The causes are very numerous, but fall into a few main groups:

(a) When due to *intra-abdominal disease* it is usually preceded by nausea. In pyloric obstruction the vomiting may be projectile, the gastric contents being ejected from the patient's mouth with great force, and frequently very large quantities of vomit are produced containing recognisable food taken many hours previously. In intestinal obstruction the reverse peristalsis throughout the gut may eventually cause faeculent vomiting.

(b) *Cerebral vomiting* occurs in patients with raised intracranial pressure and there is often no preceding nausea. Labyrinthine disturbances are also common causes of vomiting, as in patients with acute vertigo or travel sickness.

(c) *Psychological vomiting* is also common. Some people vomit from sudden fear or horror, as for example if they see an accident in the street; others do so for less obvious and more deep-seated psychological reasons. Repeated persistent vomiting without loss of weight is nearly always of this type.

3. Heartburn

A burning pain behind the sternum is a symptom common in many alimentary disorders and is therefore not very helpful in diagnosis. It is perhaps most commonly found in patients with peptic oesophagitis due to gastro-oesophageal regurgitation; these patients may also have *acid regurgitation*, complaining that from time to time a bitter-tasting fluid rises up into the throat.

4. Waterbrash

Waterbrash is filling of the mouth with a tasteless fluid (saliva) and nearly always indicates the presence of a duodenal ulcer.

5. Diarrhoea

(a) *Acute Diarrhoea* is usually due to dietetic indiscretion, food poisoning, infections such as bacillary dysentery, or an exacerbation in one of the causes of chronic diarrhoea.

(b) *Chronic diarrhoea* occurs:

(1) after operations such as gastrectomy and vagotomy,
(2) from lesions of the small intestine such as regional ileitis (Crohn's disease) and the malabsorption syndromes,
(3) in diseases of the colon, such as carcinoma, diverticulitis, amoebiasis and ulcerative colitis.

Apart from alimentary disorders such as the above, chronic diarrhoea may be due to general causes, such as thyrotoxicosis or anxiety neurosis.

6. Constipation

Many men and nearly all women when asked about their bowels reply that they have always tended to be rather constipated. They mean that instead of having a daily bowel action, which the patent medicine advertisements have taught them is essential for normal health, their bowels move only once every two or three days. They have therefore fallen into the habit of taking a purgative every day or once or twice a week, and they believe that continuing with this ritual is essential to their well-being. In fact, however, variations in the normal rhythm of the colon are quite wide, and to evacuate the bowel twice a week is not constipation; it may be just as normal and healthy as to evacuate it twice a day. On the other hand, the taking of regular evacuants seldom does any actual harm and when a patient with a lifelong dependence on one of them comes into hospital with an organic complaint, undoubtedly the most sensible plan is to continue prescribing his usual laxative. The time is not appropriate to attempt re-education of bowel function, which in any case would be most unlikely to succeed.

Normal regular movement of the bowels is not to be expected in febrile dehydrated patients who are taking little or no solid food and a dose of cascara or senna or a simple enema every few days is all that is needed. Greater care must be taken to ensure a regular evacuation in weak, elderly patients, in whom impaction of a mass of faeces in the rectum tends to occur.

Dyschezia is constipation due to functional sluggishness of the bowel, due mainly to persistent failure to answer the call to stool. It is treated by patient re-training of a regular bowel habit, helped in the early stages by a mild aperient such as senna or by glycerine suppositories.

THE MOUTH AND THROAT

Inspection of the mouth and throat in a good light is an essential part of every medical examination for, apart from purely local conditions which will not be discussed here, it occasionally reveals evidence of some general disorder.

Furring of the tongue is too common to be of much help in diagnosis and is often seen in smokers who are in good health. The 'black hairy tongue' due to alteration in the normal flora of the mouth is mainly seen in patients who have been treated with broad spectrum antibiotics. The thickly coated tongue and uriniferous breath of the uraemic patient contrast sharply with the clean dry tongue and sweetish ketotic breath of the severe diabetic.

Atrophy of the filiform papillae of the tongue, making the normal velvety surface smooth and shiny, is seen in *iron deficiency,* when it appears first round the edge of the tongue; in *vitamin B_{12} deficiency,* when it is usually first seen on the dorsum; in *riboflavin and nicotinic acid deficiency,* in this country usually the result of some intestinal disorder and sometimes associated with cracking at the angles of the mouth; and occasionally after the oral administration of antibiotics.

Brown pigmentation on the lips and on the buccal mucosa lining the cheeks is an important sign of Addison's disease, but is also seen in normal people of mixed racial origin.

Sloughing ulceration of the mouth and throat is an important sign of agranulocytosis and acute leukaemia and in the monocytic variety of the latter disease there may also be swelling and infiltration of the gums and occasionally of the tongue.

THE OESOPHAGUS

Peptic Oesophagitis. The squamous epithelium of the oesophagus is not designed to resist the digestive action of acid gastric juice and it frequently becomes inflamed and eroded in patients with gastro-oesophageal reflux. Such reflux occurs particularly, but not exclusively, in association with hiatus hernia. It should be noted too that other patients with hiatus hernia, with or without radiologically demonstrable reflux, suffer no ill-effects whatever.

Two important *symptoms* may arise from peptic oesophagitis. The commoner is *substernal pain,* similar in quality and distribution to angina pectoris; it is brought on, however, not by effort but by positions which encourage gastro-oesophageal reflux, mainly lying flat and stooping after a meal. The second symptom is *bleeding,* rarely presenting as haematemesis but sometimes causing severe and at first obscure anaemia.

Diagnosis. *Barium meal* examination in the Trendelenburg position demonstrates the gastro-oesophageal reflux and usually an associated hiatus hernia and the inflammation and erosion of the oesophageal mucosa can be confirmed by *oesophagoscopy.* Reproduction of the pain by introducing 0·1N hydrochloric acid into the lower oesophagus (*Bernstein's test*) or even by drinking a hot cup of tea is useful confirmatory evidence.

Treatment. (1) *Medical.* Most patients can be treated successfully by a simple regime designed to minimise gastro-oesophageal reflux and to neutralise any gastric acid which finds its way into the gullet. These ends are achieved by sleeping in a 'head up' position, either well propped up on pillows or with the head of the bed blocked, by avoiding stooping, taking small frequent meals and between them sucking milk-alkali tablets such as 'Nulacin' or 'Prodexin'. A preparation of the consistency of tooth-paste, containing bismuth oxycarbonate and tragacanth, taken in doses of half an ounce before meals is often helpful in relieving heartburn.

(2) *Surgical* repair of the oesophageal hiatus in the diaphragm usually gives excellent results in those patients in whom severe symptoms persist in spite of a reasonable trial on the above regime.

Achalasia of the Cardia

Achalasia of the cardia is due to a disorder of motor function of the oesophagus. Essentially there is an absence of peristalsis through the lower two-thirds of the oesophagus and a failure of the cardia to relax. Normal peristalsis may be replaced by slow ring-like contractions. The oesophagus becomes dilated and its muscle wall is hypertrophied. Because it cannot empty properly the oesophagus may contain food residue. In severe cases these residues may spill over into the lungs to produce recurrent attacks of pneumonia.

Achalasia of the cardia is due to degeneration of the cells of Auerbach's plexus. This is most marked in the dilated portion of the oesophagus and results in denervation of the oesophageal muscle. At the cardia some innervation appears to persist, but it seems likely that the nerves which cause relaxation of the cardia have disappeared.

Clinical Features. Achalasia of the cardia may occur at any age, but is more common in middle age and in women. The chief symptoms are *dysphagia* and *regurgitation*. They may be gradual in onset or may start suddenly, sometimes following an emotional upset. The dysphagia is often worse when the patient is emotionally upset or worried. In the early stages of the disease radiographic examination with a barium swallow will show delay at the cardia and often considerable oesophageal activity in the form of spasm and ring contraction, but no proper peristalsis. Some patients complain of discomfort behind the sternum when the oesophagus becomes distended with food. X-ray of the oesophagus in advanced cases shows it to be grossly dilated and filled with food residue; when the level of barium in the oesophagus reaches a certain level the cardia opens momentarily to let little through into the stomach. It is at this stage that spill over into the lungs occurs and the patient develops recurrent attacks of pneumonia which may finally lead to severe lung damage. Other complications include the development of carcinoma of the oesophagus and of multiple arthritis. In the early stages of achalasia of the cardia the patient's general health remains remarkably good and there is no weight loss. When the condition becomes more severe weight loss may occur.

Treatment. Inhalation of octyl nitrite relaxes the cardia, but this effect lasts for only one or two minutes and treatment giving more permanent relief is always needed. Dilatation with an instrument such as the Starke dilator, which causes forcible rupture of muscle fibres at the cardia, is often very effective. If this fails, or if the gullet is obviously dilated, cardiomyotomy (Heller's operation) should be performed. Results are excellent except in patients with gross dilatation and tortuosity of the gullet who require more extensive surgical procedures.

Carcinoma of the Oesophagus

This condition, which is much commoner in men than in women, should be suspected in any patient of middle age or beyond who develops dysphagia. The growth may occur in any part of the oesophagus and usually, though not invariably, the patient can indicate fairly accurately the level at which his food appears to stick. The dysphagia is steadily progressive, so that whereas at first there is difficulty only in swallowing solid food such as meat, within a month or two semi-solids and eventually fluids are affected also. The other striking symptom is rapid loss of weight.

Diagnosis. Barium swallow shows an area of narrowing which is rigid and may be irregular. Oesophagoscopy enables a biopsy to be taken for histological confirmation of the diagnosis.

Treatment. In general the prognosis is extremely bad, but carcinoma at the lower end of the oesophagus can occasionally be successfully resected. Alternatively, a Mousseau-Barbin tube, inserted at operation, may delay complete obstruction in swallowing for a month or two. Radiotherapy is usually ineffective, but occasional palliation of symptoms occurs after use of the supervoltage techniques available with the linear accelerator or cobalt unit.

THE STOMACH AND DUODENUM

Acute Gastritis

Acute gastritis is due to an irritant such as excessive alcohol or food poisoning, or occasionally to an acute specific infection such as influenza. The symptoms are loss of appetite, nausea, vomiting and abdominal discomfort; diarrhoea often occurs too, due to an associated enteritis. The vomited material is occasionally blood-stained. The symptoms subside spontaneously within a few days and usually all that is needed in the way of treatment is to keep the patient warm and comfortable and avoid any further irritation of his stomach. Occasionally, however, severe haematemesis necessitating transfusion occurs from acute superficial gastric erosions; sometimes these follow the taking of aspirin, of which even the soluble forms are common causes of minor gastric bleeding, but more often the aetiology is unknown.

Chronic Gastritis

Although chronic gastritis is a diagnostic label frequently attached to middle-aged and elderly patients with dyspeptic symptoms, it has no clear-cut pathology or clinical picture. The best-known variety is that due to chronic alcoholism. The patient complains of loss of appetite and nausea, particularly in the early morning, and frequently vomits mucus which has collected in the oesophagus and stomach during the night. He does not feel well until he has had another drink or two and so the vicious circle goes on. The only treatment of any value is complete and permanent abstention from alcohol. Chronic gastritis in people who are not alcoholics is of unknown cause; in some patients so diagnosed the symptoms are probably mainly of psychological origin. Thickening of the gastric rugae and evidence of excessive secretion of mucus can, however, sometimes be demonstrated by barium meal. Improvement sometimes follows the eradication of septic foci in the teeth or upper respiratory tract and a course of morning gastric wash-outs.

PEPTIC ULCER

Peptic ulcers may be acute or chronic. They occur in the lower oeso-phagus, stomach or duodenum, or occasionally in the upper jejunum or at a gastro-enterostomy stoma.

Acute ulcers cause little in the way of symptoms and are seldom diag-nosed unless they cause serious bleeding or perforation. They usually heal rapidly but often recur. Aspirin is a gastric irritant and may cause super-ficial gastric erosions which bleed.

Chronic peptic ulcers nearly all occur in the stomach or duodenum; when they co-exist the gastric ulcer usually develops second. A hereditary factor in gastric and duodenal ulcer has long been suspected from their frequent occurrence in several members of a family; furthermore, both types of ulcer have a higher incidence in persons of blood group O and are also more common in those who are unable to secrete their blood group sub-stances in the saliva and gastric juice. This is a genetically determined factor; non-secretors number about 20 per cent of the general population and 30–35 per cent of the ulcer population.

Patients with duodenal ulcer as a group have twice as many parietal cells in their gastric mucosa as healthy people or patients with gastric ulcer and in general the further an ulcer is from the cardia the more hydrochloric acid is secreted by the stomach. Patients with duodenal ulcer also secrete more pepsin and have a tendency to nocturnal hypersecretion of acid. Gastric ulcers on the other hand tend to be associated with a low or normal acid secretion and with a gastric mucosa affected histologically by chronic gastritis; whether the latter is cause or effect is not known.

Chronic peptic ulcers occur at any age but are particularly common in middle life; gastric ulcers tend to arise in rather older people than duodenal ulcers. The sex incidence of gastric ulcers is almost equal; duodenal ulcers are 3–4 more times common in men than in women. Duodenal ulcers are evenly distributed throughout the social classes, but gastric ulcers are more common in social classes IV and V. There is no firm evidence to show that psychological factors, physique or personality are important in the cause of ulcer, but anxiety, overwork and stress of various kinds often lead to exa-cerbation of symptoms.

Oesophageal peptic ulcers arise in patients with hiatus hernia and gastro-oesophageal reflux. **Stomal ulcers** are particularly common in patients with gastro-enterostomy in whom no procedure to reduce acid secretion, such as vagotomy, has been performed. **Upper jejunal ulcers,** usually at the duodeno-jejunal flexure, are associated with gross hypersecretion of gastric juice, which is produced continually at a maximal rate. This is the Zollinger-Ellison syndrome (p. 76).

Clinical Features. The principal and often the only symptom is *pain*, which is usually accurately localised to the centre of the epigastrium. It has two very characteristic features. The first is its *time-relation to food*: duodenal ulcer typically causes a hunger pain, which comes on when the stomach is empty and is relieved by the taking of food; in gastric ulcer the timing is often less regular, but the pain tends to come on about half to one hour after meals. The pain of duodenal ulcer often wakes the patient up about 2 a.m., but curiously there is seldom pain before breakfast. Though typically localised to the epigastrium, the pain is occasionally referred to the lower abdomen, to the chest or to the back. The second very characteristic feature is the *periodicity*. Apart from treatment the history invariably tells of remissions, with complete freedom from symptoms for weeks or months, and subsequent relapses which are particularly liable during the winter months.

Mechanism of the pain. For many years there has been debate between those who believe that the pain is due to spasm and those who ascribe it to irritation of the ulcer by acid, but neither of these theories is entirely satisfactory. It has been shown that pain is dependent on the presence of acid in the stomach, but it is also dependent on inflammation in the ulcer. From time to time a chronic peptic ulcer becomes inflamed and sensitive and at these times the action of acid, and other stimuli, cause pain; at other times they do not, even though the ulcer is still demonstrable by X-ray or gastroscope. The cause and mechanism of these episodes of inflammation constitute one of the basic unsolved problems of the disease. It is clear, however, that the state of tone in the stomach and duodenum and the acidity of their contents are largely incidental in the production of pain and that the administration of antispasmodics and antacids at times when the ulcer is in a quiescent phase is unlikely to serve any useful purpose.

Other symptoms include vomiting, a common event in patients with severe pain, when it is followed by relief, and in those with pyloric obstruction from either spasm or cicatricial stenosis; and water brash, or the filling of the mouth with tasteless watery saliva.

Physical signs are of minor importance. The 'pointing sign' is probably the most helpful: the patient when asked where his pain is places his finger tip on the centre of the epigastrium. There may also be some epigastric tenderness.

Diagnosis depends on *barium meal* screening of the patient by an experienced radiologist. The great majority of gastric ulcers occur in the middle third of the lesser curvature and are quite easily demonstrated in profile as a niche projecting from this aspect of the stomach. Ulcers occur only in the first part of the duodenum, referred to by the radiologist as the duodenal bulb or cap, and are much more difficult to demonstrate, being identified with certainty in little more than half the cases. They are more often seen '*en face*' than in profile, appearing as a round pool of barium a millimetre or two in diameter surrounded by a clear halo, and sometimes mucosal rugae can be seen radiating from this area. Frequently, however, the only signs are irregularity, irritability and tenderness of the duodenal cap.

Gastroscopy is helpful in the diagnosis only of gastric ulcers, and there are some areas of the stomach which are difficult to visualise.

Tests for occult blood in the stools are usually positive in patients with active peptic ulcer.

Complications

(1) **Haemorrhage.** Slight bleeding always takes place from the raw surface, but if the ulcer is a deep one it may erode into an artery in the wall of the stomach or duodenum and lead to massive haemorrhage. The patient may vomit a large quantity of blood (this is a *haematemesis*) and it is obvious at once that serious bleeding is in progress, but if the blood goes the other way down through the intestines the diagnosis must be made first on the signs of internal haemorrhage and later on the appearance of a large amount of altered blood in the stools making them black and tarry. The latter event is a *melaena*. Internal haemorrhage should be suspected in any patient who complains of sudden faintness and is found on examination to be pale and sweating, with a fast thready pulse and a low blood pressure.

(2) **Perforation** is the most dangerous complication and is almost confined to men. The discharge of acid gastric or duodenal contents into the peritoneal cavity causes severe generalised abdominal pain and board-like rigidity of the abdominal muscles. The patient lies quite still, because any movement aggravates his pain, and he shows signs of shock (pallor, sweating, fast pulse and low blood pressure). The diagnosis is usually easily made from this striking clinical picture and emergency operation to close the perforation should be done without delay.

(3) **Pyloric stenosis** is a complication of ulcer in the duodenum or rarely in the pyloric canal itself and results from contraction of scar tissue laid down in the base of the ulcer. In many patients, however, the syndrome of pyloric obstruction is due mainly to spasm in association with an active ulcer and clears up as the ulcer heals. Obstruction at the pylorus leads to distension of the stomach, which is evacuated from time to time by vomiting, which is often copious and projectile; and if the vomit contains recognisable articles of food, such as tomato skins, known to have been eaten many hours previously, this provides clear evidence of delay in gastric emptying. Patients with pyloric stenosis lose weight and become dehydrated and the alkalosis resulting from loss of hydrochloric acid may lead to tetany, either overt (carpo-pedal spasm) or latent (positive Chvostek and Trousseau's signs). The only satisfactory treatment for pyloric stenosis is gastro-enterostomy.

(4) **Hour-glass stomach** is the result of scarring from a chronic lesser curve ulcer and is usually simply an incidental X-ray finding. It is nearly always seen in women and its incidence seems to be diminishing.

Treatment of Peptic Ulcer

(1) Medical Treatment

The only two factors which have been shown to have a beneficial effect on the healing of duodenal ulcer are admission to hospital, which implies *bed rest*, and *giving up smoking*; and although a light diet given in two-hourly feeds in the early stages of a period of strict medical treatment probably does hasten the relief of symptoms, there is no evidence that it does anything more than this and it is quite a good plan to make this point clear to the patient. Many ulcer subjects becomes slaves to an unnecessarily strict diet to no purpose, so denying themselves many of the simple pleasures of life and becoming a continuous nuisance to their wives and families.

The patient should be kept in bed, though allowed up for toilet purposes, for a minimum period of two weeks, and sometimes it may be wise to insist on four or even six weeks of bed rest. Until he is free of symptoms (usually only a few days) he is given a *diet* of two-hourly milky feeds supplemented by junkets, jellies, baked custard, arrowroot, puréed vegetables and melba toast. As soon as the pain has gone such items as egg, fish, chicken and minced meat may be added and within a week or two he should be gradually put back on to a more or less normal diet, including meat, fruit and vegetables but avoiding highly spiced or recooked dishes and foods which he knows from experience will upset him. Throughout this time he should continue taking a few ounces of milk half way between the main meals and last thing at night. Patients whose pain is unusually severe and persistent may be given a continuous milk drip through a nasal catheter, the flow being adjusted so that about five pints are administered in 24 hours. This procedure is sometimes remarkably effective in relieving previously intractable pain.

Drugs. If the patient is very active and restless a mild *sedative* such as amylobarbitone 60 mg. twice or three times daily may be given with advantage.

Antacids. Although it can be shown that antacids taken by mouth have a very temporary effect in reducing gastric acidity, they are effective in relieving pain and are usually given three times daily after feeds and last thing at night. Quickest pain relief is obtained with sodium bicarbonate, but if such an absorbable alkali is taken over a long period there is a danger of alkalosis or even of the 'milk-alkali syndrome', hypercalcaemia and renal impairment. This danger has probably been over emphasised, but most physicians prefer to prescribe non-absorbable antacids such as magnesium trisilicate or aluminium hydroxide. Proprietary tablets containing milk powder and antacids (e.g. Nulacin or Prodexin) if sucked between feeds help to keep the acid concentration low. Olive oil is sometimes prescribed in doses of 30g three times daily before meals for its inhibitory effect on the secretion of acid.

Antispasmodics. Drugs of the belladonna group, which inhibit acetylcholine, are given to reduce the motor activity of the stomach and also reduce that part of the gastric secretion which depends upon vagal impulses. Tincture of belladonna 1–2 ml. or tab. hyoscyamine sulphate 0·5 mg. three or four times daily are commonly given for this purpose and are probably as effective as any of the newer synthetic analogues. Dosage may have to be reduced if dryness of the mouth or blurring of vision become troublesome.

Carbenoxolone has proved effective in promoting healing in *gastric* ulcers. It is an anti-inflammatory agent but its exact mode of action is unknown. It is given in doses of 100 mg. t.d.s. In the elderly or in those with cardiac insufficiency, it should be avoided or used in smaller doses as it causes sodium and water retention.

After Care. The great majority of ulcers heal on the above regime, but few escape subsequent relapse. Although there is no known way of preventing recurrence, it is probably wise for the ulcer subject to continue having small regular meals and particularly to avoid long spells of work without food. He should abstain from smoking if he can do so without too much distress. Perhaps even more important, he should make a point of having two or three days in bed, with two-hourly milky feeds, at the first indication of recurrence of his pain, as this may prevent a major relapse.

The Treatment of Massive Bleeding. A patient who has had a large haematemesis or melaena is always an anxious and difficult problem in treatment. In the hope that the bleeding will stop spontaneously he must be kept as quiet as possible; an injection of morphine 15–20 mg. is therefore given on admission and repeated in a few hours if restlessness returns. Blood is taken for grouping and for haemoglobin estimation and an hourly pulse and blood pressure chart is started. The haemoglobin level does not reflect the severity of the bleeding until several hours later, so that the pulse and blood pressure give a better immediate indication. *Transfusion* may not be necessary if the patient is young and the haemorrhage relatively slight, but an elderly patient who has bled severely must be given at least two pints of blood without delay. For a patient whose bleeding is thought to have stopped transfusion at the rate of one pint in four hours is satisfactory, but the blood must be run in much more quickly if the bleeding is continuing. In addition to the obvious immediate risk to life, two serious hazards of failing to replace lost blood may be mentioned: in the elderly, severe anaemia may lead to cardiac failure by inducing an increase in cardiac output; and very occasionally recurrence of bleeding in a severely anaemic patient leads to permanent blindness. A good rule to follow is: 'When in doubt, transfuse.' At one time these patients were given only ice to suck, in the mistaken idea that this would rest the stomach. An empty stomach is in fact much more active than a full one and it is wiser to give the patient a *diet* corresponding to the first stage of the usual ulcer regime as soon as he can take it. Emergency *operation* may be needed if the bleeding continues or recurs, but carries a high mortality in these severely ill patients;

the decision whether to operate, and when, calls for a high degree of clinical judgment on behalf of both physician and surgeon and cannot be made according to any hard and fast rules.

(2) Surgical Treatment

Surgery is very frequently demanded by the patient himself, who naturally thinks that if only he can have his ulcer cut out that will be the end of it and he need have no more tedious weeks in hospital and irksome diets. Unfortunately, however, the matter is not as simple as this. Partial gastrectomy may be performed for either gastric or duodenal ulcer, though for the latter many surgeons now prefer vagotomy with a drainage operation on the stomach. Many patients do very well after these procedures, but a proportion have persistent diarrhoea after vagotomy or various ill-effects (listed below) after gastrectomy. Severe post-gastrectomy syndromes are particularly common in young adults and the operation should seldom be performed before early middle age. With this proviso, the *indications for surgery* may be stated as:

 (1) Failure of the symptoms of a duodenal ulcer to remit, or failure of a gastric ulcer to show radiological evidence of healing, after an adequate period of efficient medical treatment.

 (2) Pyloric obstruction.

 (3) Severe bleeding, particularly if this has recurred and the patient is above middle age.

 (4) Doubt whether a gastric ulcer be malignant. Duodenal ulcers are never malignant.

 (5) Enormous ulcers and those invading the pancreas.

 (6) Perforation is of course an immediate indication for operation.

Post-Gastrectomy Syndromes

(1) Malnutrition

 (a) Most patients either lose weight or fail to gain weight. This may be partly due to inadequate food intake, the stump of the stomach being able to accommodate only a small meal, but some patients also develop steatorrhoea, in part due to poor mixing of food with pancreatic juice and possibly also to intestinal hurry and to bacterial contamination of the small bowel, which is normally sterile.

 (b) Iron deficiency anaemia develops in about 20–30 per cent of the patients and may require parenteral iron therapy for its correction. Macrocytic anaemia is less common; usually due to folic acid deficiency.

 (c) Very occasionally vitamin B and C deficiency develops.

(2) **Post-Prandial Attacks.** These are of two types:

 (a) *The Dumping Syndrome.* Symptoms start either during a meal or within half an hour, with abdominal fullness and sensations of 'rolling' or 'churning', nausea, palpitations, dizziness, and faintness. Soon afterwards the patient usually complains of weakness, fatigue, or exhaustion which may persist for up to three hours. Severe attacks may be precipitated by large meals or less often by sweet foods and drinks. The symptoms are probably the result of excessive jejunal stimulation: they can be reproduced by various abnormal jejunal stimuli such as the entry of iced water, hypertonic solutions, or distension by a balloon. Barium meal shows precipitate gastric emptying, the meal leaving the stomach within 10 minutes. Inadequate handling of a glucose load, with a lag type of glucose tolerance test and a reduction in plasma volume have been demonstrated and sodium tolbutamide 0·25–1·0 g. ten to thirty minutes before meals may help to prevent attacks. Dry meals rich in protein and poor in carbohydrate and lying down after eating are other helpful measures.

(b) *Late hypoglycaemic attacks* are due simply to functional post-prandial hyperinsulinism. The patients are frequently rather nervous unstable people who have been subject to similar but milder attacks even before the operation. They require treatment by reassurance, correction of malnutrition if necessary, and should take small frequent meals with a low carbohydrate content.

CARCINOMA OF THE STOMACH

Carcinoma of the stomach is one of the commonest forms of cancer, and occurs slightly more often in men than in women.

Clinical Features. Early diagnosis is of the utmost importance if the patient is to have any chance of radical cure, and to this end the possibility of malignant disease of the stomach should be borne in mind when a patient of early middle age or beyond develops for the first time dyspeptic symptoms which persist for more than two or three weeks. The symptoms are very variable, but the most common are anorexia and epigastric pain which usually does not show the clear-cut relation to food seen in patients with peptic ulcer. Within a few months most patients show obvious loss of weight and anaemia, though occasional very slowly growing gastric cancers may cause only very vague symptoms for as long as two years. Frequently a good deal of bleeding occurs from the surface of the carcinoma, and the vomiting of altered blood which looks like coffee grounds is a characteristic feature. On the other hand, negative tests for occult blood in the stools do not exclude this diagnosis, for the infiltrating type of growth (causing the 'leather-bottle stomach') may extend widely in the wall of the stomach without causing surface ulceration. Some patients develop symptoms and signs of pyloric obstruction; less often a fundal tumour obstructs the cardia and the patient complains that his food appears to stick at the lower end of the gullet. In some unfortunate patients the earliest symptoms are those due to metastases in the liver or elsewhere.

Physical signs are usually present only in patients whose disease has advanced beyond the reach of curative surgery. Common findings at this stage are a hard fixed mass in the epigastrium and evidence of secondary deposits; important among the latter are an enlarged irregular liver, a hard lymph-node above the clavicle (described by Virchow), deep-vein thrombosis in the leg (Trousseau's sign), or on rectal examination bilateral Krukenberg tumours in the ovaries or a hard mass in the rectal pouch from trans-coelomic spread. The only sign sometimes found in early cases is slight epigastric tenderness.

Diagnosis depends mainly on the *barium meal* examination, which classically shows a filling defect and failure of peristaltic movements over the affected part of the stomach. It is now thought that not more than about 1 per cent of peptic ulcers of the stomach undergo malignant change; in this group a very large ulcer and a suggestion of filling defect at one end of it are signs arousing suspicion of carcinoma. A leather-bottle stomach is small, indistensible and inactive and the barium runs straight through it into the duodenum. *Gastroscopy* by an expert may give helpful information. There is usually a *hypochromic anaemia* and a raised *sedimentation rate* but both of these may also be found in patients with simple gastric ulcer.

Treatment. Radical surgery provides the only opportunity for cure, but the prognosis is among the worst for all forms of carcinoma and five-year survivals are few. Even in advanced cases the primary growth should be resected whenever possible, for apart from possible prolongation of life symptomatic relief makes the procedure worth while.

DISORDERS OF THE INTESTINES

The Malabsorption Syndromes

These disorders are characterised by failure of absorption of essential food factors by the small intestine, with consequent chronic diarrhoea and malnutrition. All somewhat rare, the more common members are coeliac disease in children, idiopathic steatorrhoea, and tropical sprue. Similar effects may result from resection of part of the small gut, especially when a blind loop has been formed, from regional ileitis, from pancreatitis, from drugs such as neomycin or phenindione and from the very rare Whipple's disease (intestinal lipodystrophy).

Tropical Sprue

Sprue is endemic in certain countries in the Far East, notably India, Ceylon, Indo-China, and the East Indies. It occurs also in the West Indies but is apparently rare in Africa. It particularly affects Europeans living temporarily in an endemic area, though usually not until after many years residence. The gut shows abnormal or atrophic villi but the cause of the disease is obscure; at present the most popular theory for the failure of intestinal function is an alteration of the normal bacterial flora following recurrent dysenteric infection.

Idiopathic Steatorrhoea (Non-tropical sprue)

This is probably the adult counterpart of coeliac disease (which will not be described here) and sometimes the symptoms can be traced through a series of remissions and exacerbations back to childhood. It was noted in Holland after the second world war that children with coeliac disease who had been making good progress under conditions of near starvation during the German occupation began to deteriorate when wheat and rye were introduced into the diet. Further investigation soon confirmed that there was an intolerance to gluten, the protein part of the wheat or rye germ, but curiously enough not to the glutens in other cereals. It is probable that intolerance to wheat and rye glutens is also the cause of idiopathic steatorrhoea. The cause of this intolerance is probably deficiency of the enzyme which normally hydrolyses the toxic peptide part of the gluten.

Clinical Features of Sprue and Idiopathic Steatorrhoea. There is usually an insidious onset of looseness of the stools, general weakness, and loss of weight. The diarrhoea is persistent, though most patients have exacerbations from time to time followed by remissions in which the stools become temporarily almost normal. During exacerbations the stools typically are pale, bulky, frothy, and greasy; but they may be fluid and not obviously fatty, though analysis will usually reveal an excess of fat. Flatulence is usually severe and the distension of the abdomen contrasts with the progressive emaciation of the rest of the body. Clubbing of the fingers occasionally develops. Other symptoms and signs result from failure of absorption of essential food factors:

Factor Deficient	Clinical Effect
Iron	Hypochromic anaemia
Vitamin B$_{12}$ Folic acid	Macrocytic anaemia

(The anaemia is usually of mixed type)

Vitamin B complex aneurine (thiamine)	Peripheral neuritis (rare)
riboflavin nicotinic acid	Glossitis Stomatitis
Vitamin D Calcium	Tetany Osteomalacia
Vitamin K	Haemorrhagic tendency
Potassium	Weakness, apathy and mental disturbance

Diagnosis. Confirmation of malabsorption of fat is essential but analysis of a casual stool specimen for fat is useless. On a ward diet which contains about 70 g. of fat per day a 3–5 day collection should be made; a loss greater than 6–7 g. daily is abnormal. If this is done a formal fat balance is usually unnecessary. The radio-active iodine labelled fat excretion test is not so accurate probably because the isotopic label becomes detached from the fat in the small bowel. Glucose tolerance test shows a flat blood sugar curve, but has been replaced by the xylose tolerance test in which impaired absorption of xylose is revealed by reduced excretion in the urine. Barium follow through, using 350 ml. of a flocculable barium sulphate suspension, shows a typical small intestine pattern; the mucosal markings are thickened and the barium is clumped in elongated masses. In idiopathic steatorrhoea and tropical sprue peroral small intestinal biopsy with a special capsule reveals that the normal epithelium with slender villi has been replaced by a flat or ridged mucosa; this is almost diagnostic. Occasionally a radio-active B_{12} absorption test or estimations of serum B_{12} and folic acid provide helpful additional data.

Treatment of Idiopathic Steatorrhoea. Although most patients respond completely to a strict gluten-free diet within a few weeks, some require supplements of iron, vitamin B_{12}, folic acid, calcium or vitamin D. A few continue to have diarrhoea or relapse, usually from failing to keep to the diet; it should be made clear from the outset, therefore, that wheat gluten will probably have to be avoided for life.

Treatment of Sprue. Europeans who develop sprue in the tropics usually recover spontaneously when they return to a temperate climate. Sometimes a course of tetracycline, 250–500 mg. six-hourly for five days, is of benefit, probably by altering the bacterial flora of the gut. It is usual to give a diet rich in protein and vitamins and low in fat and roughage. Vitamin B_{12} is given intramuscularly, starting with 100 μg. on alternate days and gradually increasing the interval between injections during recovery. Folic acid 10–20 mg. three times daily is given by mouth. Other vitamin and mineral deficiencies are corrected as necessary.

Other Causes of Malabsorption

Obstructive jaundice impairs the digestion of fats and in long standing cases the resulting steatorrhoea may lead eventually to osteomalacia. In *chronic pancreatitis* lack of pancreatic digestive enzymes impairs the digestion of fat and protein and leads to steatorrhoea and heavy loss of nitrogen in the stools; absorption of glucose, iron, folic acid, and vitamin B_{12} is usually normal.

Extensive resection of the small gut may be followed by malnutrition, but in organic disease of the small intestine malabsorption results not from loss of absorbing surface but from bacterial activity. The normally sterile small gut may be invaded by coliform organisms, as a result of stasis, either above a *stricture* (as in Crohn's disease) or in a *blind loop* formed by a fistulous communication or surgical by-pass, or as a result of direct access through a *gastro-colic fistula*. In the very rare *Zollinger-Ellison syndrome*, probably as a result of gastrin secretion by the pancreatic tumour always present, there is heavy and continuous outpouring of gastric juice and the usual clinical presentation is severe and intractable peptic ulceration, but sometimes the contents of the small intestine are rendered acid and steatorrhoea results from inactivation of the pancreatic enzymes. Another very rare cause of steatorrhoea and progressive wasting is *Whipple's disease* or intestinal lipodystrophy; the cause is unknown and the diagnosis can be made with certainty only by biopsy of the small intestine to show large foamy macrophages, filled with an unidentified glycoprotein, in the tunica propria, and lipogranulomatosis in the mesenteric lymph-nodes. The disease is progressive, but temporary remission of symptoms may be induced by corticosteroid therapy.

Disaccharide Intolerance

Digestion of disaccharides such as lactose, sucrose and maltose takes place within the mucosal cells. If one of the enzymes lactase, sucrase or maltase is lacking the corresponding disaccharide accumulates and may cause diarrhoea and malabsorption. Patients with *lactase deficiency* may give a history of diarrhoea after drinking milk; the diagnosis is supported by demonstrating a flat blood sugar curve after a loading dose of lactose. The deficiency may be an inborn error or the result of various diseases affecting the small intestine. Symptoms are relieved by a milk-free diet.

Regional Ileitis (Crohn's disease)

In this disease of unknown aetiology there are single or multiple sharply demarcated areas of intestine, usually in the lower reaches of the ileum, which become grossly thickened by lymphoid hyperplasia, ulceration, oedema, and secondary infection. Complications include cicatricial stenosis of the bowel, localised perforation, abscess, and the formation of fistulae. The sex incidence is approximately equal and symptoms usually begin in the twenties or thirties.

Clinical Features. Symptoms usually develop very gradually and there are often long natural remissions so that the history commonly extends over several years by the time the diagnosis is made. Most patients present with attacks of colicky pain round the umbilicus or in the right iliac fossa, with associated mild diarrhoea and general weakness. Loss of weight is usual and there is often low fever. The most helpful and important *physical sign* is a tender fixed mass, usually in the right iliac fossa, and the *barium 'follow through'* examination demonstrates gross filling defects and narrowing of the lumen of the affected segments of intestine. The blood count shows anaemia and some leucocytosis and a high sedimentation rate. Fistulous *complications* may lead to peri-anal abscess and fistula-in-ano, dysuria and passage of wind *per urethram* from ileo-vesical fistula or abscess in the abdominal wall. An associated granular proctitis is common.

Treatment. The patient should be confined to bed during febrile exacerbations and should be advised at all times to avoid exhaustion from either physical or mental overstrain. Improvement does sometimes seem to follow the resolution of emotional problems and worries, but in the individual patient it is seldom that any useful action can be taken in this connection. A course of phthalylsulphathiazole 1–2 g. six-hourly or tetracycline 250 mg. six-hourly for five to seven days may help in combating secondary infection. The diet should be low in roughage and high in protein and vitamin supplements should be given as in other causes of malabsorption (see sprue, p. 74). Rapid relief of symptoms often follows treatment with cortisone, but the improvement is not always maintained and it is probably wise to reserve steroid therapy for the control of exacerbations. A suitable course would be prednisolone 40–60 mg. daily for a few days until the fever and other symptoms have subsided, then a maintenance dose of about 20 mg. daily for two or three weeks, after which the dosage should be gradually tailed off. Operation should be avoided if possible during the stage of active ulceration but frequently becomes necessary for the relief of complications such as perforation, cicatricial obstruction or fistulae. Resection of the affected segment of bowel is the treatment of choice.

Ulcerative Colitis

This is a serious and chronic disease of the colon and although temporary remission of symptoms is common, relapse nearly always follows after a variable interval of months or years and complete recovery is very rare. The cause of ulcerative colitis is unknown. Its acute stage is very similar to bacillary dysentery, which suggests that an infection might be responsible, but no specific organism has ever been isolated. Some authorities have been very struck by the characteristic personality of many of these patients, who are often extremely fussy, tidy, meticulous people, emotionally immature and showing an abnormal dependence on one or other parent, and by the fact that the onset of the illness or exacerbations in its severity quite often appear to be precipitated by an emotional crisis associated with marriage, childbirth, or the death of a parent or near relative. It has therefore been suggested that the changes in the bowel are secondary to some psychological disturbance. Other physicians, and most surgeons, take the view that these psychological factors simply aggravate the disease or indeed that they are the result of it.

Clinical Features. It usually starts in early adult life and is slightly more common in women than in men. The principal symptom is *diarrhoea*, which continues in some degree throughout the whole course of the illness. During acute relapses the stools are greatly increased in number and contain *blood and mucus*, abdominal pain is often severe, the temperature is raised and the patient becomes very weak, anaemic and emaciated; in remissions the general health becomes more or less restored, but there is nearly always some persistent looseness of the stools. The severity of the disease varies greatly in different patients. There is an acute fulminating variety which renders the patient gravely ill, even moribund, within a few weeks; at the other end of the scale is a mild type which causes only relatively trivial inconvenience; and between these extremes the majority of patients require admission to hospital from time to time over many years and are always more or less severely disabled by their disease.

Physical signs are few, though there is usually some tenderness over the affected part of the colon. The blood count reveals *anaemia* which is sometimes severe and usually a *leucocytosis*. The *sedimentation rate* is very high during relapses and seldom falls completely to normal even during remissions. *Sigmoidoscopy* shows a very red, granular, bleeding, and superficially ulcerated mucosa. The *barium enema* in moderately severe or advanced cases shows the affected bowel to be shorter and narrower than normal and to have a rather fuzzy outline devoid of the normal haustral markings; these appearances are particularly helpful in assessing how much of the colon is involved.

Complications. Stricture of the bowel, peri-anal abscess, perforation leading to abscess or peritonitis, severe haemorrhage and the development of carcinoma in the diseased colon are complications particularly to be feared in the younger patients with severe ulcerative colitis. Opinions differ about the frequency of malignant change, but it certainly occurs sufficiently often in patients who have had a severe form of the disease for ten years or more to be a powerful argument in favour of treatment by colectomy.

Treatment. There is no specific therapy and during the acute stages undoubtedly the most important measure is a period of complete *rest* in bed. The *diet* should be high in protein and in total calories but low in roughage, and very hot or very cold drinks should be avoided as these tend to stimulate the bowel. Vitamin supplements should also be given. For the relief of anaemia fresh *blood transfusion* is the most effective treatment and in addition often seems to be of benefit to the patient's general condition. *Iron* is indicated too and should be given parenterally (see p. 468 for details) if oral preparations appear to aggravate the diarrhoea. To control the diarrhoea tab. codeine phosphate 30–60 mg. three or four times daily or tincture of opium 0·3–1·3 ml. three or four times daily are the most useful preparations and tincture of belladonna in doses up to 2 ml. three or four times daily may help to relieve colic.

It is now usual to give oral *sulphasalazine* in doses of 1 g. 4–6 times daily, since a number of controlled trials have shown that it exerts a beneficial effect. This treatment must be continued over many weeks or months; its toxic effects include haemolytic anaemia. In addition, many patients improve greatly after a course of prednisolone hemisuccinate retention enemas. Only if severe symptoms persist in spite of these measures, or for a very acute fulminating form of the disease, should systemic steroid therapy be instituted. *Prednisolone* is given by mouth in initial daily dosage of 40–60 mg. which is gradually reduced as soon as improvement in the patient's condition permits; a gratifying remission of symptoms is often induced, but all too often relapse quickly ensues when the drug is withdrawn. Long-term maintenance therapy with prednisolone in lower dosage (preferably not more than 10 mg. daily) is therefore often necessary.

Many patients need surgery but there is no general agreement about the *indications for operation*. The procedure employed is total colectomy, and although it is occasionally possible to join the ileum to the rectal stump, most patients are left with a permanent ileostomy. With modern techniques, however, patients with this disability are able to lead almost normal lives. The present tendency therefore is not to regard surgery as the final desperate gamble for an almost moribund patient, but to advise operation after a reasonable trial of medical treatment. The improvement in health is usually well worth the price of the ileostomy and, as mentioned above, the risk of malignant change and other complications is a further incentive to relatively early surgery.

Protein-losing Enteropathy

In some gastro-intestinal diseases, notably ulcerative colitis, regional ileitis, idiopathic steatorrhoea and carcinoma of the stomach, exudation of plasma occurs into the lumen of the gut. The faecal nitrogen is not increased, since most of the plasma is digested and reabsorbed; but hypoproteinaemia and resulting oedema may develop in view of the liver's limited reserve capacity to synthesize albumen.

Diverticulitis

The presence of diverticula in the colon is known as *diverticulosis*, a condition which causes no symptoms and requires no treatment. Though uncommon in childhood and early adult life, it is an incidental finding on X-ray or at autopsy in about 5 per cent of people over middle age. It is rather more common in men than in women and has a higher incidence in fat people. The diverticula are found particularly in the descending colon and pelvic colon.

Diverticulitis, or inflammation of a segment of colon containing diverticula, occurs in only a small percentage of those with diverticulosis.

Clinical Features. The main symptom is colicky *abdominal pain* usually, but not always, referred to the lower abdomen. Some patients remain otherwise well, but those with severe acute inflammation of the bowel have fever and general malaise. There may also be constipation or diarrhoea. Rectal bleeding is uncommon in diverticulitis and should always lead to suspicion of carcinoma, but occasionally diverticulitis presents with a haemorrhage more profuse than is usual in patients with colonic cancer.

Abdominal or rectal examination usually reveals *tenderness* and often a tender *inflammatory mass* in relation to the affected segment of bowel. Leucocytosis is common. The diagnosis is established by *barium enema*, which shows diverticula with distortion of the mucosal pattern and gross deformity of the outline of the colon in the affected area.

Treatment. Most patients can be treated satisfactorily by *medical measures* alone. During an acute febrile attack the patient should be kept in bed, warmth should be applied to the abdomen with a hot-water-bottle and he should be given a course of antibiotic; penicillin 500,000 units and streptomycin 0·5 g. by intramuscular injection twice daily for 5 to 7 days is usually satisfactory. Avoidance of constipation is important in prophylaxis against subsequent inflammation and for this the patient may be given liquid paraffin 10 ml. two or three times daily.

Surgical treatment by colostomy and perhaps subsequent resection of the affected segment of colon is needed only for the relatively rare cases in which intestinal obstruction develops or where perforation of the bowel has led to peritonitis, local abscess formation or the development of fistulae between the colon and other viscera. The most common of these is vesicocolic fistula, which is indicated by the passage of urine containing gas or faecal material.

JAUNDICE

Definition. Jaundice is an increase in the amount of bilirubin in the blood resulting in yellow discoloration of the sclerotics of the eyes, the skin, mucosae, and certain body fluids.

Physiology of Bile. After circulating in the blood for about 120 days red corpuscles are removed and broken up by cells of the reticulo-endothelial system, mainly in the liver, spleen, and bone marrow. The haemoglobin is split into two fractions, an iron-containing part which is returned to the bone marrow for re-synthesis into haemoglobin and an iron-free porphyrin fraction from which the pigment bilirubin is derived. When liberated into the blood for transport to the liver this bilirubin is insoluble in water; it is therefore unable to pass into the urine and it gives an indirect van den Bergh reaction. The bilirubin is taken up by the liver cells, where it becomes conjugated through its carboxyl groups with glucuronic acid to form water-soluble bilirubin-glucuronides which give a direct van den Bergh reaction. In this form bilirubin passes down the bile duct to the duodenum, where it is converted into stercobilinogen, the pigment responsible for most of the normal colour of faeces. Some of this is absorbed (as urobilinogen) from the small intestine into the portal bloodstream; and though nearly all of this fraction is removed again by the liver cells and returned to the biliary passages, traces of it usually escape through the liver into the general circulation and are excreted in the urine.

Causes of Jaundice. It is obvious that jaundice may result either because too much bilirubin is liberated into the blood from excessive breakdown of red corpuscles (*haemolytic jaundice*) or because too little bilirubin is removed from the blood in its passage through the liver. The latter disorder can occur in two ways: the function of the liver cells may be deranged, so that they cannot take up the bilirubin from the blood (*hepatic jaundice*); or obstruction in the common bile duct may dam the flow of bile, so that the bilirubin-glucuronides excreted by the liver diffuse back into the blood (*obstructive jaundice*).

Haemolytic Jaundice. This is the least common of the three main types of jaundice and the yellow discoloration of the skin and other tissues is seldom more than slight. The *urine* contains *no bilirubin* since the bilirubin in the blood is insoluble in water; but as more bile pigment than normal is being produced and consequently an excess of urobilinogen is formed in the duodenum, more of this pigment is absorbed into the portal bloodstream than the liver cells can remove and an *excess of urobilinogen* passes through into the urine. The stools retain their normal colour and chemical analysis shows that they too contain an excess of urobilinogen (sometimes called stercobilinogen in this context). The causes of haemolytic jaundice are discussed under haemolytic anaemia (p. 471).

Obstructive Jaundice. When the common bile duct is obstructed the rising pressure in the biliary system causes bile to flow back into the perilobular lymphatics and by this route into the bloodstream. The bile salts produced in the liver also accumulate in the blood and are probably responsible for the pruritus and bradycardia often found in patients with obstructive jaundice. As explained above, the *bilirubin* in these patients is soluble in water and when its concentration in the blood rises above the renal threshold of about 2 mg. per 100 ml. *it passes freely into the urine*; the latter contains *no urobilinogen*, however, since none is being formed, and for this reason too *the stools are very pale*. Liver function tests which depend on qualitative changes in the serum proteins (and which are therefore manifestations of hepatocellular damage) are negative; these include the thymol flocculation, thymol turbidity, and colloidal gold tests. The level of the serum alkaline phosphatase, however, is raised and usually continues to rise in parallel with the level of the serum bilirubin, and in long-standing cases there is often a rise in the level of the total serum cholesterol.

The common causes of occlusion of the common bile duct are gallstones and carcinoma of the head of the pancreas or of the ampulla of Vater; see *A Short Text-book of Surgery*, pp. 336 and 349. A rare cause is chronic pancreatitis (p. 93).

Hepatic Jaundice. In this group the jaundice is due primarily to difficulty in the transport of bilirubin through the hepatic cell, and possibly in its conjugation; but the pattern of bile-pigments in the serum is in fact identical with that which follows occlusion of the bile duct, and the jaundice must be due partly to regurgitation from the bile canaliculi. In addition, diminished red cell survival is found in all these patients and adds a haemolytic component to the jaundice. There is usually a stage in the disease in which the stools are pale and the urine contains bilirubin but no urobilinogen, as in obstructive jaundice; there may also be a misleading rise in the serum alkaline phosphatase. Positive empirical liver function tests (such as the thymol flocculation, thymol turbidity and colloidal gold reaction) which depend on serum protein changes, and raised serum transaminase levels, are the characteristic biochemical findings. The total serum cholesterol is usually decreased.

Cholestatic Jaundice is the condition in which the clinical and biochemical picture of obstructive jaundice is found in the presence of patent bile-ducts, and liver biopsy reveals stasis of bile in the liver cells and canaliculi. It is seen as a toxic effect of certain drugs, notably chlorpromazine (incidence 1 per cent), less commonly promazine, trifluoperazine, P.A.S., chlorpropamide, thiouracil, nitrofurantoin and methyl testosterone. A similar picture is seen in the rare recurrent jaundice of pregnancy, which appears in the third trimester and clears up in the puerperium. All patients in this group have a good prognosis, with the occasional exception of those with so-called primary biliary cirrhosis.

Familial Hyperbilirubinaemia

This condition, of which a number of varieties have been described in recent years, causes few if any symptoms and is usually detected on routine blood examination, so that in published cases there has been a high incidence in doctors and other hospital workers. The most common type is that described by Gilbert; there is a defect in the transport of bilirubin to its site of conjugation in the liver cell and non-conjugated (water-insoluble) bilirubin accumulates in the blood. Liver function tests are normal, needle biopsy shows normal hepatic structure, there are no complications and prognosis is excellent. The importance of the condition lies in distinguishing it from haemolytic jaundice and progressive hepatic disease. In the rarer Dubin-Johnson variety the hold-up occurs after conjugation and the clinical picture is that of obstructive jaundice; liver biopsy reveals a dark brown pigment in the liver cells. Diagnosis is important so that these patients may be reassured that they are not suffering from serious liver disease.

DISEASES OF THE LIVER

Infectious Hepatitis

There are two strains of virus causing acute hepatitis and differing mainly in their mode of transmission and incubation period. Virus A has an incubation period of about a month (20–40 days) and is present in the patient's stools, being transmitted by faecal contamination of food or water. Where hygienic standards are high only sporadic cases are seen, but where large groups of people live under relatively primitive conditions in a warm climate widespread epidemics may occur. Thus, during the war there were large outbreaks among troops in India and the Middle East. Under these conditions flies are important agents in the spread of the infection.

Virus B hepatitis (associated with Australian (Au) antigen in the blood) and usually called serum hepatitis, has an incubation period of about three months (60–160 days) and is found only in the patient's blood. Some healthy people harbour this virus in their blood for prolonged periods (perhaps indefinitely) and people found to be Au-antigen positive should be excluded from service as blood donors. Transmission to susceptible individuals occurs through transfusions or injections containing plasma, or even from the use of inadequately sterilised syringes or needles. Patients presenting with infectious hepatitis should therefore always be asked if they have been given any injection during the preceeding four months. Au-positive hepatitis is a particular hazard in dialysis units treating patients with chronic renal failure.

After recovery the patient usually has lifelong immunity, but only to infection with the same strain of virus. Furthermore, there is some evidence that the virus of infective hepatitis causes only a mild gastro-enteritis in young children and that those who acquire the more severe illness in adult life are those who have escaped childhood infection and consequent immunisation. This is known to apply to some other virus infections, such as poliomyelitis, which are more serious in adults than in children.

Clinical Features. The illness starts with fever, general malaise, aching in the back and limbs, nausea, and loss of appetite; arthralgia and urticaria are common prodromal symptoms of serum hepatitis not seen in infectious hepatitis. *Anorexia* is a very constant symptom and its occurrence for a few days before the appearance of icterus is one of the most important points distinguishing hepatitis from other causes of jaundice. Clinical jaundice usually becomes manifest within a week and about the same time the temperature settles and the patient starts to feel better. At this stage the liver is usually somewhat enlarged and tender and in about 20 per cent of patients the spleen can be felt too. In the pre-icteric phase the *urine* usually contains an excess of urobilinogen; then when intrahepatic biliary obstruction occurs the urobilinogen disappears, bilirubin is found in the urine (which is consequently dark in colour) and the stools become pale; and finally during recovery after bilirubin has disappeared from the urine there may be a temporary return of urobilinogen in excess before the urine reverts to normal. The great majority of patients are jaundiced for only a week or two and then make a complete recovery. Very occasionally, however (less than 0·5 per cent), fulminating infection may cause death even before the appearance of jaundice; or, equally rarely, recovery is incomplete and slowly progressive hepatic damage leads eventually to cirrhosis. Very mild cases never develop clinical jaundice (infective hepatitis sine ictero) and usually escape recognition except during epidemics. Raised serum transaminase levels are a sensitive index of hepatocellular damage; they are found even in anicteric patients (and are helpful in tracing the course of an epidemic) and if persistent indicate the need for further bed rest and observation.

A long convalescence is advisable after this illness, since depression and tiredness are often rather persistent and it may be some months before the patient recovers his full mental and physical vigour. Abstention from alcohol for about three months is also a wise precaution.

A small number of patients with chronic hepatitis have been found to carry the Australian antigen in the blood. These patients are clinically similar to those with chronic active hepatitis (see below) but do not usually have evidence of multisystem disease. This finding suggests that chronic liver damage can occur as a result of the persistence of the Australian antigen.

Treatment. There is no specific treatment for infective hepatitis. The most important measure undoubtedly is rest and as a general rule the patient should be kept in bed until the temperature has settled, his appetite has returned, bilirubin has disappeared from his urine and his liver is no longer tender. Particular care should be taken in the disposal of excreta and the washing of hands after attending the patient. Diet should be regulated by the patient's appetite rather than the physician's fancy.

A short course of prednisone, starting with 40–50 mg. daily and tailing the dosage off over about a week, may be tried in patients who continue to be deeply jaundiced after six weeks or more and sometimes appears to hasten recovery. If the patient is so ill that he cannot tolerate 1,000 calories by mouth the regime for acute hepatic failure (p. 88) should be instituted. Human gamma-globulin 0·06–0·12 ml. per kg. body weight, given not later than 6 days before the onset of symptoms, modifies the disease and its administration may be considered for specially debilitated patients at risk.

Chronic Active Hepatitis (Lupoid Hepatitis)

In some patients, usually but not invariably young women, hepatitis may persist and may proceed ultimately to a lobular cirrhosis. This type of hepatitis is frequently associated with disorders of other systems including renal tubular acidosis, Sjørgren's syndrome, arthropathy, alveolitis, and colitis.

Investigation may show impaired hepatic function; in addition the plasma gamma globulin is usually increased and in about half the patients antinuclear factors and antibodies to smooth muscle are found in the plasma. Liver biopsy shows liver cell necrosis with infiltration by lymphocytes and plasma cells.

Most patients die within five years. Treatment with steroids particularly if started early in the disease may induce a remission and there is evidence that it may prolong life.

Cirrhosis of the Liver

The word cirrhosis means tawny and was introduced by Laënnec because of the slightly icteric tinge sometimes seen in the livers of patients who have died of this disease. Later it became realised that a much more characteristic feature than the tawny colour is the presence of a great deal of fibrous tissue and cirrhosis has come to mean diffuse hepatic fibrosis. This may be the result of a number of different pathological processes, so that cirrhosis should be regarded as analogous with pulmonary fibrosis rather than as a disease entity.

Clinical Features. *Laënnec's cirrhosis* occurs most often in the forties and fifties and the alcoholic variety is commoner in men than in women. The disease is usually brought to light by the discovery of splenomegaly, hepatomegaly, jaundice, gastro-intestinal bleeding, or ascites. In alcoholics there is usually a history of epigastric discomfort, loss of appetite—particularly for breakfast—and morning sickness with vomiting of mucus, symptoms attributable to alcoholic gastritis; but patients with idiopathic cirrhosis have frequently had no symptoms up to the time of diagnosis. Furthermore, in about one third of cases seen at autopsy the disease has been unsuspected in life.

The clinical features arise from two main causes, hepatocellular failure and portal hypertension:

Hepatocellular failure may have many different effects. *Low-grade fever* often with leucocytosis is seen in about half the patients. More common is the development of *vascular spiders*, each consisting of a central dilated arteriole from which a number of tiny vessels radiate; these appear on the face, neck, upper half of the trunk and upper limbs. Their cause is not known; it is probably not the high blood oestrogen level, as once thought. Erythema of the thenar and hypothenar eminences and of the pads of the fingers ('*liver palms*') is also common. Mental and physical *fatigue, loss of weight* and vague *indigestion* are the rule. *Foetor hepaticus*, which can be detected in the breath and urine is a common sign; it is presumably due to a substance from the gut which is normally detoxicated by the liver. It is a sweetish somewhat faeculent smell which is usually likened to that of a freshly opened corpse. It is a grave sign, often quickly followed by hepatic coma, in patients with severe hepatocellular failure, though in patients with extensive porta-caval venous anastamoses it may be present intermittently for quite long periods and does not necessarily imply such a bad prognosis.

Hepatic coma is probably related to failure of the liver to convert ammonia to urea and the blood ammonia level is raised. It is more common in patients with porto-caval connections and may be precipitated by a high protein diet, by the taking of nitrogenous compounds, or by gastro-intestinal haemorrhage, intercurrent infection or the rapid removal of ascitic fluid. Coma is preceded by a stage of lethargy with mental confusion, irrational behaviour and a typical 'flapping' tremor of the outstretched hands.

Jaundice in cirrhosis, due to failure of the liver cells to excrete bilirubin, is not very common and usually slight; when present it implies a bad prognosis.

Portal hypertension in cirrhosis is due to the combined effect of diminution in the portal vascular bed, the result of both fibrosis and the pressure of regenerating nodules of liver tissue against small portal venous radicles, and of the increased transmission of hepatic arterial pressure to the portal venous system. It leads to congestive *splenomegaly* and to the opening up of porta-caval anastamoses. The two situations in which these distended veins are of clinical importance are:

(a) the abdominal wall, since here they are readily seen and are helpful in diagnosis. Portal blood passes to the umbilicus through the paraumbilical veins to reach collaterals of the caval system. There are usually only one or two distended veins, the classical 'caput medusae' being rare, but it can be demonstrated that the flow of blood is radially away from the umbilicus. This helps in the distinction from inferior vena caval obstruction in which the blood in the distended abdominal veins always flows from below upwards.

(b) Varicose veins in the *oesophagus and fundus of the stomach* are the most dangerous effect of portal hypertension, since bleeding from this source is always serious and often fatal. They may be demonstrated by barium swallow, using a thin emulsion to delineate the delicate mucosal pattern, though negative findings on X-rays do not exclude their presence.

The spleen is almost invariably palpable in patients with portal hypertension and, as in any condition associated with splenomegaly, *pancytopenia* is frequently found in the peripheral blood (see hypersplenism, p. 478).

Ascites develops in cirrhosis from the combined effect of portal hypertension and the reduced plasma osmotic pressure which follows hepatocellular failure and diminished albumen synthesis. Accumulation of fluid in the peritoneal cavity reduces the effective body fluid volume and compensatory mechanisms to retain fluid in the body come into operation and lead in turn to increase in the ascites; they include increased secretion of anti-diuretic hormone from the neuro-hypophysis and of aldosterone from the adrenal cortex.

Clinical features of obscure origin, sometimes seen in cirrhosis, include *clubbing of the fingers, gynaecomastia,* and *scanty or absent body hair.* In acute hepato-cellular failure the circulation is overactive, as shown by a rapid collapsing pulse, high pulse pressure, warm extremities and increased jugular venous pressure. The *diagnosis* of cirrhosis is difficult to establish in the early stages. The first biochemical test to show abnormal results is usually the bromsulphalein (B.S.P.) retention test; later the serum albumen is reduced, the globulin raised and the empirical sero-flocculation tests positive. Sometimes the serum bilirubin level is slightly raised. In early cases the diagnosis can be made with certainty by needle biopsy, but the indications for this procedure must be carefully assessed for each patient as it incurs a slight risk of haemorrhage which is occasionally serious.

Treatment. Whatever the aetiology of the cirrhosis the patient must abstain completely from alcohol for the rest of his life. An adequate mixed diet is important, but there is no advantage in giving protein supplements. Special indications are as follows:—

(a) For **oedema and ascites** give a diet containing no added salt and mersalyl rather than thiazide diuretics as the latter may precipitate hepatic coma. Spironolactone 100 mg. four times daily is sometimes a helpful addition. Paracentesis should be avoided if possible.

(b) **Haematemesis and/or melaena.** Many cirrhotics have a duodenal ulcer and the cause of the bleeding must always be considered and an emergency barium meal done if necessary. Bleeding from varices is usually better controlled by intravenous pitressin than by the inflatable balloons of a Sengstaken tube. If bleeding continues emergency operation (porto-caval anastomosis, or Tanner's operation if the portal vein is not patent) may be considered unless there is hepato-cellular failure or gross ascites.

(c) **Coma** from **acute hepatic failure.** Neuro-psychiatric symptoms of incipient coma are an indication for reducing the protein content of the diet. In established coma enough calories must be given as intravenous glucose, if necessary by intracaval catheter, to minimise endogenous protein catabolism; ammonium absorption from the gut is reduced by giving oral neomycin 1 g. four times daily and if necessary pitressin to cause evacuation of melaena stools; paracentesis, thiazide diuretics and sedative drugs must be avoided; and it may be necessary to give potassium if the serum level is reduced due to secondary aldosteronism.

Special Types of Cirrhosis

(1) Obstructive Biliary Cirrhosis

Some patients with chronic extra-hepatic cholestasis, usually due to stone in the common duct, carcinoma of the head of the pancreas, compression from peri-biliary lymph-nodes or surgical injury to the common duct, eventually develop diffuse hepatic fibrosis which in turn may lead to portal hypertension and hepato-cellular failure. This sequence of events occurs particularly in patients with long-standing partial or recurrent obstruction complicated by cholangitis and the clinical course is often punctuated by bouts of rigors and pyrexia (Charcot's 'biliary remittent fever'). The only effective treatment is surgical relief of the obstruction.

(2) Primary Biliary Cirrhosis

In this rare disease the primary disorder appears to be diffuse intra-hepatic biliary obstruction of unknown cause. Most of the patients are middle-aged women. Insidious onset of itching of the skin is slowly followed by the appearance of jaundice of obstructive type without fever or abdominal pain. The spleen is palpable at an early stage and later the liver becomes greatly enlarged; eventually signs of portal hypertension and hepato-cellular failure develop. Pigmentation and skin xanthomata are quite often seen. The prognosis is better than in Laënnec's cirrhosis; some patients recover and others run a very prolonged downhill course. A remission sometimes follows treatment with cortisone and this may be given a trial in patients who seem to be doing badly.

(3) Haemochromatosis

The primary lesion is probably an inborn metabolic defect which results in the absorption of a slight excess of iron. There is no mechanism by which this extra iron can be eliminated from the body and it is laid down in various tissues and organs, where eventually functional and structural changes may be induced. Symptoms rarely appear before early middle age. The disease is extremely rare in women (5–10 per cent of cases) and in them appears at a later age than in men, probably because the loss of iron in menstruation and pregnancy delays or prevents the clinical expression of the disease. Cirrhosis is a constant feature and the diagnosis should be considered in patients found to have a very enlarged firm liver and greyish pigmentation of the skin, notably over exposed parts. Impotence and general weakness are early symptoms and testicular atrophy with absent or scanty body hair are found much more commonly than in other forms of cirrhosis. Diabetes develops in about two-thirds of the patients. Death usually results from hepato-cellular failure or heart failure, the result of impregnation with haemosiderin of the liver cells and of the myocardium. The *diagnosis* may be confirmed by serum iron studies; the combination of a raised serum iron level with complete or almost complete saturation of the serum iron-binding capacity is almost pathognomonic. If any doubt remains needle biopsy of the liver will settle the matter. *Treatment* is by regular bloodletting; in most patients a pint a week can be taken for many months before early signs of iron deficiency appear in the blood picture. Thereafter a pint should be removed every month or two to prevent re-accumulation of iron in the tissues.

(4) **Syphilitic cirrhosis** (hepar lobatum) is now extremely rare but may be suspected in patients with hepatomegaly and gummata elsewhere in the body. Serological tests for syphilis are positive and the diagnosis is confirmed by the favourable response to anti-syphilitic treatment.

(5) **Cardiac Cirrhosis** (see p. 110).

(6) **Hepato-lenticular Degeneration** (Wilson's disease; see p. 433).

Drug Induced Liver Damage

There are a variety of drugs which may produce liver damage.

(1) **Toxic Hepatitis.** Certain substances including the *chlorinated hydrocarbons (carbon tetrachloride) benzene derivatives (trinitrotoluene, dinitrophenol)* are liver poisons and will produce necrosis of liver cells. This is probably due to direct action of the toxic agent on the liver. Industrial workers exposed to such hepatic poisons should be examined regularly for enlargement or tenderness of the liver and the urine should be tested weekly for bilirubin or urobilinogen.

Other substances only occasionally produce liver necrosis, which when it occurs however may be severe and fatal. This group includes some of the *amine-oxidase inhibitors (iproniazid)* and *cincophen*. The cause for this type of change is unknown but it may be some form of hypersensitivity reaction.

(2) **Cholestasis.** This produces a picture resembling obstructive jaundice without evidence of extra hepatic biliary obstruction. Examination of the

liver shows dilation of the bile canaliculi and sometimes inflammation in the portal area.

This type of liver damage is found most commonly with *chlorpromazine, methyl testosterone* and *thiouracil.* Uneventful recovery is the rule.

Acute Yellow Atrophy of the Liver

This term is applied to any very severe, usually rapidly fatal, variety of acute hepatic necrosis, whether of infective or toxic aetiology. Rapid onset of hepatic insufficiency and shrinkage of the liver are characteristic. Deep jaundice with purpura and bleeding from mucous surfaces and into internal organs are soon followed by hepatic coma and death.

Liver Function Tests (See Table on p. 91).

(1) Their use in the differential diagnosis of the cause of jaundice.

In the following table are listed the typical findings in patients with hepatic jaundice and obstructive jaundice. It must be emphasised, however, that in many jaundiced patients a clear distinction cannot be based on the biochemical findings alone and that not infrequently results are obtained which appear to conflict with the rest of the clinical evidence. These anomalous findings may be partly due to the fact that in many patients with a primarily hepatic jaundice there are a number of complex factors leading to the raised serum bilirubin levels found (p. 82); and partly because in longstanding obstructive jaundice liver cell damage may eventually develop. A clearer picture of the course of events is obtained if the tests are repeated several times during the course of the illness. It is unwise to perform laparotomy on a patient with obstructive jaundice if serum transaminase levels are grossly and persistently raised and the alkaline phophatase level is less than 30 K.A. units per 100 ml.

(2) Assessment of Liver Damage in Cirrhosis

In patients with jaundice the severity of liver cell damage is indicated by the height of the serum bilirubin level, the degree of reduction in the serum albumen and of rise in the serum globulin levels, and the number of units of turbidity in the thymol turbidity test.

In patients without jaundice the *bromsulphalein* (B.S.P.) *retention test* is an accurate index of the severity of liver damage. 1 ml. of a 5-per-cent solution per 10 Kg. body weight is injected intravenously and 30 minutes later a sample of venous blood is taken from the other arm; normally the serum at half-an-hour contains only 0–10 per cent of the injected dose. This test can also be used as an accurate index of recovery after infective hepatitis; it cannot be used, however, when the serum bilirubin is above 2 mg./100 ml.

Thrombosis of the Portal Vein

Cirrhosis accounts for about half the cases of portal vein thrombosis, but it is a rare complication seen in only about 1 per cent of cirrhotics.

Test	Normal Range	Hepatic Jaundice	Obstructive Jaundice
Serum bilirubin	0·4–0·9 mg./100 ml.	Raised	Raised
Serum albumen	3·5–4·5 gm./100 ml.	Reduced	Normal
Serum globulin	2–3 gm./100 ml.	May be raised	Normal
Sero-flocculation tests: 1. Thymol turbidity 2. Thymol flocculation 3. Colloidal gold precipitation	0 0 0	1–4 units + to +++++ + to +++++	0 0 0
Serum glutamic oxaloacetic transaminase (S.G.O.T.)	8–30 units	Raised	Normal or only slightly raised
Serum Isocitric Dehydrogenase (S.I.C.D.)	2–8 Units	Raised	Normal
Serum alkaline phosphatase	3–13 King-Armstrong units	Usually less than 30 units	Usually over 30 units
Urobilin in urine	0 to trace	Increased in early hepatitis	0
Bilirubin in urine	0	Often present for a few days after the stage of urobilinuria	Present

Other causes are malignant disease, portal phlebitis secondary to cholangitis, pancreatitis, or appendicitis, and increase in blood platelets (thrombocytosis) such as occurs in polycythaemia vera and after splenectomy. The clinical features are abdominal pain, splenomegaly, haematemesis, and ascites and distinction from intrahepatic portal obstruction is difficult. Absence of hepatomegaly and signs of hepatic failure are sometimes helpful but the diagnosis can be established with certainty only by splenic venography (which can be performed by percutaneous injection of the dye). The only practical importance in recognising the condition is that it precludes porta-caval anastamosis.

Hepatic Vein Thrombosis (Budd-Chiari syndrome)

This very rare condition is usually a complication of renal or hepatic carcinoma, thrombophlebitis migrans or polycythaemia. It causes sudden vomiting, enlargement of the liver, slight jaundice and ascites which is very resistant to treatment. Anticoagulant therapy should be instituted, but it is difficult to be sufficiently sure of the diagnosis for this to be done. The prognosis is very bad.

DISEASES OF THE PANCREAS

Acute Pancreatitis

The cause of this relatively common disease is not known, but about half the patients also have disease of the biliary tract and many of them are alcoholics or morphine addicts. An acute attack may occur during or soon after an alcoholic bout. It is thought that the characteristic lesions are produced by pancreatic enzymes which have escaped from their normal channels. They include necrosis and haemorrhagic oedema of the gland and plaques of fat necrosis on the mesentery and peritoneum as well as on the pancreas.

Clinical Features. The main symptom is extremely severe and persistent pain in the epigastrium or left upper quadrant of the abdomen passing through to the back, with vomiting and sometimes profound shock. There is deep epigastric tenderness and frequently some abdominal distension. A serum amylase level of 500 Somogyi units or higher (normal range 40–140) is practically pathognomonic of the disease, though smaller increases in the level may be the result of spasm of the sphincter of Oddi induced by morphine and are occasionally found in other intra-abdominal diseases.

Treatment. Unless there is doubt about the diagnosis laparotomy should be avoided as it incurs a high mortality. If pethidine 100 mg. intramuscularly every few hours fails to relieve the pain, morphine 15-20 mg. may need to be given in spite of its tendency to cause spasm of the sphincter of Oddi. Shock must be combated by restoration of normal fluid and electrolyte balance, antibiotics such as penicillin 500,000 units with streptomycin 0·5 gm. twice daily are given to prevent secondary infection of the damaged pancreas, and pancreatic secretion is minimised by giving nothing by mouth and administering a vagal blocking agent such as atropine sulphate 0·6 mg. intramuscularly every three or four hours. Aprotinin (Trasylol) is said to inhibit trypsin and may be of value if given in the first 24 hours. A million units are given I.V. followed by 100,000 units hourly for 3–4 hours.

Chronic Pancreatitis

Chronic pancreatitis is the term applied to the extensive fibrosis and atrophy of the acinar and islet tissue which may follow repeated attacks of acute or subacute pancreatitis and which may lead eventually to pancreatic insufficiency and diabetes mellitus. The condition is usually seen in middle-aged men. The *clinical history* starts with recurrent epiodes of upper abdominal pain as described above; a stage may then be reached in which attacks recur every week or two or pain may become almost continuous and extremely demoralising; and finally diabetes mellitus and/or pancreatic insufficiency may develop. Occasionally the final stage may be reached without any history of severe pain. Pancreatic insufficiency is characterised by loss of weight and the passage of bulky fatty stools. Calcification of the pancreas seen on X-ray strongly favours chronic pancreatitis but estimation of the serum amylase level is less helpful than in the acute disease, though it is usually somewhat raised.

Treatment. The fat content of the diet should be restricted to 70 gm. or less, but enough protein and carbohydrate must be given to ensure an adequate calorie intake. Strong Pancreatin powder B.N.F. 0·25–2 g. should be given with each meal. Alcohol should be forbidden. In patients with severe intractable pain sphincterotomy or even partial or complete resection of the pancreas may have to be performed, but no operation gives consistently good results and the mortality is high. Diabetes if present is controlled in the usual way.

FURTHER READING

Sherlock, Sheila, *Diseases of the Liver and Biliary System*, 4th edition. Blackwell, Oxford (1968).

Truelove, S. C., and Reynell, P. C., *Diseases of the Digestive System*. 2nd edition. Blackwell, Oxford (1971).

Card, W. I., and Creamer, B. (Editors), *Modern Trends in Gastroenterology*, Series 4 (1970).

Hawkins, C. F., *Diseases of the Alimentary Tract*. William Heinemann, London (1963).

CHAPTER FOUR

THE CARDIOVASCULAR SYSTEM

INTRODUCTION

Diseases of the cardiovascular system are the commonest cause of death. With an ageing population it seems likely that there will be further increases in the incidence of those varieties of cardiovascular disease which occur in both middle and advanced age, namely coronary artery disease and hypertension.

THE EXAMINATION OF THE CARDIOVASCULAR SYSTEM

(1) Cyanosis

The colour of a part in terms of its redness or pallor depends on the amount of blood in the capillaries of that part and the thickness of the overlying tissues—where that tissue is thin, e.g. lips and conjunctivae, the colour may be very deep. The colour of blood depends on its haemoglobin and therefore the state and amount of the haemoglobin also influence the colour of the part.

When the capillary blood contains an excess of reduced haemoglobin, it looks blue and produces a blue shade in the skin and mucosae. This is cyanosis. Five grams of reduced haemoglobin per 100 ml. are required to produce detectable cyanosis.

Cyanosis may be of two kinds:

(a) *Peripheral cyanosis*, which is due to stagnation of blood in the capillaries, is best seen in the extremities and the lips and is often associated with coldness of the part. It may be abolished by warming the part. It is not seen in the tongue or mouth. It may occur in heart failure or be due to local causes such as poor circulation in the hands or feet. Normal people who are "blue with cold' have this type of cyanosis.

(b) *Central cyanosis* is due either to inadequate uptake of oxygen in the lungs secondary to pulmonary disease or to a right to left cardiac shunt which results in deoxygenated blood bypassing the lungs and passing directly to the systemic circulation. It is characterized by cyanosis which affects the mouth and tongue as well as the extremities, which are warm.

(2) Temperature of the Extremities

Coldness of the extremities is due to vasoconstriction or obstruction of the superficial blood vessels so that the blood supply to the skin is reduced. In heart disease it is often due to the peripheral vasoconstriction which is consequent upon the fall in cardiac output. Conversely, in conditions with a high cardiac output the peripheral vessels are dilated and the skin is very warm.

(3) Clubbing of the Fingers

Clubbing of the fingers may occur in cardiac disease. In congenital cyanotic heart disease it is related to the degree of cyanosis and is often very marked, the fingers having a drumstick-like appearance. It is also seen in patients with cor pulmonale and in bacterial endocarditis. The possibility of other causes, including chronic lung suppuration, carcinoma of the bronchus, ulcerative colitis, the malabsorption syndrome, and cirrhosis of the liver must not be forgotten.

(4) The Arterial Pulse

(a) *Rate*. During the first year of life the normal pulse rate is about 100–110 per minute. As the child grows up the pulse becomes slower and by puberty it has slowed to the adult rate, which is usually between 65–85 per minute. Athletes, however, may have a resting rate of 50 per minute or less. Increase in pulse rate is called *tachycardia* and may be due to emotion, exertion, fever, thyrotoxicosis, bleeding, intrinsic heart disease, paroxysmal tachycardia, atrial flutter or atrial fibrillation. Sleep eliminates emotion and exertion and therefore the sleeping pulse rate may be a valuable observation.

Undue slowing of the pulse is called *bradycardia* and is much less common; it may be due to sinus bradycardia as in hypothyroidism, obstructive jaundice or raised intracranial pressure and is quite commonly found in young fit people; it may also be due to heart block. Digitalis overdosage may produce either effect.

(b) *Rhythm*. Abnormalities of rhythm are considered on page 115.

(c) *Tension*. Measurement of the systolic blood presure by digital compression of the pulse is misleading. It can only be accurately measured by the use of a sphygmomanometer.

(d) *Volume*. The pulse volume is dependent on the pulse pressure. It is better appreciated at the carotid artery than at the wrist. A small pulse volume means a small stroke volume and is often associated with peripheral vasoconstriction. A large pulse volume is usually associated with a large stroke volume and a low peripheral resistance.

(e) *Pulse Wave*. There are a number of variations in the pulse wave which may be helpful in diagnosis. They are best appreciated by feeling a large artery, for example the carotid rather than the radial.

(1) *Collapsing Pulse* (Water hammer pulse). This is detected by lifting the patient's arm and grasping the wrist with the whole hand, when the pulse wave can be felt as an abrupt but forcible tap. It is associated with a wide pulse pressure with an abrupt rise and fall in the pulse wave. It is found most markedly in free aortic incompetence and may also be present in patients with patent ductus arteriosus, peripheral arteriovenous aneurysms, or a rigid arteriosclerotic aorta.

(2) *Plateau Pulse*. This type of pulse is characterised by a wave which is slow rising, flattened, and more prolonged than normal. It is found in severe aortic stenosis.

(3) *Pulsus Bisferiens*. Pulsus bisferiens is a double pulse wave and is found in patients with combined aortic stenosis and regurgitation or in pure aortic regurgitation.

(4) *Pulsus Alternans*. Pulsus alternans consists of alternate weak and strong pulse waves. It may be appreciated on palpation of the pulse, but is more easily shown with the sphygmomanometer. It is found in left ventricular failure.

(5) *Pulsus Paradoxus*. Pulsus paradoxus is found in constrictive pericarditis and pericardial effusions. Normally inspiration sucks blood into the right ventricle with a corresponding rise in right ventricular output to fill the expanded pulmonary vascular bed. If the right ventricle cannot expand due to rigidity or a surrounding effusion, this compensating rise in right ventricular filling cannot occur and cardiac output falls. It can also occasionally occur in asthma where there is a sharp fall in intrathoracic pressure on inspiration.

5) The Venous Pulse

The neck veins should be examined in the recumbent patient with the head and shoulders raised 30° from the horizontal. At this angle the column of blood in the jugular system should reach the level of the clavicle. The normal jugular venous pressure is measured with reference to the sternal angle and is usually recorded in cm. of blood. In normal individuals the range is between +3 and −6 cm. with the subject horizontal. Where precise measurement is required a catheter may be introduced into the atrium for continuous monitoring of pressure which is then sometimes called *central venous pressure*, but which really indicates right atrial pressure. An elevation of jugular venous pressure is found in *heart failure* and in certain conditions associated with a high cardiac output. It is also raised in superior vena caval obstruction when pulsation is absent. Finally minor degrees of elevated venous pressure may occur in conditions with increased intra-abdominal pressure such as pregnancy. The external jugular vein may be compressed as it passes through the cervical fascia; this can usually be relieved by varying the position of the shoulder or head. It is rare for both external jugulars to be so affected.

With the normal jugular *venous pulse* it is possible to observe 'a' and 'v' waves. The 'a' wave is caused by contraction of the right atrium and is seen just before the carotid pulsation. It is followed by the 'x' descent due to relaxation of the right atrium. Pressure recordings in addition show a notch on the 'x' descent which is called the 'c' wave and is probably due to transmitted carotid pulsation. Following the 'x' descent the 'v' wave represents the rise in pressure which occurs when the right atrium fills with the tricuspid valve closed. Finally the tricuspid valve opens in ventricular diastole causing a fall in atrial pressure which is seen in the venous pulse as the 'y' descent.

Large 'a' waves are seen in tricuspid stenosis or when there is increased rigidity of the right ventricle due to hypertrophy such as occurs in pulmonary stenosis or with pulmonary hypertension. Very large 'a' waves or *cannon waves* are seen when the right atrium contracts against a closed tricuspid valve. This occurs regularly in nodal rhythm and nodal tachycardia, and irregularly in complete heart block and rarely with ventricular ectopic beats.

Large waves corresponding to ventricular systole occur in tricuspid incompetence due to the systolic pulse being transmitted to the right atrium.

A deep and abrupt 'y' descent is found in constrictive pericarditis and is due to the ventricular walls being sprung apart early in ventricular diastole. It may also occur in right ventricular failure due to rapid ventricular filling early in diastole.

(6) The Liver

With a rise in venous pressure such as occurs in congestive cardiac failure the liver becomes congested and enlarged. It may be painful and tender on palpation if the enlargement is rapid. Expansile pulsation in the liver is found in tricuspid incompetence. Chronic congestion may lead to some interference with liver function and result in slight jaundice and even cardiac cirrhosis.

(7) Hepatojugular Reflux

Continuous pressure over the liver or abdomen increases the filling of the right atrium and ventricle; in the normal heart this can be accommodated without raising jugular venous pressure but in right ventricular failure the neck veins become distended.

Dyspnoea, orthopnoea, and *oedema* are discussed on page 107.

THE BLOOD PRESSURE

Introduction. The intermittent rise and fall of pressure within the arteries depends on the ejection of blood from the left ventricle. The peak pressure developed is called the systolic pressure and the lowest pressure the diastolic pressure. The difference between systolic and diastolic pressures is called the pulse pressure.

The height of the blood pressure depends on the cardiac output and the peripheral resistance to blood flow. An increase in cardiac output causes a rise in mean blood pressure, the systolic pressure being more affected than the diastolic pressure. A rise in resistance to flow or a rise in pulse rate causes a rise in mean blood pressure, the diastolic being more affected than the systolic pressure.

The rise in blood pressure which occurs on exercise or with emotion is predominantly due to a rise in cardiac output and this may often be associated with a fall in peripheral resistance. In essential hypertension, however, the cardiac output is normal and the elevated blood pressure is due to increased resistance to blood flow.

Another factor which modifies the blood pressure is the elasticity of the arteries. In youth when the arteries are elastic the pulse pressure tends to be low, even in the face of a high peripheral resistance. With increasing age the arteries become less elastic and the pulse pressure increases and may result in the development of so-called benign systolic hypertension of the aged, with a blood pressure in the region of 200/90 mm. Hg. This type of raised blood pressure is of less significance than that due to an increased peripheral resistance.

Measurement of Blood Pressure. When measuring the blood pressure the subject must be at rest both physically and mentally as both recent exercise and anxiety may cause a transient rise. It is customary to take the blood pressure in the right arm, although, except where there is obstruction to the arterial supply to one limb, there is not usually more than a few millimeters of pressure difference between the two arms. It is important to ensure that the sphygmomanometer cuff is firmly and evenly applied. The cuff is fully inflated and then deflated and the pressure at which the brachial pulse returns is determined by palpation. This gives a rough guide to the systolic pressure. The cuff is then reinflated and the stethoscope applied over the brachial artery. The systolic blood pressure is the pressure at which sounds appear.

The diastolic pressure is customarily taken as the pressure at which there is a change from loud clear sounds to muffled sounds. The point of total disappearance of sounds is a better indication of the true diastolic pressure but has not yet been fully accepted in this country.

As the sphygmomanometer cuff is deflated, there is sometimes a pressure range between the systolic and diastolic pressures when no sound is heard. This is called the 'silent gap' and if the blood pressure is being measured by the auscultatory method, the return of sounds at the end of the silent gap may be mistaken for the true systolic pressure. This mistake is avoided if the systolic pressure is first determined by palpation.

THE HEART

Inspection. The apex beat may be visible and its position should be noted. A search should be made for other pulsations. A characteristic 'lift' can sometimes be seen between the apex and the left sternal border in patients with right ventricular hypertrophy, and if the pulmonary arteries are dilated this may extend up to the second or third left intercostal spaces. Aneurysm of the first part of the aorta produces pulsation in the second right intercostal space.

Palpation. The position of the *apex beat* should be confirmed; if it is difficult to locate, palpation should be carried out with the patient sitting forward and expiring fully. Normally the apex beat is in the 5th intercostal space just internal to the midclavicular line. It may be displaced either by shift of the mediastinum or by cardiac enlargement. In left ventricular hypertrophy the apex beat is displaced downwards and to the left and is of a characteristically localised and thrusting nature; if hyptertrophy is combined with dilatation the apex beat feels more diffuse. With right ventricular hypertrophy a forceful impulse can be felt just to the left of the lower end of the sternum; if hyptertrophy is minimal but there is a large flow through the right ventricle as in atrial septal defect the impulse has a tapping character.

Careful examination must be made for *thrills*. These are vibrations which may be appreciated by the hand and are really palpable murmurs. Systolic thrills can be felt in the appropriate areas in both aortic and pulmonary stenosis and in mitral incompetence. A systolic thrill can also be felt over ventricular septal defects and aortic aneurysms. A diastolic thrill may be felt in mitral stenosis. The presence of a definite thrill is always abnormal, and must be distinguished from the slight vibrations which may be felt over a forcibly beating heart.

If pulsations have been found on inspection their presence should be confirmed.

Percussion. It is doubtful whether percussion affords any more information than can usually be found on palpation, but it is customary to percuss out the left and right borders of the heart. By this means the cardiac area can be roughly outlined and percussion may occasionally be useful in the diagnosis of a pericardial effusion or of an aneurysm of the ascending aorta.

Auscultation. Auscultation must be carried out over the whole praecordium and not merely in the classical mitral, aortic, pulmonary, and tricuspid areas.

(A) **Heart Sounds.** There are four groups of heart sounds.

    (1) Sounds produced by valve closure—namely the first sound, caused by closure of the tricuspid and mitral valves, and the second sound from closure of the aortic and pulmonary valves.

    (2) Sound produced by valves opening—namely the opening snap of the mitral valve.

    (3) Sound produced by rapid ventricular filling.

    (4) Extra cardiac sounds.

Some of the sounds may be heard in both normal and abnormal hearts; others only occur in the diseased heart.

(1) *Sounds of Valve Closure.* The *first heart sound* is produced by the closure of the mitral and tricuspid valves. In health it is either single or closely split. In right, and left, bundle branch block the splitting may be quite wide due to the asynchronous closure of the mitral and tricuspid valves.

The *loudness* of the first heart sound depends on the position of the A-V valves at the beginning of ventricular systole. If they have been forced well down into the ventricular cavity by the flow of blood from the atria they have a long way to snap back when systole begins and the first

HEART SOUNDS

sound is therefore loud. This occurs particularly with a short P-R interval, and in mitral stenosis. In the latter condition it is probable that the rather prolonged blood flow through the stenosed mitral valve together with shortening of the chorae tendinae keeps the valve deep in the ventricle until systole starts. Loud first heart sounds are also heard in nervous people with tachycardia, in thyrotoxicosis and in anaemia and are due to the rapid ventricular contraction forcibly closing the A-V valves.

The *second heart sound* at the base of the heart is composed of the closure of the aortic and pulmonary valves. In most children and in many adults the second sound in this area can be heard to be closely split, the first element of the split being due to aortic valve closure and the second element to pulmonary valve closure. Normally this split increases with inspiration, probably due to a momentary increase in the stroke volume of the right ventricle with a prolongation of systole. In *right bundle branch block* the split is wide and widens on inspiration, in *atrial septal defect* the split is wide and fixed.

(2) *Sounds produced by valves opening.* The most important of these sounds is the *opening snap of the mitral valve.* It is best heard between the apex beat and the lower sternum. It is a sharp, high-pitched snap and occurs in early diastole. It is almost, but not quite, diagnostic of mitral stenosis; it is rarely heard in mitral incompetence.

(3) *Sounds produced by rapid ventricular filling (Triple rhythm).* These

extra sounds are probably produced by rapid distension of the ventricles. They are low pitched and can thus be readily distinguished from the sounds of valve opening and closure.

The *third heart sound* is produced by rapid ventricular filling with distension. It is frequently heard at the apex in normal young adults, but in people over the age of 40 it is often associated with heart failure. It is heard best at the left sternal edge in right ventricular failure, and at the apex in left ventricular failure.

The *fourth heart sound* is produced by rapid filling of the ventricles associated with forceful atrial contraction and occurs just before the first heart sound in late diastole. It is best heard a little way inside the apex beat and is found particularly in hypertension and aortic valve disease. It does not necessarily mean that there is left ventricular failure but indicates left ventricular overload. It is never heard in the normal heart and cannot be present if there is atrial fibrillation. If the heart is beating rapidly the three sounds may assume the cadence of a horse's hooves when galloping. This is called *gallop rhythm*.

Sometimes both third and fourth heart sounds may be present and if the heart rate is rapid these additional sounds may blend to produce what is sometimes called a *summation gallop* or *canter rhythm*. It is always of serious significance and suggests gross failure of ventricular function.

(4) *Extra-cardiac Sounds.* These sounds are usually heard in the latter half of systole. They are of a scratchy or crunchy nature and often sound rather superficial. They alter in intensity with respiration and position. They have a variety of causes and are usually innocent.

A *systolic click* is sometimes heard over the pulmonary area—it usually indicates dilatation of the pulmonary artery and is frequently associated with pulmonary hypertension.

A special type of extracardiac sound is the *pericardial friction rub*. It may be heard at the base or apex of the heart and may be systolic or diastolic in timing or sometimes both. It is a scratchy or crunchy sound. There is usually other clinical evidence to suggest pericarditis.

(B) **Heart Murmurs** are caused by eddies set up in blood as it passes from a narrow to a wider channel. They may be caused by pathological narrowing of valves, by their incompetence, or by undue distension of channels. Eddies may also be produced by the unduly rapid passage of blood through the heart as in thyrotoxicosis. When describing murmurs the following points should be noted:

(1) Site and radiation.
(2) Timing.
(3) Loudness. This is usually graded 1–6 for systolic and 1–4 for diastolic murmurs, grade 1 being very soft and grade 6 very loud.
(4) The pitch of the murmur.
(5) The presence or absence of a thrill.

Murmurs can be classified:

(1) Systolic murmurs.
(2) Diastolic murmurs.
(3) Continuous murmurs.

(1) *Systolic Murmurs.*

(*a*) *Ejection Murmurs* are caused by the ventricles forcing blood through a narrowed orifice usually a stenosed aortic or pulmonary valve, or through a normal orifice into a dilated vessel such as an aortic aneurysm or a dilated pulmonary artery. They can also be produced by rapid flow through a normal valve (see below).

Characteristically this type of murmur commences after the first sound, rises to a crescendo in mid-systole and dies away before the second sound.

(*b*) *Pansystolic murmurs* are due to incompetence of the mitral or tricuspid valves or to a ventricular septal defect. They last throughout systole up to the second sound, they are more or less constant in intensity with sometimes a late systolic crescendo.

Systolic murmurs are usually high pitched.

Innocent Systolic Murmurs. A great many systolic murmurs are not due to organic disease. The cause of such murmurs is not fully understood but many of them may be associated with a high velocity of blood flow and

Aortic Stenosis

Pulmonary Stenosis

Atrial Septal Defect

Mitral Incompetence
Tricuspid Inc   nce
Ventricular Septal Defect

Innocent Murmur

SYSTOLIC   MURMURS

can be considered to be attenuated ejection murmurs. They are particularly liable to occur with pregnancy, anaemia, or fevers. They are commonly heard along the left sternal border or at the apex and they are rarely very loud. Their timing varies but they are usually of short duration. They nearly always begin in early systole and finish by mid-systole but there is a group which starts in mid-systole and continues until the second sound.

They usually vary considerably with changes of position and
tion. Their differentiation from organic systolic murmur
partially on the character of the murmur and partially on t
absence of other evidence of cardiac disease.

VENTRICULAR FILLING MURMURS

Mitral Stenosis (in sinus rhythm)

Tricuspid Stenosis

Opening
snap

Mitral Stenosis (atrial fibrillation)

Tricuspid Stenosis

Opening
snap

REGURGITANT MURMURS

Aortic Incompetence
Pulmonary Incompetence

DIASTOLIC MURMURS

(2) *Diastolic Murmurs.*

    (*a*) *Ventricular Filling Murmurs.* These murmurs are due to the
flow of blood through stenosed mitral or tricuspid valves.
They are separated from the second heart sound by a short
gap of variable duration. In patients in sinus rhythm the
murmur rises to a crescendo just before the first heart sound
due to the contracting atria causing a momentarily increased
rate of flow through the narrowed atrio-ventricular valve.
These murmurs are always low-pitched and rumbling.

    (*b*) *Regurgitant Diastolic Murmurs.* They are soft and high
pitched and are due to regurgitation of blood through the
aortic or pulmonary valves. They start immediately after the
second heart sound, are loudest at their onset and die away
before the end of diastole.

(3) *Continuous Murmurs.* Certain murmurs continue throughout systole
and diastole. They are found when there is blood flow between high and
low pressure vessels, most commonly when a patent ductus connects the
aorta with the pulmonary artery.

Patent Ductus Arteriosus

CONTINUOUS MURMURS

THE ELECTROCARDIOGRAM

    The electrocardiogram records the electrical changes produced by the
depolarisation and subsequent repolarisation of the heart muscle, associated respectively with systole and diastole. These changes are amplified

_ recorded on moving paper. The potential changes are recorded by ₋ectrodes attached in various combinations to the body. Each of these attachments is known as a 'lead'.

There are two main groups of leads, known as bipolar and unipolar.

Bipolar leads record the potential changes between two points of the body surface, the leads in common use being:

Lead 1—which records the potential difference between the right and left arm.

Lead 2—between the right arm and left leg.

Lead 3—between the left arm and left leg.

Unipolar leads record potential change at one position on the body's surface. This is done by connecting the leads from both arms and the left leg, the potential change from these three leads being zero. A further electrode is then placed at various positions on the body's surface and the potential changes at these positions recorded. The most usual positions are the chest leads which are numbered V1–6 and the limb leads which are designated aVR (which is the right arm), aVL (left arm) and aVF (left foot).

Tracings from all parts of the body have certain common characteristics. The first wave, which is usually upright, but may be inverted, is called the P wave and represents atrial contraction. The next wave is a small downward deflection known as the Q wave and this is followed by an upright deflection, the R wave, and a further downward deflection, the S wave. This QRS complex represents ventricular contraction.

The P-R interval, measured from the beginning of the P wave to the beginning of the R wave, represents the time taken by the wave of excitation to pass down the bundle of His and should not exceed 0·2 second in the normal subject. The duration of the QRS complex represents the time taken for the wave of excitation to spread through the ventricle and should not exceed 0·1 second in the normal subject. The QRS complex is followed by a short interval and then by a deflection which is usually upright. This is the T wave and represents the recession of the wave of excitation through the ventricle. Changes in the S-T segment and T wave area are of importance in the diagnosis of damage to the heart muscle.

In normal people the basic deflection in each lead is of one of three types. This depends on whether the electrode faces the right ventricle, the left ventricle, or the ventricular cavity. If the heart is in the normal position, leads aVF and Vs 1 and 2 have complexes arising from the right ventricle. Leads aVL and Vs 4, 5, and 6 have complexes arising from the left ventricle and lead aVR has complexes arising from the ventricular cavities. The *right ventricular lead* is characterised by a small R and large S waves and the absence of Q waves, *the left ventricular lead* by a small Q wave followed by a large R wave and small or absent S wave. In the *ventricular cavity lead* the P wave is inverted, the QRS complex consists of a negative deflection and the T wave is also inverted.

If the heart is in an abnormal position, then of course the distribution of these complexes is changed.

In reading an electrocardiogram the following points should be noted:

(1) Heart rate.
(2) Heart rhythm.
(3) Nature and direction of the P waves.
(4) The duration of the P-R interval.
(5) The direction of the main deflection and general shape of the QRS complex.
(6) The width of the QRS complex.
(7) The size of the complexes.
(8) Any depression or elevation of the S-T segment.
(9) The direction and character of the T waves.

RADIOLOGY OF THE HEART

The heart can be examined by chest radiography, by fluorescent screening or by introducing radio-opaque substances into the heart which is then photographed by X-rays—this is known as angiocardiography.

In a plain radiograph of the heart, the right side of the cardiac silhouette is made up of the right atrium, the ascending aorta, and the superior vena cava. The left border is formed by the aortic arch, the pulmonary artery and the left ventricle. When the heart is examined by X-ray screening it should also be viewed in the left and right anterior oblique positions. If a little barium emulsion is swallowed the back of the heart is outlined and slight enlargement of the left atrium can easily be seen, especially in the right anterior oblique position.

Cardiac Enlargement. A general idea of the size of the heart can be obtained by measuring the maximum transverse diameter of the heart and the maximum transverse diameter of the chest; normally the heart diameter should not be more than half that of the chest.

Enlargement of individual heart chambers can also be demonstrated radiologically. Left ventricular enlargement causes rounding of the left lower border of the heart shadow on P.A. view, and in the L.A.O. position the left ventricle can be seen bulging backwards and overlying the spine. Right ventricular enlargement causes increase in the transverse diameter of the heart and there is often straightening of the left border of the heart caused by enlargement of the outflow tract of the right ventricle. Left atrial enlargement is best seen in the R.A.O. position when it can be seen to indent the oesophagus following a barium swallow. In the P.A. view the enlarged left atrial appendage appears on the left border of the heart, below the pulmonary artery. Right atrial enlargement produces a bulge at the lowest part of the right cardiac border.

A pericardial effusion also produces an increase in the cardiac shadow which is usually pear-shaped with clear-cut margins and the lung fields frequently appear clear. It is not always easy to differentiate between enlargement of the heart and a pericardial effusion so that aspiration may be necessary to settle the diagnosis.

By radiological methods it is also possible to assess the great vessels leaving the heart and to demonstrate calcification of the heart valves.

CIRCULATORY FAILURE

Failure of the circulation occurs when the heart is unable to maintain an adequate output. It can be of both acute and chronic forms which produce differing clinical pictures.

Acute Circulatory Failure

In this condition there is a sudden fall in cardiac output. It may be due to acute myocardial failure, commonly after cardiac infarction, or it may be due to hypovolaemia causing an inadequate venous return to the heart as occurs after haemorrhage or sometimes in septicaemias. The clinical distinction between myocardial failure and hypovolaemia may be clear from the history and physical signs. In cases of doubt and to monitor progress, measurement of central venous pressure (see page 96) can be useful. It will be low in uncomplicated hypovolaemia and raised in myocardial failure. However it must be remembered that myocardial failure and hypovolaemia can coexist, in which case central venous pressure will be misleading.

Clinical Features. The picture is one of adrenergic overactivity with pallor and cold extremities due to vasoconstriction, sweating and tachycardia. The blood pressure is low. In severe cases perfusion of vital organs is impaired causing confusion, acute renal failure (see page 366), and acidosis due to overproduction of lactic acid.

Treatment. This depends on the cause. If it is primarily myocardial failure digitalis (see page 112) may help, but usually the prognosis is bad. In hypovolaemia, circulating volume should be restored by infusion of plasma expanders such as dextran (or blood if due to haemorrhage), using central venous pressure as an index of adequate replacement. Causative factors such as infection should be treated vigorously with antibiotics which may be combined with 500 mg. hydrocortisone I.V. six-hourly.

Heart Failure (Chronic Circulatory Failure)

Heart failure is a chronic failure of the ventricles to maintain an adequate output of blood for the needs of the body. This failure leads to disturbances of the circulation which are responsible for the clinical syndrome recognised as heart failure. The symptoms and signs arise in these ways:

(1) **Oedema**

    (a) A fall in the blood flow to the kidneys leads to retention of sodium chloride and water which in turn causes a rise in circulating blood volume and the appearance of excess fluid in the tissue spaces; the distribution of this fluid is influenced by gravity so that it collects mainly around the ankles, or, if the patient is in bed, over the sacrum. It is known as dependent or cardiac oedema and characteristically pits on pressure. Sometimes ascites or pleural effusions develop.

(b) A rise in venous pressure (*vide infra*) at the venous end of the capillary further increases the amount of tissue fluids by preventing reabsorption.

(c) Increased production of aldosterone also leads to retention of salt and water.

(2) **Increased Venous Pressure.** The rise in venous pressure which is found in heart failure is due to:

(a) The rise in circulating blood volume.

(b) In the normal heart a rise in ventricular volume at the end of diastole results in a rise in stroke volume and in cardiac output so that the diastolic volume is returned to normal. An essential feature of the failing heart is its inability to respond in this way. This impairment of ventricular function is reflected in the venous pressure so that in heart failure a rise in venous pressure is not followed by an increase in cardiac output as in the normal heart. The vicious circle of rising venous pressure and falling output can be broken either by increasing the output with digitalis or by decreasing blood volume and lowering venous pressure by diuretics or venesection.

(3) **Dyspnoea,** which is usually a prominent feature of cardiac failure, is due to a number of factors most prominent of which is oedema of the lungs which interferes with gaseous exchange. In addition the increased 'stiffness' of the lung due to oedema leads to an increased sensitivity of the lung stretch reflexes.

Patients with cardiac failure, except for a small group without pulmonary congestion, become dyspnoeic on lying flat (*orthopnoea*). This is due to the increase in amount of blood in the lungs which develops in the horizontal position and which leads in turn to an increase in pulmonary venous congestion. Changes in position may also affect cardiac output, but this probably plays a lesser part in the genesis of orthopnoea.

(4) **Cyanosis.** This is peripheral and results from the slowing of the circulation with consequent venous stagnation of blood.

(5) **Tiredness and Weakness** are common symptoms associated with the low cardiac output.

(6) **The Valsalva Manoeuvre.** The failing heart is unable to respond to changes in filling pressure. This can be demonstrated by forced expiration against a closed glottis or by blowing up a column of mercury, the arterial pressure being recorded continuously.

In normal individuals the rise in intrathoracic pressure decreases venous return to the heart and leads to a fall in stroke volume and blood pressure. This in turn causes reflex vasoconstriction. When the forced expiration is released there is a rise in blood pressure above resting levels, with bradycardia (overshoot phase) due to the increased stroke volume and output and persisting vasoconstriction.

In cardiac failure reduction in venous filling does not decrease output by the overloaded ventricles. There is thus a little rise in arterial pressure during the period of forced expiration ('square wave'), and no 'overshoot' with bradycardia and raised blood pressure after the forced expiration is released.

(7) **Cardiac Enlargement.** Heart failure is associated with cardiac enlargement; this is usually due to hypertrophy of the myocardium, caused

THE VALSALVA MANOEUVRE
1 Normal Subject
2 Cardiac failure
  A = Start of forced expiration
  B = Fall in stroke volume and BP
  C = Release of forced expiration
  D = Overshoot phase

by increased work, and dilation when the ventricles fail to empty properly in systole and become chronically distended.

(8) **The Heart Rate** is usually raised in untreated cardiac failure. This is due to increased adrenergic activity with increased 'drive' to the failing heart. If this adrenergic 'drive' is removed as by adrenergic blocking agents cardiac failure is made worse.

(9) **Water and Electrolyte Disorder in Heart Failure.** In mild or moderate heart failure there is retention of sodium and water, so that although the total body content of sodium rises, the concentration of sodium in the blood remains normal. In severe and prolonged heart failure, particularly if diuretics have been used vigorously, there is a tendency for the body to retain water rather than saline so that the plasma sodium concentration falls. This is often associated with considerable potassium depletion due to both diuretics and possibly leakage of potassium from chronically hypoxic cells. The result is a patient who is oedematous due to extracellular overhydration and yet suffers from intracellular dehydration due to potassium deficiency.

It is customary and useful to divide heart failure into left and right ventricular failure for although in most cases of left ventricular failure the right ventricle will sooner or later fail as well, there is often at first only failure of one ventricle.

LEFT VENTRICULAR FAILURE

The chief causes of left ventricular failure are:

(1) Hypertension.
(2) Coronary artery disease.
(3) Aortic valvular disease.
(4) Mitral incompetence (*Rare*).
(5) Acute pulmonary oedema may also complicate mitral stenosis but is due to left atrial and not left ventricular failure.

When the left ventricle is called upon to do increased work it responds by undergoing hypertrophy and this process enables it for a time to maintain an adequate circulation. Eventually, however, the ventricle can no longer maintain an adequate output and pressure rises in the left atrium and the pulmonary veins, leading to pulmonary venous congestion and oedema.

Clinical Features. Left ventricular failure may develop gradually or suddenly. When it is of slow onset the patient usually complains first of dyspnoea on effort. In addition, his sleep is disturbed. At first he is restless when lying flat and is relieved by two or three pillows (*orthopnoea*); later sleep is broken by *paroxysmal nocturnal coughing*, relieved by sitting up and hanging the legs out of bed; later still, *paroxysmal nocturnal dyspnoea* or *cardiac asthma* appears. Left ventricular failure of *abrupt* onset, almost invariably due to coronary thrombosis, may present with cardiac asthma without preceding symptoms. In the fully developed attack of paroxysmal nocturnal dyspnoea the patient goes to sleep and awakens an hour or two later in a state of great alarm, with a sense of suffocation and fighting for breath. He sits up and may throw open the windows. In severe attacks copiously frothy sputum is expectorated, which may be bloodstained and which is due to pulmonary oedema. After an hour or so the attack passes off and the patient sleeps until morning. Rarely does a first attack prove fatal.

It is not entirely clear why these attacks occur at night, but a number of factors including the recumbent position, which increase the extent of the pulmonary venous congestion, are operative.

Examination at the time of the attack shows *tachycardia*, and on auscultation *gallop rhythm* may be heard. *Fine rales* from pulmonary oedema are heard at the lung bases. If the attack is severe, there may be a fall in the systolic blood pressure. *Pulsus alternans* (p. 96) may be detected; when the difference in the systolic pressure exceeds 15–20 mm. of mercury, and particularly when the alternation persists after the tachycardia has subsided, it is of grave prognostic significance.

The *electrocardiogram* always shows some evidence of S-T or T wave changes over the left ventricle. A chest radiograph will show the hazy shadows of pulmonary oedema spreading out from each hilum into the lung fields.

Prognosis. It used to be said that the prognosis after an attack of cardiac asthma was poor, most patients dying within a year or two. With improved methods of treatment this is no longer entirely true and some patients may do quite well, particularly if the underlying disease, such as hypertension, is amenable to treatment.

RIGHT VENTRICULAR AND CONGESTIVE FAILURE

The chief causes of right ventricular failure are:

> (1) Following left ventricular failure.
> (2) Mitral valvular disease.
> (3) Pulmonary heart disease.
> (4) Certain types of congenital heart disease.
> (5) Following pulmonary embolism.
> (6) Thyrotoxicosis.

Tricuspid stenosis and constrictive pericarditis can also cause marked systemic venous congestion.

Clinical Features. Right ventricular failure is usually seen in patients who already suffer dyspnoea and orthopnoea from pulmonary congestion due to left ventricular failure or mitral valvular disease, and it is then often called *congestive cardiac failure.* When right ventricular failure occurs without pulmonary congestion or pulmonary disease, marked dyspnoea or orthopnoea is not usually a prominent feature although usually present to some degree. Other symptoms include tiredness, weakness, and loss of appetite.

The main signs of right ventricular failure are found in the systemic venous system. In a normal subject reclining at 30°, the neck veins are empty above the clavicles. In right ventricular failure, the *increased venous pressure* causes distension of the veins above this level. The pulsation in the distended veins can readily be distinguished from that of the carotids by the diffuse nature of the venous pulse, in which it is usually possible to distinguish at least two elements, and by the fact that the venous pulse can easily be obliterated by the finger. With severe right ventricular failure, there is stretching of the tricuspid ring leading to functional tricuspid incompetence and a consequent large systolic venous wave which can be seen in the neck and may be felt over the liver. It may disappear with treatment. Distension of the liver with blood, which follows right ventricular failure, may give rise to pain in the right hypochondrium. Palpation shows that the *liver is enlarged and tender.* If the congestion is of long duration the liver may be damaged, resulting in slight jaundice. Dependent *oedema*, for reasons already stated, occurs in right ventricular failure. If the oedema is severe it may be associated with ascites and pleural effusions. *Cyanosis* is common, partly due to poor oxygenation of the blood passing through the oedematous lungs and partly due to peripheral stagnation. Examination of the heart may show evidence of the disease causing the failure. In heart failure, the urine is usually diminished in volume, of high specific gravity, and may contain protein.

TREATMENT OF CARDIAC FAILURE:

Acute Left Ventricular Failure.

(1) The patient is best kept upright supported by pillows; if possible the legs should be dependent to allow as much oedema fluid as possible to drain away from the lungs.

(2) *Morphine* 15–20 mg. should be given intramuscularly. The action of morphine in this condition is not fully understood, but its good effect is probably due largely to its sedative action which decreases anxiety and reduces hyperventilation. It is undoubtedly life saving.

(3) Reduction in blood volume lowers venous pressure, relieves over-filling of the heart and leads to a rise in cardiac output and disappearance of oedema. It is usually achieved by a diuretic and *frusemide* 20 mg. I.V. is effective. Alternatively one pint of blood may be withdrawn from the antecubital vein or blood may be temporarily trapped in the limbs by means of cuffs inflated to just above the diastolic pressure.

(4) *Aminophylline* 0·5 g. intravenously is useful particularly in relieving Cheyne-Stokes respiration.

(5) Pure oxygen should be given if available.

(6) The patient will probably require digitalisation but this is not usually an emergency measure.

With these measures it is usually possible to relieve the patient of an acute attack. Thereafter he should be treated as for congestive failure with rest, digitalis and diuretics (see below). If the underlying cause is amenable to treatment, this should be dealt with. For the next few nights, many patients have difficulty in sleeping and a mixture containing chloral hydrate 1·0 g. and tincture of opium 0·6 ml. is useful.

Treatment of Right Ventricular and Congestive Failure

(1) *Rest* is extremely important in the treatment of heart failure. The patient is nursed in bed and may find breathing easier if he leans forward resting his arms on a bed-table. This upright position allows the oedema fluid to drain away from the lungs and relieves dyspnoea. If an adjustable bed is available the patient will be able to sit with his legs lowered which, by *reducing* the venous return to the heart, further relieves pulmonary congestion. An excellent alternative is a high-backed armchair; many patients find this very comfortable and so rest and sleep more easily. Every effort must be made to spare the patient unnecessary strain; all save the most gravely ill patients should be allowed up daily to the commode or toilet.

(2) *Diet* should be light and easily digestible. There is no reason to restrict fluid intake but salt should be reduced to 1·0 g. per day for a least the early stages of treatment. In severe or refractory cases it should be reduced to 0·5 g. per day, but at this level care must be taken that salt deficiency does not develop.

(3) *Digitalis* is the single most important drug in the treatment of heart failure. It is one of a group of drugs collectively known as the cardiac glycosides which are extracted from a variety of plants. Digitalis is obtained from the foxglove and there are several different preparations in use. They are all similar in their pharmacological action, but differ in the speed of onset and duration of effect and in the proportion of the oral dose which is absorbed. The following is a list of commonly used preparations.

Preparation	Route of Administration	Maximum effect	Duration of effect	Percentage absorbed by oral route
Digoxin	I.V.	2 hours	1 week	
	oral	6 hours	1 week	50–70%
Digitoxin	I.V.	6 hours	3 weeks	
	oral	12 hours	3 weeks	100%

After absorption, some of the digitalis becomes attached to various tissues including heart muscle, skeletal muscle, liver and kidney and it is only very slowly released from these sites, so that accumulation of the drug may easily occur. Digoxin is partially excreted by the kidney so that accumulation can also occur with impaired renal function.

Actions of Digitalis

In therapeutic doses digitalis has no effect on the normal heart but in heart failure the following occur:

(1) Increased force of contraction of the ventricles.

(2) Slowing of the heart by an effect on the sino-atrial node which is partly direct and partly mediated through the vagus.

(3) Depression of conduction in the bundle of His, so that in atrial fibrillation less impulses pass from the atria to the ventricles and the ventricular rate is therefore slowed.

These result in a rise in cardiac output and a fall in venous pressure. The increased renal blood flow causes a diuresis. Digitalis can be used in all types of heart failure. It is, however, not very helpful in the high output state which complicates anaemia nor in heart failure due to acute myocarditis, particularly diphtheria.

Dosage. There are many schemes of dosage of digitalis. They all aim at giving a loading dose fully to saturate the heart muscle with the drug followed by maintenance doses to replace the daily loss of the drug.

Two schemes of dosage are given below.

(a) *Routine Digitalisation*

1st day	Tablets of digoxin		0·5 mg. t.d.s.
2nd day	,,	,,	,,	0·5 mg. b.d.
3rd day	,,	,,	,,	0·25 mg. t.d.s.

This dosage should be continued until the ventricular rate falls to between 70 and 80 per minute; it should then be reduced to 0·25 mg. b.d. and further adjustment in dosage may become necessary to maintain this ventricular rate.

Elderly patients are often very sensitive to digitalis and overdosage is common. Digoxin tablets containing 0·0625 mg of digoxin are available and may be useful in such cases.

Equivalent amounts of prepared digitalis can be used (tablets of digitoxin 0·1 mg. = digoxin 0·25 mg.)

The treatment's aims are relieving the symptoms and signs of heart failure and keeping the patient's resting heart rate at about 70 per minute.

(b) *Emergency Digitalisation.* This is rarely required and is not without risk. Digoxin 0·5 mg. is given slowly intravenously and is followed by digoxin 0·5 mg. orally after four hours and then digoxin 0·25 mg. t.d.s. until a satisfactory response is obtained.

Intravenous digoxin should not be given to a patient who has received digitalis within the last two months. Nearly as rapid a result can be obtained if the initial dose of digoxin is given orally.

Signs of Overdosage. The most important signs of overdosage are:

(1) *Coupled beats.* This is due to increased excitability of the ventricles leading to ventricular premature systoles which occur after every normal beat. If overdosage is allowed to continue ventricular tachycardia or fibrillation may occur.

(2) *Undue slowing of the pulse*—a resting pulse below 65 per minute suggests too much digitalis.

(3) *Atrial tachycardia* with atrio-ventricular block may sometimes occur.

(4) *Nausea, vomiting,* and diarrhoea. Overdosage with digitalis can cause central vomiting—but it should be remembered that vomiting is sometimes a feature of heart failure itself.

(5) *Xanthopsia.*

It is usually sufficient to omit the drug for a day or two to abolish these effects.

Potassium and Digitalis. The presence of potassium ions decreases the effects of digitalis and vice versa. This means that overdosage of digitalis can be temporarily reversed by giving potassium salts. It will also be found that patients who are losing potassium ions (for instance, due to treatment with chlorothiazide) may become more sensitive to digitalis and develop evidence of overdosage.

Digitalis and Cardiac Arrhythmias. Digitalis has a complex effect on atrial arrhythmias due to its double action on atrial muscle; this is partially direct and partially vagal.

    (a) In atrial paroxysmal tachycardia, digitalis may abolish the arrhythmia by virtue of its vagal action.

    (b) In atrial flutter, the flutter is often converted to fibrillation.

    (c) The rate of atrial fibrillation will be increased although the ventricular rate is slowed due to the A-V block.

(4) **Diuretics** are extremely useful in patients with heart failure for they lead to decrease in extra-cellular fluid volume and lower venous pressure.

    (a) *The Benzothiadiazines.* This group of diuretics prevent the reabsorption of sodium, potassium and water by the renal tubule. They are given orally. There are several drugs in this group with similar actions but differing in dosage.

Chlorothiazide	0·5–2·0 g.
Hydrochlorothiazide	50–200 mg.
Hydroflumethiazide	50–200 mg.
Bendrofluazide	5·0–10 mg.
Cyclopenthiazide	0·5–2·0 mg.

Their diuretic action lasts about twelve hours.

They are given orally usually on three or four days each week. Chlorthalidone in doses of 50–200 mg. is similar, but its action lasts up to forty-eight hours.

In the upper dose ranges these diuretics will produce some potassium depletion. This is important as it potentiates the effects of digitalis and may lead to signs of digitalis overdosage. Patients on diuretics should therefore receive potassium supplements. The benzothiadiazines also have some blood pressure lowering action and therefore increase the effect of hypotensive drugs.

Side effects are not common, but benzothiadiazines cause some uric acid retention and may precipitate an acute attack of gout. Rarely they produce diabetes mellitus, which however usually recovers when the drug is withdrawn.

    (b) *Frusemide* is a more powerful diuretic than the benzothiadiazines. Orally in doses of 40–120 mg. either daily or on alternate days it produces a diuresis lasting about six hours. It is also very effective intravenously in doses of 10–40 mg., producing an intense diuresis lasting about two hours.

Ethacrynic acid is similar to frusemide, and is given orally in doses 50–100 mg. daily. Both diuretics will produce potassium depletion and supplements will be required. Care must be taken when using these diuretics as they can cause such an intense diuresis that collapse may occur due to sudden salt and water loss.

(c) In addition *spironolactone,* which antagonises the action of aldosterone, has been used in patients with obstinate oedema. It acts on a different site in the renal tubules to the usual diuretics and can be useful. The dose is 100 mg. four times daily and it must be combined with another diuretic.

(d) *Triamterene* increases the excretion of sodium and water but reduces that of potassium. It is most effective when combined with one of the benzothiadiazines, the dose being 200 mg. daily. *Amiloride* is similar to triamterene but is rather more powerful. The dose is 10–40 mg.

Amiloride, spironolactone and triamterene can cause potassium retention and for this reason must be used with great care in renal failure.

(5) *Sedation* is important in these patients as they are often restless and anxious. In the early stages a mixture containing chloral hydrate 1·0 g. and tincture of opium 0·6 ml. is useful last thing at night and later on a barbiturate hypnotic such as butobarbitone 100 mg. can be used.

(6) *Oxygen* may be required in patients with severe heart failure and may be given either by a Ventimask or by an oxygen tent. The indications are marked cyanosis or distress.

(7) If the oedema is very severe, or if there are collections of fluid in the chest or abdomen, recourse must be made to tapping the chest or abdomen (*paracentesis*) or making multiple incisions in the skin of the legs (*acupuncture*) to allow the oedema fluid to drain away.

Bed rest treatment should continue until the evidence of cardiac failure has disappeared, usually about three weeks. Thereafter the patient should be allowed gradually to return to activity, but his ultimate mode of life will be conditioned by the limits imposed by his disease.

ABNORMALITIES OF RHYTHM

(1) EXTRASYSTOLES

Extrasystoles, or more accurately premature systoles, are due to the cardiac impulse arising in an ectopic focus which may be in the atria, the atrio-ventricular node, or in the ventricles. As the contraction is premature the ventricles are only partially filled so that the resulting pulse wave is diminished or even impalpable at the wrist. The subsequent normal impulse falls in the refractory period, so that there is a compensatory pause during which more blood enters the ventricles than normal and the next beat is unusually forceful.

Extrasystoles are extremely common and most people have them at some time in their lives. Their incidence increases with age; they may occur only occasionally or may be as frequent as every alternate beat, this rhythm being known as pulsus bigeminus or coupled beats. They are often noticed when the patient is lying in bed at night, and though they disappear during exercise they may appear after exertion. They are often more frequent when the patient is tired or worried or during a feverish illness. In some people they may also be related to over-indulgence in tobacco, coffee, or alcohol. Extrasystoles may also occur in heart diseases.

Many patients fail to notice their own extrasystoles. Others complain of a thump in the chest which is due to the powerful contraction after the compensatory pause. Sometimes patients notice the compensatory pause and complain of a 'dropped beat'.

Extrasystoles can usually be diagnosed by the pulse, when a premature beat followed by a pause is felt. Multiple extrasystoles can be confused with atrial fibrillation; the former will, however, disappear on exercise, whereas atrial fibrillation will become more marked. Some confusion may also result if the extrasystoles cannot de detected at the wrist. They can, however, always be heard on careful auscultation of the heart.

Prognosis and Treatment. Extrasystoles by themselves are of no significance. Their presence calls for a careful examination and if no abnormality is found reassurance should be vigorous. If extrasystoles are found at a routine examination in an otherwise normal heart it is usually best not to tell the patient.

Occasionally in subjects with heart disease multiple extrasystoles may herald the onset of a more serious arrhythmia; e.g. the occurrence of ventricular extrasystoles after a coronary thrombosis is sometimes followed by ventricular paroxysmal tachycardia. In those taking too much digitalis, ventricular extrasystoles cause coupled beats and indicate that the drug should be discontinued for a day or two.

Drug treatment is rarely required for extrasystoles; reassurance and the avoidance of obvious precipitating factors are usually sufficient. and if the extrasystoles are very frequent and distressing, quinidine in doses of 200 mg. three times daily or practolol 100 mg. three times daily will sometimes abolish them within a few days.

(2) PAROXYSMAL TACHYCARDIA

Paroxysmal tachycardias are usually classified as ventricular, nodal or atrial according their apparent site of origin. Ventricular tachycardia arises from an ectopic focus and drives the ventricles at a rate, usually between 160–200 beats per minute. Ventricular paroxsymal tachycardia usually occurs in patients with severe disease of the ventricular muscle.

Atrial tachycardia is the commonest form; it is currently believed that in most cases it arises from a circus movement involving the bundle of His. This becomes established if the impulse from an atrial premature beat reaches the A-V node when one pathway in the bundle is still refractory; the stimulus is conducted down another pathway and by the time it reaches the ventricle the previously refractory pathway may have recovered so that the stimulus may be conducted back to the atria whence the whole cycle may be repeated. In most cases the existence of such dual pathways in the bundle of His is not associated with any apparent abnormality of the heart.

Paroxysmal tachycardia may occur at any age, but more usually starts in youth. In this age group there is rarely any associated heart disease. When attacks start later in life it is more frequently but by no means always associated with heart disease, particularly coronary artery disease. It may also occur in thyrotoxicosis, digitalis poisoning, in association with acute fevers, over-indulgence in alcohol and in certain rare forms of congenital heart disease, namely the Wolff-Parkinson-White syndrome (see page 123) and Ebstein's syndrome.

Clinical Features. An attack of paroxysmal tachycardia starts suddenly. The patient may remember the moment when his heart began to beat rapidly. The tachycardia may be described as palpitations or as a fluttering in the chest. It is always quite regular. Sometimes the attacks may start without warning and on other occasions they may be precipitated by a sudden movement or emotion. The attacks last any time from a few seconds to a day or two and then stop quite suddenly and normal rhythm is resumed; sometimes they are followed by extrasystoles. They may recur every few hours or only once or twice in a lifetime.

The degree of constitutional upset varies. Some patients are not disturbed by the attacks whereas others are anxious, feel faint or may complain of discomfort or even an anginal type of pain across the chest. Rarely patients may develop signs of heart failure during the attack, particularly if it lasts more than a day or so and more particularly if there is underlying heart disease.

Prognosis and Treatment. The prognosis in paroxysmal tachycardia, both of the acute attack and of subsequent events, depends on the presence or absence of underlying heart disease. If the heart is healthy the outlook is extremely good, though the paroxysms may cause a good deal of worry and distress.

In treating an attack of paroxysmal tachycardia it is important to know whether it arises from atrial, nodal or a ventricular focus. This is best determined by an electrocardiogram. Occasionally physical signs help. Rapid venous 'cannon waves' (p. 97) caused by the atria contracting against a closed atrioventricular valve, suggest a nodal tachycardia. Sudden slowing produced by carotid sinus stimulation suggest an atrial origin.

Atrial and nodal tachycardia can often be stopped by some trick which results in vagal stimulation, for example tickling the back of the throat, pressure on the eye-balls, or stimulation of one carotid sinus. If these manoeuvres fail and the heart is otherwise healthy it is often best to sedate the patient and wait for a spontaneous return to normal rhythm. If further treatment is required practolol either intravenously or orally (see below) may be successful. If these measures fail full digitalisation is effective. D.C. cardioversion is only indicated in resistant cases.

In *ventricular tachycardia* intravenous lignocaine is the drug of choice. If this fails propranolol or phenytoin is sometimes successful (see below).

In patients who do not respond to drugs and in those whose general condition suggests that rapid restoration of sinus rhythm is necessary electrical cardioversion should be used.

Drugs used to Decrease Cardiac Excitability

β adrenergic blocking drugs are used in cardiac arrhythmias. *Practolol* is a pure *β* blocker and most effective in atrial arrhythmias. *Oxprenol* is similar to practolol. *Propranolol* has in addition a direct depressing effect on the myocardium which makes it particularly useful in ventricular arrhythmias. Drugs can be given intravenously—

Propranolol 2·0–5·0 mg.
Practolol 5·0–10 mg.

Given in this way they cause bradycardia, a drop in cardiac output and hypotension. These can be minimised by giving atropine 0·6 mg. I.V. Blockers can also be given orally to prevent attacks or where emergency treatment is not required.

Propranolol 10 mg. q.i.d.
Practolol 100 mg. t.d.s.
}and increased if necessary.

Propranolol by reducing the adrenergic drive to the heart and by its depressing effect on the myocardium may exacerbate heart failure. It may also precipitate bronchospasm in the asthmatic. Practolol appears less likely to produce these side effects and may therefore be preferred.

Lignocaine is particularly useful in ventricular arrhythmias. It is given intravenously as a single dose of 50–100 mg. or as an infusion at the rate of 1·0 mg. per minute. It may cause bradycardia and should not be used in heart block or when the heart depends on a low nodal or ideoventricular pacemaker.

Procainamide can be given orally in doses of 250 mg. q.i.d. to prevent arrhythmias. It can also be given intravenously, 250 mg. being injected over five minutes. It may cause considerable myocardial depression and hypotension and prolonged use may produce lupus erythematosus, which however is reversible on withdrawal of the drug.

Phenytoin is useful in both ventricular and atrial arrhythmias—either given orally in doses of 100 mg. t.d.s. or as a single intravenous dose of 125 mg. given over five minutes.

Quinidine is now rarely used in acute arrhythmias. It is sometimes effective in preventing arrhythmias in doses of 200 mg. t.d.s. by mouth.

If antiarrhythmic drugs are given intravenously continuous ECG monitoring is essential except in extreme emergencies.

(3) ATRIAL FLUTTER

Atrial flutter is less common. It is nearly always associated with heart disease, commonly rheumatic, hypertensive, or coronary disease. The mechanism of flutter is not entirely settled. Until recently it was thought to be due to a wave of contraction circling round the atria, but more recently it has been suggested that it is due to an excitable focus in the atria, discharging at a high rate, usually between 210–300 per minute. The ventricles are unable to respond at this rate so that there is usually some degree of partial atrio-ventricular block, the ventricles only responding to every second, third, or perhaps fourth atrial contraction.

The *symptoms* of atrial flutter are variable. The patient may complain only of symptoms due to the underlying heart disease and the flutter may be found on examination. Sometimes there may be a complaint of palpitations of sudden onset. Examination may show little, especially when there is a considerable degree of heart block so that the ventricular rate is perhaps only 70 per minute. Sudden change in the degree of heart block resulting in doubling or halving of the pulse rate is characteristic of flutter. Halving of the pulse rate can sometimes be induced by pressing on one carotid sinus. In some patients, continuous variation in the degree of A-V block leads to complete irregularity of the pulse, which feels similar to that of atrial fibrillation. The rather unstable rhythm in atrial flutter may be troublesome to the patient and in most cases an effort should be made to induce a more stable rhythm.

Prognosis and Treatment. The prognosis of flutter depends largely upon the underlying heart disease and is, therefore, variable. Flutter is treated by giving full doses of digitalis; this usually converts the flutter to atrial fibrillation. If the digitalis is then stopped about 40 per cent of patients will revert to sinus rhythm. The remainder will either continue to fibrillate or return to flutter. The decision whether to continue digitalis indefinitely or to try to restore sinus rhythm (see below) depends on the underlying heart disease (see atrial fibrillation).

(4) ATRIAL FIBRILLATION

Atrial fibrillation is a common and important cardiac arrhythmia. Each small muscle bundle in the atria contracts independently at a rate between 400–500 per minute. These contractions can be seen as the '*f*' waves in the electrocardiogram. The result of this disordered atrial activity is that there is no co-ordinated atrial contraction and the ventricles are stimulated in an irregular and often rapid fashion. This in turn throws a greater strain on the ventricular myocardium and may precipitate failure in an already damaged heart.

Atrial fibrillation is usually associated with heart disease, classically with mitral stenosis or thyrotoxicosis; it is, however, also very common in coronary artery disease, in hypertension and it occasionally occurs with acute fevers. It may also be seen in constrictive pericarditis and carcinoma of the bronchus involving the myocardium. Sometimes it follows alcoholic excess or very heavy smoking and it is frequent after thoracotomy. Occasionally it occurs without any apparent cause. It may be paroxysmal or permanent. Atrial fibrillation is rare in aortic valve disease and in most forms of congenital heart disease.

Clinical Features. The onset of atrial fibrillation may pass unnoticed by the patient. More commonly he will complain of palpitations and may notice the irregularity of the pulse. Occasionally the onset is more dramatic, with fainting and collapse, and followed perhaps by acute cardiac failure. The *diagnosis* can be confirmed by feeling the pulse, which is characteristically completely irregular in force and rhythm. Exercise makes the arrhythmia more obvious (cf. extrasystoles p. 115). Further examination will usually show evidence of underlying heart disease.

Paroxysmal Atrial Fibrillation and Lone Atrial Fibrillation. Although atrial fibrillation is usually associated with heart disease, it is sometimes found when the heart is otherwise normal. These patients may either have paroxysms of atrial fibrillation or permanent fibrillation. Follow-up studies of these patients indicate that their prognosis is excellent, except for a number who develop the arrhythmia later in life and who may subsequently show evidence of underlying heart disease.

Treatment of this group consists of abolishing the attacks when they arise (see below). Quinidine may be used prophylactically. When the attacks of arrhythmia are very frequent or when it appears permanent, digitalis is useful in controlling the heart rate, although in these cases the ventricular rate is often surprisingly slow and no drug treatment may be required.

Treatment of Atrial Fibrillation. The majority of patients with atrial fibrillation have heart disease, perhaps with associated heart failure, and are best treated with digitalis.

In a small group of patients with atrial fibrillation an attempt should be made to restore sinus rhythm. This applies when there is no underlying heart disease, when thyrotoxicosis has been relieved and following a successful mitral valvotomy. Cardiac failure, any degree of cardiac enlargement or other evidence of severe heart disease all contra-indicate the use of quinidine. The presence of atrial fibrillation for more than a few months is said to increase the risk of embolism when sinus rhythm is restored.

The method of choice in restoring sinus rhythm is cardioversion by direct current shock. Drugs are now rarely used.

Direct Current Shock for Cardiac Arrythmias. Cardiac arrythmias due to ectopic foci can be reverted to sinus rhythm in most patients by direct current shock. The widest experience is in treating atrial fibrillation. Cardioversion is performed under short duration anaesthesia, and the shock is delivered synchronously with the down stroke of the R wave of the electrocardiogram. It depolarises the heart muscle and allows the sinoatrial node to resume as the cardiac pacemaker. Although cardioversion is successful in some 80% of patients, about 60% of them relapse over the next year despite maintenance treatment with quinidine, procainamide or phenytoin.

HEART BLOCK

There are three degrees of heart block:

(1) Prolongation of the P-R Interval

This degree of heart block can only be diagnosed with certainty from an electrocardiogram.

(2) Increasing P-R Interval with Dropped Beats (Wenckebach's Periods)

The P-R interval increases with each beat until finally a beat is dropped. With the next beat the P-R interval returns to normal and the cycle is repeated.

Clinically this type of block can be diagnosed by noting regular dropping of the heart beats. It requires electrocardiographic confirmation.

(3) Complete Heart Block

The atria and ventricles contract in complete dissociation, the stimulus to ventricular contraction arising in an ectopic focus which may be ventricular or nodal. This type of heart block is recognised by a slow pulse, usually between 30 and 40 per minute, and a wide pulse pressure; by dissociation between the atrial elements of the jugular venous pulse (a waves) and the carotid pulse; and by the presence of occasional "cannon" waves in the jugular pulse which occur when the atrium contracts against a closed tricuspid valve. The heart is usually slightly enlarged. With careful auscultation it is sometimes possible to hear the sound produced by the contracting atria and the first heart sound varies in intensity owing to the varying intervals between the atrial and ventricular contractions (see p. 100).

Heart block is a relatively rare type of arrhythmia. It occurs most frequently in association with coronary artery disease although previous myocarditis of unknown aetiology may be an important cause. It can also occur in diphtheria, in rheumatic fever and digitalis poisoning. It is found rarely in syphilitic heart disease. In about 10 per cent of patients with complete block the disorder is congenital.

Prognosis and Treatment. The prognosis of heart block depends upon the underlying causes. In congenital heart block the outlook is very good and it does not influence expectation of life. In patients developing heart block with pre-existing heart disease the prognosis should be guarded. Generally speaking, no treatment is required for heart block provided it is not producing symptoms. If it is associated with heart failure, digitalis can be used, but should be given with care as it may turn a partial into a complete block while artificial pacing is useful in resistant cases.

Stokes-Adams Attacks. These are attacks of unconsciousness from cerebral anoxia resulting from circulatory standstill. 50 per cent are caused by cardiac arrest, 25 per cent by ventricular tachycardia and 25 per cent by ventricular fibrillation. All cause effective pumping by the heart to cease.

When due to cardiac arrest they are associated with acquired heart block, particularly when the rhythm is unstable and is fluctuating between partial and complete block; circulatory arrest is due to a delay in ventricular contraction when complete block develops suddenly. In the attack the patient falls suddenly to the ground, blue and pulseless and breathing increasingly deeply; if the asystole lasts more than a few seconds convulsions occur. With the commencement of the heart beat, the patient develops a characteristic flush and consciousness returns.

Attacks may occur with varying degrees of frequency and any one may prove fatal.

Treatment

The Acute Attack (*Circulatory Arrest*). The following treatment is used in patients with heart block whose Stokes-Adams attacks are so prolonged as to threaten life. It should also be used when ventricular fibrillation or ventricular asystole complicates unstable rhythms, which are particularly liable to occur after cardiac infarction (p. 159).

The immediate signs of ventricular asystole or ventricular fibrillation are:—

(a) Loss of consciousness

(b) Absent pulses, the carotid being the best artery to palpate.

(c) Cessation of respiration.

(d) Dilated pupils, which occur within thirty seconds.

Resuscitation must be started at once as irreversible damage to the cerebral cortex may occur in two minutes. The immediate treatment is aimed at maintaining circulation and ventilation.

(a) The patient must be laid supine on an unyielding surface and external cardiac massage applied by sharp compression of the lower end of the sternum about eighty times a minute.

(b) The airway must be cleared and the lungs inflated. This can be done by either mouth to mouth respiration or better by an inflating bag (e.g. the Ambu bag) connected to air or oxygen.

(c) As soon as possible 100 ml. of 8·4% sodium bicarbonate should be given intravenously to reduce the rapidly developing acidosis, and repeated as required.

At this stage it is important to take an ECG record to reveal whether there is asystole or ventricular fibrillation or whether normal rhythm has returned, but further resuscitation, if required, should not be delayed when no record is available.

If the heart is in ventricular fibrillation D.C. defibrillation at 200–300 joules may restore sinus rhythm but if the fibrillation continues after five shocks lignocaine 100 mg. I.V. should be given and defibrillation repeated.

When the heart is in asystole, the shock may restart it, but if asystole persists ventricular fibrillation should be provoked by giving 10 ml. of 1:10,000 adrenaline and 10 ml. of 10% calcium chloride I.V. Sinus rhythm may then be restored with the defibrillator. If normal rhythm has not returned after ten minutes of maintained circulation recovery is unlikely.

Preventative. Stokes-Adams attacks can sometimes be prevented by giving slow release isoprenaline ('Saver ine') 30 mg. eight-hourly by mouth, or ephedrine 30 mg. t.d.s. Prednisolor may occasionally be effective particularly in the period following a cardiac infarct, when it reduces oedema and inflammation around the bundle.

If Stokes-Adams attacks are not controlled, artificial pacemaking should be used. This can be temporary to tide the patient over a crisis, when the electrode can be wedged against the endocardium of the right ventricle by cardiac catheterisation, or permanent when it is implanted in the myocardium. The stimulating current is usually provided by a battery.

Bundle Branch Block. Bundle branch block is due to an interruption of conduction in one or other branch of the atrio-ventricular bundle. The wave of excitation passes down the normal branch and stimulates the corresponding ventricle, then passes across to the other ventricle whose contraction is delayed.

Either branch of the bundle may be blocked. *Left bundle branch block* occurs only with heart disease, commonly coronary artery disease, hypertension and aortic valvular disease. *Right bundle branch block* is found in coronary artery disease, congenital heart disease, especially atrial septal defects, and occasionally in otherwise normal hearts.

Clinical Features. Bundle branch block by itself produces no symptoms. Examination shows evidence of the underlying heart disease, if present, and in addition right bundle branch block leads to wide and fixed splitting of the second sound in the pulmonary area.

Bundle branch block can usually only be diagnosed with certainty from an electrocardiogram.

Prognosis and Treatment. The prognosis of bundle branch block depends on the underlying heart disease. No treatment is required for bundle branch block, but the associated heart disease may require therapy.

Wolff-Parkinson-White Syndrome. This usually occurs in young subjects with otherwise healthy hearts. It consists of shortening of the P-R interval on the electrocardiogram with widening of the QRS complexes. It is due to an accessory bundle between the atria and the ventricles. Its main clinical importance is that it may be associated with recurrent episodes of atrial arrhythmias.

HYPERTENSION

It is impossible to define the normal blood pressure for the term in this sense is without meaning. It is possible to find the average blood pressure for a group of healthy people and this average pressure is found to increase with age, being about 120/80 at the age of twenty, rising to 160/90 at the age of sixty. Within this apparently healthy group of people, however, is a wide range. For the purposes of life insurance and similar medical examinations 150/90 is usually taken as the upper limit of normal pressure, although this is probably a little high in the young and a little low in the elderly.

Causes of Hypertension. When a blood pressure which is above the usual level for the patient's age group is discovered the possible causes should be considered. They are the following:

(1) Essential hypertension (80 per cent).

(2) Hypertension associated with renal disease (20 per cent).

(3) Rare causes:

> (a) Hypertension associated with endocrine disease i.e.:
> > (i)   Cushing's syndrome
> > (ii) Phaeochromocytoma
> > (iii) Primary Aldosteronism.
> (b) Coarctation of the aorta.

The discovery of a raised blood pressure calls for full clinical examination, particular attention being paid to the cardiovascular system, including the femoral pulses, the retinae and examination of the urine. If there is any suspicion of a renal cause the urinary tract should be further investigated. Endocrine causes should also be remembered and can usually be diagnosed by specific tests.

ESSENTIAL HYPERTENSION

The cause of essential hypertension is unknown. There is at present a widespread opinion that patients with essential hypertension merely represent the extreme uppermost limit of normal variation in blood pressure in the population. There is little doubt that heredity plays a part and it is common to find evidence of hypertension in the patient's father or mother. Essential hypertension is more common in women than in men.

Clinical Features. The blood pressure may remain raised for many years without producing any symptoms or signs; in fact if a blood pressure of over 150/90 is considered abnormal, quite a large proportion of the older people of this country have essential hypertension which in the majority of cases causes them no harm for many years. Many such subjects die in old age of some other complaint.

The symptoms and signs of hypertension are really due to the effects of the raised blood pressure on the cardiovascular system. These complications are particularly liable to occur when the diastolic pressure is high and when hypertension develops at a relatively early age; they are more common in men than in women. The cardiovascular system and the kidneys are most commonly involved.

(1) *The Heart.* The heart is the organ most frequently affected by hypertension. The left ventricle must work against an increased resistance and may in time fail. The *symptoms* are those of left ventricular failure:

dyspnoea on effort and paroxysmal dyspnoea at night. *Examination* in a fully developed case shows a full pulse with some thickening of the wall of the radial artery. The heart is enlarged and the apex beat is of the left ventricular type. In at least 50 per cent of patients there is a triple rhythm with a presystolic (atrial) extra sound best heard at the apex. Although the triple rhythm is common in the more severe hypertensives, it does not necessarily imply a failing left ventricle and is not of great prognostic significance. The aortic component of the second sound is loud. A systolic murmur either at the apex or base is quite common; it is usually due to flow through the aortic valve and only rarely to aortic stenosis or a functional mitral incompetence. Eventually the left ventricular failure may progress to congestive failure with raised venous pressure and perpheral oedema.

(2) *The Blood Vessels.* The increased pressure within the blood vessels leads to thickening of the walls of the medium-sized arteries and this change may be palpable in the radial artery at the wrist. Hypertension also predisposes to atheroma with an increased incidence of coronary artery disease.

Hypertensive Retinopathy. The arteries of the retina may show a series of changes which have been subdivided:

Grade I.   Narrowing and increased tortuosity of the retinal arteries.

Grade II. Arterial changes more marked and nipping of the veins at the arterio-venous crossing due to the thickened arterial wall pressing on the vein.

Grade III. Grades I and II with the addition of haemorrhage and/or exudates.

Grade IV. Previous grades with papilloedema.

Cerebral Arteries. The cerebral arteries are affected in hypertension. Headaches, usually worse in the morning, are often found in severe hypertension. These headaches must be distinguished, however, from anxiety headaches commonly found in patients who know they have hypertension. In severe hypertension attacks of cerebral oedema occur, producing the clinical syndrome of *hypertensive encephalopathy* with blinding headaches, fits, unconsciousness, and transient palsies.

Frequently an artery gives way under the strain with a resulting cerebral haemorrhage which may well be fatal; thrombosis may also occur.

(3) *The Kidney.* In the majority of patients with essential hypertension there is no evidence of serious interference with renal function and death from renal failure is rare. The urine may, however, contain a little protein, particularly in the more severe cases. In malignant hypertension (see below), there are marked changes in the blood vessels of the kidney, particularly fibrinoid necrosis of the afferent artery to the glomerulus, and in these cases there is a progressive decrease in renal function and death may occur from renal failure.

Investigations

The *electrocardiogram* may show evidence of left ventricular hypertrophy. In addition, if the myocardium is beginning to fail there will be S-T depression and T-wave inversion in left ventricular leads. The presence and degree of change in the electrocardiogram is a useful index of the amount of damage to the heart which is resulting from the hypertension.

Radiography may show enlargement of the left ventricle with some dilatation of the aorta. If left ventricular failure has developed, there will in addition be fluffy shadows spreading out from the hilar region due to pulmonary venous congestion.

Malignant Hypertension

Malignant hypertension, which is relatively uncommon, may be regarded as the most severe grade of essential hypertension, although this view is not universally accepted. It is characterised by a high diastolic pressure (usually over 140 mm./Hg.), by marked arterial changes in the retina with papilloedema, and by progressive renal failure. It arises most commonly in men of early middle age.

A proportion of these patients develop secondary hyperaldosteronism. The plasma potassium concentration is low but in contradistinction to primary hyperaldosteronism (Conn's Disease, page 449) the plasma sodium concentration is also reduced and the plasma renin level is raised. It is suggested that the damaged kidneys liberate large amounts of renin and this leads to increased aldosterone production via the angiotension system.

Prognosis of Hypertension

The prognosis of essential hypertension is very important for it largely determines the management of the patient. There are now a large number of follow-up studies of hypertensives and although much evidence is conflicting, a general pattern is emerging.

Generally speaking the factors which influence prognosis are:

(1) Sex of the patient—women have a better prognosis than men.
(2) The height of the diastolic blood pressure. A diastolic pressure of over 130 mm./Hg. usually carries a bad prognosis.
(3) The degree of arterial change (particularly the retinal changes).
(4) The degree of change in the heart.
(5) Evidence of renal involvement.

It would seem that the majority of patients with mild or moderate essential hypertension, particularly middle-aged or elderly women, will live for ten or twenty years or longer; but in those with high pressure and evidence of marked arterial or cardiac change the prognosis is considerably worse. Most patients with untreated malignant hypertension are dead within three years.

Treatment

General Measures. Most patients with hypertension require some *reassurance.* Their mode and tempo of life may require modification, but they should lead as normal a life as possible. There is no evidence that *diet* plays any part in the genesis of hypertension, but if the patient is overweight this should be corrected as loss of weight may cause some fall in blood pressure.

Low sodium diets such as the Kempner rice diet have been used successfully in lowering blood pressure, but they are trying to take over long periods and are not used very frequently.

Sedation should be used in those patients who are unduly anxious. Chlordiazapoxide 10 mg. three times daily is usually satisfactory.

Drug Treatment. There is now evidence that lowering the blood pressure decreases the mortality and morbidity from hypertension, particularly if it is severe. There is however, no evidence that it is possible to decrease those complications due to coronary artery disease. There is as yet no drug which is entirely satisfactory and free from side effects. Drug treatment is therefore usually confined to those with a bad prognosis although some experts would also treat the milder grades of hypertension, particularly in younger patients. Generally speaking patients over sixty-five do not do very well with these drugs. If the blood urea is over 80 mg. per 100 ml. due to renal damage, lowering of the blood pressure may well precipitate acute renal failure.

The drugs available are:

(1) *Sympathetic Blocking Group*

    (a) *Guanethidine* blocks the post-ganglionic fibres of the sympathetic system without affecting the parasympathetic system. The initial dose is 10 mg. daily and it may take several days until the full effect is seen. The dose is therefore increased every five days until a satisfactory fall in blood pressure is produced: the controlling dose is usually between 30–60 mg. daily. The fall in blood is postural so that the blood pressure must be measured both standing and lying.

    Side effects are:

    (i) Diarrhoea is common and can be controlled by codeine phosphate 30 mg. b.d. or by combining guanethidine with a small dose of pempidine.

    (ii) Other side effects are nasal stuffiness, bradycardia, parotid pain, muscle tremors and failure of ejaculation.

    (b) *Bethanidine* blocks the adrenergic neurone. The initial dose is 10 mg. b.d. which is increased until a satisfactory response is obtained. It is given up to 4 times a day as its duration of action is short. This means that a more flexible control is possible than with guanethidine.

(c) *Debrisoquine* is similar to bethanidine. It is relatively short acting. The initial dose of 20 mg. daily is increased as required.

(d) *Methyldopa* blocks the action of noradrenaline and adrenaline by competing at receptors after conversion to methyl noradrenaline. It also probably has a central action. The intial dose is 250 mg. four times daily. The full effect is not seen for about five days, so dosage is increased gradually until control is satisfactory. (The usual dose is 1·0–1·5 g. daily.) Methyldopa is not as powerful as guanethidine and symptoms from postural hypotension are not common. Some patients complain of drowsiness early in treatment, also dry mouth and occasionally pyrexia. Water retention may occur but responds to diuretics.

(e) *Clonidine* lowers blood pressure by both central and peripheral actions. It is similar both in its actions and side effects to methyldopa. The initial dose is 50 μg. three times daily and increased as required. It should not be stopped suddenly as this may result in a sudden rise in blood pressure.

(2) *Diuretics.* The benzothiadiazine group (p. 114) are satisfactory. Their mode of action is not clear. They produce a transient fall in blood volume but their hypotensive effects seems to depend on other factors. They are very effective when combined with blood pressure lowering drugs, particularly the sympathetic blocking group or rauwolfia, both of which tend to cause salt and water retention. Satisfactory diuretics are:—

Bendrofluazide 2·5–5·0 mg. daily.
Chlorthalidine 50 mg. daily or on alternate days.

Potassium supplements are not normally required provided the patient is on a full mixed diet.

(3) *Rauwolfia.* Although it has some sympathetic depleting action it can be considered separately. The purified extract *reserpine* is usually used. It produces a mild hypotensive action which takes several days to appear and is probably due to a central action. The fall in blood pressure is not postural. The daily dose should not exceed 0·25 mg., and at this level side effects including nasal stuffiness, bradycardia and most important, mental depression, are not usually troublesome.

(4) *Propranolol* (p. 118) lowers blood pressure by decreasing cardiac output, and flattening the rises in bl od pressure which accompany periods of sympathetic activity. It takes several weeks to produce its full effect. The initial dose is 10 mg. four times daily and this is increased. It must not be used in patients with heart failure or asthma.

(5) *Ganglion Blocking Group.* These drugs interfere with transmission at

all autonomic ganglia, reduce the sympathetic tone of the arterioles and thereby diminish the peripheral resistance. Unfortunately there are several side effects with this group of drugs.

(a) The fall in blood pressure is postural; fainting may occur on standing and can be relieved by lying down. Blood pressure readings of the patients on these drugs must always be taken both standing and lying.

(b) Interference with the autonomic supply to the gastro-intestinal tract leads to a dry mouth and to constipation. The bowels must be kept open with an aperient or intestinal ileus may develop.

(c) Paralysis of accommodation can occur and may require reading glasses.

(d) Difficulty with micturition is sometimes troublesome.

The important drugs in this group are:

Mecamylamine in doses of 2·5 mg. three times daily or *pempidine tartrate* in doses of 2·5 mg. three times a day increased until a satisfactory fall is produced.

Use of Hypotensive Drugs

Opinions differ as to the relative efficacy of these drugs in hypertension, but is usual to start with a sympathetic blocker, i.e.

Methyldopa 250 mg. q.i.d. is frequently satisfactory or
Bethanidine 10 mg. twice daily may be required in severe cases.

When treatment is started the blood pressure should be recorded at least four times daily and this may require admission to hospital. The dose is then adjusted until a satisfactory fall is produced. It is usually best not to try to lower the blood pressure to normal, but to aim at a level of about 160/100–170/105; this prevents low levels when the patient may feel faint. If control is not very steady on this regime a diuretic should be given in addition to try and smooth out the swings in blood pressure. In less severe hypertension reserpine 0·25 mg. with a diuretic is sometimes effective, producing few side effects, or even a diuretic alone may be sufficient. The patient then returns home but continues to be seen regularly by his doctor and the dose of the drug is modified as required.

Hypertensive Crisis

It may be necessary to lower the blood pressure rapidly in a hypertensive crisis. For this purpose pentolinium tartrate 0·5 mg. I.V. is effective. It acts rapidly and if there is no response within five minutes the dose may be doubled and increased until a satisfactory fall is observed. Pentolinium is a ganglion blocker and the patient must therefore be nursed as upright as possible, as the fall in blood pressure is largely postural. It must also be remembered that it is excreted via the kidneys and accumulation will occur in renal failure.

If a less rapid fall in blood pressure is required methyldopa 1·0 g. I.V. is effective within about six hours.

RHEUMATIC HEART DISEASE

Acute Rheumatic Fever

Acute rheumatic fever is a disease affecting connective tissue, particularly that of the heart and its valves and the joints.

Aetiology. It is a disease of childhood and adolescence, about 90 per cent of cases occurring between the ages of eight and fifteen. It is common in temperate climates, as for example in the British Isles, and it affects the poorer classes, its incidence probably being increased by bad housing and overcrowding. The exact cause of the disease is unknown, but in many patients it follows about two or three weeks after a sore throat due to infection with haemolytic streptoccocus (Lancefield Group A). It is possible that other organisms or viruses may play a part. There has been a sharp decline in the incidence of the disease in this country in the past two decades, possibly related to an improvement in social conditions.

It seems very probable that the lesions represent an allergic reaction to exotoxins from the haemolytic streptococcus in an individual who has already been sensitised.

Clinical Features. The attack of rheumatic fever nearly always follows seven to twenty days after a streptococcal throat infection. Typically but not invariably, the illness starts suddenly with fever, pain, stiffness, and sometimes swelling in one or more of the larger joints, namely the elbow, wrist, shoulder, hip, knee, or ankle. After a day or two the pain leaves the joint first affected and appears in another one; this *flitting from joint to joint* is unusual in other forms of arthritis and is a useful pointer to the diagnosis. Small joints are rarely affected. Skin rashes are sometimes seen in rheumatic fever; the most typical is *erythema marginatum* which consists of red rings of irregular size and shape which have slightly raised edges and normal centres. They tend to coalesce, and come and go rather quickly. In parts of the body where bones lie immediately under the skin, particularly shins, forearm, elbows, wrists, ankles, and scalp—*rheumatic nodules* may be felt. They are not tender, usually about the size of a pea and are not attached to the overlying skin.

In some children the rheumatic process takes a much milder and more insidious form which can easily be overlooked, though it is as likely as the more obvious type of rheumatic fever to be associated with active heart disease. Thus about half the patients who are later found to be suffering from chronic rheumatic heart disease give no history of rheumatic fever or chorea.

Evidence of Cardiac Involvement. The following findings may be taken as evidence of cardiac involvement:

(1) *Tachycardia.* Patients with active rheumatic carditis nearly always have a raised sleeping pulse rate and awaking pulse disproportionate to the degree of fever; that is more than 10 beats per minute rise per degree of fever.

(2) *The Development of Cardiac Murmurs.* There are two types of cardiac murmur which indicate active rheumatic carditis. The *Carey Coombs murmur*, a short mid-diastolic murmur heard at the apex is the earliest indication of involvement of the mitral valve. When the rheumatic process resolves this murmur may disappear or if the valve is sufficiently damaged it may develop the typical presystolic accentuation of mitral stenosis. The typical rumbling murmur of mitral stenosis results from scarring of the valve, and takes two years at least to appear.

Similarly the *soft early diastolic murmur* heard best down the left or right border of the sternum is typical of aortic incompetence and is the earliest sign of involvement of the aortic valve.

Isolated apical systolic murmurs are difficult to interpret in rheumatic fever because they are common in healthy children, but generally it can be said that the louder, rougher and more prolonged the murmur the more likely it is to indicate active carditis. It must however be emphasised that both systolic and diastolic murmurs may disappear when healing of the rheumatic process occurs.

(3) *Cardiac Enlargement.* The development of cardiac enlargement indicates active carditis. It may be due to dilatation of the heart or to the presence of a pericardial effusion, or both.

(4) *Pericarditis.* The finding of a pericardial friction rub indicates active heart involvement.

(5) *Heart Failure.* The appearance of heart failure in acute rheumatic fever indicates a severe myocarditis. Rheumatic myocarditis may also be responsible for patients with established rheumatic heart disease developing heart failure.

Laboratory Investigations. The blood shows a moderate leucocytosis with some anaemia and a raised E.S.R. The antistreptolysin titre in the blood is raised. A figure above 200 Todd units is considered significant, though it must be realised that this merely indicates a recent streptococcal infection and is not diagnostic of rheumatic fever. The electrocardiogram shows no specific abnormality, but there may be various conduction defects.

Treatment. The seriousness of this disease lies in the risk of carditis occurring at some time in the illness and resulting in chronic rheumatic heart disease.

The most important principle in the treatment is *rest*. The patient should be semi-recumbent on a firm mattress with two or three pillows. Sweating may be profuse. If the joints are very painful they may be supported by pillows and the pressure of bedclothes relieved by a cradle.

The diet should be light and fluid intake must be high.

The specific drugs in the relief of rheumatic fever are the *salicylates*. High dosage is essential and should aim at producing a blood salicylate level of 30–40 mg./100 ml. Soluble aspirin 1–2 g. four hourly for an adult should be given until symptoms are relieved or until deafness, tinnitus, nausea, and perhaps vomiting occur, when the dose should be slightly decreased. With this treatment the fever and joint pains should be relieved in two to three days.

Prednisolone 40 mg. daily is useful in the severely ill patient who is not responding to salicylates.

Whether the use of salicylates does more than relieve the symptoms of rheumatic fever is still open to doubt, but there is some evidence that adequate treatment with this drug does decrease the subsequent incidence of rheumatic valvular disease.

A course of *penicillin* should be given to eradicate any residual streptococcal infection, but it does not alter the course of an acute attack. It should also be used to prevent further streptococcal infections (see below).

Duration of Treatment

Complete rest must be enforced until all evidence of active disease has gone, which means the disappearance of all signs of infection and the return of the E.S.R. to normal. It must be remembered that high blood salicylate levels cause acceleration of the E.S.R.: conversely it is reduced if heart failure appears. Consequently the E.S.R. must be interpreted in the light of the whole clinical picture. It rarely requires less than six weeks to return to normal and patients may have to be confined to bed for many months. Thereafter a graduated return is made to normal activity, a careful watch being kept for recrudescence of acute rheumatism.

After Care. On return to normal life the child should not be fussed over, but exposure to cold and dampness should be avoided as much as possible. Because of the danger of further damage to the heart from relapses, streptococcal throat infections should be prevented by giving sulphadimidine 0·5 g. daily or phenoxymethylpenicillin 250 mg. twice daily, continuing until the age of eighteen in childhood rheumatic fever or for five years if the disease starts after the age of thirteen.

Prognosis. Approximately half the children who have acute rheumatic fever develop rheumatic valve disease. The older the child at the time of the acute attack the less likely are the valves to be permanently affected. Some 95 per cent of those with no evidence of cardiac involvement when treatment is started have no residual heart disease. The incidence of permanent valve damage increases with increasing evidence of carditis and is more common after recurrent attacks.

RHEUMATIC CHOREA (Sydenham's Chorea)

Chorea may be considered as a manifestation of the rheumatic process in which the brain is affected. About 20 per cent of patients with chorea develop chronic rheumatic heart disease identical with that found after rheumatic fever. In a certain number of cases there may also be other manifestations of the rheumatic process. Chorea commonly occurs in childhood and adolescence, but a particularly severe though rare type of chorea is associated with pregnancy. It is commoner in girls.

Clinical Features. The child developing chorea is first noticed to be very restless and fidgety and some time may elapse before it is appreciated that her jerkiness and clumsiness indicate illness rather than original sin. All four limbs are usually affected though occasionally the disorder may be confined to one arm or leg or one side of the body (hemichorea). When the disease is at its height the *involuntary movements* are the most prominent feature. The child is constantly grimacing and making sudden, jerky, and ever varying movements of the limbs; these movements cease in sleep. In doubtful cases it is a useful test to ask the child to grasp one's hand, as she is unable to maintain a steady pressure and the intensity of her grip will be found to be always waxing and waning. The *muscles are weak* and have a *poor tone*, so that the joints can be moved through an abnormally wide range, and typically the outstretched hands are held with the wrists slightly flexed and the fingers hyperextended at the meta-carpo-phalangeal joints. These movements must be differentiated from nervous tics, the most important points being that unlike tics they are not purposive and never repetitive. *Emotional changes* are common, consisting of depression, weeping, uncontrolled laughter, and hysteria. Examination of the cardiovascular system may show evidence of cardiac involvement similar to that described under rheumatic fever. The E.S.R. is usually normal unless the heart is involved.

The average *duration* of the disease is about two months, though occasionally chorea may last up to six months or longer. After apparent full recovery odd choreiform movements may persist and be particularly noticeable when the child is under stress. These movements are often considered hysterical, but recently it has been suggested that they represent residual brain damage.

Treatment. *Rest* is the most important part of the treatment of this disease, in order to prevent or limit permanent heart damage. To achieve complete rest in this type of patient is not easy. Some children are happier in a single room, others prefer the company of a general ward. The cot or bed should have sides to prevent the child falling out and there should be padding to prevent injury. One or two pillows are satisfactory and great care should be taken of the child's skin and cleanliness. Feeding may be difficult and great patience will be required by the nurse or mother.

There is no specific treatment for chorea. Soluble aspirin 0·3 g. t.d.s. and phenobarbitone 60 mg. t.d.s., during the day and a mixture containing chloral hydrate 0·3–1·0 g. at night is useful for sedating the patient. Occasionally in very severe cases (*manic chorea*) paraldehyde 3–5 ml. intramuscularly can be given.

Following an attack of chorea prolonged convalescence is required with efforts to improve general health as far as possible. About one-third of patients with chorea will have a further attack. *Prophylaxis* similar to rheumatic fever is recommended.

CHRONIC RHEUMATIC HEART DISEASE

Following acute rheumatic fever or chorea, the heart may return to normal; but if damage to the valves is severe enough, they will become deformed and scarred and thus unable to function properly.

The incidence of involvement of the various valves is approximately:

Mitral valve	80% of cases
Aortic valve	45% of cases
Tricuspid valve	10% of cases
Pulmonary valve	1% of cases
Mitral valve alone	50% of cases
Mitral and aortic valves together	20% of cases

The *natural history* of the condition starts with the acute rheumatism, usually between the ages of eight and fifteen. There may have been one or several attacks. There is then usually an asymptomatic period of 15–20 years until the patient begins to notice dyspnoea.

By about the age of thirty many patients have had their first attack of congestive cardiac failure, which is often precipitated by the onset of atrial fibrillation or perhaps some extra strain such as ill-advised pregnancy. The attacks of cardiac failure become less and less amenable to treatment and death usually occurs in the mid-thirties. It must be realised that the foregoing account is merely an average course of events. In some patients the course is even shorter, whereas others may live to middle or even old age without developing any symptoms from their heart lesion.

ACQUIRED LESIONS OF THE HEART VALVES

MITRAL STENOSIS

Mitral stenosis is the commonest valve lesion and is always due to previous rheumatic inflammation. It occurs more commonly in women than in men. It is probable that at the time of the acute rheumatic affection the mitral valves fuse at the point of insertion of the chordae tendinae. At first there may be little interference with the flow of blood from the left atrium to the left ventricle, but subsequently there is gradual contraction and narrowing of the mitral orifice and if the orifice is reduced below a size of about 1×0.5 cm. the passage of blood into the left ventricle is seriously obstructed.

There is thus a rise in pressure in the left atrium, which is transmitted back to the pulmonary veins, the pulmonary capillaries, and finally the pulmonary arteries, leading to pulmonary congestion. This passive rise in pressure is not very great, the pulmonary artery pressure being usually about 40 mm. Hg., but it would be sufficient to force fluid from the pulmonary capillaries into the alveoli and thus produce pulmonary oedema. This is prevented in two ways:

(1) There is a certain amount of thickening of the alveolar walls which become less susceptible to oedema.

(2) In a proportion of patients there is active vasoconstriction of the smaller branches of the pulmonary artery which 'protects' the pulmonary capillaries from the pressure developed by the right ventricle. The active pulmonary vasoconstriction, although lowering capillary pressure, causes a considerable rise in pulmonary artery pressure which is often about 80/40 mm. Hg.

Sometimes these protective mechanisms fail. This is liable to occur in the early stages of the disease when alveolar thickening has not developed and when the pulmonary artery vasoconstriction suddenly relaxes. Such patients develop attacks of *acute pulmonary oedema* which are always serious and may be fatal. In the majority of patients, however, the passive pulmonary congestion runs parallel with alveolar thickening. Such patients do not develop active pulmonary vasoconstriction or have attacks of pulmonary oedema. The *pulmonary congestion* does, however, lead to increased 'stiffness' of the lungs which plays a large part in causing dyspnoea which is a leading symptom of mitral stenosis. The changes in the walls of the alveoli also interfere with oxygen uptake.

Finally the right ventricle fails and the fully developed picture of congestive cardiac failure emerges.

Clinical Features. *Dyspnoea* is the commonest presenting symptom of mitral stenosis. It may be of two types:

(1) *Dyspnoea on effort* which becomes progressively more severe and is sooner or later accompanied by *orthopnoea*. This dyspnoea is due to increasing pulmonary congestion.

(2) A small proportion of patients with mitral stenosis present with attacks of *pulmonary oedema* similar symptomatically to those found in acute left ventricular failure. The mechanism of the oedema is considered above. These attacks frequently follow some undue excitement such as a dance or other unusual exertion; they may also be precipitated by pregnancy.

Pulmonary congestion is also responsible for two other symptoms of mitral stenosis, *bronchitis* and *haemoptysis*. The former is usually more marked in the winter but may be troublesome throughout the year.

Haemoptysis may be confined to mere blood streaking of the sputum but sometimes takes the form of a frank haemoptysis presumably due to rupture of a congested blood vessel.

The low cardiac output which is often found with mitral stenosis of any severity is probably responsible for the general symptoms of *weakness* and *tiredness* which are found in the developed condition.

Sooner or later most patients with mitral stenosis develop *congestive cardiac failure*. This may occur insidiously, but common precipitating factors are:

(1) The development of atrial fibrillation.
(2) Intercurrent infection.
(3) Further acute rheumatic carditis.
(4) Subacute bacterial endocarditis.
(5) Pregnancy.
(6) Anaemia.

Complications. There are three complications of mitral stenosis which are not uncommon and which may seriously affect the patient's prognosis. *Thrombi* commonly form in the left auricle of patients with mitral stenosis, particularly in those with atrial fibrillation. Clots may break off from these thrombi and passing out into the systemic circulation obstruct arteries and produce a variety of symptoms and signs. Thrombi may also form in the deep veins of the legs leading to *pulmonary infarcts*; these are sometimes very intractable and precipitate cardiac failure which may be irreversible. Finally patients with mitral stenosis may develop *subacute bacterial endocarditis*; this is, however, uncommon if atrial fibrillation is present.

Physical Signs. The patient with mitral stenosis typically, although by no means invariably, has a slight cyanotic flush on the malar region of the cheeks (*mitral flush*). If heart failure has supervened the patient will be orthopnoeic and slightly cyanosed. The pulse will be small and may show atrial fibrillation. The blood pressure is usually on the low side with a narrow pulse pressure.

Examination of the neck veins may show evidence of heart failure and in addition a small group of patients who are in sinus rhythm will show a large 'a' wave indicating pulmonary hypertension or co-existing tricuspid stenosis.

The *apex beat is tapping* and the lift of the *enlarged right ventricle* can be felt between the apex and the left border of the sternum. A *diastolic thrill* may be palpable at the apex.

The first heart sound at the apex is loud. Careful auscultation at the lower end of the sternum will also show a sharp, clear sound following the second heart sound; this is the *opening snap of the mitral valve* and is a useful confirmatory sign of mitral stenosis. The pulmonary component of the second sound is loud and may even be palpable.

The typical *murmur of mitral stenosis* is a low-pitched, rumbling diastolic murmur, localised to the apex (ventricular filling murmur). It is best heard with the patient lying on the left side and is accentuated after exercise. It is due to the blood rushing through the narrowed mitral valve and if the patient is in sinus rhythm there will be a presystolic accentuation due to the left atrium contracting and forcing the last portion of the blood even more rapidly through the mitral valve. The presystolic accentuation disappears with atrial fibrillation. In severe mitral stenosis the murmur extends from the opening snap to the first heart sound; in less severe stenosis it is shorter. If severe pulmonary hypertension develops the mitral diastolic murmur may become brief and insignificant due to the associated low cardiac output.

Very rarely there may be heard a pulmonary diastolic murmur down the left border of the sternum (*Graham-Steell murmur*) due to pulmonary incompetence subsequent upon dilatation of the pulmonary artery; it must be stressed, however, that such a murmur is very much more commonly due to associated aortic incompetence.

An *electrocardiogram* may show large wide P waves or atrial fibrillation; there may also be right ventricular hypertrophy. A *radiograph of the heart* will confirm the enlargement of the right ventricle and in addition will show a small aorta and enlargement of the left atrium best seen in the right oblique position. Calcification of the mitral valves may be seen but this can also occur in mitral incompetence. The pulmonary arteries are often dilated. The lung fields will be congested if heart failure has supervened.

Normally the flow of blood through the lungs is higher in the lower than the upper lobes. In mitral stenosis there is constriction of the arteries to the lower lobe and thus a redistribution of the pulmonary circulation, so that pulmonary congestion affects both upper and lower lobes. In addition dilated lymph channels will show as fine horizontal lines in the costophrenic angles (Kerley's Lines).

Left heart catheterisation is useful in that it allows the left atrial pressure and the gradient across the mitral valve to be measured. Right heart catheterisation is rarely necessary but gives information as to the pulmonary artery pressure and the pulmonary wedge pressure (indirect left atrial pressure).

Treatment. Minor degrees of mitral stenosis, producing no symptoms and without evidence of cardiac enlargement, are no contraindication to leading a normal life, although extreme effort must be avoided.

Cardiac failure, with or without atrial fibrillation, should be treated as outlined previously (p. 111).

The risk of subacute bacterial endocarditis can be greatly diminished by giving benzyl penicillin 1·0 mega unit just before dental treatment or tonsillectomy followed by phenoxymethyl penicillin 250 mg. q.i.d. for five days. In patients sensitive to penicillin, erythramycin is an adequate substitute.

The indication for operation is the onset of significant symptoms in particular dyspnoea, attacks of pulmonary oedema, or evidence of pulmonary hypertension. Mitral valvotomy also decreases the risk of systemic emboli. It is a mistake to wait until cardiac failure has developed.

If the symptoms, signs and investigations suggest the patient has pure mitral stenosis with a mobile valve, the closed operation is satisfactory, with a mortality rate of less than 5% and about 80% of patients obtain a satisfactory result. With calcified valves or with a significant degree of mitral incompetence open operation will be necessary, the mortality is higher and the results less satisfactory.

Restenosis can occur, probably in about 10% of patients and its frequency depends on the state of the valve and the success of the previous valvotomy.

MITRAL REGURGITATION

Mitral incompetence may be due to dilatation of the mitral ring which is caused by general dilatation of the left ventricle and found in such conditions as aortic valvular disease or hypertension.

This group accounts for the loud apical murmur which may be heard with gross dilatation of the left ventricle and which will sometimes disappear when the associated heart failure is successfully treated.

It may also be due to rheumatic affection of the mitral valve.

RHEUMATIC MITRAL REGURGITATION

Rheumatic mitral regurgitation is slightly more common in men. The essential lesion is contraction and fibrosis of the chordae tendinae and thickening of the valve cusps so that the normal valve mechanism is unable to function. When the left ventricle contracts blood regurgitates into the left atrium so that the left ventricular stroke volume increases and the left ventricle dilates and hypertrophies. Left atrial pressure rises rapidly in ventricular systole but is not sustained and so pulmonary pressure is rarely as high as in mitral stenosis.

Clinical Features. Symptoms usually develop some years after the attack of rheumatic fever and generally a little later in life than in mitral stenosis. The presenting symptom is dyspnoea due to pulmonary congestion in which left ventricular failure will sooner or later play a part. The enlarged left ventricle may bulge into the right ventricle (Bernheim effect) producing some right ventricular obstruction and this may be partially responsible for producing the congestive failure which ultimately develops. The course is then usually rapidly downhill.

Sinus rhythm is more common than in mitral stenosis. The apex beat is hyperdynamic and suggests left ventricular enlargement. A third heart sound is often present. The first sound at the apex is not accentuated, the typical harsh pansystolic murmur is heard best at the apex and spreads towards the axilla, it is loud and may be associated with a thrill.

A short mitral diastolic murmur is quite common in mitral regurgitation. It is due to a rapid flow of blood through the rigid mitral orifice and is brief because pressure equalisation between left atrium and ventricle occurs rapidly.

Radiography shows left ventricular enlargement and often considerable dilatation of the left atrium perhaps with expansile pulsation in ventricular systole.

Treatment. The treatment is that of heart failure when it supervenes; bacterial endocarditis should be avoided as for mitral stenosis.

Surgical treatment consisting of valve replacement or refashioning has so far not proved very successful.

MIXED MITRAL STENOSIS AND REGURGITATION

In many patients with rheumatic mitral disease there is a mixture of stenosis and regurgitation and the physical signs show features suggestive of both these lesions.

INNOCENT APICAL SYSTOLIC MURMURS

It must be clearly understood that the majority of apical systolic murmurs are not due to mitral valvular disease. A small proportion are transmitted from other areas: for example, they may be aortic systolic murmurs which can quite commonly be heard at the apex. The majority are benign murmurs due to a variety of physiological causes. These benign murmurs are not associated with other evidence of cardiac disease, such as cardiac enlargement or thrills, they may disappear at various phases of respiration, they alter considerably in intensity with changes in posture and they are usually neither harsh nor loud. If a murmur shows these characteristics it can usually be disregarded.

TRICUSPID VALVE DISEASE

Tricuspid Regurgitation

Tricuspid regurgitation may be due to dilatation of the tricuspid ring in association with right ventricular failure. It is common in the late stages of mitral stenosis and may occur in pulmonary heart disease and with various congenital lesions. Organic tricuspid regurgitation is always rheumatic.

Clinical Features. The patient will nearly always have the symptoms and signs of congestive heart failure. In addition, the effects of the direct transmission of right ventricular systole to the veins is apparent. Gross pulsation of the cervical veins is seen, both superficial and deep, so that if the neck is viewed from the front in silhouette it widens perceptibly with each beat. The lobes of the ears are moved by this forceful deep pulsation. Expansile pulsation of the liver may be felt, and even superficial veins in the back of the hands can be seen to pulsate (sign of Levine). If tricuspid regurgitation is not rapidly relieved then *cardiac cirrhosis* of the liver results, and prolonged renal congestion may cause heavy *proteinuria*. The combination results in markedly reduced serum albumen levels, with generalised oedema. There is a systolic murmur lasting throughout systole and best heard over the lower end of the sternum. It becomes louder during inspiration.

Treatment is along the general lines for congestive cardiac failure.

Tricuspid Stenosis

Tricuspid stenosis is nearly always rheumatic and is associated with rheumatic lesions of other valves.

Clinical Features. It is characteristic that these patients do not complain of much dyspnoea or orthopnoea, because the stenosed tricuspid valve guards the lungs against congestion. The main symptoms as the disease advances are weakness due to the low cardiac output together with peripheral venous congestion with liver enlargement and oedema.

There is a raised pressure in the neck veins and if the heart is in sinus rhythm a large presystolic wave ('a' wave) is present due to the right atrium contracting against the narrowed tricuspid valve and resulting in a sharp rise in pressure in the atrium and great veins. On auscultation a diastolic murmur similar to that of mitral stenosis can be heard over the lower end of the sternum. It is sometimes more marked on inspiration.

Treatment is along the usual lines for congestive cardiac failure.

AORTIC VALVE DISEASE

AORTIC STENOSIS

The commonest cause of aortic stenosis is probably *rheumatic* inflammation. It can also occur in the elderly as a result of extensive *atheroma* of the aortic valves or it may be *congenital* in origin. The exact frequency with which these three causes operate is still debatable because the end result, whatever the initial lesion, is a scarred, deformed valve, with deposits of atheroma, so that identification of the original aetiology is very difficult.

If, however, aortic stenosis is combined with mitral stenosis it can be presumed to be rheumatic and if it is diagnosed in infancy it is obviously congenital in origin.

When the aortic valve orifice is reduced to about one quarter its normal size the flow of blood is so restricted that the left ventricular pressure begins to rise above the aortic pressure. This is followed by hypertrophy of the left ventricle and finally heart failure.

Clinical Features. Aortic stenosis may produce no symptoms, but in the majority of cases sooner or later the strain on the left ventricle produces first hypertrophy and then dilatation and failure. This may present as *dyspnoea on effort*, often with attacks of acute left ventricular failure causing pulmonary congestion with *paroxysmal nocturnal dyspnoea*. Once heart failure develops the downhill course is progressive and death usually occurs within five years.

The narrowed aortic valve reduces the cardiac output, which cannot be increased to meet the demands of the body on exercise. This may lead to *fainting on effort* and *angina of effort.*

The *pulse* in aortic stenosis is typically small, with a slow rise and a low pulse pressure; it may, however, be normal. In a fully developed case the heart shows evidence of *left ventricular hypertrophy.* There is a *systolic thrill in the aortic area.* A *harsh systolic murmur* which is maximal in mid-systole (an ejection murmur) can be heard extending from the aortic area up into the neck and often also down to the apex.

In addition there is sometimes a short blowing early diastolic murmur best heard down the left border of the sternum; it is due to minimal aortic regurgitation and is caused by the damaged valves failing to close completely. The second sound at the base is absent or greatly reduced.

Not all patients with aortic stenosis show all the signs enumerated above. Sometimes the diagnosis may be suspected on the grounds of a harsh systolic murmur transmitted to the neck, without obvious abnormalities of the pulse or the presence or a thrill, but it must be remembered that innocent systolic murmurs at the base of the heart are very common and a diagnosis of aortic stenosis should only be made if the murmur is loud and quite characteristic and does not disappear with changes of posture or during different phases of respiration.

An *E.C.G.* shows left ventricular hypertrophy usually with a vertical heart. *Radiography* of the heart confirms the left ventricular hypertrophy and careful screening may show *calcification of the aortic valves.*

Left heart catheterisation shows a considerable gradient across the valve often in excess of 50 mm. Hg.

Treatment. Asymptomatic cases of aortic stenosis require no treatment except for the avoidance of undue physical effort; they may otherwise lead a completely normal life. Dental extractions and E.N.T. operations should be covered with penicillin as in mitral stenosis (p. 137). When heart failure develops it should be treated along the usual lines (p. 111).

Several surgical procedures are now available to relieve aortic valve disease. The indication for surgical treatment are:

    (1) Severe angina of effort.
    (2) Developing cardiac failure.
    (3) Syncopal attacks.

In aortic stenosis it may be possible to perform a simple valvotomy, but for severely damaged or calcified valves, or if there is aortic regurgitation, some form of valve replacement is required. This may be either a homograft aortic valve, or some form of prosthesis, of which the Starr-Edwards ball valve is probably the most satisfactory at the present time. In the best hands the operative mortality is down to about 10%, although there may be a further 10% of deaths within the next year. The principal post-operative complications are infection or thrombosis on the prosthesis, or residual valve leak with homografts.

AORTIC REGURGITATION

Aortic regurgitation may result from the following conditions:

(1) *Rheumatic valvular disease*, which commonly gives rise to a combination of regurgitation and stenosis.

(2) *Syphilitic aortitis* affecting the aortic valve ring, which becomes stretched and renders the valve incompetent.

(3) *Subacute bacterial endocarditis.*

(4) *Rupture of an atheromatous aortic valve cusp.*

(5) A small proportion of patients with *severe hypertension,* especially those with coarctation of the aorta have some degree of aortic regurgitation.

(6) *Bicuspid aortic valves* may become incompetent when associated with subacute bacterial endocarditis or with coarctation of the aorta.

If the aortic valve is incompetent blood flows back from the aorta to the left ventricle during diastole. This produces certain signs in the peripheral circulation and also imposes a strain on the left ventricle. The freer the regurgitation the more striking are the peripheral signs and the greater the left ventricular strain.

Clinical Features. The commonest presenting symptoms of aortic regurgitation are those of developing left ventricular failure, namely *dyspnoea on effort* and perhaps attacks of *cardiac asthma*; once heart failure develops the downhill course is usually rapid and death ensues within two or three years. Aortic regurgitation, particularly if due to rheumatic infection, can, however, exist for many years before heart failure develops.

Aortic regurgitation may be complicated by *angina of effort* because the low diastolic pressure found in this condition leads to poor filling of the coronary arteries. When angina occurs in aortic incompetence due to syphilitic aortitis an additional factor may be the involvement of the mouths of the coronary arteries by the gummatous process.

The *pulse in aortic regurgitation* is typically collapsing in nature, due to the rapid flow of blood forwards through the dilated peripheral arterioles and backwards into the left ventricle during diastole. It is best appreciated if the patient's wrist is grasped by the whole hand, when it can be felt as a distinct tap, which has been likened to a water-hammer. For similar reasons pulsation can sometimes be seen in the peripheral capillaries, particularly those of the nail bed, lips, and forehead. Marked pulsation can also be seen in the carotid arteries. There is a large pulse pressure, the systolic pressure being slightly raised and the diastolic very low. These peripheral signs are not present if there is only a slight leak back through the aortic valve.

The heart usually shows evidence of *left ventricular hypertrophy*, particularly if there is free regurgitation. The typical *aortic diastolic murmur* is soft and blowing and is not associated with a thrill. It is best heard with the patient sitting upright and with his breath held in expiration. It may be loudest down the left or right sides of the sternum or even at the apex. It is maximal immediately after the second sound and dies away through diastole.

There may in addition be an aortic systolic murmur, which is not due to aortic stenosis but to the greatly increased blood flow through the aortic value.

If there is gross enlargement of the left ventricle it may be possible to hear a rumbling diastolic murmur at the apex, similar to that found in mitral stenosis. This may be due to blood passing through normal mitral valves into the dilated left ventricle or to eddies produced by the regurgitant stream of blood around the medial cusp of the mitral valve. It is known as *Austin Flint murmur*.

The chief complications of aortic regurgitation are heart failure and bacterial endocarditis.

Treatment. Surgical treatment for aortic disease is considered on page 141. Complications should be treated as they arise. If the incompetence is syphilitic in origin, the syphilis should be treated, but this will not cure the leaking valve. Generally speaking the physical activities of patients with aortic incompetence should be limited. Penicillin must be used to cover dental extractions and E.N.T. operations.

SYPHILITIC AORTITIS

Syphilis attacks the aorta in the tertiary stage of the disease, so that symptoms do not appear until many years after the infection has been acquired. Most patients are men in their fifties or sixties.

The essential lesion is an endarteritis obliterans of the vasa vasorum supplying the aorta, which leads to the replacement of the media of the aorta by fibrous tissue. Stretching of the aortic ring results so that the aortic valve is no longer competent. Sometimes a particularly weak part of the aortic wall balloons out into a saccular aneurysm. Syphilitic aneurysms are found most commonly in the ascending part of the aorta and in the aortic arch. They are rarely found in the descending thoracic aorta and very rarely in the abdominal aorta.

Syphilitic aortitis also causes thickening of the endothelium of the aorta and when this occurs round the mouths of the coronary arteries it reduces the coronary blood flow and causes angina pectoris.

Clinical Features. The substernal pain of *angina pectoris*, coming on when the patient exerts himself, and relieved by rest, is a common symptom of syphilitic aortitis. Other patients remain symptom-free until the strain imposed on the left ventricle by co-existing aortic regurgitation leads to *left ventricular failure* (p. 109).

When an *aneurysm* is present it may compress important structures which lie close to it in the chest and so produce groups of symptoms and signs. An aneurysm of the ascending aorta may erode the anterior chest wall, producing severe local pain and tenderness, and in addition may press on the superior vena cava causing obstruction.

It may be possible to percuss out the aneurysm to the right of the upper part of the sternum; and the aneurysm may finally appear on the surface as a pulsatile swelling which ultimately ruptures. It is common to find a harsh systolic murmur and thrill over the aneurysm. There may also be the typical murmur of aortic regurgitation.

An aneurysm of the arch of the aorta may compress the *trachea* and left bronchus causing a typical brassy cough and sometimes collapse of the lung, the *oesophagus* causing difficulty in swallowing, the *recurrent laryngeal nerve* causing paralysis of the left vocal cord and a hoarse voice, and the *sympathetic chain* causing Horner's syndrome (p. 251). When the aneurysm expands during systole it may push downwards on the trachea and left main bronchus causing a downward *tug on the trachea* and larynx which is best felt by standing behind the patient and palpating the cricoid cartilage. It may involve the origins of the great vessels and cause *inequality of the pulses.*

Aneurysms of the descending aorta rarely produce dramatic signs, but may cause *pain in the back and chest* wall by pressure and erosion of the spine and ribs. The fourth thoracic vertebra is most usually affected.

A radiograph will confirm the presence of aneurysmal dilatation arising from the aorta. Theoretically, on screening it should be easy to see expansile pulsation of the aneurysm, but this is not always so, partially because it may be confused with transmitted pulsation from the heart and partially because the sac of the aneurysm may be lined with blood clot which prevents pulsation. *Calcification* of the ascending aorta is suggestive of syphilitic aortitis. The *blood W.R. and Kahn* reactions are positive in 85 per cent of cases. Occasionally, however, they may revert to negative before the disease becomes apparent, so that a negative W.R. does not rule out syphilitic aortitis. If the syphilitic process is active the E.S.R. is raised.

Treatment. The patient should be at rest in bed during the anti-syphilitic treatment and he should first be given a course of potassium iodide 0·6 g. t.d.s. for three weeks with the object of resolving the gummatous infiltration of the aortic wall and thereby reducing the chances of a Herxheimer reaction (p. 548). In this reaction there is local inflammation with swelling of the gummatous tissue which may occlude the mouth of the coronary arteries.

Penicillin should then be given, 1·0 million units daily for fourteen days. The E.S.R. and W.R. should return to normal over the next month or so, and if they are not normal after three months the treatment should be repeated.

The patient may also require treatment along the usual lines for his cardiac failure or his anginal pain.

DISSECTING ANEURYSM OF THE AORTA

This relatively rare complaint occurs in an aorta already damaged by *atheroma* or by *cystic medial necrosis* of unknown cause. There is, however, an association with scoliosis. The blood forces its way between the layers of the aortic wall and splits it for a variable distance, often occluding various branches of the aorta. The blood in the false passage may re-enter the lumen, leaving the patient with a 'double-barrelled aorta', but more often it ruptures externally into pericardium, mediastinum, or retroperitoneal space and the patient does not long survive.

Clinical features. The patient is seized by a sudden severe pain usually in the chest and often extending to the back. The attack is associated with collapse and may prove rapidly fatal. Examination usually shows a severely ill patient in great pain and a clue to the diagnosis may be provided by finding absent or unequal radial or femoral pulses. If the dissection involves the thoracic aorta it may produce acute aortic incompetence or a left-sided bloody effusion. Occlusion of the spinal arteries may cause focal neurological signs.

The E.C.G. shows no specific change. If the patient survives the acute episode radiological examination shows widening of the aorta.

Treatment. Treatment consists of bed rest with morphine at frequent intervals to relieve the pain. If the patient survives the acute attack the prognosis must be guarded as the process may recur, although there have been some remarkably long survivals.

ANEURYSM OF THE ABDOMINAL AORTA

An aneurysm of the abdominal aorta is nearly always due to atheroma. It may cause abdominal pain which is often quite severe and is due to pressure on the vertebral column and neighbouring organs. The diagnosis can be confirmed by palpation. Some such aneurysms can be treated by resection and replacement by an arterial graft. Death may occur from rupture of the aneurysm.

CARDIOMYOPATHY

Cardiomyopathy occurs in several diseases and affects primarily myocardium, although the endocardium or pericardium are also sometimes involved. It may complicate such generalised diseases as amyloidosis, scleroderma, systemic lupus erythematosus or leukaemia, or may appear as an isolated phenomenon. One well-defined variety is due to *endomyocardial fibrosis*, which is a common cause of cardiac failure in East Africa. Its aetiology is obscure.

There are two main types:—

> (1) *Congestive Cardiomyopathy*. This is essentially a dilatation of the heart with failure of the myocardium. The main clinical

features are left ventricular failure rapidly followed by congestive failure. The heart is enlarged, often with a triple rhythm and sometimes functional mitral and tricuspid incompetence.

(2) *Hypertrophic Cardiomyopathy.* The essential feature is hypertrophy without dilatation. This leads to resistance to filling of the ventricles in diastole and to obstruction to outflow in systole producing a picture similar to aortic stenosis. The clinical course may be prolonged over many years but sooner or later congestive failure develops. Sudden death is not uncommon.

Attempts have been made to relieve outflow obstruction by using β blockers which decrease left ventricular contraction.

Alcoholic Cardiomyopathy. Prolonged and heavy drinking can damage the heart muscle. Early symptoms are dyspnoea on effort and palpitation. There are no specific physical signs but tachycardia and ectopic beats are common and the electrocardiogram may show T wave changes. At this stage the condition is probably reversible. If drinking continues, a state similar to beri-beri may develop with oedema and cardiac enlargement and with signs of a high cardiac output.

THE HEART AND THYROID DISEASE

THYROTOXICOSIS

Thyrotoxicosis frequently affects the heart, particularly in the older age groups. The action of increased thyroid hormone is to raise the cardiac rate and output. In young subjects tachycardia with a full bounding pulse, high pulse pressure, warm extremities and an over-active heart are the chief signs in the cardiovascular system. In older patients these signs may be complicated by various arrhythmias, particularly atrial fibrillation, and by heart failure. The heart failure and atrial fibrillation of thyrotoxicosis are difficult to control adequately with digitalis and the thyrotoxicosis itself should be treated as quickly as possible. After this is relieved the heart usually returns to normal and if atrial fibrillation persists it can nearly always be easily reversed by quinidine.

MYXOEDEMA

Myxoedema may also have effects on the heart. Bradycardia, sometimes extreme, is not uncommon. Patients with myxoedema have a high incidence of coronary artery disease. In addition, myxoedema is occasionally complicated by a pericardial effusion, the cause of which is not clear.

The *electrocardiogram* is characteristic, showing low-voltage QRS complexes in all leads, with flat T waves.

HEART DISEASE AND PREGNANCY

Pregnancy produces a number of changes in the circulation which throw an increased strain on the heart and which may be wrongly interpreted as evidence of heart disease.

These changes begin during the second month of pregnancy, increase until about the thirty-second week and then diminish. The chief changes are:

(1) An increase in cardiac output.
(2) Some retention of sodium and water.

Clinically there is tachycardia, a full pulse and warm, flushed and pulsating extremities. There may be some ankle oedema, although this may also be a sign of toxaemia. The apex beat is rather forcible and may in the later months of pregnancy be displaced a little to the left. The jugular venous pressure is slightly raised. The increased cardiac flow produces pulmonary and aortic systolic murmurs. A physiological third heart sound is not uncommon due to rapid ventricular filling.

Fitness for Pregnancy. The decision as to whether a patient with heart disease is fit for pregnancy is not always easy and when there is any doubt expert advice should be sought.

Generally speaking the following rules will be found useful:

(1) Patients with no symptoms or evidence of cardiac enlargement will usually go through a pregnancy without trouble.
(2) Patients who have had heart failure or who have severe effort intolerance should be advised against pregnancy; if they have already conceived, the pregnancy should be terminated in the first three months.
(3) The middle group present the main difficulty. This includes those with moderate dyspnoea on effort and some cardiac enlargement. Each of these cases will have to be judged on its own merits.

Cardiac Surgery and Pregnancy. If the patient has some lesion which can be corrected surgically this should be done before pregnancy or, if the patient is already pregnant, within the first three months.

General Management during Pregnancy. All patients with heart disease should be carefully observed by both physician and obstetrician.

Patients who have symptoms before pregnancy or those who develop some dyspnoea during pregnancy must have a full night's rest and in addition should rest during the afternoon. The earliest signs of cardiac failure are the development of pulmonary congestion with râles at the bases of the lungs and X-ray evidence of congestion. Filling of the neck veins and the presence of slight ankle oedema are often misleading as these may occur normally in pregnancy.

If failure develops it should be treated in the usual way (p. 111).

Management of Labour. In most patients natural delivery assisted perhaps by forceps in the second stage is quite satisfactory. Caesarian section is rarely required except perhaps in coarctation of the aorta where there is a risk of rupture.

Post-Partum Period. Rest is important in the post-partum period and the long-term problem of looking after a child and a home must be considered before embarking on a further pregnancy.

Mitral Stenosis in Pregnancy. The vast majority of patients with heart disease and pregnancy have rheumatic heart disease, usually mitral stenosis.

The main danger in these patients is the rapid development of pulmonary congestion with attacks of pulmonary oedema, which may be fatal. This usually starts early in pregnancy and is an indication for an emergency mitral valvotomy. In addition, atrial fibrillation may start in pregnancy and produce a rapid onset of cardiac failure.

CONGENITAL HEART DISEASE

Congenital heart disease may be classified as follows:

Acyanotic
Without shunt
Coarctation of the aorta
Dextrocardia
Bicuspid aortic valves
Pulmonary stenosis
Congenital aortic stenosis

With shunt (left to right)
Persistent ductus arteriosus
Atrial septal defect
Ventricular septal defect

Cyanotic
With right to left shunt
Fallot's tetralogy
Pulmonary atresia ⎫
Transposition of the ⎬ Very rare
   great vessels ⎭

This list is by no means exhaustive, but covers the commoner congenital lesions.

ACYANOTIC GROUP

COARCTATION OF THE AORTA

In coarctation of the aorta there is a narrowing of the aorta usually just below the origin of the left subclavian artery.

The narrowed aorta is partially bypassed by a collateral circulation between branches of the subclavian and axillary arteries and the intercostal and superior epigastric arteries.

Clinical Features. The condition may remain asymptomatic in early life and adolescence. It may present as hypertension; as heart failure, which usually develops between the ages of thirty and forty years; or as a subarachnoid haemorrhage due to rupture of a congenital berry aneurysm of the circle of Willis, which is a common (15%) associated condition.

Examination shows a raised blood pressure in the arms; the mean blood pressure in the legs is usually normal, but with a low pulse pressure. The *femoral pulses* are either absent or feeble and delayed. There is often conspicuous *arterial pulsation in the neck*. The heart may show evidence of left ventricular enlargement and there is a widespread *systolic murmur* heard over the praecordium and at the back. This murmur is due to blood passing through the coarctation and also through the collaterals. A small number of cases are complicated by bicuspid aortic valves and these may have the characteristic murmur of aortic regurgitation. Careful examination will show pulsation in *collateral vessels*, particularly around the scapula. A radiograph of the chest will often show *notching of the ribs* due to erosion by the large and tortuous intercostal arteries.

Prognosis and treatment. The prognosis is variable, but few patients with coarctation live beyond middle age. The possibility of resection of the coarctation should therefore be remembered when the abnormality is diagnosed, the optimum age for operation being between seven and fifteen years.

DEXTROCARDIA. Dextrocardia is often associated with transposition of the abdominal viscera. It is of no importance clinically except that if its presence is unrecognised it may lead to misdiagnosis.

BICUSPID AORTIC VALVES. These may remain symptomless throughout life, but are especially liable to severe atheromatous change and to subacute bacterial endocarditis. They may be associated with coarctation of the aorta and may become incompetent.

CONGENITAL AORTIC STENOSIS is considered under aortic stenosis (p. 140).

PULMONARY STENOSIS. Simple congenital pulmonary stenosis is usually valvular and rarely infundibular.

Clinical Features. In mild pulmonary stenosis there may be no symptoms and the diagnosis is suggested by finding a systolic ejection murmur and thrill over the pulmonary artery, usually in the second or third left intercostal space.

Severe cases usually develop cardiac failure by early adult life. The venous pulse in the neck shows a large 'a' wave; there is evidence of right ventricular hypertrophy with a systolic ejection murmur and thrill in the pulmonary area. The second sound in the pulmonary area is usually single, because the pulmonary component is delayed and often inaudible.

If the foramen ovale is patent and the pressure rises in the right atrium during the course of severe pulmonary stenosis, there will be a shunt from the right to the left atrium with the subsequent development of central cyanosis.

An *E.C.G.* shows evidence of right ventricular hypertrophy, and an X-ray shows diminished vascularity of the lung fields with post-stenotic dilatation of the pulmonary artery.

Prognosis and Treatment. Severe cases of pulmonary stenosis rarely reach middle age and all cases run the risk of bacterial endocarditis. All but the mildest cases should be offered relief of the stenosis by valvotomy.

PERSISTENT DUCTUS ARTERIOSUS. The ductus joining the left pulmonary artery and aorta usually closes at birth or soon afterwards. If it persists, there is a shunt from the aorta to the pulmonary artery, with a consequent increase in pulmonary artery flow and in the output of the left ventricle.

Clinical Features. The condition is often symptomless when it is discovered. Subacute bacterial endocarditis develops in about one third of the patients who reach middle age. Cardiac failure is another complication which is found in the third and fourth decades, although in a proportion of patients with a large ductus it may occur even in infancy.

Examination may show a *collapsing pulse* with a low diastolic blood pressure. The apex beat is forcible and suggests some left ventricular hypertrophy. The *'machinery' murmur* which is characteristic of persistent ductus is best heard in the second left intercostal space. It is more or less continuous, starting in early systole, becoming louder in late systole and dying away towards the end of diastole. It may be associated with a thrill.

In addition over a third of subjects with a persistent ductus have a *mitral diastolic murmur* which is presumed to be due to increased blood flow through the mitral valve.

A proportion of patients with a persistent ductus arteriosus develop pulmonary hypertension, with reversal of the blood flow through the duct and the development of peripheral cyanosis.

An *E.C.G.* may show some left ventricular hypertrophy and radiography some enlargement of the pulmonary vessels with a well-marked aortic knuckle.

Prognosis and Treatment. Persistent ductus arteriosus is amenable to surgical closure and this should be advised for all patients except those with pulmonary hypertension.

ATRIAL SEPTAL DEFECT

Atrial septal defect is commonly due to a failure of development of the septum secundum. More rarely the septum primum fails to fuse and this defect is usually accompanied by a deficiency in the mitral valve causing mitral regurgitation. Half or more of the blood which enters the left atrium passes through the defect into the right atrium and thus back through the pulmonary circulation. Usually the increased flow can be accommodated by the pulmonary circulation without a rise in pulmonary artery pressure.

Rarely changes occur in the pulmonary vessels with a rise in pressure and a reversal of the atrial shunt.

Clinical Features. Atrial septal defect does not as a rule produce much in the way of symptoms until middle age when it usually presents as cardiac failure. *Examination* will show some right ventricular enlargement. The apex beat is not obvious and is sometimes described as 'tapping' in quality. The increased pulmonary blood flow may be detected as marked pulsation in the enlarged pulmonary artery, palpable in the second and third left intercostal space. The majority of patients have a *systolic murmur* in the pulmonary area due to increased blood flow from the right ventricle into the dilated pulmonary artery. The *second sound* in the pulmonary area is *widely split*. This split is not altered by respiration and is due to delay of the pulmonary element and is an almost constant feature of the disorder. Sometimes a diastolic murmur is present at the lower end of the sternum and is due to a very high flow rate through the tricuspid valve in diastole, and occasionally a pulmonary regurgitant murmur can be heard if pulmonary hypertension is present.

On a *radiograph of the chest* there is marked dilatation of the pulmonary arteries, which can be seen to pulsate on screening (hilar dance). The right ventricle is enlarged and the aortic knuckle is small.

The *E.C.G.* shows some evidence of right ventricular enlargement with characteristically an RSR pattern (right bundle branch block) in Lead V1.

If pulmonary hypertension develops there may be reversal of the shunt through the defect leading to venous blood entering the left side of the heart and producing cyanosis.

Prognosis and Treatment. Most patients with atrial septal defect eventually develop cardiac failure, which should be treated along the usual lines. Surgical repair of the defect should be undertaken if possible.

VENTRICULAR SEPTAL DEFECT

The volume of the shunt between the left and right ventricles depends on the size of the defect and the pulmonary artery pressure and may vary considerably. It may be an isolated defect or may be complicated by other defects (see Fallot's tetralogy).

Clinical Features. *Small Defect* (*Maladie de Roger*). A small defect gives rise to no symptoms unless bacterial endocarditis supervenes. It is suggested by finding a *systolic murmur and thrill* in the third or fourth left intercostal space.

The prognosis is good and the patient should live his normal span.

Large Defect. If the left to right shunt is large so that the pulmonary blood flow may be three or four times the systemic flow there is overloading of the pulmonary circulation and the output of the left ventricle is increased. Heart failure may present in middle age, or more commonly pulmonary hypertension may develop with reversal of the shunt and consequent central cyanosis. The heart is enlarged, with a forcible left ventricular type of apex beat. Marked pulsation over the pulmonary artery in the second and third interspaces will be palpable. A systolic murmur and thrill in the third and fourth interspaces will be found.

An *E.C.G.* may show evidence of some left ventricular hypertrophy and if pulmonary hypertension is present some right ventricular hypertrophy as well.

A *radiograph of the chest* may show dilated pulmonary arteries, which will be seen to pulsate on screening.

Prognosis and Treatment. Few patients with a large ventricular septal defect reach middle age. Surgical treatment is now advisable in patients with large defects provided severe pulmonary hypertension has not developed.

CYANOTIC GROUP

FALLOT'S TETRALOGY

Fallot's tetralogy is the commonest cause of cyanotic congenital heart disease. The tetralogy consists of pulmonary stenosis (valvular or sub-valvular), ventricular septal defect, over-riding of the aorta so that it lies over both ventricles, and right ventricular hypertrophy. As a result of the obstruction of outflow from the right ventricle due to the pulmonary stenosis venous blood passes into the aorta. The size of the shunt will depend on the severity of the pulmonary stenosis and the pressure in the aorta.

Clinical Features. *Central cyanosis*, with polycythaemia and clubbing of the fingers, is usually present from birth or soon after. In severe cases the patient is under-sized. *Dyspnoea* is a prominent symptom. The patient often adopts a characteristic *squatting position* which decreases the right to left shunt by increasing the peripheral resistance and thus the pressure in the aorta.

The heart usually shows minimal right ventricular enlargement and the apex is tapping in quality. There is a *systolic murmur*, often accompanied by a thrill, in the second or third left intercostal space. The pulmonary second sound is single.

An *E.C.G.* shows marked right ventricular hypertrophy.

On *radiography of the heart* the cardiac apex is often elevated with a deep pulmonary bay, giving rise to the classical 'cœur en sabot'. The *lung vascular markings are much reduced.*

Prognosis and Treatment. Patients with Fallot's tetralogy rarely reach adult life. Operative treatment is now available, either the Blalock operation which aims at increasing the pulmonary blood flow by an anastomosis between a systemic artery and the pulmonary artery, or preferably by the Brock operation which directly relieves the pulmonary stenosis. More recently total correction of the deformity has been undertaken with relief of the stenosis and repair of the septal defect. This will probably become the treatment of choice ultimately.

There are a number of other causes of cyanotic congenital heart disease but they are rare and will not be discussed.

CONGENITAL HEART DISEASE AND SUBACUTE BACTERIAL ENDOCARDITIS

Practically all forms of congenital heart disease are prone to develop bacterial endocarditis, but it is very rare in atrial septal defect. When, therefore, there is any risk of a transient septicaemia such as may occur with dental manipulation, extraction, or tonsillectomy, these patients should be given benzyl penicillin 1·0 mega unit just before operation followed by phenoxymethylpenicillin 250 mg. four times daily for five days.

ISCHAEMIC HEART DISEASE

The following conditions may cause cardiac ischaemic pain:

(1) Coronary artery disease.
(2) Aortic valve disease.
(3) Syphilitic aortitis.
(4) Severe anaemia.
(5) Paroxysmal tachycardia (occasionally).

CORONARY ARTERY DISEASE

One of the most striking changes in the twentieth century in the pattern of disease which affects the Western world has been the emergence of coronary artery disease as one of the most common causes of death, particularly amongst middle-aged men. The reason for this increase is not clear, but several factors may be involved, including a high intake of animal fat, lack of exercise, and excessive smoking.

Coronary artery disease starts with narrowing of the arteries by plaques of atheroma. Obstruction of the blood flow eventually becomes so severe that when exercise increases the oxygen consumption of heart muscle, not enough blood can pass through to supply it. The muscle, therefore, becomes ischaemic and produces the characteristic pain of angina of effort.

The next stage of the disease is the development of a thrombus on the plaque of atheroma, which cuts off the blood supply to an area of heart muscle and produces a cardiac infarct. This may be fatal, but often healing occurs with fibrosis and scar formation. If collateral circulation is good, however, the muscle will survive. It can be seen therefore that thrombosis is not necessarily followed by infarction, although the terms coronary thrombosis and myocardial infarction are often used synonymously.

It must be realised that some atheroma of the coronary arteries is universal over the age of forty and that the coronary circulation has great powers of opening collateral channels and thus circumventing narrowed arteries. Whether or not symptoms develop depends on the rate of progress of the atheromatous process and the ability of the coronary circulation to open up adequate collateral circulation.

The Background to Coronary Disease. It seems probable that clinical coronary disease is the result of a number of factors and processes. Many of these factors are now known, although the whole picture is not complete. A knowledge of these factors may be important in that some of them can be avoided, and therefore it may be possible to diminish the risk of developing coronary disease.

The most important factors so far discovered are:

(1) *Hyperlipidaemia.* Increase in blood lipids, both cholesterol and triglycerides, is associated with an increased incidence of coronary disease. The mechanism is probably a complicated one including both effects on the arterial walls and on coagulation. Hyperlipidaemia is essentially a disorder of lipoprotein metabolism but is considerably influenced by several factors in the diet. It is considered in detail on page 424. Communities living on a diet which includes a high intake of animal fat usually have a higher level of blood lipids than those whose fat intake is low. However in a community such as the United Kingdom with a high fat intake, and with a high incidence of coronary disease, the actual variations of fat intake do not seem so important. More recently a high intake of sucrose has also been implicated, the excess carbohydrate being converted to triglyceride by the liver. Finally, a relative deficiency of unsaturated fatty acids (found in vegetable and fish oils) may also be a factor. How far these findings are applicable to the management of coronary disease is not clear. Lowering the serum cholesterol levels by dietary means or by such drugs as *clofibrate* in those who have had a coronary thrombosis may improve the prognosis of these patients. It is possible, moreover, that prophylactic modification of the diet in those at special risk due to hyperlipidaemia may be even more successful.

(2) *Hypertension.* A raised blood pressure carries with it an increased risk of coronary disease. The problems of treating hypertension are considered on page 127.

(3) *Cigarette Smoking.* There is a correlation between smoking and coronary disease, particularly in the younger age groups. The risk decreases if smoking is stopped.

(4) *Exercise and Obesity.* There is an increased incidence of coronary disease in the under-exercised and overweight.

Epidemiological studies suggest therefore that moderation in diet, avoiding excessive amounts of animal fat and sugar, regular exercise, weight control, and no cigarette smoking, plus lowering of a raised blood pressure if possible, should reduce the incidence of coronary disease, although proof of this is still incomplete. It would seem reasonable that they should also be applied to those who have had a coronary thrombosis.

ANGINA OF EFFORT (Angina Pectoris)

Clinical Features. The patient with angina of effort usually has few complaints apart from his pain. This is described as constricting, or as a heavy feeling, a pressing feeling, an ache or tightness. It is usually substernal and may radiate down the inside of the left arm or both arms or up into the neck or jaw. It may be felt only in the back. *It is brought on by effort and relieved within a few minutes by rest.* It is more easily provoked in cold weather, after a heavy meal, or with emotional upsets.

The onset of the attacks of pain may be gradual or it may appear quite suddenly one day. A sudden onset of severe angina of effort should always

E.C.G. IN ANGINA OF EFFORT.
A: Normal at rest; B: Ischaemic changes on exercise.

raise the suspicion that the complaint has gone beyond a narrowing of the coronary arteries and that an actual coronary thrombosis with infarction has occurred. The course of the disease is variable. The symptoms may become progressively more severe, they may remain stationary or rarely they may improve. At any time a coronary thrombosis may supervene and this may be fatal.

Examination of the patient with angina of effort rarely shows any sign diagnostic of the disease. There may be evidence of associated hypertension but this does not help in the diagnosis, which depends entirely on an accurate history.

The *electrocardiogram* may be very useful in confirming the diagnosis. The following may be found:

    (1) There may be evidence of actual infarction (see p. 155).
    (2) There may be evidence of cardiac ischaemia with depression of the S-T segment over the left ventricular leads.
    (3) The E.C.G. may be normal at rest, but after effort show ischaemic changes.
    (4) The E.C.G. may be normal even after effort.

The last finding is unusual in practice and the diagnosis should be carefully reconsidered before any final conclusion is reached.

Prognosis and Treatment. Depression and anxiety often follow a patient's discovery that he has angina, which is understandable since the probability of sudden death at a relatively early age is common knowledge. Considerable reassurance is therefore required as many of these patients live full and useful lives for ten, fifteen or more years.

The patient's mode of life must be organised to fit both his disease and his temperament. Strenuous exercise must be prohibited, but moderate exercise is not harmful provided it does not produce pain and it may perhaps be beneficial. The patient should if possible continue in his occupation, but overwork or work which keeps him under continued pressure must be avoided. If he is overweight then weight must be reduced. Smoking undoubtedly reduces coronary blood flow and all patients with angina should be advised to abstain from it. Some patients improve remarkably on giving it up.

Nitrites are the most useful drugs for relieving the attacks of pain. *Glyceryl trinitrate* in doses of 0·5 mg. should be sucked or chewed and will relieve angina within two to three minutes. The drug should be used whenever the pain occurs but is more effective if used to prevent attacks of pain when some effort is required.

Long-acting coronary vasodilators can be used particularly in patients who have frequent attacks of angina; pentaerythritol tetranitrate 30 mg. is given three or four times daily.

Propranolol may be useful in angina by decreasing the sympathetic drive to the heart. The initial dose of 10 mg. t.d.s. is increased up to a dose of 200 mg. four times daily or until relief is obtained. It should not be given to patients in heart failure or those with a history of bronchial asthma.

There have been many attempts to improve coronary circulation by *surgical measures*. Until recently these have proved disappointing but the introduction of coronary angiography has given fresh stimulus to various forms of graft operation which appear promising.

MYOCARDIAL INFARCTION

In subjects with coronary atheroma, there is always the danger that a clot may form on the atheromatous plaque, thus suddenly cutting off the blood supply to an area of heart muscle; in other words, a coronary thrombosis may occur leading to myocardial infarction.

When a large coronary artery is obstructed by thrombosis the patient may suddenly fall down dead; indeed this is the only cause of really sudden death. More often, however, the patient survives, and over the next few weeks the dead heart muscle is absorbed and replaced by a fibrous scar. This scar may be firm and strong, but occasionally, particularly if the infarct has been a large one, the scar may become stretched and produce an aneurysm of the heart wall. The functional ability of the heart may be near normal after an infarct, but sometimes after a large infarct, the loss of infarcted muscle so encroaches on the reserve power of the heart that congestive failure occurs, or the patient may be left with crippling angina of effort.

Clinical Features. A coronary thrombosis may occur at any time of the day or night, at rest or on exercise. The onset is usually sudden with severe substernal pain, of the same type and distribution as angina pectoris. It can be distinguished from angina by the fact that it often comes on when the patient is at rest, and, unlike angina, which is relieved by a few minutes' rest, it persists for several hours. Some patients will have noted that for a few days before the acute attack they have had mild and short-lived attacks of substernal pain, the so-called 'warning pains', while in other patients the only complaint may be the rather sudden onset of severe angina.

Rarely, other symptoms may overshadow the chest pain, for example sudden onset of left ventricular failure, abrupt loss of consciousness due to transient cardiac arrest or arrhythmia, or severe vomiting. These may all be presenting symptoms and only careful questioning will elicit a history of substernal pain. Generally speaking, however, the history is typical and the diagnosis obvious.

Examination in typical cases shows the patient to be anxious, pale, sweating, and with a rapid pulse and low blood pressure. In milder cases these signs may be missing and it is worth remembering that the blood pressure may not fall markedly for some hours after the acute attack. Cardiac arrhythmias of any type may occur with a coronary thrombosis, one of the most common being ventricular extrasystoles; these may herald the onset of a dangerous ventricular tachycardia or even ventricular fibrillation. Auscultation of the heart shows a triple rhythm in about half the cases. If the heart is examined daily after the acute attack it is often possible to hear a pericardial friction rub on about the third or fourth day. Pericarditis should also be remembered as a cause of persistent chest pain after a cardiac infarct.

During the first week there is often a rise in temperature, a polymorphonuclear leucocytosis, and a rise in the sedimentation rate, all indications of the inflammatory reaction around the damaged myocardium.

The serum levels of glutamic oxaloacetic transaminase (aspartate transaminase S.G.O.T.) and glutamic pyruvic transaminase (alanine transaminase S.G.P.T.) are raised in most patients after an infarct. The enzymes are released by breaking-down heart muscle and the serum levels are elevated from the first to the fourth day after infarction. The serum levels of lactic dehydrogenase are similarly elevated but for a longer period. Upper limits of normal are S.G.O.T. 35 Karmen units, S.G.P.T. 25 Karmen units. The serum levels of these enzymes are also raised in damage to the liver, pancreas, kidneys and skeletal muscle.

The E.G.G. should be used to confirm the diagnosis and define the position and extent of the infarct. The following changes may be found:

(1) *The Classical Picture of a Cardiac Infarct*—

    (a) *Anterior infarction* produces a large Q wave and raised S-T segment in Lead I and in the anterior chest leads with S-T depression in Lead III. This changes during the next few

ANTERIOR MYOCARDIAL INFARCTION.
A: Immediate; B: After some weeks.

weeks to a Q wave with marked T-wave inversion in Lead I
and the anterior chest leads and the return of the S-T shift
to the iso-electric level.

(b) *Posterior infarction* with a large Q wave and raised S-T segment in Leads II and III and aVF with S-T depression in

POSTERIOR MYOCARDIAL INFARCTION.
A: Immediate; B: After some weeks.

Lead I. This also changes in the next few weeks to Q wave with marked T-wave inversion, in Leads II and III and aVF and return of the S-T shift to the iso-electric level.

(2) *Lesser Changes*

Symmetrical inversion of T waves without large Q waves or S-T segment shift.

A number of other minor changes in the electrocardiogram have been described which alone do not necessarily indicate myocardial infarction, but taken in conjunction with such a history as outlined above, are good enough evidence of an infarct.

It must be remembered that a full 12-lead electrocardiogram must be taken and must be repeated at frequent intervals as the changes after a small infarct may be confined to one lead and may be quite transitory.

Complications of Cardiac Infarction

(1) *Cardiac Failure.* This is most commonly found after a large infarct. It may resolve as the infarct heals, but some patients may be left in chronic failure.

(2) *Cardiac Arrythmias.* Some 80% of patients develop some type of arrythmia after cardiac infarction. These may be transient and last no more than a few seconds, or may be prolonged and may seriously decrease cardiac output. The arrythmia may be of any type. They tend to disappear as the infarct heals, although atrial fibrillation and varying degrees of heart block may persist indefinitely.

(3) *Thrombo-embolic phenomena.* Patients lying immobile after a coronary thrombosis are very liable to deep vein thrombosis in the calf veins with the attendant risk of pulmonary embolism. A thrombus may form on the endocardium over the infarcted area. A piece of clot may break off and obstruct arteries in the systemic circulation, particularly those of the brain.

(4) *Hypotension.* Hypotension may complicate cardiac infarction; it may be due to a fall in cardiac output when it is associated with peripheral vasoconstriction, cold extremities and mental clouding. If this state is prolonged oliguria will develop. Sometimes, however, the cardiac output may in fact be higher than normal, but the peripheral resistance is lowered by vasodilation. These patients usually have extremities of normal colour and temperature.

It is not uncommon for patients to develop vasovagal attacks with bradycardia, sweating, hypotension and nausea, and in some but not all such patients these symptoms appear to be precipitated by the administration of morphia. Finally, any prolonged arrythmia may aggravate or cause a hypotensive state.

(5) *Rupture of the Heart.* Sudden exertion in the week immediately after

an infarct may cause a fatal rupture of the heart. This risk can be diminished by strict bed rest.

Treatment. Until the cardiac infarct has healed firmly it is important to avoid any sudden rise in pressure within the ventricles which may cause rupture of the heart. In addition cardiac failure may develop. The patient must, therefore, be kept at *complete rest* in bed for about four weeks; in the elderly this may be reduced to two or three weeks.

Severe pain is often a prominent feature immediately after the infarct and *morphine* 15–20 mg., according to the size of the patient, will be required to relieve the pain and mental anguish and may have to be repeated several times in the first twenty-four hours. Morphine may produce vomiting and hypotension, though this can sometimes be helped by combining it with cyclizine. *Pentazocine* 30 mg. by injection is also used but can cause a rise in pulmonary artery pressure and thus further embarass the circulation.

All unnecessary effort must be avoided, particularly in the first few days. If the patient is worried by constipation a small enema may be given after 48 hours and repeated every two or three days. If the patient is not too severely ill, a commode may be less exhausting than a bed-pan. To prevent thrombosis in the deep veins of the lower limbs, passive exercises should be given from the start, followed in the third week by active exercise. The diet should be light and easily digestible.

The value of *anticoagulants* after cardiac infarction has never been wholly accepted, and they are now used much less than they were. The theoretical reason for using these drugs is to prevent the development of thrombi in the deep veins of the legs and on the endocardium. It is possible that with less severe restriction of movement in the immediate post-infarction period and with regular leg exercises the danger of deep vein thrombosis has been reduced. It seems probable that in the future they will no longer be given after cardiac infarction and their use is considered under pulmonary embolism on page 167.

Many patients are anxious and worried in the weeks following a cardiac infarct and sedation with chlordiazapoxide 10 mg. three times daily may be useful. If cardiac failure, with or without atrial fibrillation, develops it should be treated in the usual way with digitalis and diuretics. Digitalis may somewhat increase the risk of ventricular arrhythmia developing and must, therefore, be used with caution.

Monitoring, the Treatment of Arrhythmias and Hypotension. It is now realised that arrhythmias are a frequent cause of circulatory failure and death after cardiac infarction. If the patient is continuously monitored by ECG in the two or three days after infarction, these arrhythmias can be diagnosed immediately and with appropriate treatment the mortality rate can be halved.

(a) *Prevention of Arrhythmias.* The use of various drug regimes to prevent the development of arrhythmias after infarction has not proved useful and at present it is best to treat arrhythmias as they arise.

(b) *Treatment of Developed Arrhythmias.*

(1) Ventricular ectopics, propranolol 10 mg. q.i.d. or phenytoin 100 mg. t.d.s. by mouth. If multiple, lignocaine I.V. (see below).

(2) Ventricular tachycardia—lignocaine 50–100 mg. I.V., followed, if necessary, by infusion at the rate of 1·0 mg. per minute. If this fails d.c. cardioversion should be used (see p. 120).

(3) Ventricular fibrillation—Electrical defibrillation (see p. 122).

(4) Atrial fibrillation—the patient should be cautiously digitalised.

(5) Heart block—steroids rarely help. Electrical pacemaking may be required.

(6) Sinus bradycardia—atropine 0·6 mg. I.V.

(c) *Hypotension.* This may be due to vagal overactivity perhaps exacerbated by morphine, or to low cardiac output with circulatory failure. Vagal overactivity will respond to atropine (see above). In circulatory failure the foot of the bed should be raised provided this does not precipitate pulmonary oedema. Most of these patients have a low arterial oxygen saturation due to disorganisation of ventilation and perfusion in the lungs and should be given oxygen 2 litres per min. by M.C. mask (approx. 40–60%). The patient should be digitalised to try and raise the cardiac output, and if hypotension persists 200 mg. of hydrocortisone should be given intravenously and repeated as required. Vasoconstrictor drugs are rarely used for they raise the blood pressure at the expense of peripheral organ perfusion. Prolonged hypotension carries a bad prognosis.

Subsequent Management

When the period of rest has finished the patient is gradually allowed up, but should not return to work for at least three months after the acute attack. If possible the patient should return to his normal employment. If, however, his job is exceptionally heavy or if he is severely crippled by cardiac failure or angina of effort, then some change will be necessary. Overweight patients should be dieted until they reach normal levels. Heavy meals, especially those containing large quantities of fat, must be avoided. Otherwise the patient should lead a normal life, but avoid excesses of all kinds.

In patients who are having recurrent infarcts the possibility of long-term anticoagulants should be considered. When the patient has been stabilised on one of the oral anticoagulants it may only be necessary to estimate the prothrombin time once or twice a week.

BACTERIAL ENDOCARDITIS
ACUTE BACTERIAL ENDOCARDITIS

This usually occurs in the course of septicaemia due to organisms of high virulence. The endocardium is affected and the heart valves may be spared.

SUBACUTE BACTERIAL ENDOCARDITIS

Subacute bacterial endocarditis is due to infection of the endocardium by organisms of moderate virulence. The most common infecting organism is the streptococcus viridans which is often an inhabitant of the mouth and throat of normal people. However, in recent years there has been an increase in bacterial endocarditis due to other organisms, particularly the streptococcus faecalis, the micro-aerophilic streptococcus and the staphylococcus.

Subacute bacterial endocarditis starts on the heart valves, usually the aortic valve. It most commonly occurs on valves damaged by previous rheumatic fever. It may complicate various congenital lesions including ventricular septal defect, pulmonary and aortic stenosis, persistent ductus arteriosus and bicuspid aortic valves and may develop on various types of artificial valves. It is very rare in syphilitic aortitis and atrial septal defect. There is a group of patients, usually over fifty, who appear to develop subacute bacterial endocarditis on an apparently normal heart. The infecting organism is frequently the streptococcus faecalis. It is a curious fact, as yet without explanation, that subacute endocarditis very rarely begins in a heart with atrial fibrillation.

The starting point of bacterial endocarditis is often a transient bacteraemia. This may follow dental extraction or filling, when the organism is usually streptococcus viridans; or after operations on the urinary tract or bowel, when infection with streptococcus faecalis is more common. This emphasises the need for penicillin 'cover' if these operations are performed in a patient with damaged heart valves. The bacteria settle on the damaged valve, set up an inflammatory reaction which is followed by deposits of fibrin and the formation of a vegetation which often spreads from the valve to adjacent endocardium.

Clinical Features. The most constant clinical feature is a persistent *low grade fever*, and this diagnosis should be considered in any patient with rheumatic heart disease who develops a pyrexia for which there is no other obvious cause. Increasing *malaise, tiredness*, and *breathlessness* are common symptoms. In some patients sweating and vague joint pains may suggest a recurrence of rheumatic fever. After the first week or two *anaemia* develops and the patient begins to lose weight. The fingers become *clubbed* and in patients left untreated generalised pigmentation occurs; this combined with the anaemia causes a characteristic coloration, sometimes described as the '*café au lait*' appearance.

From time to time small fragments of the vegetation growing on the heart valve break off, are swept into the general circulation and cause emboli in different parts of the body. These multiple emboli are responsible for some of the most characteristic features of the disease. Minute emboli to the skin cause small, tender, red, slightly raised areas most commonly seen on the pads of the fingers and lasting 24–48 hours; they are called *Osler's nodes*. Emboli in the small vessels under the nails produce small 'splinter' *haemorrhages*. The kidney may be affected; sometimes large emboli occur causing infarcts, but more commonly there is a diffuse focal nephritis (probably toxic) producing the pathological picture of the 'flea-bitten' kidney and leading to an increased number of *red cells in the urine*. Rarely is the kidney so severely damaged as to produce renal failure. Emboli may occur elsewhere; in the retina they cause the typical 'boat-shaped haemorrhage'. *Purpuric spots*, often most noticeable over the chest and neck, are common and are probably due to toxic damage to the capillaries. In 30 per cent of cases larger vessels are acutely obstructed, causing major infarcts in the brain, liver, spleen, intestines, or limbs.

The *spleen* is usually moderately enlarged, from the chronic septicaemia which is a feature of the condition. Infarction may lead to an acute attack of pain in the splenic area.

The *heart* shows signs of the underlying valve lesion, and rarely changes in the character of the murmurs can be detected. Heart failure may develop.

When bacterial endocarditis occurs in congenital heart disease with a left to right shunt such as a patent ductus arteriosus, the emboli are swept into the pulmonary circulation and lead to infarcts of the lung. This produces rather a different clinical picture, with recurrent episodes of fever, pleurisy, and patchy consolidation of the lungs, so that an erroneous diagnosis of recurrent pneumonia may be made.

Special Investigations. Examination of the blood reveals a moderate anaemia with a slight leucocytosis. The sedimentation rate is nearly always raised. The urine in the great majority of cases shows an increased number of red cells, although these may be only detected on microscopy.

The *diagnosis* is confirmed by isolation of the organism on *blood culture*. At least three samples of blood must be taken for culture before antibiotic treatment is started and incubation should continue for three weeks. If organisms are isolated, their sensitivity to various antibiotics must be determined. It is best if blood for culture is taken at the height of the fever. If the patient is very ill and the diagnosis is suspected on clinical grounds, the blood cultures should be taken at short intervals so that the onset of treatment is not delayed. There is rarely need to await the report on the blood cultures before giving antibiotics.

Complications. (1) *Rupture of a Valve*. The aortic valve may be weakened and finally rupture during the course of bacterial endocarditis. When this occurs it may lead to sudden death or to the rapid development of cardiac failure. Examination shows the characteristic, loud, regurgitant murmur (*cooing dove*).

(2) *Mycotic Aneurysm*. Mycotic aneurysms may develop due to small emboli in the vessels supplying the walls of the large arteries. They may require surgical treatment.

Treatment. The patient must be in bed and be given full nursing care. The specific treatment will depend on the infecting organism.

(a) *Streptococcus Viridans*. 2·0 mega units of benzylpenicillin intramuscularly four times daily, is usually adequate if the organism is sensitive. It is sometimes possible to use large doses of oral phenoxymethylpenicillin, but careful observation is required. If there is no response, or if the organism proves to be partially resistant to penicillin the dose can be increased to 20 mega units of penicillin or more daily. Owing to the bulk of the injection, it is necessary to give it by continuous intravenous drip. Blood levels can also be increased by giving probenecid 0·5 g. four times daily.

(b) *Streptococcus Faecalis.* 2·0 mega units of benzylpenicillin q.i.d., plus 0·75 g. of streptomycin b.d. The dose of antibiotics should be modified according to response and sensitivity tests.

(c) *Staphylococcus Aureus.* The antibiotic programme will depend on sensitivities. Usually two antibiotics will be required and benzylpenicillin or cloxacillin plus streptomycin or gentamycin are useful combinations.

Treatment should aim at abolishing the fever, stopping all embolic phenomena and restoring the E.S.R. and urine to normal. Blood cultures should of course be negative after treatment. The earlier treatment is started in the course of the disease, the better the chance of effecting a cure. Antibiotic therapy must be given for at least 6 weeks.

With these measures it is possible to eradicate infection in the great majority of patients with subacute bacterial endocarditis. In some, however, the disease has caused considerable damage to the heart valves and in these subjects chronic failure and death may ensue although the infection has been cured. All patients must be carefully followed up as relapse or reinfection may occur.

PERICARDITIS

The following types of pericarditis may be encountered:

(1) Benign.
(2) Rheumatic.
(3) Pyogenic.
(4) Tuberculous.
(5) Malignant.
(6) Subsequent to a cardiac infarct.
(7) Associated with uraemia.
(8) Systemic lupus erythematosus.

Pericarditis may be dry or may be associated with an effusion.

DRY PERICARDITIS

Clinical Features. Dry pericarditis may occur from any of the above causes. Pain is a frequent, but not a constant, symptom. It may be praecordial or referred to the shoulder or neck region. It may be constant or made worse by movement or by respiration. The patient may also complain of symptoms which are related to the disease underlying the pericarditis.

Examination will usually show a pericardial friction rub; this may be either loud or soft; it usually sounds rough and rather superficial. It may be heard anywhere over the praecordium and may be either systolic and/or diastolic in timing.

E.C.G. Changes. In the early stages the electrocardiogram shows elevation of the S-T segment, the elevated segment being concave upwards. This is followed by the return of the S-T segment to the iso-electric line and flattening or inversion of the T waves. These changes, unlike those of cardiac infarction, can be recorded from both the anterior and posterior aspects of the heart at the same time.

PERICARDIAL EFFUSION

The symptoms and signs of a pericardial effusion depend on the underlying cause and on the size of the effusion. Small effusions may be indistinguishable from a dry pericarditis. When the size of the effusion increases rapidly the pressure within the pericardial sac rises, interfering with the venous return to the heart, a state known as *cardiac tamponade*. This in turn reduces the cardiac output and thus seriously interferes with cardiac function.

Clinical Features. The patient often appears restless and ill and complains of praecordial discomfort and dyspnoea. If the effusion is large, examination will reveal *pulsus paradoxus* (p. 96). The venous pressure will be raised, and the apex beat may be felt within the outer limit of cardiac dullness to percussion, which is increased. A pericardial friction rub can often be heard on auscultation, in spite of the presence of an effusion.

A radiograph of the heart shows a pear-shaped cardiac shadow with sharper margins than usual; this is because they have moved less during exposure of the film.

Treatment. Effusions large enough to endanger life are rare. A high venous pressure and low arterial pressure are indications for tapping the effusion. It must be remembered that the high venous pressure found with pericardial effusions is necessary to maintain diastolic filling of the heart and attempts should not be made to lower venous pressure by venesection or by diuretics. Otherwise the treatment is that of the underlying condition.

Benign Pericarditis. Benign pericarditis can probably be caused by several viruses including coxsackie, mumps and influenza. It is most common in young adults and there is often a history of a recent upper respiratory tract infection. The onset is sudden with fever, malaise, and pericardial pain. Small effusions sometimes develop. Recovery is the rule within a few weeks, but a number of cases relapse.

Treatment is symptomatic.

Rheumatic Pericarditis. Pericarditis develops during the course of acute rheumatic fever in about 10 per cent of patients and provides definite evidence of cardiac involvement. It may or may not be associated with an effusion. Treatment is as for rheumatic fever.

Pyogenic Pericarditis. Pericarditis may occur as a complication of pneumonia or may complicate a septicaemia. It should be vigorously treated with antibiotics. Surgical drainage is rarely required.

Tuberculous Pericarditis. Tuberculous pericarditis is not common. It usually presents as a subacute pericarditis with effusion and some general malaise with evening fever. The effusion is a clear yellow fluid, occasionally bloodstained, and may be found on culture to contain tubercle bacilli.

Treatment consists of prolonged rest, with streptomycin, isoniazid, and para-aminosalicylic acid (see p. 227).

If the effusion is large, aspiration may be required and streptomycin 0·5 g. should then be injected into the pericardial sac.

A number of patients subsequently develop constrictive pericarditis (see below).

Cardiac Infarction. A pericardial friction rub can often be heard transiently over the infarcted area within a few days of a coronary thrombosis.

Uraemia. A pericardial rub may be heard in the terminal stages of uraemia (see page 375).

Malignant Pericarditis. Involvement of the pericardium by new growth may give rise to an effusion which may require tapping. This is a common terminal complication of bronchial neoplasms.

CHRONIC CONSTRICTIVE PERICARDITIS

Chronic constrictive pericarditis is due to previous tuberculous pericarditis. The heart is encased in a shell of fibrous tissue which may be calcified, and as a result the heart is unable to expand in diastole and venous filling is greatly impeded.

Clinical Features. The patient is usually in adult life and complains of some dyspnoea on effort associated perhaps with oedema of the ankles and swelling of the abdomen. Orthopnoea is not a feature and the degree of dyspnoea is often slight in comparison with the evidence of gross venous congestion.

Examination sometimes shows a pulsus paradoxus and there often is atrial fibrillation. The venous pressure is high, but falls sharply during diastole (the y descent) when the tricuspid valves open. The heart is not usually much enlarged and auscultation is not helpful. Enlargement of the liver, ascites, and oedema of the ankles are often present. Long-standing disease may have caused chronic hepatic congestion sufficient to end in cirrhosis of the liver.

A radiograph of the heart usually shows a normally sized or slightly enlarged heart and calcification may be seen in the pericardium in about half the cases, provided lateral as well as postero-anterior radiographs are taken.

An *electrocardiogram* usually shows decreased voltage in the QRS complexes with widespread flattening or inversion of T waves.

Treatment. Treatment consists of surgical removal of the constricting pericardium. The operation is a major undertaking, but the results are usually satisfactory.

ADHERENT PERICARDIUM

Occasionally following rheumatic pericarditis the heart may become attached to surrounding structures. This may be diagnosed clinically by systolic retraction of the lower left ribs posteriorly (Broadbent's sign), fixation of the apex beat and systolic retraction of intercostal spaces. There is no evidence that an adherent pericardium has any effect on cardiac function and if heart failure supervenes in these cases it is due to the associated valve disease.

PULMONARY HEART DISEASE

PULMONARY EMBOLISM

A pulmonary embolus arises most commonly from deep vein thrombosis in the leg (p. 173). Rarely it may arise from an intracardiac thrombosis following atrial fibrillation or cardiac infarction. Phlebothrombosis in the legs occurs particularly in obese middle-aged or elderly patients who have been confined to bed, usually with heart disease, but also with other medical conditions, pregnancy, or after major surgical operations. Occasionally it occurs in apparently healthy people, particularly women taking an oral contraceptive.

Clinical Features. A large pulmonary embolism causes dilatation of the right ventricle with a drop in right ventricular output, and a rise in systemic venous pressure. This results in a fall in cardiac output which is accompanied by peripheral vasoconstriction. A massive embolism may cause sudden death but more commonly the patient complains of the sudden onset of substernal tightness, or pain, dyspnoea and a sudden call to stool. He is sweating, pale and slightly cyanosed. The pulse is small and rapid, the blood pressure low, the cervical venous pressure is raised and frequently there is a gallop rhythm.

The ECG is variable. It may show a deep S wave in Lead 1 with a Q or inverted T wave in Lead 111. The chest leads may show T wave inversion in Lead V1-V3, or more rarely there may be a right bundle branch block pattern. The changes are usually transitory.

Smaller pulmonary emboli cause pulmonary infarction, the symptoms of which are often so slight that it is the most commonly overlooked serious respiratory lesion. When the infarct extends to the surface of the lung there may be acute pleuritic pain, and about 40 per cent of patients have a haemoptysis; but frequently the only clinical features are sudden shortness of breath or unexplained rise of temperature and/or pulse rate.

It should also be remembered that repeated small pulmonary emboli may seriously obstruct the pulmonary vascular bed and lead to pulmonary hypertension and right ventricular failure.

Treatment. A patient who has had a pulmonary embolus should be nursed fairly flat in bed because the cardiac output and blood pressure may be low. In severe cases oxygen should be given by mask or by a tent.

If the patient is in pain or distress a small dose of morphine 10 mg. can be given but there is a danger of respiratory depression. If morphine is used or if there is evidence of respiratory depression nikethamide 500 mg. intravenously can be given and repeated as required. Digitalis is not very helpful in the acute stage but if chronic heart failure ensues the patient should be digitalised (p. 112). *Anticoagulants* should be started with heparin 10,000 units six hourly intravenously. Clotting time estimations are only required if treatment with heparin is prolonged, when the dosage is adjusted to increase the clotting time to twice normal. The anticoagulant effect of heparin is almost immediate.

At the same time treatment should be started with an oral anticoagulant. This group of drugs acts by suppressing the formation in the liver of prothrombin and factor VII, which are necessary for the coagulation of blood. Among those commonly used are:—

Drug	Maximum Effect	Duration of Effect	Dose	
			Initial (1st day)	Maintenance (daily)
Phenindione	24–36 hrs	48 hrs	200 mg.	12·5–50 mg.
Warfarin	24–36 hrs	48 hrs	30–60 mg.	5–10 mg.
Dicoumarol	36–48 hrs	72 hrs or more	300 mg.	25–100 mg.

The dosage of these drugs is controlled by estimation of the patient's prothrombin time which is kept between two and three times the normal.

The most important side effect of these drugs is bleeding from overdosage, a common site being the urinary tract. If this occurs the drug must be stopped. The coagulability of the blood can be restored by giving vitamin K_1 (mephyton) intravenously, it is important to use the smallest effective dose or there may be an abrupt fall in prothrombin time with further clotting. The dose usually lies between 10–50 mg.

Anticoagulants should rarely be used in the very elderly and in those in whom there is a risk of haemorrhage, e.g. from a duodenal ulcer.

The following drugs should not be combined with oral anticoagulants.

    (1) Aspirin—risk of gastric bleeding.
    (2) Liquid paraffin—enhances effect by blocking vitamin K absorption.
    (3) Phenylbutazone, Clofibrate—enhance effect by decreasing plasma protein-binding.
    (4) Barbiturates—enhance breakdown of anticoagulant in the liver.

The clot can be lysed by using *streptokinase*. However its control is more difficult, although a short course at the beginning of treatment may become widely used.

Anticoagulants are usually continued for at least six weeks, and many authorities consider they should be continued up to six months or longer, particularly if there is any evidence of recurrent embolism.

Rarely in patients with massive pulmonary embolism and where facilities are available *embolectomy* may be performed within a few hours of the acute episode.

PULMONARY HYPERTENSION

Physiology

In health the pulmonary circulation is a low pressure system (range = 15/5–30/15 mm.Hg). It seems probable that at rest in the upright position the main blood flow is through the lower parts of the lungs. With increased flow as occurs on exercise, vasodilatation occurs and more blood passes through the upper zones. The pulmonary artery pressure rises only with flow rates above 15 litres per minute.

In man there is evidence that active vasoconstriction of the pulmonary arteries can occur, although its mode of production is unknown.

This may be in response to:

(1) Increased pulmonary blood flow
(2) A rise in left atrial pressure.
(3) Hypoxia and perhaps hypercarbia

Clinical Types of Pulmonary Hypertension

(1) Idiopathic (Primary) Pulmonary Hypertension

Idiopathic pulmonary hypertension is due to structural narrowing of the pulmonary arteries of obscure cause; it is probably often due to multiple small pulmonary emboli (see below).

(2) Secondary Pulmonary Hypertension

(a) Pulmonary hypertension may be due to progressive obliteration of the pulmonary arteries by repeated thrombosis or embolism. This often follows a phlebo-thrombosis in the puerperium. Early symptoms are dyspnoea on effort, cough and sometimes haemoptysis. Early diagnosis is important as at this stage the process may be reversible by anticoagulants.

(b) It may be secondary to increased blood flow through the lungs such as occurs in *atrial* or *ventricular septal defects* or with a *persistent ductus arteriosus*. In these conditions the pulmonary artery can usually accommodate the increased flow without a rise in pulmonary artery pressure.

Sometimes, however, active constriction of the pulmonary arteries eventually develops and pulmonary artery pressure may even exceed the systemic pressure, with reversal of the shunt and the development of central cyanosis.

(c) In *mitral valve disease* there is usually a small passive rise in pulmonary artery pressure transmitted back from the left atrium. In a small porportion of cases there is in addition active pulmonary vasoconstriction with a considerable rise in pulmonary artery pressure (p. 134).

(d) Pulmonary hypertension and heart failure may complicate *chronic lung diseases*, commonly chronic bronchitis or emphysema, or rarely pulmonary fibrosis due to silicosis, sarcoidosis or other causes. It is due to obliteration of the pulmonary artery bed by the lung disease; in addition there may be active vasoconstriction due to hypoxia and perhaps hypercapnia. The clinical features and management of *cor pulmonale* are considered on p. 198.

Clinical Features. Dyspnoea is common and other symptoms are cough and syncope. Early signs are evidence of right ventricular hypertrophy, a short systolic murmur and a systolic click over the pulmonary artery and a loud pulmonary element to the second heart sound. Later a giant 'a' wave in the jugular venous pulse, triple rhythm and cardiac failure with functional tricuspid incompetence may develop. The electrocardiogram shows right ventricular hypertrophy and strain.

Treatment. With repeated pulmonary emboli, long-term anticoagulant therapy may reverse the process. In mitral stenosis, relief of the stenosis will frequently release the vasoconstriction.

In those with increased pulmonary flow repair of the shunt with reduction of flow has proved disappointing.

DISEASES OF THE ARTERIES

Diseases of the peripheral vasculature may be subdivided into:

(1) Chronic obliterative arterial disease due to
    (a) Atherosclerosis
    (b) Buerger's disease.
(2) Acute obstruction to the arterial circulation by embolism or thrombosis.
(3) Venous thrombosis, which may affect either the superficial or deep veins.
(4) Raynaud's syndrome.
(5) Acrocyanosis.

CHRONIC OBLITERATIVE ARTERIAL DISEASE

ATHEROSCLEROSIS. This occurs most commonly over the age of fifty and may complicate diabetes or hypertension. The areas of narrowing or occlusion are often first found in the femoral artery below the profunda femoris branch, or may even be in the lower aorta. In more advanced cases the areas of narrowing can be found throughout the arterial tree of the leg. The arms are very rarely affected.

Clinical Features. The earliest symptom is intermittent claudication, a cramp-like pain usually in the calf or more rarely in the thigh, causing the patient to limp. It may be bilateral or unilateral, but is usually worse on one side. It is brought on by walking and quickly relieved by rest. The degree of disability is variable. With obstruction of the lower end of the aorta (Leriche's syndrome) pain may be referred to the thighs and buttocks, there may be muscle wasting, and in men failure of penile erection may occur.

In severe cases pain may occur at rest and may be particularly troublesome at night when it may become almost unbearable.

When the circulation to the limbs is severely impaired, areas of gangrene may appear. They often start following trauma, particularly round the nail bed and over the heel. In the most severe cases, gangrene of a whole foot or even of extensive areas of the leg, may occur.

Examination shows absent or reduced pulses in the limbs and in advanced cases coldness of the limbs with failure of the vasodilatation which normally occurs on warming. If the limb is elevated it blanches unduly rapidly, and cyanosis on dependence may be extreme. Both these signs indicate reduced arterial blood supply.

There is an increased incidence of coronary artery disease in those with symptoms from peripheral atherosclerosis. This is a reminder that the disease is always general, not central or peripheral alone.

Prognosis and Treatment. For the majority of patients with intermittent claudication the condition is relatively benign and symptoms may last for years without progression and without the development of gangrene. In a few patients symptoms may actually improve. For the elderly patient with a mild to moderate disability, treatment should be conservative. Patients should be told to avoid trauma to the feet and the assistance of a chiropodist should be enlisted to help with care of the toe-nails and to deal with callouses, etc. Undue heat or cold should be avoided as far as the feet are concerned, but the body should be kept warm to produce as much reflex vasodilatation as possible. Various vasodilator drugs are used to try and improve the peripheral circulation; tolazoline in doses of 25 mg. t.d.s. is one of the best, but the clinical effect is often disappointing. Alcohol may be of value in moderate doses.

Tobacco reduces peripheral blood flow and should be avoided by all patients with vascular disease.

In the younger patient and those seriously disabled, an attempt should be made to define the extent of the arterial block by arteriography. If there is only a local block and the patient is otherwise fit, arterial grafting may be possible. When a longer segment of artery is obstructed it is sometimes possible to divert the blood through an Orlon bypass.

In a few patients, lumbar sympathectomy may be successful, but it is difficult to predict which patients will be helped by this operation. Finally, if gangrene supervenes amputation may become necessary.

BUERGER'S DISEASE

Buerger's disease is very rare. It occurs almost exclusively in men and usually starts between the age of twenty-five and forty-five. The lesions begin in the small arteries in the feet and lead to progressive obliteration from the periphery of the arteries of the lower limbs. Involvement of arteries in the arms and elsewhere is very rare.

Clinical Features. Intermittent claudication is the main symptom, but in this disease it usually starts in the foot. Later it spreads up the leg and gangrene of the extremities may occur. In addition, a number of cases have recurrent episodes of phlebitis.

Treatment. Treatment consists of care of the extremities, giving vaso-dilator drugs, and avoiding tobacco. Anticoagulants should be used for acute thrombophlebitis. Sympathectomy may produce prolonged relief of symptoms, particularly in the earlier stages of the disease. Amputation may be necessary in advanced cases.

ACUTE ARTERIAL OCCLUSION

Acute arterial occlusion may be caused by an embolus arising from the left side of the heart, usually in a patient with mitral stenosis or subacute bacterial endocarditis. Mural thrombi overlying infarcted areas may similarly become detached. Alternatively, thrombosis on an atheromatous plaque may occur *in situ* as a complication of chronic obliterative arterial disease.

Clinical Features. The onset is sudden with severe pain, pallor, coldness, loss of sensation, and weakness in the affected limb. The arterial pulses disappear below the level of the obstruction.

If embolectomy is impossible or too long delayed the patient must be treated conservatively. Full anticoagulant therapy should be given; the limb should be kept cool to reduce its oxygen requirements to a minimum; the rest of the body must be kept warm; and a careful watch must be maintained for the appearance of gangrene. Amputation may sometimes be required.

RAYNAUD'S SYNDROME

This is produced by spasm of the digital arteries. It may be the result of a variety of causes.

(1) *Raynaud's disease*, believed to represent hypersensitivity of the digital vessels to cold.

(2) *Auto-immune disorders*, especially systemic lupus erythematosis and scleroderma.

(3) *Occupational* in butchers, fishmongers, and people handling vibrating tools.

(4) *Other arterial diseases*, atheroma, Buerger's disease.

(5) *Blood disorders*, polycythaemia vera, haemolytic anaemias.

(6) *Thoracic outlet syndromes*, cervical ribs, prefixed plexus.

(7) *Diseases of the nervous system*, syringomyelia.

(8) *Phaeochromocytoma*.

Clinical Features. Most common in young women. It begins distally and spreads proximally. First the fingertips, then the fingers and even the hands become cold, white, and pulseless, and sensation and fine movement are impaired. Recovery is in the reverse order, and causes painful paraesthesiae in the affected areas, which become patchily discoloured red, white, and blue. It may be followed by reflex vasodilatation, so that the hand is red and warm, and the pulse bounding. Rarely the nose and more frequently the toes may be affected. Early in the disease there is no evidence of permanent changes but after some years gangrene of the tips of the fingers may develop.

Treatment. The patient should avoid exposing the hands to cold and the whole body should be kept as warm as possible to promote reflex vasodilation. Vasodilator drugs are sometimes useful and tolazoline, 25 mg. t.d.s., is the most satisfactory. Sympathectomy is indicated if medical treatment fails.

ACROCYANOSIS

This is a condition of unknown cause found in young people, characterised by painless cyanosis of the hands and feet, sometimes with swelling. The condition is harmless and treatment is unsatisfactory.

VENOUS THROMBOSIS

Deep Vein Thrombosis (Phlebothrombosis)

There are many factors which lead to a deep vein thrombosis, including venous stagnation, dehydration, and the rise in platelets which follows operation. It is particularly liable to occur after operation or during the course of a severe medical illness. Studies using phlebography and measuring the uptake by the thrombus of ^{125}I-labelled fibrinogen suggest that up to 35% of patients have venous thrombosis after major surgery, although nearly all of them show no clinical evidence of disease. It may be symptomatic of a hidden neoplasm (particularly carcinoma of the pancreas or bronchus) or of Buerger's disease. Rarely it occurs for no apparent reason. The danger of a deep vein thrombosis is that a portion of the clot may break off and be swept through the right side of the heart to the lungs to produce a pulmonary infarct (p. 167).

Clinical Features. The symptoms of a deep vein thrombosis are often slight. There may be a slight rise of temperature with a leucocytosis and the patient may complain of pain in the calf. Examination will show perhaps slight swelling of the ankle, tenderness of the calf and dorsiflexion of the ankle will be painful (Homan's sign). Sometimes a pulmonary embolism will be the first indication of a deep vein thrombosis.

Treatment. Deep vein thrombosis should be prevented if possible by encouraging the patient to move his legs at frequent intervals and by avoiding dehydration.

If it does occur the patient and the affected limbs should be rested. Active movements are best avoided in the early stages in case a clot is dislodged, but gentle passive movements are allowed to prevent stagnation of blood. As soon as the acute stage has settled a crepe bandage should be firmly applied to the leg and the patient should be encouraged to walk.

Anticoagulants should be given whenever facilities for prothrombin estimation are available and continued until one week after all the signs have disappeared and the patient is ambulant.

Superficial Vein Thrombosis

Thrombosis may occur in the superficial veins, particularly of the lower limbs. The vein becomes painful and on examination the thrombosis can be palpated as a tender cord. The skin over the thrombosis may be red. Superficial vein thrombosis may occur as a result of injury or as a complication of varicose veins. It should be remembered that it occasionally indicates a deep-seated neoplasm. There is little risk of pulmonary embolism.

Treatment consists of firmly bandaging the limb and allowing the patient to walk as much as is comfortable. Phenylbutazone in doses of 100 mg. three times daily for a few days will often reduce inflammation and discomfort.

Iliac Vein Compression

Obstruction of the venous return from the lower limbs by the right common iliac artery has recently been recognised as an occasional cause of swollen legs. Usually in such patients the left common iliac vein is compressed (68%) but the lower end of the inferior vena cava (16%) and the right common iliac vein (16%) may also be affected. The condition is twice as common in women as in men, and is believed to be a major factor in the occurrence of acute venous thrombosis after childbirth or surgical operations (p. 173), which may be followed by lifelong oedema of one or both limbs. In other patients no such acute episode is recorded, the patient presenting with aching and swelling of one or both legs.

Swelling occurs three times as commonly on the left as the right, and the whole of the affected limb is swollen. Pain in the limb on exertion is the rule, and has been termed 'venous claudication'. It differs from arterial claudication (p. 171) in that it takes longer to appear and is less quickly relieved by rest. It usually affects the calf, but may spread to the thigh. Sometimes there are recurrent episodes of thrombosis, and chronic varicose ulcers may occur.

The diagnosis is proved by combined phlebography and arteriography, and treatment is surgical.

Thrombosis of the Axillary Vein

This occasionally occurs in young, fit adults, particularly following trauma to the vein such as produced by carrying a rucksack. There is a swelling of the arm and the axillary vein is tender. An embolism is rare and the arm should be rested until the condition subsides.

FURTHER READING

Lowe, R. D., and Robinson, B. F., *A Physiological Approach to Clinical Methods.* J. & A. Churchill, London (1970).

Wood, P., *Diseases of the Heart and Circulation*, 3rd Edition. Eyre and Spottiswoode, London (1968).

Pickering Sir George, *High Blood Pressure* 2nd edition. J. & A. Churchill, London (1968).

Lown, B., *Modern Concepts of Cardiovascular Disease*, 33, No. 7, 1964.

Shillingford, J. P., *Second Symposium on Advanced Medicine*, Pitman Medical Pub. Co. (1966).

Schrire, V., *Clinical Cardiology*, 2nd Edition. Staples Press, London (1966).

CHAPTER FIVE

THE RESPIRATORY SYSTEM

ANATOMY AND PHYSIOLOGY

For descriptive purposes the respiratory system is subdivided into the upper respiratory tract, consisting of the nose, nasopharynx, and larynx, and the lower respiratory tract, comprising the trachea, bronchi, and lungs. The lining membrane of the air passages has a rich blood supply which enables it to warm and moisten the inspired air. A thin film of mucus covers the whole respiratory tract, and is kept continuously moving upwards away from the lungs by the sweeping action of the ciliated mucous membrane; this is a most effective filter for removing particles of dust from the air before it reaches the lungs. The irregularity of the nasal cavity and the accessory air sinuses which open into it increase the area of mucous membrane with which the air comes into contact, and so makes the warming and filtering more efficient; on the other hand, swelling of the mucous membrane readily obstructs drainage of secretions from the sinuses and so may predispose to sinusitis. Another important defence mechanism is the cough reflex.

ANATOMY OF THE BRONCHIAL TREE

A proper knowledge of the anatomy of the bronchial tree is essential to the understanding of the localisation and spread of many diseases of the lung. Many lung infections spread via the bronchi and the distribution of the infection is determined by the segments which these bronchi supply. Unless the anatomy of the broncho-pulmonary segments is known, the correct localisation of disease within the lung, whether by means of physical signs or radiography, is impossible. Finally, treatment by postural drainage requires a knowledge of the direction of the bronchi so that the patient may be correctly positioned.

Surface Markings of the Lobes

The upper and lower lobes of the left lung are separated by the oblique fissure. The right lung is composed of three lobes and the right oblique fissure separates the lower lobe from the upper and middle lobes. On each side the oblique fissure extends from the anterior end of the 6th rib and runs upwards and backwards round the chest wall, usually along the line of the 5th or 6th rib to the vertebral column. Its surface marking roughly corresponds to the position of the medial border of the scapula when the hand is placed on top of the head. The horizontal fissure separates the right upper lobe from the middle lobe. Its surface marking starts at the fourth right costal cartilage and runs horizontally around the chest to join the oblique fissure in the mid-axillary line. The segment of the left lung which occupies the position corresponding to the middle lobe is called the lingula, and it is part of the left upper lobe.

The Broncho-pulmonary Segments

The bronchi to the separate lobes of each lung arise from the main bronchi on their respective sides. The primary subdivisions of the lobar bronchi, together with the segments of lung which they supply, form the broncho-pulmonary segments. The segments of each lobe are named after their corresponding bronchi.

The Upper Lobes. The right upper lobe bronchus divides almost immediately into anterior, apical, and posterior branches. The anterior and posterior bronchi have axillary branches which supply the lateral part of the upper lobe.

The left upper lobe bronchus quickly gives origin to the lingula bronchus which runs downwards and forwards, subdividing into superior and inferior branches. It then gives off branches to the anterior, apical, and posterior segments of the lobe, but differs from the right side in having a common apico-posterior bronchus.

The Middle Lobe bronchus is only present on the right side and runs downwards and forwards dividing into lateral and medial divisions.

The Lower Lobes. The right lower lobe bronchus gives off an apical branch which arises opposite the middle lobe bronchus and runs backwards to the apical segment of the lower lobe. The basal bronchi consist of anterior, lateral, and posterior branches and, in addition, a medial basal (or cardiac) bronchus supplies a small segment on the medial aspect of the lower lobe.

On the left side the arrangement is similar, but the medial basal is usually insignificant or absent.

LOOKING AT THE CHEST X-RAY

A chest radiograph is an integral part of the examination of a patient suspected of lung disease, and indeed in many conditions radiological abnormalities are present long before the development of physical signs.

The film should be examined in a systematic, rather than haphazard, manner. Firstly it should be ensured that the film has been taken straight by observing that the medial ends of the clavicles are equidistant from the centre of the spine. Undue rotation can produce abnormal looking appearances of the mediastinum and the hilar shadows, as well as gross differences in the opaqueness of the two lungs. The trachea should be central; displacement may be due to rotation, shift of the mediastinum (see palpation, p. 188) or due to a superior mediastinal swelling (p. 244). The diaphragms should next be examined; flattening of the diaphragms occurs

*

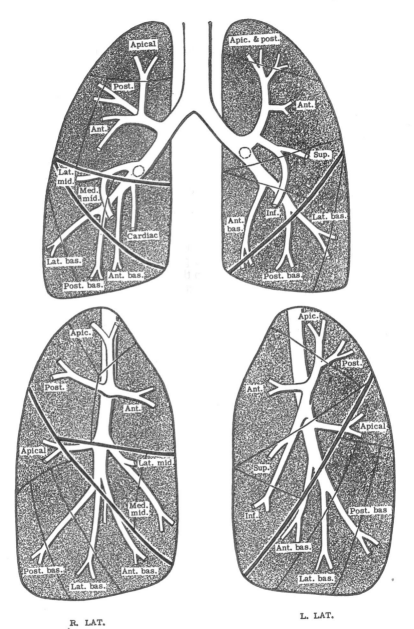

THE BRONCHO-PULMONARY SEGMENTS.

with over-inflated lungs and undue elevation of a diaphragm may be due to diminished lung volume on that side or to diaphragmatic paralysis. The right diaphragm is normally higher than the left and the costo-phrenic angle should be clear and at an acute angle, filling-in being due to fluid or pleural thickening. The lung fields are then examined by comparing one side with another; the apices of the lungs above the clavicles are first compared and then coming down the chest X-ray and using the anterior ends of the ribs as markers one interspace is compared with the other on the opposite side. In this way small focal lesions can be detected. In addition, the pulmonary vascular markings should be examined and an assessment made as to whether there is any diffuse shadowing in addition to the normal markings. The position of the horizontal fissure should be noted. The hilar regions should be examined; enlargement may be due to a prominent pulmonary artery, pathological enlargement of the pulmonary artery, enlarged lymph glands or hilar mass. Starting with the first ribs, and comparing one side with another, both the posterior and anterior parts of the ribs should be examined for abnormalities. A lateral chest X-ray will be necessary for full interpretation of a lesion and for correct anatomical localization (see bronchopulmonary segments p. 177), and in addition a lateral film is essential for a suspected lesion in the left lower lobe as it may be obscured in the straight X-ray by the heart shadow.

RESPIRATORY FUNCTION TESTS

INTRODUCTION

Tests of respiratory function aid the clinical assessment of a patient, for they provide an objective method of estimating the respiratory ability. They may be helpful, for example, when thoracic surgery is being considered, and serial recordings are of value both in assessing the effectiveness of a form of treatment and in following the progress of a disease.

Some tests are easy to perform and others require skill and complicated apparatus. Each has its limitations and it may be necessary to test several aspects of function before reaching a satisfactory conclusion. It is proposed to discuss the principles involved, rather than the technical aspects.

TESTS OF VENTILATION

The diagram, which is self-explanatory, illustrates the various subdivisions of the lung volumes. The *Tidal Volume* is the volume of air breathed in or out at rest and the *Resting Expiratory Level* is the most satisfactory reference point on the spirometer tracing as it is the most constant. The *Minute Ventilation* is the product of the Tidal Volume and the number of respirations per minute.

The *Vital Capacity* is the largest ventilatory volume that a patient can achieve. It is measured on the spirometer as the volume of a maximal unhurried expiration following a maximal inspiration. Normal figures for the Vital Capacity can be predicted from tables, the values being larger in males, increasing with size and, in adults, diminishing with age. As a single test of respiratory function, it has many limitations. The predicted normal values have a wide range of $\pm$ 20 per cent, and this means that reduction in the Vital Capacity has to be gross before it becomes significant. It is therefore unsuitable for measuring mild to moderate ventilatory defects. In addition, the degree of reduction in the Vital Capacity does not necessarily correlate with a patient's disability and neither does it indicate the nature of the ventilatory defect or the underlying disease. It can be

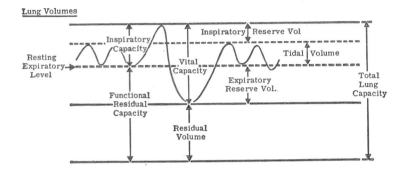

Tests of Pulmonary Ventilation

reduced in practically any disease of the lungs, pleura, or thoracic cage. Its most useful application is that of serial measurement in an individual patient.

The *Residual Volume* (RV) is that volume of gas remaining in the lungs after a maximum expiration. It can be estimated indirectly by subtracting the *Expiratory Reserve Volume* from the more easily measured *Functional Residual Capacity*. The Residual Volume (RV), like the Vital Capacity, has a wide normal range, but its proportion to the *Total Lung Capacity* (TLC) is fairly constant. Up to the age of thirty years, it forms 20 to 25 per cent of the Total Lung Capacity. It increases further with age, rising to some 40 per cent in elderly people. The RV/TLC ratio is abnormally increased in conditions where there is over-inflation of the lungs, such as *obstructive emphysema, asthma,* and *kyphoscoliosis,* and reduced in *pulmonary fibrosis.*

Obstructive airway disease, such as occurs in emphysema and asthma, is best revealed when the Vital Capacity is determined with reference to speed. The *Forced Vital Capacity* (FVC) is the volume of a maximal expiration carried out *as rapidly as possible* following a maximal inspiration. The volume expired during the first second of the FVC is termed the

$FEV_{1.0}$ (*the Forced Expiratory Volume in one second*). The percentage of the FVC expired during this first second is termed the FER (*Forced Expiratory Ratio*), and is normally 75 per cent or more. Reduction in both the $FEV_{1.0}$ and the FER occurs with expiratory obstruction and is particularly useful in detecting airflow obstruction from asthma, chronic bronchitis and emphysema. The response of asthma to the inhalation of a

$$FER = \frac{FEV_{1.0}}{FVC} \times 100$$

TIMED VOLUME STUDIES

bronchodilator is best detected by an improvement in the $FEV_{1.0}$ and this change distinguishes reversible airflow obstruction (asthma) from irreversible airflow obstruction (chronic bronchitis and emphysema).

The *Maximum Breathing Capacity* (MBC) or *Maximum Voluntary Ventilation* (MVV), can be estimated directly by measuring the ventilation when a patient is made to breathe maximally over a period of 15 seconds; it is expressed in litres per minute. This method is often distressing to the patient and it has been shown that the MBC can be calculated simply and accurately by multiplying the $FEV_{1.0}$ by 35. As with the Vital Capacity, predicted figures for the MBC can also be obtained from tables, and there is the same normal range of $\pm$ 20 per cent. The MBC is a test of the overall function of pulmonary ventilation. Provided a diffusion defect is not present, a normal value means that dyspnoea is not respiratory in origin. It is **reduced** in all respiratory diseases causing *impairment of ventilation*, but particularly in those where there is *airway obstruction*.

The *Peak Flow* is the maximum expiratory flow rate achieved during a forced expiration. The Wright 'Peak Flow Meter' is one instrument designed for measuring this and has the advantage of being small, portable, and easy to operate. Although the Peak Flow and the $FEV_{1.0}$ measure rather different aspects of pulmonary ventilation they are **reduced** by the same circumstances, namely *airflow obstruction* or general *reduction in ventilatory function*. Normal values for Peak Flow are also influenced by sex, age, and size. For example, a man aged thirty-five years, 5 ft. 11 in. tall and weight 11 st. 7 lb. should have the following predicted mean values:

Forced Vital Capacity (FVC)	5·1 litres
Forced Expiratory Volume in one second ($FEV_{1.0}$)	4·1 litres
Peak Flow	545 litres/min

Mixing of Gases

Efficient ventilation ensures that the inspired air is evenly distributed throughout the lungs. In one test, after a full inspiration of pure oxygen, the patient breathes out fully, and the concentration of nitrogen at the mouth level is measured continuously with a nitrogen meter. During expiration there is a brief period during which the air passages are cleared of the Dead Space oxygen. The nitrogen concentration then rises sharply and by the time 750 c.c. have been exhaled it has reached the steady level of alveolar gas. In the normal, further rise in the alveolar nitrogen concentration during the period of 750 to 1,250 c.c. of expiration should not exceed 2 per cent. This figure is increased in conditions where there are poorly ventilated air sacs and uneven ventilation, and the test has its greatest value in the assessment of **emphysema.**

Blood Gas Analysis

Measurements of the oxygen saturation and the carbon dioxide pressure in arterial blood can be used to assess the efficiency of alveolar ventilation. Normally, the partial pressures of CO_2 (P_{CO2}) and O_2 (P_{O2}) in arterial blood are 40 mm.Hg. and 100 mm.Hg. respectively, and the normal arterial oxygen saturation is not less than 95 per cent.

Alveolar hypoventilation leads to arterial oxygen desaturation and retention of carbon dioxide in the blood. This state of affairs may be precipitated by any complication producing severe impairment of ventilation, such as *poliomyelitis* or *respiratory depression from drugs,* or it may be persistent in patients with chronic chest disease. The arterial oxygen saturation is also reduced in conditions producing severe impairment of gas transfer and in intracardiac right-to-left shunts.

In chronic anoxic states the respiratory centre depends on the anoxia for its stimulation. Relief of severe anoxia by oxygen therapy is an important part of the treatment of cor pulmonale for example, but this may release the respiratory centre from its 'drive' and depress respirations further. The patient may thus be relieved from anoxia, but the additional reduction in alveolar ventilation leads to further retention of carbon dioxide in the blood with acidoses. Mental disturbance usually occurs when the arterial pH is less than 7·2 or the P_{CO2} higher than 100 mm.Hg., and coma usually supervenes with arterial levels of pH below 7·1 or the P_{CO2} above 120 mm.Hg. Serial estimations of the P_{CO2} in arterial blood or the mixed venous blood by the Campbell rebreathing technique are thus very valuable in ensuring the proper control of oxygen administration to such patients.

GAS TRANSFER

In certain conditions the predominant physiological defect is one of impairment of the transfer of gases across the alveolar-capillary membrane, and other aspects of ventilatory function may be within normal limits or only moderately reduced. This occurs in such diseases as fibrosing alveolitis, asbestosis, infiltration of the lungs with sarcoid granulomata, carcinomatosis lymphangitis, and pulmonary oedema. In these examples of the so-called 'alveolar-capillary block' syndrome impairment of the transfer of carbon dioxide does not occur, as this gas is about twenty times more diffusable than oxygen. Hyperventilation is often present even at rest, and this may indeed produce increased excretion of carbon dioxide by the lungs with reduction in its arterial partial pressure (P_{CO_2}). According to the severity of the condition the arterial oxygen saturation may be normal or reduced at rest, but after exercise it falls sharply with perhaps further reduction in P_{CO_2}.

There are various methods of measuring the *Transfer Factor*, and normal figures vary according to the techniques and the gases used. In one method, carbon monoxide, which is slightly less diffusible than oxygen, is breathed in low concentration and its uptake by the lungs measured. Gas transfer can be shown to be *impaired* in the '*alveolar-capillary block*'-syndrome and it may also be impaired when there is a reduction in the area available for transfer of gases, as in *emphysema or multiple pulmonary emboli*.

THE WORK OF BREATHING AND COMPLIANCE

The measurement of the work involved in breathing requires the summation of various complicated physiological processes. These include such aspects as the oxygen requirements of the respiratory muscles and the mechanical effects of overcoming airway resistance, tissue resistance and lung elasticity. Most of these are difficult to test, but lung elasticity, or *lung compliance*, can be measured fairly simply by recording the negative intrathoracic pressure through an oesophageal catheter at the same time as ventilatory volumes. The lung compliance is the inspiratory volume which is produced by a change in negative pressure of 1 cm. H_2O, and in the normal is 0·09 to 0·33 litres/cm.H_2O. The normal values have been related to the Functional Residual Capacity, as they are influenced by the size of the lungs. The compliance is *reduced* in conditions which produce abnormally stiff lungs. Examples of such conditions are pulmonary venous congestion from *mitral stenosis* or *chronic left ventricular failure*, and *diffuse fibrotic or infiltrative lesions of the lungs*.

BRONCHOSPIROMETRY

At times it is of value to assess the function of each lung separately by bronchospirometry. This may be the case when lung disease appears to be unilateral or when pneumonectomy is contemplated and adequate function in the opposite lung is in doubt. By passing a double-lumen catheter down the trachea it is possible to record ventilation and to collect gas samples for analysis from both lungs separately.

SYMPTOMS AND SIGNS OF LUNG DISEASE

Types of Cough and Sputum

A cough is a forced expiration against a closed glottis. A high pressure of air is built up in the trachea and bronchi and the sudden opening of the glottis is followed by explosive discharge, producing the characteristic barking noise. This removes collections of mucus and foreign particles from the air passages. The cough reflex is stimulated by irritation of nerve endings in the larynx, trachea, bronchi, and even the pleura.

In the early stages of respiratory tract infections, inflammatory swelling of the mucous membrane causes the cough to be dry and unproductive. With the later development of inflammatory exudate, the cough produces clear or whitish, sticky sputum. In *whooping cough* the exudate is particularly tenacious. The patient gives a series of quickly repeated coughs during one expiratory movement in an effort to dislodge the sputum, and this is followed by an inspiratory 'whoop' through a partially closed glottis. The cough typically occurs in paroxysms and is not always associated with a 'whoop'.

A yellow or greenish colour to the sputum signifies that it is purulent. This occurs with secondary pyogenic infection during respiratory tract infections. Purulent sputum is also expectorated in patients with *bronchiectasis*. With change of posture when waking in the morning, the patient coughs up the infected sputum which has collected in the dilated bronchi during the night. The quantity of sputum depends on the degree of infection and extent of the disease. It may amount to several ounces per day and is sometimes very offensive in smell due to the action of putrefactive bacteria. Purulent sputum tends to be more fluid than other types as enzymes from the pus cells liquefy the mucus.

The cough in *bronchial carcinoma* is at first persistent and unproductive due to invasion of the mucous membrane. With increase in size of the growth, secretions collect distal to the partially obstructed bronchus so that mucopurulent, often bloodstained, sputum is then produced.

In *pulmonary tuberculosis* there may be no sputum in the earlier stages of the disease. If sputum is produced it is clear or white and very sticky, so that it remains in separate lumps in the sputum mug (nummular sputum).

During the early stages of *pneumococcal pneumonia* the patient may cough up very viscid sputum tinged with blood which gives it a rusty colour.

Cardiac asthma (p. 109) is due to acute engorgement of the lungs with blood. In extreme cases oedema fluid exudes into the alveoli and the attack is associated with the expectoration of a large quantity of clear, frothy sputum, which is sometimes pinkish in colour due to the presence of red cells. In *bronchial asthma*, however, the sputum consists of firm, whitish pellets, which can sometimes be unravelled in water into spiral ribbons (Curschmann's spirals). These represent casts of the bronchial tubes in which they have formed.

Haemoptysis

The coughing up of blood must be distinguished from haematemesis, the vomiting of blood.

(1) Blood from the lungs is usually bright red, frothy, and mixed, with sputum. That from the stomach is usually dark in colour, having been altered to acid-haematin by the hydrochloric acid; it is often mixed with food.

(2) Many patients can state definitely whether the blood has been coughed up or vomited.

(3) Often there will be symptoms or signs which point to disease of the lungs or the alimentary tract.

The common causes of haemoptysis are:

Respiratory	*Cardiovascular*
Carcinoma of the bronchus	Pulmonary infarct
Pulmonary tuberculosis	Mitral stenosis
Acute or chronic bronchitis	Acute left ventricular failure
Bronchiectasis	
Lung abscess	

Although there may be an isolated haemoptysis in carcinoma of the bronchus, characteristically the ulcerated area leads to repeated daily blood-streaking of sputum. An early lesion of pulmonary tuberculosis sometimes presents with an haemoptysis of an ounce or more of bright-red blood, not associated with sputum. Blood-streaking of sputum is very common in respiratory tract infections and ulceration of the mucosa in bronchiectasis sometimes produces severe haemoptysis.

Every patient presenting with haemoptysis should be fully examined and have a chest radiograph, particularly to exclude bronchial carcinoma and pulmonary tuberculosis. A normal chest radiograph does not exclude an early bronchial carcinoma, and ideally bronchoscopy should be performed to exclude this possibility. However, unless there are good clinical grounds for suspecting a bronchial carcinoma, bronchoscopy is often not justified at this stage and it is sufficient for the patient to be followed-up carefully with fairly frequent chest radiographs. The majority of such patients do not develop any serious disease and in nearly half of all patients presenting with a small haemoptysis, no definite cause is found.

Pain in the Chest

Acute pleuritic pain from pleurisy is sharp and stabbing in character and aggravated by coughing or deep breathing. The pain is usually localised to the site of the pleurisy, but it may be referred to the abdominal wall and be confused with an acute abdominal condition. With diaphragmatic pleurisy the pain is referred to the tip of the shoulder, as the skin in this situation has the same sensory nerve supply (C3, 4, and 5).

Lesions of the chest wall, such as fractures or secondary deposits in the ribs, may cause severe local pain and tenderness. The aetiology of *Tietze's syndrome* is uncertain, but it is a painful condition, usually involving one of the upper costo-chondral junctions. Chest pain may also be referred from the thoracic spine. The seventh cervical nerve supplies the pectoralis major and pain referred from this root may be felt in that muscle as well as in the arm. Intrathoracic structures, other than the lungs, can produce pain in the chest, common examples being the pain from coronary thrombosis and hiatus hernia.

Types of Respiration

Respiration in men is mainly diaphragmatic in type and in women it is mostly costal. Inspiration is a more powerful muscular movement than expiration, the latter depending on elastic recoil of the lungs and relaxation of the diaphragm and intercostal muscles. Obstruction to the large air passages produces a prolonged inspiratory phase with stridor, as inspiration is the more powerful movement. The bronchi and bronchioles normally dilate on inspiration and narrow on expiration, so that obstruction of the smaller air passages, as in asthma, leads to prolonged, wheezy, and difficult expiration.

Respirations in *pneumonia and pleurisy* are rapid and shallow, the inspirations being abruptly stopped, often with an audible grunt, as soon as the pleuritic pain is felt. Normally, expiration immediately follows inspiration and there is then a pause before the next breath. In pneumonia this rhythm is sometimes reversed, the pause taking place between inspiration and expiration.

The acidosis which occurs with uraemia and diabetic ketosis causes very deep breathing, known as *air hunger*, or *Kussmaul's breathing*, due to marked stimulation of the respiratory centre. *Cheyne-Stokes breathing* is a characteristic respiratory arrhythmia occurring when the respiratory centre has a diminished sensitivity to carbon dioxide in the blood. The amplitude of respiration progressively deepens until a maximum is reached and then diminishes until there is a period of apnoea. During the period of apnoea, the carbon dioxide in the blood rises to a level high enough to stimulate the respiratory centre. There is then an exaggerated response producing the period of hyperventilation, which washes the carbon dioxide out of the blood until the stimulus to respiration is removed and apnoea occurs. The whole cycle lasts two or three minutes and is then repeated.

This type of breathing occurs with left ventricular failure and with various cerebral causes of depression of the respiratory centre.

Clubbing of the Fingers

The earliest change is a filling in of the angle between the skin at the base of the nail and the base of the nail itself, the skin becoming swollen and shiny. Later increased curvature of the nails occurs and finally the pulps of the fingers become enlarged. Clubbing has many unrelated causes:

Cardiovascular

(1) Bacterial endocarditis
(2) Cyanotic congenital heart disease.
(3) Arteriovenous communications in the arm.

Respiratory

(1) Carcinoma of the bronchus
(2) Chronic suppuration in the chest, such as bronchiectasis, lung abscess, and empyema.
(3) Chronic fibrosing alveohtis

At times clubbing is familial and there is no underlying disease. More rarely it is associated with cirrhosis of the liver, steatorrhoea, or polyposis of the colon.

EXAMINATION OF THE CHEST

Inspection

(1) *The General Contours*

(a) *Kyphosis* and *kyphoscoliosis* may be developmental in origin. If gross, they may in later years give rise to severe impairment of lung function and heart failure. Abnormalities of spinal curvature may also occur secondary to intra-thoracic disease.

(b) *Funnel-shaped depression of the sternum* (pectus excavatum) may occur in varying degrees. Deep depression may displace the heart to the left and lead to the erroneous diagnosis of cardiac enlargement.

(c) *Over-inflation of the lungs,* such as occurs with asthma and emphysema, leads to increase in the antero-posterior diameter of the chest and the shoulders are held high.

(d) *Unilateral flattening* of the chest occurs with long-standing pulmonary or pleural fibrosis.

(2) *The Respiratory Movements*

(a) The respiratory rate is increased in many conditions, including acute and chronic lung disease, cardiac failure, and anxiety.

It is decreased with depression of the respiratory centre, as in narcotic poisoning and with various cerebral lesions.

(b) The accessory muscles of respiration may be used if there is severe respiratory distress, as in an asthmatic attack.

(c) Decreased movement on one side of the chest indicates disease of the lung or pleura of that side.

(d) The respiration may have a special character (see p. 186).

Palpation

The position of the mediastinum is assessed by determining the position of the apex beat and the trachea. Shift of the mediastinum towards the side of the lesion indicates shrinkage of the lung due to collapse or fibrosis. Displacement away from the lesion occurs with fluid or air in the pleural cavity. Displacement of the trachea alone is more likely with contraction of an upper lobe and shift of the apex beat alone in a lesion of a lower lobe.

Tactile vocal fremitus (TVF) is decreased with air or fluid in the pleural cavity and with pulmonary collapse. Increased tactile vocal fremitus occurs with conditions which also produce bronchial breathing.

Percussion

Normally the lungs are resonant to percussion and there are areas of dullness over the heart and liver. In emphysema and pneumothorax, hyper-resonance is sometimes found and cardiac and liver dullness are either diminished or absent. Impaired resonance is found over consolidated, collapsed, or fibroid lung, or with pleural thickening. A flat, dull note is found over pleural fluid.

Auscultation

(1) *The Breath Sounds*

The normal breath sounds are rustling, with a long inspiratory phase followed by a short expiratory phase. Over the lung roots the normal breath sounds take on a bronchial character. The breath sounds are diminished or absent with fluid or air in the pleural cavity and with impaired inflation of the lung, as in emphysema and collapse. In *bronchial breathing*, the breath sounds have a harsher quality and the expiratory phase is longer than the inspiratory, with a short gap between the two. Bronchial breathing is heard in the normal by listening with a stethoscope over the larynx or trachea. When bronchial breathing is heard over the lungs, it indicates a pathological process which is enhancing the transmission of the tracheal sound to the chest wall. It occurs with pneumonic consolidation, with fibroid lung (fibrosis plus bronchiectasis), and over a large cavity. It also occurs sometimes above the upper level of a pleural effusion and over a large pneumothorax. Bronchial breathing is always accompanied by whispering pectoriloquy and by increased T.V.F. and bronchophony.

Condition	Inspection	Palpation	Percussion	Auscultation
*CONSOLIDATION	Respiration rate increased. Movement decreased on affected side.	Mediastinum central T.V.F. increased over consolidation.	Dullness over consolidation.	Bronchial breathing, Bronchophony, W.P., Fine or medium râles. } Over consolidation.
ABSORPTION COLLAPSE	Movement diminished on affected side.	Mediastinum shifted to affected side. Absent T.V.F. over collapsed segment.	Dullness over collapsed area.	Breath sounds diminished or absent. Voice sounds diminished or absent.
FIBROSIS	Flattening of the chest and diminished movement on affected side.	Mediastinum shifted to affected side. Increased T.V.F. over fibrosis.	Dullness over fibrosis.	Bronchial breathing, Bronchophony, W.P. } Over fibrosis. Frequently coarse râles due to concomitant bronchiectasis.
FLUID	Movement diminished on affected side.	If large, mediastinum shifted to opposite side. T.V.F. absent over fluid.	Stony dullness over fluid, the line tending to rise in the axilla with moderate effusions.	Absent breath sounds and voice sounds over fluid. Sometimes bronchial breathing, W.P., and aegophony above upper level of fluid.
PNEUMOTHORAX	Movement diminished on affected side.	If large, mediastinum shifted to opposite side.	Normal or hyper-resonant. Diminished cardiac dullness on the left and liver dullness on right.	Breath sounds and voice sounds diminished or absent. Sometimes if large, bronchial breathing, W.P., and positive coin sound.

* These signs are only heard over a considerable area of consolidation. With small patches of pneumonia, or when the pneumonic process has not reached the surface of the lung, signs may be scanty and are often confined to a small area of crackling râles.

(2) *The Voice Sounds*

Normally, when the stethoscope is placed over a peripheral part of the lungs the spoken voice comes through in a modified form so that the consonants are blurred and indistinct; the whispered voice cannot be heard at all. Transmission of the spoken and whispered voice in an unmodified bronchial form (such as can be heard in the normal subject by listening over the trachea, though it is not necessarily as loud as this) is called respectively *bronchophony* and *whispering pectoriloquy* (W.P.). They occur under the same circumstances as bronchial breathing.

Aegophony is the peculiar nasal quality to the voice sounds heard above the upper level of an effusion.

(3) *Rhonchi*

A rhonchus is a musical squeak due to air passing through a narrowed bronchus. It is low-pitched if the bronchus is large and high-pitched with small bronchi. Rhonchi are most marked on expiration and may be cleared by coughing. The narrowing is commonly due to bronchial spasm or mucosal swelling or exudate. A bronchial neoplasm may produce a persistent low-pitched rhonchus.

(4) *Râles*

Râles are popping noises due either to air bubbling through fluid or to the sound of alveolar walls opening. The râles are coarse if the fluid is in large bronchi and fine if the bronchi are small. *Crepitations* are very fine râles due to fluid in the bronchioles or alveoli. They are sometimes heard at the bases of the lungs in normal people who have been breathing quietly, when they are due to the noise of the partially closed alveoli opening, but they should disappear after a few deep breaths. If the râles are associated with bronchial breathing, they become very clear-cut (*consonating râles*). Râles are most marked towards the end of an inspiration. There are coarse, crackling râles in bronchiectasis, medium râles in bronchitis, and crepitations in pulmonary oedema, pneumonia or fibrosing alveolitis.

DISEASES OF THE UPPER RESPIRATORY TRACT

HAY FEVER AND PERENNIAL RHINITIS

These are allergic disorders characterised by bouts of sneezing, profuse watery nasal discharge, and smarting and watering of the eyes. Hay fever is due to sensitivity to grass pollens and occurs during the months of May to August; perennial rhinitis is due to sensitivity to a variety of allergens, such as house dust, and may occur throughout the year.

Treatment. *Hay fever:* A course of desensitisation injections may be given if skin testing (p. 205) reveals specific allergens. Starting in January, weekly injections continue until 14 days before the hay fever usually begins.

Alternatively, less frequent injections of a depot vaccine may be used. At least three yearly courses are required for a prolonged effect. *Antihistamines* are of considerable value during an attack. Usually one preparation can be found to suit the patient. Among the most valuable are chlorpheniramine, 4·0 mg. twice daily or promethazine, 25 mg. once or twice daily; the latter often causes troublesome drowsiness which may be counteracted with amphetamine sulphate, 2·5–5·0 mg. in the morning. *Betamethasone* (0·1 per cent) nose drops also give good symptomatic relief. *Disodium cromoglycate* inhaled into the nose is a promising new treatment for hay fever.

Perennial rhinitis: Precipitants such as house dust, pets, or feathers should be avoided. Skin testing is seldom helpful as the patient is often sensitive to many allergens. Antihistamines may be tried, but are not usually as successful as in hay fever. Surgical treatment, e.g. submucous resection, should be avoided unless there is a very definite indication.

VIRUS INFECTIONS OF THE RESPIRATORY TRACT

The following are some of the viruses which affect the respiratory tract;

Rhinovirus
Adenovirus
Influenza virus
Parainfluenza virus
Respiratory syncytial virus
Coxsackie ⎱ Enteroviruses
ECHO ⎰

All the above viruses have a nucleic acid content of RNA, with the exception of the adenovirus which is DNA containing. An increasing number of serotypes are being identified with some of the above viruses; for example, there are more than 90 serotypes of the rhinovirus and 28 of the adenovirus. The enteroviruses, ECHO and Coxsackie A and B, also produce respiratory infections as well as other illnesses such as pericarditis and meningitis (p. 507). The influenza virus consists of types A, B and C; influenza A virus is the cause of pandemics and major epidemics, B virus causes smaller epidemics and is a less virulent type of infection and influenza C is principally endemic producing a fairly trivial respiratory infection. Major changes in the antigenic nature of influenza A virus occur about every ten to fifteen years, but minor changes may occur during the intervening years— the so called 'antigenic drift'. For this reason effective vaccines against influenza should contain type B virus and the latest strain of type A, at the present time A2/Hong Kong/68. The development of effective vaccines against the other respiratory viruses has not been possible because of the large number of viruses involved and because there would be no cross-protection between the different serotypes in the same group.

Generally speaking each type of acute respiratory illness can be produced by a number of different viruses. A cold, for example, can be caused by the rhinovirus and the adenovirus, and the latter virus may also be responsible for a sore throat, an influenza-like illness or pneumonia.

CORYZA (The Common Cold)

Coryza is an infection of the mucous membrane of the nose and naso-pharynx. The majority of cases are due to infection with the rhinoviruses, but any of the other respiratory viruses may be responsible—in particular the adenoviruses. It is spread by droplet infection, particularly in crowded places such as buses, trains, and cinemas. There is a high level of endemic infection during the autumn and winter and chills and dampness seem to be predisposing factors. After sneezing and profuse watery nasal discharge for a few days, secondary bacterial infection often occurs and the secretions become thick and yellow. Infection may spread causing:

(1) *Acute sinusitis*, with fever, headache or pain in the face, and localised tenderness may be present over the frontal or maxillary sinuses. Chronic sinusitis may result.
(2) *Acute otitis media* with fever, deafness and earache.
(3) *Tracheitis, bronchitis, or pneumonia.*

Treatment. A day or two in bed usually cuts short the course and prevents complications. It also helps to limit spread of the infection to others.

Soluble aspirin 0·6 g. six-hourly, often alleviates the minor discomforts. Inhalation of tinct. benzoin and menthol, one teaspoonful in a jug of hot water, may relieve the nasal congestion.

ACUTE LARYNGITIS AND LARYNGOTRACHEOBRONCHITIS

Acute laryngitis occurs with the common cold and in young children with parainfluenzal virus infection. Tracheitis and bronchitis often occur at the same time. The throat is sore, the voice is at first hoarse and then reduced to a whisper and there is a dry, painful cough. In small children, swelling of the mucous membrane of the larynx may cause serious obstruction, the condition known as 'croup'; breathing becomes noisy and laboured and alarming paroxysms of coughing occur.

Treatment. If feverish the patient should be in bed in a warm room where the atmosphere is not too dry. The dryness of central heating, electric and gas fires should be prevented by using a steam kettle. The patient must not talk, since the larynx needs rest. Smoking is forbidden. Steam inhalations containing tinct. benzoin co., one teaspoon to one pint of boiling water, given for ten minutes three times a day, often give great relief; hot gargles and frequent hot drinks make the throat more comfortable. Linctus codeine, 4·0 ml., will suppress an irritating cough.

CHRONIC LARYNGITIS

It is more common in men than in women and is particularly liable to occur with untrained over-use of the voice. Hence the term 'clergyman's throat', though costermonger's throat would be more apt, as excessive use of tobacco and alcohol are often predisposing factors. Chronic sinus infection may also play a part.

Clinical Features. The voice is hoarse and weak. Examination of the larynx shows congestion with thickening of the vocal cords, either generalised or confined to the posterior third.

Persistent hoarseness for more than three weeks demands expert examination of the larynx. It may be due to papilloma, carcinoma, laryngeal palsy, or more rarely tuberculosis or syphilis.

Treatment. Complete rest of the voice is important. The patient should not speak above a whisper for several weeks. Nasal infection should be treated if present and tobacco and alcohol forbidden.

DISEASES OF THE BRONCHI

ACUTE TRACHEITIS AND BRONCHITIS

Acute tracheitis and bronchitis may complicate colds, influenza, measles, and other virus infections, and are particularly liable to occur in cold, damp and foggy weather. After the first few days, secondary bacterial invasion commonly occurs. Broncheolitis in infants is due to the respiratory syncytial virus.

Clinical Features. Acute tracheitis causes a dry, painful cough with soreness behind the sternum. Spread of infection to the bronchi produces tightness of the chest, with wheezing and difficulty in breathing. At first there is a little sticky, mucoid sputum, but secondary bacterial infection soon makes it yellow and more profuse. The severity and duration of the fever and of the general malaise are very variable; usually the illness is a mild one, lasting a few days. It may be serious and lead to pneumonia in young children, in the elderly or debilitated, or in patients with chronic bronchitis.

The signs of acute bronchitis are moderate fever, raised respiratory rate, particularly in children or in those with underlying lung disease, widespread rhonchi and often râles.

Treatment. The patient should be kept in bed. The room should be warm and the atmosphere not too dry. A steam kettle or steam inhalations reduce the soreness and aid expectoration. A dry, troublesome cough is helped by linctus codeine 4–8 ml. t.d.s. or elixir diphenhydramine 4 ml.; the latter also aids sleep.

After a few days the fever settles and the cough disappears. Convalescence is advisable after an attack of acute bronchitis, as early return to work with exposure to cold and a smoky atmosphere may delay complete recovery. Antibiotics are not required in mild, uncomplicated acute bronchitis. They are required where the risks of bronchopneumonia are greater:

(1) In a patient with severe bronchitis.
(2) In children and in the elderly and infirm.
(3) In the presence of complicating disease, such as heart disease.
(4) In patients with chronic bronchitis or bronchiectasis.

In these circumstances ampicillin or tetracycline (250 mg. four times daily), or trimethoprim-sulphamethoxazole combinations (Bactrim or Septrin) two tablets twice a day are usually effective.

CHRONIC BRONCHITIS

Great Britain has a higher mortality rate from chronic bronchitis than any other country in the world. It is a major cause of chronic disability and death, particularly in men over middle age. It is related to air pollution, cigarette smoking and the liability to viral respiratory tract infections, and is most common in outdoor manual workers in urban districts. It is a complication of the pneumoconioses (p. 231), and obesity is an aggravating factor.

In the early stages there is hypertrophy of the mucous glands of bronchi, even when there is no inflammatory cell infiltration of the mucosa. In addition goblet cells replace the normal peripheral bronchial epithelium. Later, inflammatory changes in the mucosa occur with micro-abscesses and ulceration of the alveolar walls. When the sputum is mucoid bacteriological study is unrewarding. With persistently purulent sputum, and in acute exacerbations of bronchitis, haemophilus influenzae and the pneumococcus are the most common pathogens isolated.

Clinical Features. The earliest symptom is probably the 'smoker's cough', with the early morning production of non-infected mucoid sputum. This causes no disability and the patient is unlikely to seek medical advice. Later the patient complains of a winter cough with sputum, often with wheezing. At first these symptoms may only occur in episodes after a cold, which is slow to clear. Later they persist throughout the whole winter and eventually during the summer as well. There is usually a moderate amount of sputum, which may be mucoid or purulent; the latter nearly always occurs during an acute exacerbation of bronchitis, but sometimes the sputum is persistently purulent. A large volume of sputum should arouse suspicion of concomitant bronchiectasis.

After some years increasing dyspnoea, due to diffuse airway obstruction and the development of emphysema, becomes an even more urgent symptom. The patient becomes too breathless to work and finally becomes completely disabled. There is considerable variation in the degree of disablement as many patients go throughout life with chronic cough and sputum and little dyspnoea, whereas others may become complete respiratory cripples within a few years.

Examination shows generalised rhonchi due to narrowing of the bronchi by spasm, mucosal swelling and exudate. Râles may also be heard particularly at the bases. As emphysema develops it produces additional signs (p. 197). A *chest radiograph* in chronic bronchitis may show no abnormality until emphysema is present.

Treatment. This is generally disappointing, but in certain cases considerable symptomatic improvement can be achieved. The progress of the disease may be slowed by preventing, as far as possible, acute exacerbations of bronchitis and by treating them vigorously when they occur. This is more rewarding in the early case where lung destruction is not advanced and symptoms are minimal.

General Management. The smoky atmosphere of the city and dusty work should be avoided. This ideal is difficult to achieve as most patients, for financial and social reasons, cannot move to a healthier district or change their occupation. They can give up smoking and should be strenuously urged to do so. They should be advised to sleep in a warm bedroom, with the windows closed in the winter and they should stay at home in foggy weather and when they have a cold. A cold must be taken seriously, and the patient should retire to bed and be given a prophylactic antibiotic (see below) without delay.

Bronchodilators. Some degree of bronchospasm is often present and may be relieved by ephedrine (p. 206), aminophylline (p. 206) or inhalers containing isoprenaline, salbutamol or orciprenaline.

Prednisolone may be tried is some severely disabled patients in whom persistent bronchospasm is thought to be an important feature. Eosinophils in the sputum and a family history of allergy may be useful guides. This steroid therapy should be continued only if there is striking improvement within a week; it is then given on the same lines as for chronic asthma (p. 206).

Expectorant mixtures aim at loosening and aiding the expectoration of sputum. Pharmacological evidence suggests that in the dosage usually prescribed they have no effect on the volume or characteristics of the sputum expectorated. Whether they have any effect on secretions deep in the bronchi is not settled. However, many bronchitic patients and doctors find such mixtures helpful and they continue to be prescribed. The reader is referred to the National Formulary for suitable prescriptions.

Sedative cough mixtures are used to suppress a troublesome cough at night, or to enable a patient to attend a social meeting in comfort. Examples are linctus codeine (N.F.) 4–8 ml. and linctus pholcodine (N.F.) 4–8 ml.

Prophylactic antibiotics do not prevent colds, but are used to prevent the secondary bacterial infection and to cut short, or prevent, acute exacerbations of bronchitis. In a small group of patients with persistent purulent sputum considerable improvement can be achieved by prolonged treatment with antibiotics, from November to March. However, the majority of patients are best treated by giving them a supply of antibiotics so that they can start a course, on their own initiative, at the first signs of a cold. As haemophilus influenzae and the pneumococcus are the common pathogens, tetracycline 1 g. daily, ampicillin 1–2 g. daily, or trimethoprim-sulphamethoxazole combinations (Bactrim or Septrin) two tablets twice daily, are preferred to penicillin.

Breathing exercises.

Heart failure in chronic bronchitis is quite common; it may be due to concurrent hypertension or coronary artery disease, or to true cor pulmonale (p. 198), or to a combination of factors.

EMPHYSEMA

Emphysema may be defined as a condition of the lungs in which there is pathological enlargement of the distal air spaces either from chronic dilatation or from destruction of their walls. Emphysematous bullae, which are cystic spaces of varying size, may develop and at post-mortem the lungs appear bulky as they fail to deflate. The numerous pathological classifications of emphysema are both complex and confusing. There are two main types:

Pan-acinar emphysema. There is a dilatation or destruction of the acinus. This is the lung tissue distal to the terminal bronchiole and includes the respiratory bronchioles, alveolar ducts, atria and alveoli.

Centrilobular emphysema. The dilatation or destruction is more proximal and involves the respiratory bronchioles. The emphysema is present in the centre of the lobules with the more distal part remaining unchanged. Bronchiolitis is probably the main causative factor.

Aetiology. Emphysema most commonly occurs with longstanding disease of the bronchi, namely chronic bronchitis or chronic asthma, or a combination of the two. At times it may be related to an occupational cause such as exposure to dust, and in coal miners' pneumonoconiosis (p. 231) there is characteristically a centrilobular emphysema ('focal' emphysema.). Occasionally it develops as a primary disease without any previous history of bronchitis.

The actual mechanism of production of emphysema is debated; 'air-trapping' due to widespread narrowing of the bronchioles, and weakening of the respiratory bronchioles and the alveolar walls from inflammation are both likely factors.

Effects on lung function. Emphysematous lung loses its elasticity and thus expiration requires a muscular effort on the part of the patient. Apart from the increased work involved, the forced expiration produces early closure of the diseased respiratory bronchioles and thus enhances the diffuse airflow obstruction already present. The chronic over-inflation of the lungs also leads to increase in the fixed volume of gas in the lungs, the residual volume, with the result that the mixing of inspired air in the lungs is less efficient. These two factors lead to alveolar hypoventilation. In addition, over-ventilation of the under-perfused alveoli (where there is atrophy of the pulmonary capillaries), under-ventilation of normally perfused alveoli (producing a right to left shunt) and reduction in the total surface area of the alveoli all lead to deficiency in the transfer of gases between alveoli and the pulmonary capillaries.

It is now recognised that blood gas abnormalities and cor pulmonale are less likely in 'pure' emphysema (*'pink puffers'*), but do occur if there is accompanying chronic bronchitis, being a particular feature of this disease (*'blue bloaters'*).

Clinical Features. The major symptom is dyspnoea. When emphysema is not too advanced there is likely to be only moderate shortness of breath on exertion. With progression of the disease the patient eventually becomes unable to walk more than a few steps. Quite frequently the breath is exhaled through pursed lips. The rate of progress of the disease is variable. Frequently it is slow, the patient reaching old age with only moderate disability. Sometimes it is rapid, the patient becoming a complete respiratory cripple by middle life. Occasionally the onset of severe disability is apparently sudden. This is usually precipitated by fog or a respiratory tract infection, the patient not admitting to significant symptoms beforehand.

With well-established emphysema, the chest appears over-inflated, with thoracic kyphosis, increase in the antero-posterior diameter of the chest, and horizontal ribs. Chest expansion is diminished, the chest being lifted up by the accessory muscles of respiration rather than expanded. The percussion note is hyper-resonant and the areas of cardiac and liver dullness are diminished. The breath sounds are faint, often with prolonged expiration. Rhonchi and râles may be present, indicating bronchial disease. Respiratory function tests show impaired ventilation with airflow obstruction (p. 181), increased residual volume (p. 180), uneven ventilation (p. 182), and impaired gas transfer (p. 183). In advanced cases with associated chronic bronchitis hypoxia causes cyanosis, and the presence of cor pulmonale produces additional signs (p. 198).

The *chest radiograph* may be normal unless emphysema is well developed. In such cases the lung fields appear unduly translucent with atrophy of the peripheral vessels. The main pulmonary arteries are large and the heart thin and vertical. Bullae may be visible as localised areas of increased translucency. The ribs are horizontal and the diaphragm depressed and flattened.

Treatment. (1) *To improve the airways and prevent progression of the disease.* Treatment of bronchial infection and bronchospasm are dealt with under chronic bronchitis (p. 195) and asthma (p. 204).

(2) *To make full use of the remaining lung tissue.* This is best achieved by *breathing exercises.* Most subjects with emphysema breathe with the upper part of the chest and hardly use the diaphragm at all. Exercises teach the patient to use the diaphragm and lower ribs more efficiently.

(3) *Heart failure from cor pulmonale.* For treatment see p. 199.

Compensatory Emphysema

When a section of lung contracts by fibrosis or collapse, or is removed surgically, the rest of that lung expands by over-inflation to fill the space. This is known as compensatory emphysema and is not usually associated with any defect of function.

Unilateral Emphysema

Unilateral translucency of a lung may be due to a large bulla or cyst, or be due to compensatory emphysema as a result of a totally collapsed lobe in the lung on that side. It also occurs when there is over-inflation of a lung due to partial obstruction of a major bronchus; this can produce a 'ball-valve' mechanism so that air enters on inspiration but is trapped in the lung on expiration. This is likely to be due to a bronchial neoplasm in an adult and to pressure from tuberculous glands in a child. *Unilateral emphysema* (Macleod's syndrome) may follow an obliterative bronchiolitis occurring in early childhood; this arrests development of the lung which normally proceeds until the age of 8 years. The affected lung has both diminished ventilation and poor perfusion; the chest X-rays shows attenuated vessels and an expiration film will show failure of the lung to deflate with shift of the mediastinum to the opposite side.

RESPIRATORY FAILURE

The function of the lungs may be so impaired by various diseases that oxygenation of the blood becomes seriously deficient; this is respiratory failure. It is associated with central cyanosis and with low oxygen and with high carbon dioxide tensions in the arterial blood, and with respiratory acidosis (p. 182). It may be due to *depression of the respiratory centre* by poisons, drugs, anoxia or cerebral disease; to *failure of the respiratory muscles* as in poliomyelitis, acute infectious polyneuritis and myaesthenia gravis; to *loss of functioning lung* as in extensive pneumonia, pulmonary collapse, pneumothorax or following surgical lung resection; to *obstruction of airways* as in status asthmaticus or severe bronchitis.

Patients with chronic lung disease are especially prone to respiratory failure with any of the above complications, which may occur separately or in combination.

Respiratory failure can occur independently of cor pulmonale, although it may precipitate it.

Treatment is directed at the underlying cause. *Respiratory stimulants* (p. 200) are indicated when there is depression of the respiratory centre. *Oxygen therapy* (p. 199) and some form of *assisted respiration* may be essential to maintain life. *Tracheostomy* may be required. It improves ventilation by reducing dead space and airway resistance and enables sputum to be sucked out of the air passages in a patient unable to cough adequately. It may be combined, using a cuffed endotracheal tube, with positive-pressure ventilation, but such treatment needs careful management and it is only feasible in specialised units. One of the disadvantages of assisted respiration is that it may not be possible to wean patients with chronic lung disease from the respirator or the tracheostomy.

COR PULMONALE

This is cardiovascular disease secondary to disease of the lungs. It occurs most commonly with chronic bronchitis and emphysema; also with chronic asthma and with diffuse fibrosis of the lungs due to such diseases as sarcoidosis and the pneumoconioses. It may follow the longstanding deficient ventilation of severe kyphoscoliosis or gross obesity.

It is mostly precipitated by a respiratory tract infection, which increases the severity of respiratory failure causing *hypoxia* and carbon dioxide retention (*hypercarbia*). The abnormal blood gases produce impairment of renal function with retention of sodium and water, increase in blood volume and at first a rise in cardiac output. The systemic arterioles are dilated with warm extremities and bounding pulse, and dilatation of the cerebral vessels may produce headache and even papilloedema. The effect of the hypoxia on the pulmonary arterioles, however, is to produce active vasoconstriction. This, combined with obliteration of these vessels by disease and with the increase in cardiac output, produces pulmonary hypertension. It is only in the later stages of the disease, if pulmonary hypertension becomes severe or if the heart muscle is seriously affected by anoxia, that the cardiac output falls.

Clinical Features. The patient is cyanosed, with signs of chronic bronchitis and emphysema. The extremities are warm but cyanosed, and the pulse full. The venous pressure in the neck is raised, the liver enlarged and there is dependent oedema. The heart sounds are often difficult to hear due to the overlying emphysematous lung, but it may be possible to detect triple rhythm. With gross enlargement of the right ventricle a right ventricular heave may be palpable and the systolic murmur of functional tricuspid incompetence be heard, with systolic pulsation of the neck veins. Proteinuria and a raised blood urea may be present. If the cardiac output falls, the extremities become cold and the pulse small; venous congestion and oedema increase and signs of right ventricular hypertophy and dilatation are more obvious.

An electrocardiogram shows the large sharply-pointed P-waves of right atrial hypertrophy and there may be signs of right ventricular hypertrophy. The heart is usually vertical.

Radiography shows dilatation of the main pulmonary arteries with cardiac enlargement. The lung fields may show evidence of emphysema.

Treatment is primarily directed at improving alveolar ventilation.

Bronchial infection is treated with an effective antibiotic, such as ampicillin or tetracycline 250 mg. four times daily.

Bronchospasm is best treated by aminophylline, either intravenously or by rectal suppository and a course of corticosteroids may be indicated.

Oxygen therapy is required for acute respiratory failure and highest concentrations can be achieved by using an oxygen tent or B.L.B. mask. However, in patients with cor pulmonale and chronic carbon dioxide retention the respiratory centre may depend on oxygen lack for its stimulation and treatment with high concentrations of oxygen may produce respiratory depression with increasing CO_2 retention; the patient becoming drowsy or comatose. For this reason it is best to use oxygen in a concentration of 28 per cent by a mask using the Venturi principle (Ventimask or Venturi head tent), or by using a nasal catheter with a flow rate of 4 litres/min. This method should produce a pO_2 level of above 50 mm.Hg., which is usually considered safe. Even this method of oxygen administration can cause increasing CO_2 retention during the first few days, and a watch must be kept for CO_2 narcosis; estimations of blood gases and pH are invaluable (see p. 182). If respiratory depression does occur, *respiratory stimulants* should be used. These arouse the patient, increase the ventilation and induce coughing. Nikethamide is effective, and is given intravenously, either by intermittent injections (2 ml.), or by continuous infusion; too large a dose may produce twitching or convulsions.

Physiotherapy is important to assist the patient to clear the air passages of secretions.

Assisted positive pressure ventilation with cuffed endotracheal tubes or with tracheostomy may be lifesaving for the patient with some chronic lung disease whose air passages fill with mucopurulent secretions due to an acute respiratory infusion; they should seldom be employed for uncomplicated chronic lung disease, as it may be impossible ever to wean the patient from them.

Diuretics (p. 114) should be given for dependent oedema and may improve alveolar ventilation by eliminating pulmonary oedema. *Digitalis* is disappointing in cor pulmonale but is indicated if atrial fibrillation is present.

Sedation. All hypnotics are potentially dangerous because of the liability of producing respiratory depression. Morphia is contra-indicated. Treatment should be directed at relieving anoxia which is the cause of restlessness and mental confusion. However, when these symptoms are severe chloral hydrate or intramuscular paraldehyde are the safest drugs.

BRONCHIECTASIS

The essential pathological change in bronchiectasis is dilatation of the bronchi. It usually results from pulmonary collapse or as a complication of various types of pneumonia. In many patients the disease follows an attack of pneumonia complicating one of the childhood fevers, particularly whooping cough or measles. Plugging of some of the bronchi by sticky mucus lends to absorption collapse and dilatation of the bronchi in the related portion of the lung. At this stage the process is reversible if the obstructing plugs of mucus are removed by vigorous physiotherapy, that is by firm percussion on chest wall combined with postural drainage and 'assisted' coughing. If the bronchial plugging is allowed to persist for any length of time, however, inflammatory changes develop in the walls of the dilated bronchi and lead to permanent bronchiectasis.

Bronchiectasis also develops distal to a chronic bronchial obstruction, such as bronchial carcinoma or bronchostenosis. Pressure of tuberculous nodes on a bronchus, from childhood primary tuberculosis (p. 223), may lead to bronchiectasis in later life. This most commonly affects the middle lobe, producing the *middle lobe (Brock) syndrome*.

Pulmonary infection which heals by fibrosis, particularly tuberculosis of the upper lobes, commonly leads to associated bronchiectasis.

Sometimes an infective bronchiolitis results in a progressive form of the disease in the absence of pulmonary collapse. A similar wisespread bronchiectasis commonly develops from a suppurating bronchiolitis in patients with fibrocystic disease of the pancreas.

Clinical Features. The clinical features of bronchiectasis are variable and depend on the extent of the disease and the degree of infection in the affected bronchi.

(1) *Classical Bronchiectasis.* There is a history of recurrent episodes of pneumonia in childhood—the first often occurring after an attack of whooping cough or measles. The patient has a cough productive of a considerable volume of purulent sputum which may sometimes contain blood. In the winter there are exacerbations of the condition with increased cough and sputum and with fever, and recurrent attacks of pneumonia may occur. Examination shows a thin patient who looks ill. Dyspnoea and cyanosis are present if sufficient volume of lung is involved. The fingers are often clubbed. Examination of the chest usually shows signs of fibrosis (see p. 189) and of retained bronchial secretions over the affected lobe or lobes. The physical signs may be few, perhaps only an area of persistent râles, if healthy lung separates the diseased segments from the chest wall. If the patient is encouraged to cough, large quantities of foul sputum are expectorated, and his breath may, in addition, always smell foul. Such is the picture of classical bronchiectasis, but the majority of patients with this disease present in less dramatic form.

(2) *Other Types of Bronchiectasis.* Some patients with bronchiectasis have no symptoms at all, particularly those with bronchiectasis of the upper lobes where drainage is continuous. Such bronchiectasis is frequently the result of old tuberculous infection. In others recurrent haemoptysis, sometimes profuse, is the only symptom. Sometimes infection occurs only in the winter following upper respiratory infection and for the rest of the year the patient is well. In such patients there may be no physical signs, or simply a persistent patch of râles over the bronchiectatic lobes.

Complications of Bronchiectasis. Patients are prone to recurrent attacks of pneumonia either in the affected lobe or in another part of the lung due to 'spill-over' of infected sputum. Spread of bronchiectasis and lung fibrosis may follow. Lung abscess and empyema may also occur. Haematogenous spread, from infected thrombus in a pulmonary venous radicle, may lead to cerebral abscess. If infection has been extensive and prolonged, amyloid disease may develop, but is now rarely seen.

Diagnosis. The chest radiograph may show no abnormality; more commonly there is some increased striation in the bronchiectatic lobe due to crowding of the blood vessels and cysts with fluid levels may be seen. Abnormal shadowing will be present if there is much associated fibrosis, with compensatory emphysema in the surrounding lung. The diagnosis of bronchiectasis is confirmed and its extent determined by *bronchography*. Radio-opaque iodised oil is introduced into the bronchi to make them opaque to X-rays. The right bronchial tree is outlined first and both postero-anterior and lateral views are obtained. The left lur g is then filled and an oblique view taken. The diseased bronchi appear dilated, their walls are often irregular and their outline blurred.

Treatment. Management depends on the careful assessment of the patient's history and the extent of the bronchiectasis.

Surgical Treatment. Young patients with a history of severe chronic or recurrent lung infection should be considered for surgical treatment, provided that the bronchiectasis is not too extensive, that there is no co-incident asthma and the patient is not breathless due to impaired ventilation. Generally speaking it is possible to resect an area equivalent to one lung, provided the rest of the lung is healthy. If resection is carried out it is important to remove all the bronchiectatic lung, as any residual bronchiectasis will still produce symptoms and act as a focus from which the disease can spread. Surgery is contra-indicated in patients in whom the bronchiectasis is caused by a generalised infective bronchiolitis. Removal of an affected portion of a lung will not prevent spread of the disease to other lobes.

Medical Treatment. In many cases the disease is not severe enough to warrant surgical treatment. In others the bronchiectasis is too extensive for resection, or the remaining lung is too damaged by chronic bronchitis and emphysema. Sometimes the patient's age or general health make operation impossible. In such cases medical treatment is usually remarkably effective, though clearly it cannot be curative.

The symptoms can nearly always be satisfactorily controlled and the complications largely prevented by regular and competent *postural drainage*. The patient is taught the position in which secretions will drain from the bronchiectatic area towards the main bronchi and the trachea. This enables sputum to be coughed up. The lower lobes are affected in the majority of patients. Postural drainage for this lobe is achieved by leaning face downwards over the side of the bed with the hands on the floor. Alternatively the foot of the bed is raised on 18-inch blocks, the patient lying on his face or side, according to the segments affected. Postural drainage of the right middle lobe is achieved by placing the patient on his back with a pillow under the right side of the chest and the foot of the bed is slightly raised. With upper lobe bronchiectasis, drainage will take place if the patient is sitting up, leaning towards the unaffected side. The appropriate position must be adopted for at least 10 minutes twice a day, and forcible coughing should be continued until no more sputum will come up. Drainage of the secretions can often be improved by 'clapping' on the chest over the affected lobe. The physiotherapist or the nurse may carry out this procedure, but later the patient's relatives will have to be instructed. Postural drainage should be carried out first thing in the morning as sputum collects in the dilated bronchi during the night. It should also be performed before retiring to bed and it may be necessary to repeat it before the midday and evening meals. A hot drink given before each treatment may increase expectoration.

A course of ampicillin or tetracycline, 250 mg. six-hourly, for one or two weeks may be given if the purulent sputum becomes more profuse, particularly if the patient also has fever and malaise. Sometimes continuous antibiotic treatment over the winter months may be considered. In patients with foul sputum there is often infection with the anaerobic organisms of Vincent's angina (Vincent's spirillum and the fusiform bacillus) and penicillin is the antibiotic of choice. No treatment is necessary in patients whose bronchiectasis is symptomless and without evidence of infection.

ASTHMA

Patients with bronchial asthma suffer attacks of wheezing and difficulty in breathing, due to bronchial spasm and sticky secretions. The cause of the disease is complex, and in most patients several factors contribute to its development.

In *extrinsic* (allergic) asthma both heredity and allergic factors predominate, and the condition usually starts in earlier life. A type I (anaphalactoid) hypersensitivity mechanism operates; inhaled allergen combines with reaginic antibody fixed to cells in the bronchial mucosa and damage to the cells releases histamine and various other spasmogens. Reaginic antibody has been identified with the immunoglobulin IgE. *Intrinsic* (late-onset) asthma usually occurs in later life. Allergy is usually not important and the condition is more often associated with bronchitis and psychological factors.

(1) *Heredity.* When asthma starts in childhood or adolescence there is more likely to be a family history of an allergic disorder, such as hay fever, asthma or urticaria. Migraine in a parent is common.

(2) *Allergy.* There are a large number of substances to which the asthmatic may become allergic. They may be inhaled from the atmosphere or absorbed from the gut. The inhalants are the most important. Common examples are pollen and spores from plants, moulds (such as aspergillus fumigatus and dry rot), dust of various kinds (such as house dust which contains mites which live on scales of human skin), animal hair, face powder, and dandruff. Foodstuffs are less often to blame, but eggs, milk, fish, particularly shell-fish, certain fruits, and chocolate may induce attacks.

The history is the best guide to the part that allergy plays. Eosinophilia suggests that allergy is important. If attacks occur only in the spring and early summer it is reasonable to suspect that pollens are responsible; or attacks may be induced by a particular food, by a drug, such as aspirin, or by proximity to a cat or dog. Skin tests can also be done. A drop of a specially prepared solution of the suspected allergen is placed on the skin and a superficial scratch made through it. The result is positive if a raised wheal appears within 15 minutes. Skin testing is much less helpful in the investigation and treatment of asthma than a carefully taken history. Allergy is more important in asthma starting in early life.

(3) *Infection.* When asthma starts later in life it often appears to be complicated by chronic bronchitis and allergy is much less prominent. Respiratory tract infections, however, often precipitate asthma in asthmatic patients in whom allergy is also much in evidence.

(4) *Reflex Factors.* The bronchi are supplied by the vagus nerve, and various stimuli may induce attacks by a reflex mechanism. Common examples are sudden exposure to cold air, laughing, severe exertion, and heavy meals.

(5) *Psychological Influences* play some part in nearly every asthmatic and quite often they appear to be mainly responsible, if not in starting the asthma, at least in maintaining it. Anxieties of various kinds, a sense of frustration or frequently discord and an atmosphere of tension in the home, often underly the tension in the bronchi. Treatment is not likely to be satisfactory unless these influences are appreciated and the patient handled with sympathetic understanding, tact, and firmness, and the difficulties eased as much as possible.

Clinical Features. An asthmatic attack usually starts fairly suddenly and lasts about an hour or so, but the duration varies a good deal. Many asthmatics have a bad spell lasting some weeks, when they may be continuously rather wheezy with frequent acute exacerbations, especially during the night. A severe attack lasting more than a day or so is known as *status asthmaticus.* During an attack the patient complains of tightness in the chest and difficulty in breathing. There is often cough, dry at first, but towards the end of an attack some sticky, tight little pellets of mucus are produced. The sputum is purulent when there is associated respiratory tract infection or when it contains large numbers of cosinophils. On examination the chest is over-inflated and there are widespread rhonchi, particularly on expiration.

The structure and function of the lungs return to normal between attacks. However, patients with long-standing severe asthma often develop emphysema and are then persistently short of breath.

Treatment. (a) *During Attacks.* An attack can usually be stopped by sucking $\frac{1}{2}$–1 tablet (10–20 mg.) of *isoprenaline sulphate* or by the subcutaneous injection of about 0·5 ml. of 1:1,000 *adrenaline.* These methods have been mostly supplanted by the use of pressurised aerosols, of which there are a number of proprietary preparations containing isoprenaline, orciprenaline or salbutamol and which are both more convenient and more efficient then the hand pump. The patient must be carefully instructed in its use; after breathing out fully the vapour is then inhaled and the breath held for a short period to allow absorption to take place. A single dose taken at the onset of an attack will often abort it; but patients must be warned that repeated use of the aerosol in established asthma may be extremely dangerous. Another valuable drug for severe attacks is intravenous *aminophylline* 0·25–0·5 g. in 10–20 ml. sterile water.

Severe status asthmaticus which has failed to respond to these drugs is a potentially fatal illness. Although the patient is exhausted by sleeplessness and by the effort expended on breathing, on no account must morphine or any other opium derivative be given. The resulting depression of respiration is liable to cause death. Any hypnotic is best avoided, but if restlessness is increasing the exhaustion to a dangerous extent, paraldehyde 4–8 ml. intramuscularly is the safest drug. *Steroids* may be lifesaving. Prednisolone is given 50 mg. on the first day, 30 mg. on the next day and 20 mg. subsequently. A more rapid response may be obtained by giving I.V. hydrocortisone 200 mg. three hourly. Improvement usually occurs within a day or so. It is then best to tail off the steroids as long-term treatment is best avoided unless really essential. Status asthmaticus is likely to be associated with infection, either as a precipitating factor or as a secondary feature, and an antibiotic, such as tetracycline, is indicated.

(b) *Between attacks* the treatment of each patient has to be planned after careful assessment of the various possible causative factors indicated above. The aim of treatment is prevention, for the longer the patient can be kept free of attacks the less likely asthma is to return.

The psychological handling of the patient is of the utmost importance. The doctor must be a good and sympathetic listener and an atmosphere of calm confidence must be preserved at all times.

It is advisable for the asthmatic to avoid contact with various substances to which he is or may become allergic; the bedroom should be bare and spartan, containing no cushions, curtains or other soft furnishings which harbour dust; feather quilts should be avoided, and sorbo rubber substitutes should be used in place of feather pillows and hair mattresses. When there is clear-cut allergy—for example, to pollen—specific desensitisation may be attempted. This is done by giving injections of a solution of the allergen once a week, starting with a very small dose and gradually increasing it until the patient is able to tolerate quite a large dose, or in other words has become desensitised. Alternatively, less frequent injections of a depot vaccine may be used. The patient must be kept under observation for at least half an hour after each injection. Syringes containing 1:1,000 adrenaline must be available, and an injection of 0·5 ml. of adrenaline and 10 mg. of chlorpheniramine given at once if the patient develops any reaction, such as wheezing or faintness. If a reaction occurs at the next injection the does is reduced slightly, and then steadily increased again over the following weeks. Desensitisation against pollens must be completed before the end of April, as severe and even fatal reactions may occur if injections are given when pollens are present in the atmosphere.

Regular administration of *ephedrine* is helpful for the prevention of attacks, young children being given 15 mg. twice or three times daily and older children or adults a dose of 30–60 mg. Ephedrine has a cerebral stimulating effect and if used at bedtime it may be necessary to combine it with a barbiturate to ensure sleep. It may also cause difficulty in micturition in elderly men with prostatic hypertrophy. It is best to continue ephedrine for a month or two. *Choline theophyllinate* 200 mg. four times daily is of value at times. A rectal suppository of aminophylline, 0·36 g., before sleep often prevents a troublesome attack at night. The allergy blocker *disodium cromoglycate* 1 to 4 capsules a day may be of great value in patients with *extrinsic* (allergic) asthma. It is administered by inhalation using a Spinhaler. When emotional factors are important tranquillisers may be used.

All asthmatics should be taught *breathing exercises* which should be carried out regularly.

Some patients with chronic asthma usually of late onset, are controlled only by continuous steroid therapy and in them the dangers of such treatment are outweighed by the benefits. Initial dosage of 30–40 mg. prednisolone daily is gradually reduced to the minimum effective level, usually between 5 and 10 mg.

CARCINOMA OF THE BRONCHUS

This disease has become much more common in recent years. It is now the commonest type of cancer in men, in whom it occurs four or five times more frequently than in women. The reports from the Royal College of Physicians and others have emphasised the importance of cigarette smoking as a cause of bronchial carcinoma. There is also some evidence that the incidence is higher in those who live in the polluted atmosphere of industrial areas. An increased incidence is reported in miners exposed to dust from chromium, nickel, and radioactive ores, and pulmonary asbestosis is said to increase its incidence by fifteenfold. About half the tumours arise within an inch or two of the bifurcation of the trachea. The remainder are peripheral. Histologically they are most frequently anaplastic (oat cell carcinoma) and squamous carcinoma, but adeno-carcinoma also occurs.

Clinical Features. A dry cough is the commonest early symptom. Recurrent haemoptysis may result from ulceration and sometimes this is the presenting symptom. Mucopurulent sputum occurs as increase in size of the growth produces progressive bronchial obstruction, then distal infection and shortness of breath develop with collapse of the lung segment supplied by the affected bronchus. A presistent wheeze due to the narrowed bronchus and dull deep-seated pain are common symptoms. Some patients are symptom free when the disease is discovered by mass radiography or remain so until one of the **complications** occurs. These are:

(1) *Pneumonic Infection.* The segment of lung beyond the bronchial obstruction is particularly liable to infection. Patients may present with a seg-

mental pneumonia, which either fails to resolve satisfactorily or recurs repeatedly in the same area of lung. Such events should always raise suspicion of an underlying carcinoma.

(2) *Collapse*. Complete obstruction of a bronchus by carcinoma produces collapse of the lung segment supplied by that bronchus. The collapsed lung may become infected causing fever and toxaemia, but there may be little or no sputum because of the bronchial obstruction. Collapse may be associated with a pleural effusion on the same side, with the result that there is no mediastinal shift.

(3) *Lung abscess* may develop in an area of pneumonic infection (see above). When the growth is in the periphery of the lung its centre may become necrotic and be coughed up. This produces a ragged abscess cavity with walls which are composed of carcinomatous tissue, and which characteristically are thick and irregular when seen on a radiograph.

(4) *Superior vena caval obstruction* may occur from pressure of a growth in this situation. The patient complains of fullness in the head and face and may be in acute discomfort. There is oedema of the face and upper limbs, with gross distension of the neck veins and anastomotic veins over the upper part of the chest. Other causes of this syndrome are aneurysm of the ascending aorta, malignant mediastinal glands and haemorrhage into a retrosternal thyroid.

(5) *Local Spread and Pleural Effusion*. Carcinoma cells may invade the mediastinal lymph nodes and the pleura, giving rise to a pleural effusion which is often, but by no means invariably, bloodstained.

(6) *Atrial fibrillation* may occur due to direct involvement of the atria and sometimes is a presenting symptom.

Spread of the growth to the pericardium may produce a pericardial effusion.

(7) *Distant Metastasis*. Bronchial carcinoma may metastasise to the liver, the bones, the suprarenals, the brain, the skin, and the lymphatic glands, the deposits causing symptoms and signs referable to the organs affected. When neoplasm is suspected and the primary focus is not apparent, the chest should be examined clinically and radiologically for carcinoma of the bronchus.

(8) *The Nervous System*. Tumours occurring at the apex of the lung may involve the lower part of the brachial plexus producing Horner's syndrome (see p. 251) together with pain down the arm with weakness and wasting (Pancoast's tumour). Both laryngeal and diaphragmatic palsy may occur due to invasion of the recurrent laryngeal and phrenic nerves. Carcinoma of the lung may present with cerebral metastases, and a chest radiograph should always be taken when a cerebral tumour is suspected. Occasionally patients with carcinoma of the bronchus develop neuropathies or myopathies or cerebellar degeneration (p. 312), the causes of which are unknown.

(9) *Endocrine*. Rarely Cushing's syndrome may be caused by a tumour producing an ACTH-like substance; or the tumour may produce an

'inappropriate' secretion of anti-diuretic hormone (ADH) with water retention and hyponatraemia; or a severe renal sodium-losing state may occur with profound weakness. Hypercalcaemia may also occur due to production of a parathormone-like substance.

Physical Signs. There may be no abnormal signs in the chest in spite of well-marked symptoms or obvious metastases. The changes when present may be those of collapse, pneumonia, lung abscess, or pleural effusion. A combination of effusion with collapse is very common. Clubbing of the fingers is frequent and hypertrophic pulmonary osteoarthropathy sometimes occurs; this causes pain and swelling in the fingers which may suggest rheumatoid arthritis, but the radiograph shows typical subperiostial new bone formation. The condition regresses if the carcinoma is resected. A careful examination should be made for secondary deposits in the liver and the lymphatic glands, particularly cervical and supraclavicular.

Diagnosis. A patient presenting with any of the above features should have radiological examination of the chest. This will confirm the presence of collapse, consolidation, effusion, or abscess cavity, or may show a mass spreading out from the hilum, or a peripheral mass.

If the diagnosis remains in doubt the patient should be bronchoscoped, and a biopsy of the suspected lesion removed for microscopy. Biopsy of scalene nodes or of clinically enlarged glands may confirm the diagnosis. Bronchoscopy will be essential if surgery is contemplated in order to assess the extent of the growth and its operability. Expert examination of the sputum for cancer cells is positive in 80 per cent of cases.

Treatment. The main hope of cure lies in *surgical removal* of the affected lobe or lung. Unfortunately, many patients cannot be treated in this way, either because the carcinoma has already metastasised or is too extensive, or because the patient is not fit enough to withstand the operation. With successful removal the five-year survival rate is about 20 per cent.

Radiotherapy can be used to produce a remission in patients unsuitable for surgery and for oat cell carcinoma is probably just as effective as surgery. It is extremely unlikely to destroy the growth, although occasional cures have been reported. More commonly it is used to relieve symptoms. It is of value in patients with superior mediastinal obstruction, and in those with haemoptysis, persistent cough or severe pain from bone metastases. It is best avoided in patients generally ill with advanced disease, or with large tumours, as it is likely to make them worse.

Cytotoxic drugs, e.g. cyclophosphamide, may also produce a temporary remission.

The average survival rate of patients without treatment is about nine months from the onset of symptoms.

ADENOMA OF THE BRONCHUS

Bronchial adenoma is a benign tumour either a true adenoma or more often a carcinoid tumour. It rarely undergoes malignant change. It is much less common than carcinoma of the bronchus and occurs more often in women. It may present as recurrent haemoptysis or as bronchial obstruction with lobar infection. Diagnosis is confirmed by bronchoscopy. The adenoma should be removed surgically, usually with the affected lobe.

HAMARTOMA

This benign tumour of the lung is composed of a mixture of tissues normally present in the lung, particularly cartilage. It usually produces no symptoms and is discovered on the chest radiograph as a rounded opacity with clear-cut edges. There may be areas of calcification. It is usually removed surgically as it is difficult to distinguish it radiographically from a peripheral bronchial carcinoma or a tuberculoma.

THE PNEUMONIAS

Classification can be based both on the nature of the infecting organism and on the anatomical distribution of the pneumonia.

(1) *Lobar pneumonia* is pneumonic consolidation confined to one or more lobes of the lung. It is due to infection by specific organisms such as virulent *pneumococci* and *Friedländer's bacillus*. Infections with *staphylococcus aureus* and *m. tuberculosis* may produce lobular or lobar pneumonia.

(2) *Bronchopneumonia* is consolidation occurring in patches around infected terminal bronchi. It may be confined to a small segment of lung, or with widespread bronchial involvement the infection will be scattered throughout the lungs. It is most often caused by organisms such as *streptococci, haemophilus influenzae* and non-epidemic strains of *pneumococci*. These are normally present in the upper respiratory tract and can spread down the air passages to infect the terminal bronchi. The very young, the elderly and the debilitated are particularly prone and it is often the terminal event in a seriously ill patient. Bronchopneumonia is often the result of secondary bacterial invasion following an acute viral bronchitis.

Influenza may at times cause a fulminating bronchopneumonia due to super-added infection with *staphylococcus aureus,* or less frequently with the *pneumococcus, haemophilus influenzae* or the *haemolytic streptococcus.* In the early stages, *tuberculosis* starts as a localised patch of bronchopneumonia, but widespread *tuberculous bronchopneumonia* may occur.

(3) *Acute Virus or Rickettsial Pneumonias.* Pneumonia associated with influenza or measles is usually complicated by bacterial infection. There is a further group of virus and Rickettsial infections including ornithosis, Q fever and others which cause a patchy pneumonia.

(4) *Inhalation Pneumonias.* These vary from a small patch of collapse-consolidation associated with a viral respiratory tract infection to severe suppurative infection following inhalation of infected material.

(5) *Pneumonias secondary to disease of the bronchi*, such as bronchial carcinoma (p. 206) or bronchiectasis (p. 200).

BACTERIAL PNEUMONIAS

Pneumococcal Pneumonia

Clinical Features. Pneumococcal lobar pneumonia may occur at any age; it is quite a common terminal event in the lives of the elderly or infirm, but it may equally attack people in the prime of life. It is more common in the winter months, and usually occurs sporadically. It is due to infection with virulent strains of pneumococci.

The onset is usually sudden with shivering or even a rigor and sometimes vomiting. The temperature rises abruptly and fever remains continuous. The face is typically hot and flushed and cyanosis may be marked. The respiration rate rises out of proportion to the temperature. An acute dry pleurisy develops over the affected lobe leading to severe pain on respiration, so that the breathing becomes rapid, shallow, and sometimes grunting. The development of herpes on the lips completes the classical picture. A painful cough is common at this stage of the disease and the sputum may have a 'rusty' tinge.

Examination of the chest at the onset usually shows little except diminished movement on the affected side together with reduced breath sounds, and perhaps some râles or a pleural rub. After the first 24–48 hours, the signs of consolidation appear; dullness, bronchial breathing, whispering pectoriloquy, and bronchophony over the consolidated lobe. There is a polymorphonuclear leucocytosis.

In the days before antibiotics were available recovery occurred by crisis at about the seventh day, the temperature falling quite rapidly and the patient's general condition taking a sudden turn for the better. Antibiotic treatment modifies the course of the disease and the patient's condition usually begins to improve within 48 hours of starting treatment. As the signs of consolidation disappear they are replaced by coarse râles due to the liquefying inflammatory exudate.

In the elderly, lobar pneumonia may not produce the dramatic picture outlined above. There may be little fever and the diagnosis depends on finding signs of consolidation.

Chest radiography confirms the presence of lobar consolidation.

Complications

(1) *Delayed Resolution.* The time taken for the lung to return to normal, with disappearance of physical signs and radiological clearing, varies a good deal in different patients. If resolution is delayed for more than two or three weeks the possibility of some underlying condition such as carcinoma or bronchiectasis must be investigated. Alternatively the pneumonia may be due to organisms resistant to the antibiotic in use, such as the tubercle bacillus. This will require careful and perhaps repeated examination of the sputum. Bronchoscopy and bronchography may be required. Pneumonia responds slowly to treatment in patients with diabetes, cirrhosis, chronic alcoholism, or nephritis.

There remains a small group of patients in whom the pneumonia instead of resolving proceeds to fibrosis and chronic suppuration. Postural drainage and inhalations should be used, but the affected lobe may require surgical resection.

(2) *Effusions.* Since the advent of chemotherapy, empyemata have become uncommon but serous pleural effusions appearing about one to two weeks after the onset of the pneumonia continue to occur. Treatment is by daily aspiration with infusion of 500,000 units of benzylpenicillin into the pleural cavity until the fluid subsides. The pleural fluid should be cultured for organisms and systemic antibiotics should be continued. The site of the aspiration is determined by the position of the physical signs and by radiography. The majority of serous effusions subside within a week or so of treatment.

(3) *Empyema.* In a small proportion of patients the effusion becomes purulent and the patient's condition deteriorates. Fever recurs and becomes remittent in type. The patient looks ill and suffers from anorexia, malaise, and drenching sweats. Examination of the chest reveals signs of fluid (p. 189). A white count shows considerable polymorph leucocytosis. The diagnosis is confirmed by aspirating pus from the pleural cavity. Empyema is considered further on page 240.

(4) *Heart Failure.* Cardiac failure complicated perhaps by cardiac arrhythmia, particularly atrial fibrillation, may occur in elderly patients. For treatment see page 111.

(5) *Other complications* include pericarditis, endocarditis, and meningitis. Certain patients have severe headache and some neck stiffness in the early stages of pneumonia, although the cerebrospinal fluid is normal. The syndrome is sometimes called meningismus.

Staphylococcal Pneumonia

Clinical Features. Staphylococcal pneumonia may occur at any age, but usually affects children and young adults. It may occur as a primary infection or as a complication of influenza. It is often part of a staphylococcal septicaemia and there may be a history of a recent boil or some other staphylococcal infection. Pulmonary infarcts may be secondarily infected with staphylococci.

The onset is often acute with malaise, vomiting, anorexia, and rigors. Pleurisy may occur. The sputum is purulent and may be bloodstained. Fever is characteristically remittent.

The *physical signs* are variable and often inconspicuous. They are often bilateral with patches of impaired resonance, reduced breath sounds and râles. Bronchial breathing may be present. *Radiography* of the chest confirms the presence of patchy consolidation and may also show cyst-like abscesses associated with the consolidation. These are distension cysts and are typical of staphylococcal pneumonia. Empyema and spontaneous pneumothorax may also occur.

It is often striking that a lung riddled with pneumonia and abscesses can resolve completely with antibiotic treatment, but residual areas of fibrosis and cyst formation are not uncommon. The lung abscesses and pleural infection rarely require surgical treatment.

At times staphylococcal pneumonia complicating influenza becomes a fulminating infection (see p. 213).

The *diagnosis* is confirmed by sputum culture. The sensitivity of the organism to various antibiotics should be determined, as it may be widely resistant.

Friedländer's Pneumonia

Clinical Features. Pneumonia due to Friedländer's bacillus (kl pneumoniae) is rare. It usually presents as lobar consolidation with severe general symptoms. The sputum is typically very sticky and purulent, with a greenish tinge. Friedländer's pneumonia has a tendency to progress to chronic suppuration with abscess formation and fibrosis. The mortality rate is high. The diagnosis is confirmed by finding the organism in the sputum.

Treatment of Specific Bacterial Pneumonias

General. Severe pleuritic pain is best treated with an injection of intramuscular pethidine 100 mg. or subcutaneous morphine 15 mg. The beneficial effects of these drugs in promoting rest far outweigh the dangers of respiratory depression. A persistent unproductive cough may be relieved by linctus pholcodine co. 4–8 ml.

If the patient becomes cyanosed, oxygen should be given. An oxygen tent or mask may frighten or distress the patient and careful explanation and reassurance are important.

Most patients can be allowed up five to seven days after the temperature has become normal, but this will be influenced by the patient's age and the severity of the illness. Breathing exercises should begin when the temperature falls and should be continued through convalescence, the length of which depends on the occupation and the home environment.

Specific Treatment. In practice it is not always easy to be sure of the nature of the organisms and culture of the sputum takes time or may be impracticable.

Pneumococcal Lobar Pneumonia responds satisfactorily to treatment with intramuscular benzylpenicillin 500,000 units 6-hourly.

Alternatively the patient may be treated from the start with ampicillin 250–500 mg. 6-hourly.

The patient usually responds within 48 hours, but treatment should be continued for one to two weeks. If clinical response is satisfactory the treatment can be changed to oral penicillin, such as phenethicillin 250 mg. six-hourly.

Other antibiotics are occasionally required when the patient is sensitive to penicillin or when the organisms are resistant to penicillin, such as may occur in pneumonia complicating chronic bronchitis or bronchiectasis. In these patients it is often advisable to use a 'broad spectrum' antibiotic, such as tetracycline 250 mg. four times a day or trimethoprin-sulphamethoxazole (Septrin-Bactrim) tablets 2 twice daily.

Staphylococcal Pneumonia. Benzylpenicillin is the most effective antibiotic and should be given in doses of 1·0 mega unit intramuscularly sixhourly. Quite frequently, however, infection is due to penicillin-resistant organisms and if the patient is severely ill, there is no time to await the result of sputum culture or the clinical response to benzylpenicillin. Under these circumstances cloxacillin 500 mg. intramuscularly six-hourly should be given in addition. Subsequent antibiotic treatment will depend on the response of the patient and the result of sensitivity tests, and it is advisable to continue treatment for several weeks because of the liability to relapse. If clinical response is satisfactory, cloxacillin can be given by mouth in the later stages of treatment.

Recovery is usual in these severe cases but when staphylococcal infection is associated with *fulminating influenzal pneumonia*, the outlook is grave (p. 209).

Friedländer's Pneumonia is resistant to penicillin but will usually respond to streptomycin 0·75 g. twice daily and tetracycline 250 mg. six-hourly. Many strains of *Kl. pneumoniae* are also sensitive to trimethoprin-sulphamethoxazole, cephaloridine, cephalexin and chloramphenicol. The sensitivity of the organism to antibiotics should be determined whenever possible. If abscess formation or fibrosis ensues, surgical treatment may be required.

Tuberculous Pneumonia

Tuberculosis may rarely present with lobar pneumonia or widespread bronchopneumonia, associated with severe constitutional symptoms. It will fail to respond to penicillin. The sputum of every patient with pneumonia which does not respond to ordinary antibiotic treatment must be examined, and the diagnosis of tuberculous pneumonia will be established by finding the organism.

Treatment is along the usual lines for tuberculosis (see p. 227).

Pneumonia Complicating Influenza

Influenza is sometimes complicated by pneumonia; this is rare when influenza is sporadic, but may become common during epidemics and accounts for the majority of deaths which occur.

Any type of pneumonia may complicate influenza. The most common is a localised aspiration pneumonia (see p. 216) and staphylococcal pneumonia also occurs. Of particular importance is the severe infection called *fulminating influenzal pneumonia*. This is an overwhelming toxaemia due to a combination of infection with the influenzal virus and the staphylococcus aureus. Haemophilus influenzae has also been implicated as the secondary invader.

Clinical Features. The onset of severe pneumonia complicating influenza is rapid, often alarmingly so. The patient has a simple attack of influenza which appears to be progressing in the usual way when over a few hours the condition deteriorates rapidly. The respiration rate becomes rapid, cyanosis appears, sometimes with a typical greyish blue colour (*heliotrope cyanosis*). There may be evidence of circulatory collapse with rising pulse rate and falling blood pressure. Pleuritic pain is uncommon. Examination of the chest shows evidence of patchy consolidation with scattered râles and perhaps an occasional area of bronchial breathing. Leucopenia is common.

Treatment. In *fulminating influenzal pneumonia* treatment must be started before the results of sputum culture are available. Antibiotics are therefore used which are active against both the staphylococcus and the haemophilus influenzae. Benzylpenicillin 1·0 mega units together with cloxacillin 500 mg. and ampicillin 500 mg. intramuscularly six-hourly should be given immediately and subsequent antibiotic treatment will depend on the response of the patient and the result of sensitivity tests. Alternatively the antibiotics may be given by I.V. drip. Most patients require nursing in an oxygen tent. Circulatory collapse with a falling blood pressure is probably due to adrenal failure and may respond to hydrocortisone hemisuccinate 100 mg. intravenously and then cortisone 200 mg. daily for the next few days; the latter should be tailed off as the patient recovers. Intravenously nor-adrenaline may be required.

VIRUS PNEUMONIAS

Most cases of so-called virus pneumonia have, in fact, an area of collapse-consolidation occurring at the time of a viral respiratory tract infection. This is the result of blockage of a bronchus with sputum with superimposed secondary bacterial infection. Infections with viruses, such as the adenovirus and influenza can affect the lungs producing pneumonia, but the roles of primary virus infection and bacterial infection are often in doubt. In these circumstances it is reasonable to give antibiotic treatment as for bacterial infection.

Mycoplasma pneumonia

The organism *Mycoplasma pneumoniae* has features of both a virus and a bacterium. Although it is small and has no cell wall, at the same time it does not require a living organism for culture and is sensitive to the tetracycline group of drugs. It is not sensitive to the penicillins as these depend on their action on the bacterial cell membrane for their antibiotic effect.

Clinical Features. The disease starts with the general symptoms of a virus infection, namely malaise, anorexia, headache, backache, and sometimes depression, followed within a day or two by cough and sometimes pleurisy. Venous thromboses may occur. Examination of the chest usually shows only a patch of râles or perhaps an area of impaired resonance and bronchial breathing. Radiography reveals an area of consolidation having a rather ground glass appearance and of varying distribution. There is no leucocytosis and the blood contains cold agglutinins and will produce non-specific agglutination of the streptococcus MG.

Treatment. Tetracycline should be given in full dosage of 500 mg. six-hourly for a few days followed by 250 mg. six-hourly.

Ornithosis (Psittacosis)

The organism (*Bedsonia*) occurs widely among many species of birds and is intermediate between a virus and a rickettsia. The illness is caught mainly from parrots, budgerigars and canaries. It is an influenza-like illness and the patient may develop patchy consolidation in the lungs. Splenomegaly is common and rose spots resembling those seen in typhoid fever may be found. At times a severe fulminating pneumonia with considerable mortality may develop.

In the early stages the organism can be cultured from the blood or sputum and at a later stage a rising titre of serum antibodies can be demonstrated.

Treamtent. The organism responds to tetracycline which should be given in full doses of 500 mg. four times daily.

Q Fever

The organism (*Rickettsia burneti*) is known to infect domestic animals such as sheep, cows and goats. Human infection probably occurs through drinking raw milk, from inhaling animal dust or from ticks. It is characterised by fever, toxaemia, cough and 'atypical' pneumonia. Q fever endocarditis may also occur.

Treatment. Tetracycline in full doses is effective but response is slow. Treatment may have to be prolonged, particularly with endocarditis when it may have to be continued for six months to a year.

INHALATION PNEUMONIAS

The aspiration of infected material into the lungs may give rise to pneumonia. The distribution of the consolidation depends on the quantity of material inhaled and its nature. If large amounts of highly infected or irritating material are inhaled, as when an anaesthetised patient inhales vomit, a widely distributed and severe bronchopneumonia involving both lungs may result. If a smaller amount of highly infected material is inhaled into a segment of lung it will result in pneumonic consolidation of that segment and unless the aspirated material is coughed up or sucked out and the infection controlled, the consolidation may proceed to abscess formation (see p. 216). Recurrent attacks of inhalation pneumonia, perhaps with abscess formation, are sometimes seen in patients with oesophageal obstruction from achalasia of the cardia or stricture, and are due to spill-over of material from the oesophagus to the bronchi when the patient is asleep.

Much more common is aspiration of infected material from the upper respiratory tract in patients with coryza, sinus infections, or other upper respiratory tract infections. This is sometimes called *aspiration pneumonia* or *pneumonitis,* and abscess formation is unusual.

Aspiration Pneumonitis

Clinical Features. This is the commonest type of pneumonia seen in general practice. It is due to bronchial obstruction by mucus, with subsequent infected lobular or segmental collapse. The mucus is *aspirated* from the upper respiratory tract at the time of a cold or sinus infection, or it may have a bronchial origin at the time of a bronchitis. The clinical picture varies considerably depending on the nature of the accompanying bacterial infection. At one extreme the pneumonitis may be discovered by chance on radiography, there being no localised or constitutional symptoms. With virulent organisms, however, the clinical picture resembles that of the specific bacterial pneumonias. Most commonly, a few days after a cold or bronchitis, the patient's general condition becomes a little worse and there is malaise, cough, continuing fever and sometimes pleuritic pain. Usually the only physical sign is a patch of râles over the affected area. Radiography of the chest shows an opacity due to an area of segmental collapse and consolidation. *Treatment* with ampicillin 500 m.g. four times daily combined with simple postural therapy is usually satisfactory.

LUNG ABSCESS

The *causes* of lung abscess are:

(1) *Inhalation of infected material* into the bronchial tree. This material usually comes from the upper respiratory tract, particularly gross paradonial infection. It is liable to be inhaled when the cough reflux is suppressed during sleep, or when the patient is in a coma or under anaesthesia. Infected pus and blood clots may also be inhaled at the time of dental extractions or tonsillectomy. The material is inhaled into a bronchopulmonary segment and leads to segmental pneumonia which breaks down to form an abscess. The contents are coughed up leaving a chronic abscess cavity usually infected with a mixed group of organisms. If they include various anaerobes such as Vincent's spirillum, the pus may become putrid and lung abscesses are classified into *putrid* and *non-putrid* on this basis. Sometimes the breakdown of lung tissue is very rapid and the state is sometimes called *gangrene of the lung.* Inhalation of foreign bodies or vomit may also cause lung abscesses.

(2) Secondary to breakdown of peripheral carcinoma or to bronchial obstruction from carcinoma or other causes.

(3) Abscesses may develop in the course of various *specific pneumonias*, namely staphylococcal pneumonia, Friedlander's pneumonia and tuberculosis.

(4) Rare causes include extension of an amoebic abscess of the liver through the diaphragm, actinomycosis, infected hydatid cyst, and abscesses developing during the course of a pyaemia.

(5) In a small proportion of patients with lung abscess, *no cause* can be found.

The site of the inhalation lung abscess is influenced by gravity. As the unconscious patient lies usually on his side or back the most dependent segments in these positions are those most frequently affected. These usually include the segments supplied by the axillary branches of the upper lobe bronchi and the apex of the lower lobe.

Clinical Features. These depend on the underlying cause of the abscess. With 'putrid' lung abscess onset of symptoms is usually acute. There may be a history of coma or an anaesthetic in the presence of parodontal infection, or of dental extraction or some other operation on the upper respiratory tract one to three weeks previously. The patient complains of fever, shivering, night sweats, malaise, and anorexia. Pleurisy is quite common. There is usually a cough with mucoid sputum; after some days, the abscess discharges into a bronchus and the patient coughs up large quantities of foul purulent sputum. This may be preceded by a foul smell to the breath and is pathognomonic of lung abscess.

When the abscess has discharged, the patient's general condition may improve but unless adequate treatment is given he continues to cough up large quantities of purulent sputum sometimes mixed with blood. If the abscess is allowed to become chronic there is the risk of cerebral abscess, of blocking of the abscess cavity with rapid deterioration in the patient's condition, and amyloid disease. The abscess may rupture into the pleural cavity leading to an empyema.

Clubbing of the fingers develops. The *signs* over a lung abscess are variable. Usually there is impairment to percussion together with râles and sometimes bronchial breathing; a pleural rub may also be heard. Both postero-anterior and lateral chest radiographs must be taken; the exact segment of lung involved will then be apparent. In the early stages the affected segment is opaque, but when discharge of the abscess has occurred a cavity can be seen containing a fluid level and sometimes a slough. The radiograph of a breaking-down peripheral carcinoma is characteristic, the walls of the abscess cavity being thick and irregular.

The white count shows a polymorphonuclear leucocytosis. The sputum should always be examined bacteriologically as the lung abscess may be secondary to a specific bacterial infection, such as the staphylococcus aureus, Friedländer's bacillus, or m. tuberculosis.

Treatment. Treatment is initially by antibiotics and correct postural drainage. It is usual to start with intramuscular benzylpenicillin 0·5 to 1 mega unit six-hourly, but this may have to be changed depending on the result of the sputum examination or if there is a poor clinical response. The position for postural drainage is determined by the site of the affected segment; treatment must be intense, 4–6 times daily, and the patient must sleep so as to give the abscess dependent drainage.

With this treatment the lung abscess usually resolves. When the response is not satisfactory or when drainage is not occurring freely, bronchoscopy is required to exclude any obstruction to drainage, such as a carcinoma of the lung. External drainage is rarely required.

In the small proportion of patients in whom the abscess fails to heal and who are left with a grossly damaged lobe, resection may be necessary.

PULMONARY COLLAPSE

Collapse of the lung may occur in two ways:

(1) *Absorption Collapse.* If a bronchus either to a whole lung or to a segment of lung becomes completely blocked, then the air in that segment is absorbed into the blood stream and the segment collapses to a smaller size. The space formerly occupied by the collapsed lung must be filled. To achieve this:

   (a) The diaphragm is elevated.
   (b) The mediastinum moves towards the side of the collapsed lung. (see 'palpation' p. 188).
   (c) The remaining lung becomes hyperinflated, a condition known as compensatory emphysema.

(2) *Pneumothorax and Hydrothorax.* If air or fluid is introduced into the pleural space then the elastic tissue in the lung will contract and the lung will collapse to a smaller size, the degree of collapse depending on the volume of air or fluid in the pleural cavity. The mediastinum may be displaced to the opposite side if the pneumothorax or effusion is large.

Absorption Collapse

Bronchial obstruction may be due to several causes; the more important are:

(1) *Bronchial carcinoma,* or rarely bronchial adenoma.
(2) *Foreign material* in the bronchial tree. Mucus or inflammatory exudate may collect following an operation, but is also found in asthma, bronchitis, bronchiectasis, measles, and whooping cough. Sometimes foreign material may be inhaled, for instance blood clot from the mouth following dental extraction, or foreign bodies such as beads, peanuts, or pieces of bone.
(3) *Compression of the bronchus from outside* may occur from enlarged lymph nodes in tuberculosis, sarcoidosis or Hodgkin's disease, or occasionally may be due to aortic aneurysm.

UPPER LOBE OF R. LUNG.

MIDDLE LOBE OF R. LUNG

LOWER LOBE OF R. LUNG

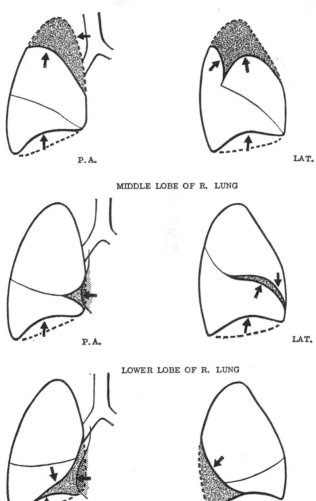

P.A.   LAT.

DIAGRAM OF RADIOGRAPHIC APPEARANCES OF LOBAR ABSORPTION
COLLAPSE.

Both bronchial carcinoma and external compression of the bronchus usually cause collapse of major segments of lung. Mucus may also cause collapse of a major segment, but if inhaled into the finer bronchi may cause multiple small areas of collapse. Absorption collapse is usually followed by some degree of infection and sometimes this may be severe enough to lead to abscess formation (see p. 216). If the lung is not re-expanded within a month, permanent changes occur and the lung does not return to normal.

Clinical Features. The symptoms of collapse depend on the extent of lung involved. They may also be overshadowed by the symptoms of the underlying lung disease.

Obstruction of a large bronchus usually gives rise to dyspnoea, some-times severe, and to a feeling of tightness across the chest. If infection occurs, there will be fever. Examination shows an increase in the pulse and respiration rate and perhaps also some cyanosis. There will be mediastinal shift towards the lesion with dullness to percussion and absent breath sounds over the collapsed area. Smaller segments of collapse may give rise to little in the way of symptoms or physical signs and can only be diagnosed by radiography. The interpretation of radiographs in this condi-tion depends on a knowledge of the anatomy of the bronchopulmonary segments; both postero-anterior and lateral films of the chest are required to localise the collapsed segment.

Treatment. This is directed towards relieving the bronchial obstruction and controlling any pulmonary infection. This in turn depends on the underlying pathology, for often it is due to carcinoma of the bronchus.

In those cases occurring with bronchitis or asthma, where bronchial obstruction is due to a mucus plug, the patient should be positioned so that drainage from the obstructed bronchus is aided by gravity. The chest wall over the collapsed lung should be percussed and the patient encour-aged to cough. Using these methods the plug is usually dislodged. Rarely, aspiration through a bronchoscope is required.

Post-operative Absorption Collapse is due to blocking of a bronchus by a mucus plug. A number of factors render this likely to occur:

(1) It is more common after abdominal and chest operations, for these make coughing painful and interfere with the clearing of mucus from the bronchi.

(2) Infections of the respiratory tract, such as a cold or bronchi-tis, increase bronchial secretions.

(3) The use of excessive amounts of atropine makes the sputum viscid and more difficult to clear from the bronchi.

Clinical Features. Post-operative collapse usually occurs within two or three days of operation. The symptoms and signs are those described under collapse (see p. 189).

The subsequent course will depend on the adequacy of treatment and the resistance of the patient, but if the condition is allowed to persist there is a danger of bronchiectasis and pulmonary fibrosis developing.

Treatment—*Preventive*

(a) No subject with an acute respiratory tract infection should be given a general anaesthetic except in an emergency.

(b) Patients with chronic respiratory infections should receive breathing exercises, postural drainage and in some cases, antibiotics, before a general anaesthetic. Smoking should be forbidden.

(c) Infected teeth and sinuses should be treated before an anaesthetic.

(d) Immediately after the operation the patient should be encouraged to clear sputum from the bronchi and his position in bed should be changed regularly to prevent stagnation of secretions in one part of the lung.

Curative

(a) The patient should be postured so that drainage of the blocked bronchus is assisted by gravity.

(b) Coughing should be encouraged. This causes pain from the operative incision which can be controlled by supporting the wound when the patient coughs, and by giving i.m. morphine 10 mg. The chest over the collapsed lung should be percussed rapidly and further coughing encouraged.

(c) If these measures are not followed by improvement in the patient's condition over the next few hours, the mucus should be aspirated by bronchoscopy.

(d) Oxygen must be given to those patients who are cyanosed and distressed.

(e) Ampicillin 250–500 mg six-hourly should be given to deal with any associated infection.

CYSTS OF THE LUNG

Cysts of the lung may be classified as follows:

(1) Congenital Cysts

Congenital cysts of the lung are due to maldevelopment of part of the primitive lung buds. They are lined with epithelium similar to that of the respiratory passages. They may be single or multiple.

Clinical Features. *In infancy* a single congenital cyst may have a valve-like connection with a bronchus so that air is sucked in during inspiration, but cannot be expired. The cyst expands until it interferes with respiration, causing distress and cyanosis. The situation can be temporarily relieved by inserting a needle into the cyst and connecting it by a rubber tube to a water seal. Further treatment is surgical.

Congenital cysts are also likely to become infected through their connection with the bronchial tree. Single cysts then present a picture similar to that of lung abscess and multiple cysts may be mistaken for bronchiectasis. Although antibiotics may control the infection and constitutional upset, postural drainage of the cyst is usually unsatisfactory due to inadequate bronchial connections; surgical excision of the infected cyst is therefore advisable when practicable.

(2) Acquired Cysts

These are much more common than congenital cysts of the lung. They have a variety of causes, but are basically due to stretching and breaking down of alveoli; they are not lined with respiratory epithelium. The chief causes are:

(a) *Acute lung infection*, particularly staphylococcal pneumonia (see p. 211).
(b) *Pulmonary tuberculosis* may lead to cavities with a stop valve connection with a bronchus. They become distended and take on the characteristics of cysts.
(c) *Emphysema.* Localised or generalised cysts of the lung may occur.

Clinical Features. Large bullæ interfere with respiratory function, for they decrease the total alveolar surface of the lung, diminish mixing of respiratory gases and may interfere with the normal stretch reflexes arising in the lung.

Generally the alveolar over-distension and cyst formation are so widespread in both lungs that no specific treatment is possible, but bullæ can occasionally be resected.

PULMONARY TUBERCULOSIS

General Considerations

Infection with the tubercle bacillus in a subject who has never previously experienced contact with the organism is called *primary tuberculosis;* reinfection after the primary lesion is called *post-primary tuberculosis*. The disease follows different courses in the two instances, the difference being attributed to the acquisition of antibodies in response to the primary lesion.

In Great Britain and the U.S.A., and most of the other countries of the Western Hemisphere, infection is almost entirely with the human bacillus. In less economically developed countries milk still serves as a vehicle for infection with the bovine organism, and primary abdominal tuberculosis and its sequelæ may occur.

The human bacillus is spread almost exclusively by droplet infection and lesions other than in the lung are uncommon. There is a wide range of susceptibility to the disease. Negroes, and dwellers in isolated communities, have little natural resistance. It is not a hereditary disease, but increased susceptibility may be inborn; if one of a pair of identical twins develops tuberculosis the other has a greatly increased chance of being affected, even if living in a totally different environment. Resistance may also be conditioned by such factors as malnutrition, overwork, and lack of sleep. The risks of infection are much increased by proximity, either from overcrowding of housing, or individual exposure, for example in dentists, and in doctors or nurses working in sanatoria.

Deaths from tuberculosis of all forms fell steadily in all civilised communities from the turn of the century. The rate of decline was so regular, with the exception of the war years, in the British Isles that it may be concluded that it was little influenced by any passing fancy in therapy and that the improvement was more likely to be due to public health measures. Since the introduction of effective chemotherapy death rates have declined precipitously.

PRIMARY TUBERCULOSIS

Characteristically the initial lesion is small and the local lymph nodes bear the brunt of the infection.

Pulmonary. A small pneumonic lesion (Ghon focus) may be situated in any part of the lungs. Lymphatic spread soon occurs and the local lymph nodes become enlarged. The radiographic appearance of a small shadow in the lung associated with hilar lymphadenopathy is known as the *primary complex*. It is accompanied by a change in the Mantoux reaction to positive (see p. 226). There is usually little upset in health and the natural tendency is to heal by fibrosis and calcification. In the past, primary tuberculosis commonly occurred in young people and up to 1950 over 95 per cent of urban dwellers had unknowingly healed such lesions before reaching adult life. Not all primary lesions heal spontaneously and without complications. As tuberculosis is now less common, an increasing proportion of children reach adult life without infection and it is these for whom protection is sought by vaccination with B.C.G. (see p. 229).

Complications. Sometimes the lung lesion increases in size to spread through the lobe, and rarely it may cavitate. This is more liable to occur in young adults, who are also prone to develop primary *tuberculous pleural effusions* (see p. 238).

In infants and young children particularly, the enlarged hilar lymph nodes may cause compression of a bronchus with segmental collapse, producing the radiographic appearance known as a *'hilar flare'*. This may lead to permanent bronchiectasis, such as in the *middle lobe syndrome* (p. 200). An infected lymph node may also rupture through the wall of a bronchus, the caseous material being discharged into the bronchial tree and causing a widespread *tuberculous bronchopneumonia* (p. 213). Alternatively, the lesions may erode blood vessels so that blood-borne tuberculosis may occur in such sites as bone, joints, kidney, epididymus, Fallopian tubes, brain, or meninges.

Miliary Tuberculosis

Miliary tuberculosis is due to widespread haematogenous dissemination. In primary tuberculosis it usually results from a caseous lymph node eroding a bronchial vessel, but it also occurs at times with post-primary lesions.

Clinical Features. The onset is usually insidious with general malaise, pyrexia, loss of weight, and sweats. Children often become listless and lose interest in their toys. Evidence of miliary spread through the lungs is not obvious early in the disease but later cough develops, with little sputum or dyspnoea. In some cases meningeal involvement is the most prominent feature and the patient presents with a tuberculous meningitis (p. 280).

Chest signs are either absent or confined to scattered fine râles. The spleen is often just palpable and careful examination of the retina may show choroidal tubercles. They are greyish-white lesions about one third the size of the optic disc. A chest radiograph shows the typical fine mottling of miliary tubercles throughout the lungs.

Treatment. This is along the usual line with chemotherapy (see p. 227). The prognosis is quite good provided meningeal involvement is not too advanced.

Primary Abdominal Tuberculosis

Bovine organisms gain access to the gut in infected milk. Small ulcers form in the small intestine and the infection spreads through lymphatics to the abdominal lymph nodes (*tabes mesenterica*). The nodes usually heal with calcification, but sometimes the infection spreads to the peritoneum (*Tuberculous peritonitis*). Miliary tuberculosis can result from involvement of abdominal blood vessels.

Tuberculous Cervical Lymphadenitis

The initial infection occurs in the tonsillar crypts and spreads to the cervical lymph nodes. These may become chronically enlarged and heal by fibrosis and calcification. They may undergo caseous necrosis, the pus tracking through the fascial planes to form a superficial cold abscess at some distance from the nodes (*'collar stud' abscess*).

Both the above are now uncommon in the United Kingdom.

POST PRIMARY TUBERCULOSIS

General Considerations. The infection is almost invariably pulmonary and usually occurs in the upper lobes or the apical segment of the lower lobe. The early lesion is a small area of tuberculous bronchopneumonia which radiographically appears as a soft shadow about 1 cm. in diameter. Spread is initially by direct extension to adjacent lung. Later *caseation* occurs and the necrotic centre of the lesion is discharged into a bronchus, producing a cavity in the lung, and cough with sputum. The infected sputum may be inhaled into other parts of either lung, producing new tuberculous lesions by *bronchogenic spread*. These may follow the same course. Peripheral lesions may cause *pleurisy*, which may progress to tuberculous *effusions* or empyema (p. 242). *Haemoptysis* occurs with erosion of blood vessels. *Tuberculous bronchitis* may produce a valvular obstruction to the bronchi draining a cavity, so that it distends to form a *tension cavity*. A *tuberculoma* is a blocked cavity with thick walls and full of inspissated material. It shows on the chest radiograph as a rounded opacity with clear-cut edges and may show areas of calcification.

The rate of progress of the disease is variable. It is rapid at times, but more commonly it is slow, the early lesion taking some years to develop into widespread tuberculosis. It depends on the extent and severity of the original infection and on the patient's resistance. The disease may become arrested at any stage, either permanently or temporarily, due to spontaneous healing by resolution, fibrosis, and calcification, or as the result of treatment. Alternatively widespread tuberculous bronchopneumonia, miliary tuberculosis, or metastatic tuberculosis may supervene. As opposed to *acute tuberculosis*, with infiltration and cavitation, a state of *chronic fibrocaseous or fibroid tuberculosis* may develop with gross fibrous contraction of the upper lobes and emphysema of the lower lobes. Respiratory reserve is then diminished and dyspnoea becomes a prominent symptom.

The expectoration of infected sputum may cause *tuberculous tracheitis, laryngitis*, or *tuberculous ulcers on the tongue*. Swallowed sputum may cause gastritis or tuberculous ulcers in the lymphoid patches of the *ileum*. The colon is usually spared, but tuberculous *fistula-in-ano* is common.

In patients with long-standing extensive disease, secondary amyloidosis may develop.

Clinical Features. Most patients with early tuberculosis of the lungs are free of symptoms but some present with haemoptysis.

The disease is usually well advanced by the time symptoms have developed. Classically they are chronic ill health, cough with mucoid sputum, low-grade fever, anorexia, tiredness, progressive weight loss, and night sweats. In advanced cases the patient appears ill, sweating and has lost weight, and the continual coughing up of infected sputum may spread infection and lead to further symptoms. Tracheitis causes retrosternal soreness, and laryngitis hoarseness and dysphagia. Tuberculous ulcers in the mouth, usually around the edge of the tongue, are extremely painful. Gastritis from swallowed sputum causes dyspepsia. As this may be a presenting symptom, pulmonary tuberculosis must always be considered in the differential diagnosis of dyspepsia. Tuberculous ileitis causes diarrhoea, and occasionally symptoms from bleeding, perforation, or obstruction. Fistula-in-ano causes a sero-sanguinous perianal discharge.

There are no abnormal signs from an early lesion. The first physical sign to appear is usually a small area of persistent fine râles at one or other apex, but by this time lung involvement is considerable. With more extensive disease there will be impairment to percussion, more widespread râles and sometimes areas of bronchial breathing if consolidation or cavities are near the chest wall. Fibrosis of an upper lobe leads to shift of the trachea towards the lesion, flattening and diminishing movement of the upper chest with impaired percussion note, bronchial breathing, and râles.

Signs of fluid will be present if there is an associated pleural effusion or empyema.

Investigations

Radiography is essential for diagnosis, to assess the extent and nature of the disease, to detect cavities and to follow progress. Both postero-anterior and lateral views are required at the start, and tomograms may be helpful to demonstrate cavities and delineate the extent of the lesion.

It is difficult to judge the activity of a lesion from a single radiograph. Cavitation means activity and soft fluffy opacities are usually of recent onset. Hard and calcified shadows suggest healing and inactivity. Serial films provide the best way of judging both the activity and progress of the disease.

There is no radiological appearance which is diagnostic of tuberculosis, although cavitating disease involving the upper lobes is extremely suggestive of it. Often the diagnosis depends on exclusion of other diseases or the confirmation of tuberculosis by sputum examination.

Sputum examination is essential in a patient suspected of having pulmonary tuberculosis. The finding of tubercle bacilli confirms the diagnosis and indicates that the disease is active and the patient infectious. Relatives and close contacts must be radiographed, sometimes repeatedly.

A random sample of sputum, stained by the *Ziehl-Neelsen technique*, may be examined by direct microscopy, or a 24-hour collection may be made, concentrated, and similarly examined. The sputum should also be cultured, as this increases the chance of finding tubercle bacilli and sensitivity tests to chemotherapeutic agents may be made. Guinea-pig inoculation is sometimes carried out, the animal being examined for tubercles after 6–8 weeks. Gastric washings, laryngeal swabs, and pleural fluid may be similarly examined. In general, the ease of finding the organism and the number found are indications of the extent of the disease.

Sedimentation Rate. A normal E.S.R. does not exclude an active lesion. A raised E.S.R. may be additional evidence of activity, and serial measurements are useful in following the progress of the disease.

Mantoux Test. Fixed antibodies to the tubercle bacillus develop in a patient with active tuberculosis, and persist after the infection has become inactive. There are rare exceptions to this; for instance, in some cases of overwhelming miliary tuberculosis. The antibodies can be demonstrated by injecting intradermally an antigen prepared from dead tubercle bacilli (tuberculin). An antigen-antibody reaction occurs in the skin, producing an area of redness and swelling and rarely ulceration. A *positive result* is judged as a papule larger than 5 mm. which appears within 2–4 days of injection. False positive results appear in the first 48 hours and last only a day or two. The test may be carried out by using a Tine skin prick test, or by hypodermic injection of a 1:10,000 solution of tuberculin; if this proves negative then in increasing strengths uo 1:1,000 and 1:100 should be used. A positive result simply indicates the presence of antibodies and implies previous exposure; it is not a measure of activity. A negative result would indicate that a radiographic pulmonary opacity is not tuberculous.

Treatment. Active disease requires treatment, whereas healed disease only requires observation. It is not always easy to decide if a lesion is active, but it must be regarded so in the following circumstances:

(a) Clinical evidence of disease, i.e. fever and weight loss.
(b) Tubercle bacilli in the sputum.
(c) Radiological evidence of spread of the disease.
(d) The presence of cavities.

The *principles of treatment* are well established and include general measure to raise resistance, specific treatment, and local measures to the lung.

(1) **General.** With effective chemotherapy prolonged bed rest is no longer required, but the patient should be kept in bed if he is ill with fever or toxaemia. It need not be absolute for more than a week or two, after which most patients can be allowed to feed themselves, later to wash themselves and to visit the lavatory. Good food is essential. This means adequate, but not excessive calories, chiefly provided by protein, with sufficient vitamin and mineral content. Iron and vitamins may be given as a supplement if necessary. The aim should be to regain, but not exceed, the normal body weight. Fresh air, bright surroundings and a cheerful atmosphere should encourage the patient towards recovery.

(2) **Chemotherapy.** The drugs of choice are streptomycin, isoniazid, and para-aminosalicylic acid (PAS), in that order. Some general principles governing chemotherapy may be stated:

(1) Chemotherapy is indicated if the disease is active.
(2) It should be continued for one to two years after all evidence of activity has gone.
(3) No drug should be given alone. Combinations of the drugs should be used to avoid the emergence of drug-resistant strains of tubercle bacilli.

Treatment should be started with *streptomycin* 1·0 *g. intramuscularly daily, isoniazid* 300 *mg. orally daily and PAS* 12 *g. orally daily.* It is safer to give streptomycin 1·0 g. on three days a week in patients over the age of 40 because of the increased danger of vestibular damage. Similarly care must be taken in patients with impaired renal function. All three drugs are given at the start of treatment so that a maximum therapeutic effect is obtained and the possibility that the organism may already be resistant to one of the drugs is covered. Sputum culture and tests of the organism's sensitivity to the drugs will subsequently determine this. Provided the bacilli are sensitive this treatment is continued until the active stage of infection is passed. After six weeks the streptomycin can be stopped if the disease is minimal, otherwise it can be continued as 1·0 g. on three days a week for a total of from three to six months depending on the severity of the disease. The patient should then continue on *PAS 12·0 g. orally daily and isoniazid 300 mg. daily* for a further long period, usually one to two years. It is best to give PAS and isoniazid in a combined preparation, for otherwise if the patient fails to take one of the drugs (usually PAS) the organisms will inevitably develop resistance to the other.

This treatment with the 'standard' drugs may have to be modified if the patient is found to have resistant organisms or develops side-effects from any of the drugs. Both PAS and streptomycin are liable to produce hypersensitivity reactions; in addition, streptomycin may produce vestibular damage and PAS may cause intolerable gastro-intestinal upset. Under these circumstances capreomycin, rifampicin or ethambutol can be used; they are more effective and less toxic than previous 'second-line' drugs such as cycloserine, ethionamide and pyrazinamide. *Capreomycin* is given by intramuscular injections of 1·0 g. in a regimen similar to that with streptomycin. *Rifampicin* has an activity comparable to that of isoniazid. It is given as a single oral daily dose before breakfast of 450 to 600 mg. (10 mg. per kg. body weight); it may well replace PAS in the primary drug treatment of tuberculosis. *Ethambutol* is given in a single oral daily dose of 25 mg. per kg. body weight for sixty days and subsequently in a daily dose of 15 mg. per kg. body weight. Visual acuity should be checked every four weeks while the patient is on the larger dose as optic neuritis has been reported; otherwise it is remarkably free of side-effects.

Corticosteroids are of value in acute tuberculosis with severe toxaemia which is not responding quickly enough to chemotherapy alone.

(3) Local Measures

(1) *Collapse therapy* for producing relaxation of the lung has been little used since the advent of effective chemotherapy. The procedures of introducing air into the pleural cavity (*artificial pneumothorax*) or into the peritoneum (*pneumoperitoneum*) have fallen into disuse. The latter was often combined with diaphragmatic paralysis, produced by crushing the phrenic nerve in the neck. Permanent collapse procedures have also been abandoned. These included the introduction of foreign bodies extrapleurally (*plombage*) and resection of ribs and allowing the chest wall to cave in (*thoracoplasty*).

(2) *Postural Retention.* A tension cavity associated with bronchial disease can sometimes be closed by positioning the patient so that the cavity is dependent. Retention of secretions in the affected bronchus may change the bronchial obstruction

from being valvular to complete, with consequent closure of the cavity.

(3) *Resection.* Surgical resection and chemotherapy were both introduced at approximately the same time. It is now realised that with adequate longer-term chemotherapy, resection is usually unnecessary; it is reserved for certain selected cases.

> (a) Patients with localised cavitation which persists in spite of adequate rest and chemotherapy.
> (b) Some cases infected with tubercle bacilli resistant to chemotherapy.

The physician may be more inclined to advise resection in patients who will not persist with rest and chemotherapy, whereas such factors as extensive disease or the greater age of the patient will influence against the decision to resect. It should be performed while continuing chemotherapy and be followed by further rest and prolonged chemotherapy.

Treatment of the Minimal Lesion

A *minimal lesion* is a small area of infiltration without evidence of cavitation, which radiographically does not extend over more than one interspace. It is usually discovered on routine radiography and the patient is symptom free. Opinions on treatment vary, but it is probably best to admit the patient to hospital for a period, for rest and assessment of activity. Thereafter the majority can be treated on an out-patient basis, leading sensible and well-ordered lives with adequate diet and rest. Initially streptomycin 1·0 g. intramuscularly daily, isoniazid 300 mg. daily and PAS 12 g. daily should be used. After six weeks the streptomycin can either be stopped or continued for a further six weeks as 1·0 g. on three days a week. PAS 12·0 g. daily and isoniazid 300 mg. daily are then usually sufficient and should be continued for at least a year. The progress of the lesion must be observed by serial radiography.

Prophylaxis

This includes measures to raise standards of hygiene and improve living conditions, and the detection of both early and infectious cases of pulmonary tuberculosis by routine radiography.

Efforts have been made to increase individual resistance by vaccinating susceptible (Mantoux negative) subjects with an attenuated strain of the tubercle bacillus (Bacille Calmette-Guerin: *B.C.G.*). An intradermal injection of 0·1 ml. of the vaccine is made, and the appearance of a papule or ulcer at the site of injection within 10–14 days indicates a successful vaccination. It may be associated with enlargement of local lymph nodes and may take as long as three months to heal. Conversion of the Mantoux reaction to positive should occur between the 6th and 8th week after vaccination.

The World Health Organisation have used B.C.G. vaccination on an enormous scale in India, Africa, and some parts of Asia with few ill effects and benefits that are already apparent. It is available at chest clinics and infant welfare centres in the United Kingdom.

OPPORTUNIST MYCOBACTERIAL INFECTION

Acid-fast bacilli distinct from *M. tuberculosis* may at times produce a lung infection which mimics an indolent form of tuberculosis. These different 'atypical' mycobacteria can be distinguished on cultures by their rate of growth and ability to produce pigment. *M. kansasii*, the commonest variety seen in this country, produces a yellow pigment when cultures grown in the dark are exposed to light.

Treatment. *In vitro* sensitivity tests invariably show these organisms to be resistant to streptomycin, isoniazid and PAS; depending on the results of the sensitivity tests, the infection is best treated with combinations of rifampicin, ethionamide and ethambutol. Response to drug therapy is slower than with tuberculosis and surgical resection may be indicated in some cases.

FUNGOUS INFECTIONS

Histoplasmosis, coccidiomycosis and *blastomycosis* are fungous diseases of the lungs occurring in the United States of America, but they are not endemic in this country.

Torulosis. Sporadic cases occur. It is due to infection with the yeast *Cryptococcus neoformans.* Pulmonary lesions may develop into cavitating granulomas, or into tumour-like masses. Infection may spread by the blood stream to the meninges mimicking tuberculous meningitis, even when the pulmonary lesions are small.

Treatment consists of surgical resection, where feasible, combined with intravenous amphotericin B. Cryptococcal meningitis has also been successfully treated with 5-fluorocytosine.

Aspergillosis. The fungus *aspergillus fumigatus* is not pathogenic to the normal respiratory tract. It may infect pulmonary infarcts, and cysts or cavities which have resulted from such diseases as staphylococcal pneumonia, tuberculosis or sarcoidosis. A solid ball of fungus (*mycetoma*) grows free in the cavity. On tomography a crescent of air may be seen above the opacity, which can also be shown to move its position when the patient is tipped. Precipitins to aspergillus can be detected in the patients blood. Recurrent haemoptyses may occur and the sputum may be thick and purulent.

A different and distinct syndrome results from hypersensitivity to aspergillus in the sputum. It produces asthma, recurrent areas of pulmonary collapse and increase of eosinophils in the blood and sputum.

Treatment. Inhalations of brilliant green or hydroxystilbamidine may be given; the latter may be given intravenously in severe infections. In patients with asthma, corticosteroids are usually the only effective form of treatment. A mycetoma does not respond to this treatment; it is usually best left untreated, or in suitable cases resected surgically.

Moniliasis. The yeast *Candida albicans* is a normal saprophyte found in the respiratory tract and in the intestines. The administration of antibiotics may encourage its growth so that it may be abundant in the sputum but not necessarily pathogenic. It may, however, invade the mucosa, causing *thrush* in the mouth and pharynx, and at times in the oesophagus and in the trachea and bronchi; it may also cause diarrhoea and ano-genital pruritus. It is debatable whether monilial infection of the lung itself occurs. Rarely, in debilitated patients and in patients on treatment with antibiotics, steroids and cytotoxic drugs (with such diseases as leukaemia and reticuloses), blood stream infection and meningitis may occur.

Treatment. Nystatin by mouth, 4 ml. t.d.s. (100,000 units per ml.), is the drug of choice. Inhalations of nystatin or brilliant green may be used for bronchial moniliasis. In the rare systemic infections intravenous amphotericin B may also be used.

DUST DISEASES OF THE LUNGS (The Pneumoconioses)

Silicosis

Silicosis is due to the inhalation of fine particles of free silica. It occurs in coal miners, and in the granite and sandstone industries, in metal foundries, in various grinding processes in which sandstone is used and in the pottery industry.

The earliest change is the development throughout the lungs of fine, fibrotic nodules around the particles of silica. As the disease develops these nodules increase in size and coalesce until finally there are large areas of fibrosis. Tuberculosis may complicate the picture.

Clinical Features. In the early stages there are no symptoms or signs and the diagnosis depends on the radiographic picture of diffuse mottling combined with a history of exposure.

The first symptom is dyspnoea on effort and later cough with mucoid sputum develops. Eventually the patient becomes severely disabled and death occurs from bronchopneumonia, tuberculosis or cor pulmonale.

Prevention consists of adequate exhaust ventilation, damping down the dust and personal protection by means of masks. All people exposed to silica dust should have regular chest radiographs.

Treatment. There is no specific treatment and those showing evidence of the disease must be removed from exposure to dust.

Asbestosis

The inhalation of asbestos fibres, which consist largely of magnesium silicate, causes a progressive diffuse fibrosis of the lungs, particularly the lower lobes. The chief symptoms are cough and dyspnoea and the clinical picture is that of fibrosing alveolitis (p. 235); *asbestos bodies*, formed of asbestos fibres and fibrin, can be found on microscopy of the sputum. Preventative measures are similar to those used in silicosis. Carinoma of the bronchus is a common complication and malignant mesothelioma of the pleura also occurs.

Coal Miners' Pneumoconiosis

A special type of pneumoconiosis affects miners who inhale coal dust, rather than rock dust which produces silicosis. In this country it is most prevalent in the South Wales coal-fields. There are two types:

(1) *Simple Pneumoconiosis*. Radiographically there is diffuse reticulation at first. Later scattered small nodules up to 5 mm. in diameter develop, often with surrounding emphysema. The disease is only progressive if the worker remains exposed to dust.

(2) *Progressive Massive Fibrosis*. Radiographically there are large dense shadows mostly in the mid and upper zones, with surrounding emphysema. It probably represents a massive fibrotic response to low grade inflammation. Although tuberculous infection or infection with atypical mycobacteria may be suspected, usually it cannot be proved. It is progressive even if the subject is no longer exposed to coal dust.

Clinical Features. There are no symptoms in the early stages. In the later etages of simple pneumoconiosis and with massive fibrosis dyspnoea on exertion is a prominent symptom. Cough and sputum, sometimes blacksned by coal dust, develop and recurrent bronchitis is common. In advanced cases the patient becomes grossly disabled and death from cor pulmonale is usual.

Prevention. Of importance are adequate ventilation and reduction of dust by damping it down with water, by wet drilling and wet cutting. Masks are not very satisfactory as they interfere with the performance of heavy work. Chest radiographs at regular intervals should be carried out on all workers at risk, and those showing evidence of pneumoconiosis should be removed from further exposure to coal dust.

Byssinosis

Byssinosis is due to exposure to dust arising from the processing of cotton. It is believed to be an unusual allergic reaction of the bronchi to cotton dust. In the early stages of the disease the patient complains of dyspnoea, tightness in the chest, and cough which characteristically occurs on Mondays when the patient returns to work. Later the dyspnoea and cough becomes permanent and finally emphysema develops. Prevention is by adequate ventilation.

PULMONARY EOSINOPHILIA

There is a group of conditions characterised by a varying degree of constitutional upset, cough, transient infiltration of the lung and eosinophilia in the blood.

The *chief causes* of this syndrome are:

(1) *Worm and Parasite Infiltration.* Pulmonary infiltration and eosinophilia may result from the migration through the lungs of the larvae of ascaris lumbricoides (see p. 528).

(2) *Asthma.* Some patients may develop patchy areas of consolidation with eosinophilia during asthmatic attacks. Sometimes this is associated with the presence in the sputum of *Aspergillus fumigatus*, to which the patient has become sensitised and antibodies may be detected in the blood.

(3) *Tropical Eosinophilia.* This is a well-defined clinical entity, occurring in tropical countries, particularly India and Pakistan, and probably due to microfilarial infestation. The symptoms may be acute or chronic with fever, cough, malaise, and attacks of dyspnoea. Radiography may show miliary mottling and there is always a high eosinophilia.

The condition usually responds to diethylcarbamazine in oral doses of 4·0 mg./kg. body weight, t.d.s. for four days.

(4) *Polyarteritis nodosa.* Transient infiltration of the lung with eosinophilia, often with associated asthma, may occur in polyarteritis nodosa.

SARCOIDOSIS

Sarcoidosis is a disease in which epithelioid cell tubercles, without caseation, are present in all the affected organs. The older lesions become converted to hyalinised fibrous tissue. A similar granulomatous lesion is sometimes seen on biopsy, for example, of skin or lymph node, in quite unrelated conditions such as carcinoma or reticuloses. This *sarcoid reaction* must be distinguished from the disease sarcoidosis.

A few patients with sarcoidosis develop frank pulmonary tuberculosis. The aetiology of sarcoidosis is not known, but tuberculosis is favoured by some authorities in this country. There is also an immunological defect present, with depression of the delayed type of hypersensitivity response in most patients.

Clinical Features. The three commonest clinical presentations are:

(1) *Erythema nodosum* with *bilateral hilar node enlargement, fever* and often *polyarthritis.*

(2) *Routine chest radiography.* The patient is commonly symptom free and an apparently healthy young adult. The radiograph may show hilar node enlargement, or hilar nodes with pulmonary mottling, or mottling alone. If the patient is breathless it is likely that longstanding fibrotic sarcoid will be present.

(3) *Iridocyclitis.* This is commonly acute and transient. It may, however, be insidious and persistent with keratic precipitates forming in the anterior chamber, adhesion of the iris to the lens and obstruction of the angle of the anterior chamber leading to glaucoma. The choroid and retina may also be involved.

Other organs which may be involved include the *spleen, lymph nodes, liver* and *salivary glands. Skin lesions* are characteristically few, sharply defined, brownish in colour with a predilection for the face. They may persist for months or even years; they are benign, do not ulcerate and involute spontaneously, leaving either no trace or a pigmented or atrophic scar. *In the nervous system* a granulomatous basal meningitis may produce pituitary lesions or cranial nerve lesions. *Cystic bone change* may occasionally occur, usually in the heads of the metacarpals. *Hypercalcaemia* may be present and probably represents an abnormal sensitivity to vitamin D. Rarely the *heart* is involved, leading to congestive failure, or sudden death.

Investigations

Chest radiograph is essential. Pulmonary involvement is one of the main features of the disease, and it can only be assessed by following the changing radiological picture.

Tuberculin reaction. A negative Mantoux reaction supports the diagnosis. However, as one third of the patients with proved sarcoidosis give a positive reaction to 10 TU (1:1000 old tuberculin), a positive reaction does not exclude it. If a patient with sarcoidosis and a negative Mantoux reaction is treated with corticosteroids, the reaction then becomes positive; this is almost diagnostic of sarcoidosis.

Plasma proteins. In approximately one third of cases there are raised a_2 and/or γ globulins present. This probably indicates activity of the disease.

Kveim Test. The intradermal injection of a saline suspension of sarcoid tissue obtained from spleen or lymph node of patients with active sarcoidosis is followed by the development of a nodule in the skin within the next six weeks. Biopsy of this nodule will show sarcoid histology. The test is positive in about 70 per cent of cases of sarcoidosis.

Biopsy of skin lesions or affected glands will confirm the diagnosis. Liver biopsy is positive in about 50 per cent of patients with sarcoidosis, even when there is no clinical evidence of involvement of the liver.

Respiratory function tests are only abnormal when there is marked pulmonary mottling, when the main defects are those of *compliance* (p. 183) and *gas transfer* (p. 183). In the later stages of pulmonary fibrosis impairment of *ventilation* may be marked.

Progress and Treatment

There is no evidence that anti-tuberculous chemotherapy influences the course of the disease.

Steroids are indicated in iridocyclitis because of the danger to sight, and local instillation of drops is usually sufficient.

Erythema nodosum and hilar node enlargement carries a good prognosis. With hilar node enlargement 70 per cent of patients improve spontaneously; the remainder develop pulmonary infiltration. With pulmonary infiltration 50 per cent of patients improve spontaneously; if this has not occurred within two years then it is unlikely to remit subsequently. The infiltration may then remain unchanged with little or no disability to the patient, but in a proportion it progresses to severe fibrosis with associated bronchiectasis and bullous change. These patients become respiratory cripples and eventually succumb to cor pulmonale (p. 198).

No specific treatment is indicated in patients with hilar node enlargement. Steroids are usually indicated in patients with pulmonary mottling showing no sign of resolution after a year. It often produces symptomatic relief and hastens resolution, and is aimed at preventing the development of severe fibrosis. Prednisolone 20 mg. daily is a satisfactory starting dose. A daily maintenance dose of 5 to 10 mg. may be required for several years, as relapse may occur if treatment is too short. Steroids have no effect on the lungs in the fibrotic stage but may help to relieve symptoms.

Once the disease has remitted it does not recur.

PULMONARY FIBROSIS

Generalised Pulmonary Fibrosis

This is relatively uncommon. The causes are:

(1) The pneumoconioses (p. 231).
(2) As an end result of infiltration of the lungs by a variety of pathological processes, including sarcoidosis (see above), and some of the generalized lipoidoses.
(3) Fibrosing alveolitis.

Fibrosing alveolitis (Chronic interstitial pulmonary fibrosis)

This is a generalised disorder of the alveolar walls in which inflammatory changes advance to progressive fibrosis. It may occur in association with the collagen diseases, such as rheumatoid arthritis and scleroderma, or be of an idiopathic variety with no known cause. Allergic forms of fibrosing alveolitis where inhalants produce a type 3 sensitivity reaction in the alveolar walls, are being more frequently recognised. *Farmer's lung* where there is sensitivity to spores in mouldy hay, and *Bird fancier's lung*, where there is a sensitivity to bird protein, are examples of this. In the latter cases precipitins to the protein of birds, such as pigeons and budgerigars, may be detected in the patient's blood.

Clinical Features. Dyspnoea is the leading symptom and cough, though usually present, is not associated with much sputum. Clubbing of the fingers is common in more advanced cases. Examination of the chest often shows fine râles, particularly at the bases, and late inspiratory rhonchi may be heard. The chest radiograph shows fine diffuse mottling most marked at the bases. Respiratory function tests indicate that the main defect is that of gaseous exchange across the alveolar membrane (see Transfer of Gases p. 183). The progress of the disease may at times be very slow, but the final outcome is death from hypoxia and right ventricular failure.

Treatment. If there are known or suspected allergens present these must be removed from the patient's environment; a course of steroids may be very effective in tiding the patient over an acute episode in the allergic variety. On the whole the treatment is not very satisfactory in the idiopathic variety or in those cases associated with collagen disease. Steroids may limit the fibrosis and relieve dyspnoea in some patients provided the fibrosis is not too advanced. Steroid therapy may have to be continued indefinitely in the smallest possible maintenance dose to maintain improvement, usually prednisolone 5 to 10 mg. daily, as severe relapse may occur when it is stopped. Advanced cases are helped by oxygen therapy in the home and by portable oxygen.

Localised Pulmonary Fibrosis

Fibrosis of the lungs is commonly localised to one or more lobes, or even a segment of a lobe. It is usually the result of inflammation and common causes are tuberculosis, unresolved pneumonia, chronic lung abscess and long-standing collapse. Bronchiectasis invariably develops in such fibrotic segments or lobes. Persistent infection is not common with fibrosis of the upper lobes because drainage is adequate.

Clinical Features. In some patients there are no symptoms, except perhaps the history of the original illness which led to the fibrosis. This is often the case with healed, fibrotic tuberculosis of the upper lobes, and no treatment is required.

In others the clinical picture is that of the accompanying *infected bronchiectasis*, both with regard to symptoms and complications (see p. 200). Diagnosis and treatment are also discussed under this section.

The physical signs of fibrosis include flattening of the chest overlying the lesion with diminished movement, impaired percussion note, bronchial breathing, whispering pectoriloquy, and bronchophony. The mediastinum is shifted towards the side of the lesion and coarse râles are present with associated bronchiectasis.

DISEASES OF THE PLEURA

PLEURISY

Inflammation of the pleura may be *dry* or associated with *effusion*, the former often proceeding to the latter.

DRY PLEURISY

It may be due to:

(1) *Pneumonia* either bacterial or viral.

(2) *Pulmonary infarct* (p. 167).

(3) *Tuberculosis.* This variety nearly always progresses to pleurisy with effusion.

(4) *Lung abscess.*

(5) *Epidemic pleurodynia* (Bornholm Disease). This is a Coxsackic virus infection which may occur in outbreaks. It affects the muscles of the chest wall and produces a primary pleurisy without lung involvement.

(6) *Injury* to the chest and lungs.

Clinical Features. The cardinal symptom of dry pleurisy is *pain,* described on p. 186.

On examination the respirations may be short and grunting, for severe pleuritic pain limits inspiration. The diagnosis is confirmed by finding a *pleural rub,* which is a superficial grating or crunching sound related to respiratory movements. It appears to arise just under the stethoscope, which indeed it does, and characteristically comes and goes. Occasionally a pleural rub may be heard in a patient who makes no complaint of pain.

Chest radiography may reveal underlying disease if present, but shows no specific sign of dry pleurisy. Screening may show diminished movement of the chest and diaphragm on that side.

Treatment. Bed rest and analgesics are required. Tabs. codeine co. 2 four-hourly, pethidine 50–100 mg. intramuscularly or hypodermic morphine 15 mg. may all be used, depending on the severity of the pain. Some patients obtain relief by applying a hot-water-bottle over the area. Specific treatment is that of the underlying lesion, and subsequent management will depend on this.

PLEURISY WITH EFFUSION

Fluid in the pleural cavity may represent a transudate or an exudate.

Transudates occur when the osmotic pressure of the plasma is reduced (the nephrotic syndrome or cirrhosis of the liver) or when the venous pressure is high (congestive cardiac failure or constrictive pericarditis). The fluid in a transudate is usually clear and of low specific gravity. It contains less than 2·0 g. protein per 100 ml.

Causes of pleural transudates are:

(1) *Cardiac failure.*

(2) *Nephrotic syndrome.*

(3) *Cirrhosis of the liver.*

Exudates occur in the presence of inflammation or neoplasm. They are of high specific gravity and contain more than 2·0 g. protein per 100 ml.

Exudates may be clear (tuberculous, neoplastic disease). Cloudiness may be due to blood (neoplasm, pulmonary infarct) or pus cells (pneumonia or lung abscess).

Causes of pleural exudates are:

(1) *Tuberculosis.*
(2) Complicating *pneumonia.*
(3) *Neoplasm.*
(4) *Subphrenic abscess*, and complicating other inflammatory lesions outside the chest.
(5) *Pulmonary infarction.*
(6) During the course of some *collagen diseases*, notably systemic lupus erythematosis.
(7) Complicating fibroma of the ovary (*Meigs' syndrome*).

Tuberculous Pleural Effusion

(1) **Effusion Associated with Primary Tuberculosis.** This is the common type of tuberculous effusion and usually occurs between the ages of fifteen and thirty and within a year of Mantoux conversion. It is believed that at this stage the tissues are sensitised to the tubercle bacillus, and if bacilli reach the pleura there is an acute inflammatory reaction with an outpouring of fluid into the pleural cavity.

Clinical Features. The onset is variable. Sometimes it is acute with fever, malaise, sweating, and severe pleuritic pain. Other patients have little pain but complain of vague ill-health and dyspnoea on effort. Occasionally an effusion may be found on routine examination or chest radiograph in a patient with no symptoms.

Examination shows the typical signs of effusion (see p. 189). If it is large there is mediastinal shift to the opposite side, with flat dullness on percussion and absent breath sounds over the effusion.

Chest radiograph shows the effusion as an opacity at the base of the hemithorax. It obliterates the costophrenic angle and rises up into the axilla. The mediastinum may be displaced to the opposite side. It is unusual to see any intrapulmonary lesion.

Diagnosis is confirmed by aspiration of a sample of fluid. It is straw-coloured and contains cells, most of which are lymphocytes, although in the early stages polymorphs may predominate. Tubercle bacilli can be isolated from the fluid by culture or guinea-pig inoculation in about 50 per cent of cases.

The *course* is usually towards resolution. There is a potential danger of the infection spreading and occasionally miliary tuberculosis, renal tuberculosis, or tuberculous meningitis occurs. Slow absorption of a large effusion may lead to pleural fibrosis, with subsequent restriction of lung expansion and contraction of the chest wall. Before chemotherapy was available about 25 per cent of patients developed frank tuberculous lesions in the lungs within five years of an effusion.

Treatment. The aims are to eradicate the infection and to prevent serious residual pleural fibrosis by encouraging rapid clearing of the effusion.

Antitubercular drugs should be given for 12 months, starting with triple chemotherapy (p. 227). Unless the effusion appears to be disappearing rapidly aspiration should be carried out every 2 or 3 days until no further fluid can be removed. Half to one litre should be removed at each aspiration. Fluid should be removed without delay if there is much mediastinal shift of if the patient is short of breath. Effusions which do not resolve, or which keep reforming in spite of these measures, may be treated in addition with corticosteroids. The steroid therapy need not be prolonged and must be combined with chemotherapy; prednisolone 20 mg. daily reducing to a maintenance dose of 10–15 mg. daily for 6 weeks is satisfactory.

Bed rest should be continued until the effusion has cleared usually a month to 6 weeks. The patient should then make a gradual return to full activity and should remain off work for 3 to 6 months. Follow-up supervision with chest radiographs is essential as with other forms of tuberculosis.

Effusion with Post-primary Tuberculosis

Effusions may develop with post-primary pulmonary tuberculosis and usually indicate severe pleural tuberculosis. They resolve more slowly than effusions associated with primary tuberculosis, being more resistant to treatment and being liable to develop into tuberculous empyemata. They occurred as a complication of artificial pneumothorax, when this was used as therapy for tuberculosis.

Treatment. 1·0 g. of streptomycin should be injected into the pleural cavity every other day. One pint of pleural fluid should be aspirated every other day until the pleural cavity is dry.

The subsequent management depends on the nature of the underlying lung disease, and will require bed rest and systemic chemotherapy (see p. 227).

Neoplastic Pleural Effusion

Malignant effusion is most commonly due to carcinoma of the bronchus. It also occurs with spread of extra-thoracic growth to the pleura, such as carcinoma of the breast, stomach, kidney, ovary, or testicle. Pleural effusions are quite common in Hodgkin's disease.

Clinical Features. The degree of general ill-health is variable and depends on the extent and nature of the primary neoplasm. The effusions are often of insidious onset, but as they usually become large dyspnoea is a common symptom. The fluid usually reaccumulates rapidly after aspiration; it is often bloodstained and may contain malignant cells.

Treatment. The patient must be kept comfortable by repeated aspiration; usually large quantities can be removed without danger. It is sometimes possible to prevent or slow down the reaccumulation of fluid by radiotherapy or by the introduction of nitrogen mustard into the pleural space.

Effusions associated with breast carcinoma may respond to hormone treatment.

Bloodstained Pleural Effusions

Bloodstained effusions are not uncommon. The chief causes are:

(1) Neoplasm, commonly bronchial carcinoma.
(2) Pulmonary infarct.
(3) Rarely tuberculosis.
(4) A haemothorax which has been diluted by a pleural exudate may have the appearance of a bloodstained effusion.

HAEMOTHORAX

Haemothorax usually follows trauma to the chest wall. It also occurs with a spontaneous pneumothorax, presumably from rupture of pleural adhesions; it is then a haemopneumothorax. Rarely an aneurysm may leak into the pleural cavity.

Blood in the pleural cavity clots rapidly and fibrin is deposited on the pleural surfaces. Pleural reaction also occurs, with outpouring of further fluid. If the blood is left in the pleura, organisation with pleural fibrosis occurs with subsequent serious interference with lung function.

Clinical Features. If the pleural bleeding is large and rapid the patient will be shocked and collapsed, with rapid pulse and respiration. There may or may not be evidence of trauma to the chest. There are *signs* of pleural fluid (p. 186) or in those cases complicating a pneumothorax the signs are those of both fluid and air in the chest.

Diagnosis is confirmed by aspiration of blood from the pleural space. It is important to distinguish between a frank haemothorax and a bloodstained effusion.

Treatment. The general treatment for internal haemorrhage should be given. Morphine may be required, the patient's blood group should be determined and a transfusion given when necessary.

The effusion should be aspirated and the pleural space kept as dry as possible by further daily aspiration. Antibiotics should be given during the period of aspirations as there is a danger of secondary infection, usually staphylococcal.

Severe bleeding or serious damage to the chest wall will require surgical treatment. Thoracotomy is also necessary when the blood cannot be evacuated by aspiration.

EMPYEMA

Empyema may be defined as a localised collection of pus in the pleural cavity. It most commonly results from a pneumonia, usually pneumococcal lobar pneumonia. It may also be due to spread of infection from a lung abscess, from a subphrenic abscess, from mediastinal sepsis and from a chest wound. Empyema may also result from tuberculous infection of the pleural cavity (see p. 242). Infected serous fluid may collect in the pleural cavity during the course of a pneumonia (*syn-pneumonic empyema*). It is not localised and it usually resolves with adequate treatment. It may, however, progress to become purulent and localised, and by this time the underlying pneumonia has usually resolved (*meta-pneumonic empyema*). When an empyema becomes loculated in the fissures between the lobes it is known as an interlobar empyema.

Clinical Features. Empyema most commonly arises one to two weeks after the start of a pneumococcal pneumonia. Instead of the temperature falling and the patient recovering, the temperature begins to rise again and takes on a remittent character. The patient looks ill, has drenching sweats and complains of malaise and anorexia. Examination of the chest shows the signs of fluid; the mediastinum will be shifted if the collection of fluid is large, but this is not usual. There is dullness over the fluid; classically the upper limit of the dull area rises in the axilla, but this is not constant and often the dullness is largely posterior. Usually there are absent or diminished breath sounds over the fluid, although particularly in children it is sometimes possible to hear bronchial breathing which may lead to an erroneous diagnosis of unresolved pneumonia.

It is important to take both postero-anterior and lateral radiographs of the chest so that the fluid may be exactly localised. The diagnosis is finally confirmed by needling the chest and withdrawing turbid fluid. In the early stages, the fluid will be thin and serous, but if a true empyema develops it will become thick and purulent. The fluid should be cultured for organisms.

With correct treatment the *prognosis* in empyema is good except (1) when it is associated with a severe infection, (2) when the patient's resistance to infection is low due to debility, and (3) in young children.

Treatment

(1) *The Stage of Infected Pleural Effusion*. The patient should be at rest in bed, propped up on pillows. The diet should be light and fluids plentiful. The infected effusion must be aspirated daily to keep the pleural cavity as dry as possible; following aspiration, 500,000 units of benzyl penicillin should be injected into the pleural cavity. At the same time systemic antibiotic treatment should be continued; benzylpenicillin, 500,000 units six-hourly is satisfactory unless the infecting organism is resistant to penicillin, when the appropriate antibiotic should be used. With this treatment most effusions will subside. Sometimes, however, the infection is not controlled and the aspirated fluid becomes more and more purulent.

(2) *True Empyema*. Treatment at this stage is surgical. Resection of a portion of a rib and the insertion of a drainage tube into the most dependent part of the empyema cavity ensures the best possible drainage. The aim is complete obliteration of the empyema cavity with the minimum of pleural scarring and fixation of the lung. It is therefore essential, once a true empyema has developed, not to delay surgical drainage or the wall

of the abscess cavity may become so thick and rigid that it cannot be obliterated.

The drain is left in the empyema cavity until this space has disappeared. If the drain falls out before the cavity has been obliterated it must be replaced gently because of the danger of causing spread of infection to the brain (resulting in cerebral abscess). Breathing exercises are given to re-expand the lung and minimise fixation. Provided treatment is correctly carried out results are good. *Failure of the empyema cavity to close* is usually due to:

(a) too long a delay before drainage,

(b) inadequate drainage with pocketing of pus; it will be neces-sary to radiograph the cavity, outlined with radio-opaque material, to determine the correct site for drainage of the most dependent part of the cavity,

(c) failure to recognise that it is a tuberculous empyema,

(d) presence of an underlying neoplasm.

(e) a foreign body in the empyema cavity.

An empyema cavity which fails to close owing to undue thickness of its wall will require permanent drainage with a tube; or surgical decorti-cation of the lung can be performed with removal of the abscess cavity.

Tuberculous Empyema

Tuberculous empyema nearly always occurs in an effusion complicating post-primary pulmonary tuberculosis, and it is very rare in a tuberculous effusion associated with a primary infection. It was a recognised complica-tion of artificial pneumothorax, but this type of treatment for tuberculosis is not used now.

Clinical Features. The degree of constitutional upset varies. Some patients appear surprisingly well considering the chest is filled with tuberculous pus. Others have evidence of toxaemia with weight loss, sweating, and fever. If secondary infection occurs, particularly with the staphylococcus aureus, the patient becomes severely ill. This is especially likely to occur if there is a bronchopleural fistula, such as may result from the rupture of a pulmonary cavity into the pleura. The signs are those of fluid in the chest. If a pneumothorax is also present the signs are those of fluid and air in the chest: an area of dullness below due to the fluid, with resonance above. It may be possible by tilting the patient to demonstrate shifting dullness.

Treatment. The patient requires the usual general treatment for tuber-culosis, including a full course of antituberculous chemotherapy (see p. 227). The chest should be aspirated every other day until it is as dry as possible and streptomycin 1·0 g. should be instilled into the pleural cavity after aspiration. Unless full expansion occurs, decortication, thoracoplasty or resection of part or all of the lung may be required.

SPONTANEOUS PNEUMOTHORAX

Air collecting in the pleural cavity as a result of some pathological process is known as spontaneous pneumothorax. The artificial introduction of air, which was used as a form of therapy for pulmonary tuberculosis, is known as an artificial pneumothorax.

The commonest cause of spontaneous pneumothorax is the rupture of a small vesicle under the visceral pleura which allows air to pass from the lung to the pleural space. This type of pneumothorax is common in young people and more common in men than women. It is not associated with any underlying lung disease. The patient is often slim with long fingers and high arched palate. In about 10 to 20 per cent of patients it recurs, sometimes repeatedly.

A spontaneous pneumothorax may also complicate lung disease such as emphysema, asthma, pulmonary tuberculosis, lung abscess, and pneumoconiosis. In addition, air may enter the pleural space from wounds of the chest wall or from a perforation of the oesophagus or trachea.

When the spontaneous pneumothorax is due to the rupture of a vesicle, the tear usually seals off rapidly and the air is absorbed from the pleural cavity over the next week or so. Occasionally a valve-like opening develops between the lung and the pleural space so that air can enter, but cannot leave the pleura; this leads to the accumulation of air in the pleural cavity and the development of a *tension pneumothorax*.

Clinical Features. The onset is usually sudden with pain in that side of the chest, and dyspnoea. The degree of constitutional upset is variable, but some patients may be quite shocked and collapsed. Occasionally the pneumothorax is found on routine examination and no history of chest pain can be elicited.

Examination of the chest may show diminished movement of the affected side. The degree to which the mediastinum is displaced away from the side of the pneumothorax is variable and depends on the size of the pneumothorax. Tactile vocal fremitus is decreased or absent. The note to percussion is either normal or hyper-resonant. On auscultation there are diminished breath sounds and absent voice sounds over the pneumothorax. An exocardial clicking sound may be heard over a small left-sided pneumothorax. A *coin sound* is sometimes present when their is a large or tension pneumothorax; this is a musical chiming heard through a stethoscope placed over the pneumothorax cavity when a coin laid on an adjacent part of the chest wall is tapped with another coin. The development of a *tension pneumothorax* is suggested by increasing dyspnoea, cyanosis, and distress. There will be signs of a pneumothorax with considerable mediastinal displacement. If the tension is not relieved, death may rapidly ensue.

Occasionally a spontaneous pneumothorax may be associated with a haemothorax (p. 240), presumably due to the tearing of pleural adhesions.

Chest radiograph shows air in the pleural cavity with a varying amount of collapse of the lung. There is rarely any evidence of lung disease.

Treatment. When a spontaneous pneumothorax is diagnosed within the first few hours after its onset, the patient is best moved to hospital if this is possible because of the slight but definite risk of a tension pneumothorax or haemopneumothorax developing. Rest at home for a short period is satisfactory if a pneumothorax has been present for a few days and is expanding satisfactorily. In the early stages some patients are shocked and in severe pain and require morphine 10–15 mg., perhaps repeated once or twice in the ensuing few hours.

No active treatment is required for a small or moderate sized pneumothorax. In all patients with a large or tension pneumothorax it is best to insert a catheter via a trochar through an intercostal space into the pleural cavity, the other end being connected to an under-water seal. The patient is intructed to cough gently and thus slowly to expel the air from the pneumothorax; expansion of the lung will then take place. In an emergency, where a patient's life is threatened by a tension pneumothorax and hospital equipment is not at hand, a needle should be pushed through a cork and into the pneumothorax; the needle can then be fixed into position with strapping and attached by a rubber tube to an under-water seal.

Occasionally the pneumothorax persists in spite of these measures or the patient may suffer from recurrent attacks of spontaneous pneumothorax. It is then necessary to produce a chemical pleurisy, usually by painting the pleural surfaces with a solution of silver nitrate and thus allowing the visceral and parietal pleurae to become adherent.

MEDIASTINAL CYSTS AND TUMOURS

(1) Swellings in the Mid-mediastinum

> (a) *Carcinoma of the Bronchus.* This is the commonest cause of a mediastinal mass. It may be composed of the growth alone or there may be associated infiltration and enlargement of lymph-nodes.
>
> (b) *Enlarged Lymph Nodes.* These may be due to carcinomatous infiltration (commonly from the bronchus), Hodgkin's disease, lymphosarcoma, sarcoidosis, or tuberculosis.

(2) Swellings in the Anterior Mediastinum

> (a) *Retrosternal Goitre.* This is usually, but not always, associated with a goitre in the neck. It lies anteriorly behind the manubrium and may compress the trachea or other structures in the superior mediastinum.
>
> (b) *Thymic tumours* lie in the upper anterior mediastinum. They are sometimes associated with myasthenia gravis. Some are malignant and may metastasise.
>
> (c) *Dermoid cysts and teratomas* usually lie anterior to the upper part of the heart. Dermoids may become infected and form

fistulae with surrounding structures. Both may undergo malignant change.

(d) *Pericardial cysts* (Spring-water cysts). These are found in the lower anterior mediastinum usually filling up the right cardiophrenic angle.

(3) Swellings in Posterior Mediastinum

Neurofibroma and ganglioneuroma. These tumours usually lie on the paravertebral gutter. They seldom cause symptoms and are found on routine radiography, appearing as rounded opacities with clear-cut edges. Occasionally they extend into the spinal canal causing compression of the spinal cord. A neurofibroma of the 1st thoracic nerve often causes Horner's syndrome (p. 251). *Aortic aneurysm* or aneurysmal dilatation of a pulmonary artery may appear as a mediastinal tumour.

Clinical Features. Mediastinal tumours and cysts may produce no symptoms and be found only on routine radiography. They may compress surrounding structures, causing a variety of symptoms and signs.

Investigation must always include postero-anterior and lateral radiographs of the chest. Tomography, bronchoscopy, and angiography may be required. Even with these investigations it is not always possible to make a definite diagnosis. Thoracotomy may be required both for diagnosis and for treatment.

FURTHER READING

Bates, D. V. and Christie, R. V. *Respiratory Function in Disease.* 2nd edn. W. B. Saunders Co., Philadelphia and London, 1971.

Brock, The Lord. *The anatomy of the bronchial tree with special reference to the surgery of lung abscess.* 2nd edn. Oxford University Press, London, 1954.

Crofton, J. and Douglas, A., *Respiratory diseases*, Blackwell Scientific Publications, Oxford and Edinburgh, 1969.

Knowles, J. *Respiratory physiology and its clinical application.* Harvard University Press, Cambridge, Mass., 1959.

d'Abreu, A. L. et al., *A Practice of Thoracic Surgery.* 3rd edn., 1971.

CHAPTER SIX

THE NERVOUS SYSTEM

THE CRANIAL NERVES

THE OLFACTORY NERVE (I)

Supplies special sensation (smell) to the superior nasal concha and the opposed part of the nasal septum. Pierces the cribriform plate of the ethmoid, and enters the olfactory bulb, which lies above the medial edge of the orbital plate. It continues as the olfactory tract which passes into the indusium griseum and sweeps anteriorly and superiorly round the corpus callosum and ends in the uncus.

It serves all smell, and all of flavour except salt, sweet, bitter, and acid. These functions may be tested with non-irritant aromatic odours, such as an orange, or a bar of scented soap, and it is the ability to separate rather than to identify them which must be shown to be intact.

Function

Smell is often temporarily upset with *acute and chronic rhinitis*; derangement may remain for weeks after the other symptoms have subsided. *Permanent bilateral anosmia* may follow *head injuries,* when the olfactory bulb is sheared from the ethmoid, or may accompany *tabes dorsalis,* and some influenza-like illnesses.

Unilateral (or bilateral) anosmia may be a sign of a *meningioma* growing in the olfactory groove.

THE OPTIC NERVE (II)

Fibres of the optic nerve pass centripetally in the stratum opticum of the retina. They are separated from the vitreous humour by the hyaloid membrane, and are closely applied to the ganglionic layer of the retina. They are so arranged that those taking origin close to the optic nerve pass into it first and are situated in its periphery, whereas those from the periphery of the retina pass over the more central fibres and enter the nerve nearer its midline. Thus the most peripheral fibres are the most superficial in the retina and the most central in the nerve.

The optic nerve passes back through the optic foramen to the optic chiasma, where the fibres from the medial sides of both retinae decussate. From the chiasma the optic tracts pass back to the lateral geniculate bodies, so that the right tract carries the fibres from the right half of *both* retinae, and therefore the image of the left visual field, and *vice versa.*

The fibres relay in the lateral geniculate body; the main central connection is through the optic radiation which passes through the temporal and parietal lobes to the occipital cortex. There is also a direct pathway through the pretectal area to the Edinger-Westphal nucleus.

In the occipital cortex macular vision is represented at the occipital pole, and peripheral vision arranged above and below the calcarine fissures, which are on the medial aspects of the occipital lobes.

Visual acuity should be tested by means of test type. The *visual fields* are examined first by direct confrontation and then if a lesion is suspected with a screen. Finally the optic nerve head and retina should be inspected directly with an ophthalmoscope.

(1) Changes in *visual acuity* are commonly the result of *refractive errors* or *lens opacities*. If these are excluded then affection of the *optic nerve* should be suspected. This may be confirmed by ophthalmoscopy.

(2) Changes in visual fields are of great localising value.

(a) *Tunnel vision* results when the superficial retinal fibres are compressed by *glaucoma*, with resultant loss of peripheral field.

(b) Loss of one field, without perception of light, occurs when the optic nerve itself is diseased.

(c) Affection of the lateral part of the optic chiasma and the posterior part of the ipselateral optic nerve causes homonymous hemianopia with ipselateral central scotoma. It may occur with *chromophobe adenomas, craniopharyngiomas, anterior communicating aneurysms, meningiomas of the medial wing of the sphenoid,* or *localised arachnoiditis*.

(d) Compression at the chiasma causes bitemporal hemianopia, which is the classical sign of *pituitary tumours*. It is not necessarily symmetrical, particularly in the early stages. In about half of the patients with a proven pituitary chromophobe adenoma, the initial field defect may be a central or paracentral scotoma.

(e) Lesions behind the optic chiasma cause homonymous hemianopia; their exact site must be identified by accompanying signs and symptoms. Quadrantic hemianopia is often associated with lesions of the radiation; upper quadrantic defects suggest that the temporal lobe is involved, lower quadrantic defects the parietal.

(3) The normal optic nerve head is seen as a pink disc, slightly paler in the temporal half, with clear margins, from which the retinal arterioles emerge and on which the veins converge.

Optic Neuritis and Papilloedema

The optic disc may be oedematous as in *optic neuritis* (or papillitis) and *papilloedema*: these conditions are easily separated clinically by the visual acuity. This is usually affected early and severely in papillitis, late and mildly in papilloedema.

The *common cause* of papillitis is *disseminated sclerosis*; other causes are *methyl alcohol poisoning, meningitis,* and *encephalitis.* Papilloedema is most commonly caused by *hypertension,* when the distinctive retinal changes make the diagnosis obvious. It may also result from *raised intracranial pressure,* when it is usually accompanied by headaches and vomiting. *Venous obstruction,* in the orbit or more proximally, may cause papilloedema; it may also occur in *severe anaemia* and *polycythaemia rubra.* It is commonly seen as a terminal phenomenon in *pulmonary heart disease* with marked carbon dioxide retention.

Optic Atrophy

The optic nerve head may be unduly pale, suggesting optic atrophy; this may sometimes be confirmed by showing reduced visual acuity. If optic atrophy is advanced, a dead white disc is seen. There may be no perception of light and the direct and consensual pupillary reflexes are lost; but if the absence of perception of light is unilateral the consensual pupillary reflex is retained.

Optic atrophy may result from *glaucoma,* when tunnel vision is found and the physiological cup is seen to be unduly excavated. Many other causes are recognised, and among the most important are *disseminated sclerosis, syphilis, toxins* (particularly *methyl alcohol, quinine,* and *tobacco*), as a sequel to *head injury* and as a *congenital affection.* It may also be the result of *repeated bleeding* or of long-standing *vitamin (B) deficiency.* Pressure on the nerve (from *Paget's disease of the skull, tumours* of the optic nerve or sheath, or meningiomas) obstruct its blood supply and so cause atrophy.

THE OCULOMOTOR NERVES

Oculomotor (III), trochlear (IV), abducent (VI)

The oculomotor nuclei lie in the midbrain (III) and pons (IV and VI). They represent the extreme cephalic extent of the somatic efferent trunk. The *oculomotor nerve* passes forward and laterally and emerges at the medial side of the cerebral peduncle. It passes through the interpeduncular fossa, and pierces the dura at the lateral side of the posterior clinoid process. It lies in the lateral wall of the cavernous sinus, and enters the orbit through the superior orbital fissure. It supplies all the eye muscles except the lateral rectus and the superior oblique. The *trochlear* nerve emerges on the posterior aspect of the pons, after decussating with the contralateral nerve. It passes round the superior cerebellar peduncle and pierces the dura just behind the posterior clinoid process, and just below the free border of the tentorium. It lies in the lateral wall of the cavernous sinus and enters the orbit through the superior orbital fissure. It supplies the superior oblique muscle. The *abducent* nerve emerges anteriorly just below the junction of the pons and medulla. It passes forward through the cisterna pontis and pierces the dura lateral to the dorsum sellae of the sphenoid. It is sharply angulated round the petrous part of the temporal bone. It traverses the cavernous sinus closely applied to the carotid artery and enters the orbit through the superior orbital fissure. It supplies the lateral rectus muscle.

The Eye Muscles

The lateral and medial recti are simple abductors and adductors of the eyeball. When the eye is adducted the inferior and superior oblique muscles act best as simple elevators and depressors respectively. When the eye is abducted it is elevated chiefly by the superior and depressed chiefly by the inferior rectus muscles.

The superior oblique is supplied by the trochlear nerve, and the lateral rectus by the abducent. All the other muscles are supplied by the oculo-motor.

Squint

Squints may be either *concomitant* or *paralytic*. Concomitant squint means congenital non-parallelism of the visual axes; it is never associated with diplopia, and both eyes have full movements if tested separately.

Paralytic squint is always acquired, and is always associated with double vision, unless the false image is suppressed, which is unusual. To discover the paralysed muscle the following points must be remembered:

(1) The false image is always the peripheral one.
(2) The false image is always seen by the affected eye.
(3) Separation of the images is always maximal in the direction of action of the affected muscle; it is laterally displaced with paralysis of adductors and abductors, vertically if elevators or depressors are affected.

Adductors and abductors should be tested with the gaze horizontal, elevators and depressors in full abduction or adduction.

Applied Anatomy

(1) *Lateral rectus palsy (VI)* causes a paralysis of abduction of the affected eye. If complete the gaze cannot be deviated beyond the midline in the affected eye.

(2) *Oculomotor palsy (III)*. There is marked ptosis. When the lid is lifted the eye is seen to be abducted (and depressed) and the pupil widely dilated and non-reactive to light or other stimuli. If complete there is a complete ptosis. The eye is abducted but *not* depressed. Integrity of the *IV*th nerve is demonstrated by torsion of the eye ball on *attempted* downward gaze.

(3) *Superior oblique palsy (IV)*. There is paralysis of depression of the gaze when the eye is adducted.

It must be realised that these are not mutually exclusive; combinations may occur, and any or all of the lesions may be partial or complete. Bizarre combinations may be seen in *myasthenia gravis*, or when the muscles themselves are diseased, as in *malignant exophthalmos* (p. 441).

(4) *Loss of conjugate deviation*. Conjugate eye movement originates in the second frontal convolution; if the descending fibres are interrupted in the lower mid-brain or upper pons, conjugate deviation of the eyes is affected. This may occur temporarily following *cerebral haemorrhage* or *thrombosis*; spasmodically in *epilepsy or post-encephalitic Parkinsonism*; permanent loss occurs with destructive lesions of the upper pons, usually *vascular* or *neoplastic*. Less commonly it follows *encephalitis* or complicates *demyelinating diseases*.

The Pupils

Consist of muscle fibres arranged concentrically (sphinctre pupillae) and radially (dilator pupillae). The blood supply is derived from an outer (circulus arteriosus major) and inner (circulus arteriosus minor) vascular circle, connected by radiating arterial vessels; it is supplied by the long anterior and posterior ciliary arteries. The nerve supply of the sphincter pupillae is by *parasympathetic* fibres (from the ciliary ganglion through the short ciliary nerves); the dilator pupillae by *sympathetic* fibres (from the nasociliary nerve through the long ciliary nerves).

The pupil should constrict with convergence and on exposure to light; and dilate if shaded. The path of both the light and convergence reflexes is the same as far as the lateral geniculate body. Thereafter the light reflex passes directly to the parasympathetic part of the oculomotor nucleus, whereas the convergence reflex passes back to the occipital cortex and then forward again to the oculomotor nucleus.

Applied Anatomy

(1) In *old people* and in the *presenile atheromatous conditions* the pupillary arteries are patchily arteriosclerotic, and will not collapse fully. For this reason many old people have small, irregular and unequal pupils.

(2) There is a condition known as *myotonic pupil* wherein the pupil reacts very slowly to light and convergence. It is frequently unilateral, and is common in young women. It may be associated with absent knee and ankle jerks (*Adie's syndrome*). The pathology is unknown, but the condition is completely benign. Neuronal degeneration has been reported in the ipselateral ciliary ganglion.

(3) *Horner's syndrome.* In lesions of the sympathetic nerve to the eye the pupil on the affected side is usually smaller and does not dilate to shade. There is some ptosis, and possibly enophthalmos. Sweating may be reduced on the same side of the face.

Horner's syndrome is an excellent lateralising sign, but a poor localising sign; lesions are always ipsilateral, but may occur anywhere on the path of the sympathetic fibres as they pass from the hypothalamus through the brain stem to the cervical cord, then emerging at the level of the first thoracic segment to join the cervical sympathetic ganglion, on to the carotid artery, with which they re-enter the skull, and finally into the globe itself. Of particular importance are lesions of the carotid artery, which may give rise to ipsilateral sympathetic paralysis and contralateral hemiplegia.

(4) *Argyll-Robertson pupils* are small, unequal, eccentric, and irregular in outline. They do not react to light, but do constrict on convergence. This implies an interruption of the light reflex between the lateral geniculate body and the oculomotor nucleus; it is believed to occur in the pretectal area.

Such pupils are almost diagnostic of *syphilis*. The only other condition in which they may occur is in hypertrophic polyneuritis which is comparatively very rare.

(5) Oval pupils, unequal pupils in otherwise healthy people, and pupils which show minor dilatation and contraction in time with the pulse are of no significance.

THE TRIGEMINAL NERVE (V)

The trigeminal ganglion lies in the *cavum trigeminale*, closely applied to the petrous temporal bone. Axis cylinders of the ganglion divide into peripheral and central branches; the central ones pass to the fifth nerve nuclei, extending through the pons and medulla, and lying posteriorly. The motor tract of the fifth nerve arises from the motor nucleus of V, which lies in the pons, just anterior to the middle sensory nucleus. From it all the muscles of mastication (except the buccinator) are supplied.

The peripheral axons are the sensory supply to the face and the anterior part of the scalp. They lie in three great bundles, the ophthalmic, maxillary, and mandibular nerves, each with sharply defined territory.

(1) Ophthalmic. Supplies anterior part of scalp as far back as the crown of the head, the forehead and the eye (including the cornea) and the antero-lateral part of the nose.

(2) Maxillary. Supplies the cheek, lower eyelid, side of the nose, • and upper lip only.

(3) Mandibular. From the side of the head, down to the cheek,

including the upper part of the ear, but missing the angle of the jaw. Also supplies the lower lip and chin.

Applied Anatomy

The nuclei may be affected in the brainstem by *syringobulbia, tumours, demyelinating* or *vascular lesions*. The ganglion may be compressed by *acoustic* or *trigeminal neuromas*, or involved in local *syphilitic meningitis. Trigeminal neuralgia* (p. 313) is of unknown aetiology and is not associated with signs in the nervous system.

FACIAL NERVE (VII)

The facial nucleus lies in the lower part of the pons, and fibres from it pass anteriorly to emerge at the junction of the medulla and pons on the ventral aspect of the brain stem. Fibres of the seventh nerve sweep round the *sixth nerve nucleus* and are so closely applied to it that both nerves are usually affected by lesions in this vicinity.

After leaving the brain stem the seventh nerve passes anterolaterally with the *auditory nerve* to the *internal auditory meatus*. Here it enters the facial canal with the eighth nerve.

In the bony canal the nerve bends through a right angle at the seventh nerve ganglion. Here the *nervus intermedius* leaves the facial nerve and passes to the lingual nerve (mandibular fifth) to supply taste to the anterior two thirds of the tongue.

The seventh nerve leaves the skull through the stylomastoid foramen and pierces the parotid gland, from which it emerges to supply the muscles of facial expression.

Applied Anatomy

The muscles of the forehead have bilateral cortical representation. Therefore they are relatively spared in upper motor neurone lesions affecting the face; moreover in such cases voluntary facial movements are affected more than involuntary ones, such as blinking and smiling.

In lower motor neurone lesions all the facial muscles are affected, and both voluntary and involuntary movements are paralysed. Associated lesions may contribute to better localisation.

(1) Brainstem—associated ipselateral VI nerve palsy.

(2) Cerebello-pontine angle—associated VIII and V nerve lesions.

(3) In the bony canal—associated VIII nerve lesions, sometimes hyperacusis (from paralysis of stapedius) and loss of taste over anterior two thirds of tongue.

Upper motor neurone lesions of the seventh nerve commonly occur in strokes involving the internal capsule. The nucleus may be affected in *tumours, vascular lesions*, or *poliomyelitis* affecting the brain stem. The classical lesion in the cerebello-pontine angle is the *acoustic neuroma*. The nerve is frequently affected in *acute infective polyneuritis* (p. 311).

Bell's Palsy is an acute lower motor neurone palsy of the facial nerve. It is of unknown aetiology, and the exact site of the lesion is not known. The nerve is believed to become oedematous within the facial canal. Occasionally there is associated ipselateral hyperacusis or loss of taste over the anterior two thirds of the tongue on the same side. Rarely it is recurrent, sometimes bilaterally, and most rarely of all is concurrently bilateral; these latter occurrences always cast doubt on the diagnosis of simple Bell's palsy.

It is abrupt in onset, and at its worst within 48 hours. Sometimes there is a little associated pain behind the ear. If at the end of a week any movement at all is visible on the affected side an assurance of eventual complete recovery may be given; this usually takes 4 to 8 weeks, but may be as long as a year. Even if no movement is seen at the end of a week prognosis should be optimistic. Full recovery may still occur after up to three months of total paralysis. If the patient is seen in the early stages prednisolone 20 mg. four times daily for five days and then rapidly tailed off reduces the incidence of residual paralysis. If paralysis is long-standing dental splits are of value in preventing stretching of the facial muscles, and if the eye cannot be closed it must be protected, especially during sleep.

The Ramsay-Hunt syndrome is an acute affection of the seventh nerve by the herpes virus. It is preceded by a sore throat, and herpetic vesicles can be seen on the soft palate and external auditory meatus on the affected side. Recovery from the facial paralysis is often incomplete.

Clonic facial spasm is almost confined to elderly women. It is nearly always unilateral. Its aetiology is unknown, and it does not recover spontaneously. Its most embarrassing feature is winking, and this may be treated by surgical section of the upper fibres of facial nerve.

Habit spasm occurs in children and less commonly in young adults. It is bilateral, and can be imitated by the observer and controlled by the child voluntarily—neither of which apply to facial myoclonus. It is associated with mounting mental tension, which is in some way relieved by the grimace.

THE ACOUSTIC-VESTIBULAR NERVE (VIII)

Separate vestibular and cochlear nuclei are situated in the upper medulla and lower pons. They lie anterolaterally and are widely connected centrally.

(a) *Vestibular* nuclei to:

    (1) ipselateral cerebellar hemisphere.
    (2) medial longitudinal bundle (hence *III*, *IV*, and *VI*).
    (3) vestibulo-spinal tract.
    (4) ipselateral lateral lemniscus (to inf. corp. quad. and superior temporal gyrus).

(b) *Cochlear* nucleus to:

(1) medial longitudinal bundle.
(2) trapezoid body (to contralateral inf. corp. quad. and auditory area of temporal lobe).

Thus hearing is represented in the contralateral and balance in the ipselateral temporal lobe.

Fibres from the nuclei pass forwards and emerge anterolaterally at the junction of pons and medulla. They pass into the internal auditory meatus and are distributed to the cochlear (shell like) organ and the vestibule. This consists of the semicircular canals and the otolith organ.

Hearing should be tested by whispering softly at about 18 inches from the ear. The patient should not look at the examiner's lips whilst repeating his words. Normally sounds heard by air conduction seem louder than when heard by bone conduction; this should be verified with a tuning fork (128 c.p.s. or higher). *Vestibular function* is tested by syringing the ears with water first 7° C. above body temperature (44° C.) and then 7° C. below (30° C.) (*Caloric Tests*). A standard technique is used, and the duration of resulting nystagmus is timed. Normally it should persist for at least 100 seconds from the start of perfusion. Failure to do so implies disease of one labyrinth.

Applied Anatomy

(1) *Cochlear Lesions*

In *conduction deafness* bone conduction sounds louder than air conduction. In *nerve deafness* acuity is reduced, but air conduction is still the better.

(a) Conduction deafness is usually a sequel to *inflammatory middle ear disease.* It may occur with *eustachian obstruction, otosclerosis* or *Paget's disease of bone.*
(b) Nerve deafness may be further localised by associated physical signs.
   (i) Lesions in the petrous temporal bone are associated with facial palsy and impaired taste.
   (ii) Lesions in the cerebello-pontine angle cause VIII, VII, and V nerve palsies.
   (iii) Nuclear lesions are associated with other brain stem palsies.

Nerve deafness may be *congenital,* or may be caused by *fractures of the temporal bone.* It may occur with *congenital syphilis,* or with *tumours* of the cerebello-pontine angle. Rarely it complicates *brain-stem lesions* (usually vascular or demyelinating) or tumours near the corpora quadrigemina.

(2) *Vestibular Lesions*

Classically cause vertigo and imbalance. Both have the same significance. Disequilibrium *with or without* subjective rotation sensation is implied.

Positional vertigo indicates disease of the otolith organ, and *directional* vertigo of the semicircular canals. Vertigo may also result from central lesions of the vestibular nucleus (especially with basilar insufficiency) or of the temporal lobe.

> (a) **Ménière's syndrome** consists of the concurrence of deafness, tinnitus, and vertigo. It may occur with many ear diseases. If these are excluded it is attributed to a functional derangement of the semicircular canals (*Ménière's Disease*). This occurs more frequently in women than in men, and usually appears in the second half of life. It is paroxysmal and intermittent. Long remissions may occur. No physical signs except deafness and nystagmus during an attack are found; there is no interval nystagmus. The semicircular canals can be shown to be impaired by caloric stimulation. The disease is progressive and may eventually lead to total deafness.
>
> (b) *Vestibular Neuronitis.* Hearing is not involved, but there is usually intense vertigo, passing off in a few days, with a liability for a few weeks to vertigo on turning the head or on sudden movement. It sometimes occurs in epidemics.

Vertigo

A feeling of disequilibrium, or unsteadiness, is a common complaint in patients suffering from anxiety, and in the absence of other evidence of disease should be treated by reassurance and sedation. When such attacks occur suddenly and last only a brief time, and particularly when they are associated with a sense of rotation, or with other symptoms such as tinnitus or deafness, they are more likely to imply disease of the vestibular apparatus, peripheral or central. Unfortunately the distinction is sometimes difficult to draw in practice, for some patients with clear evidence of such disease complain only of vaguely defined disequilibrium. It is usually possible, however, to form a reasonable opinion of the significance of the symptom.

Treatment depends upon the cause. In basilar insufficiency (p. 278) Librium (chlordiazepoxide 5–10 mg. t.d.s.) is the drug of choice. In Ménière's syndrome Stemetil (pro-chlor-perazine 10 mg. t.d.s.) may be tried or Perdilatil Forte (buphenine hydrochloride 6 mg. t.d.s.).

GLOSSOPHARYNGEAL NERVE (IX)

Motor and sensory nuclei lie in upper medulla. The nerve passes anteriorly across the petrous temporal bone, and leaves the skull through the jugular foramen. It passes between the carotid artery and the jugular vein to supply the pharyngeal constrictor muscles. It also supplies special and ordinary sensation to the posterior third of the tongue and adjacent soft palate. It is motor to the stylopharyngeal muscle and secreto-motor to the parotid gland.

VAGUS (X)

Sensory and motor nuclei are situated in the medulla. The nerve passes forwards and laterally and leaves the skull through the jugular foramen. In the neck it lies in the carotid sheath, and enters the thorax behind the great veins. The left nerve passes between the left subclavian and common carotid arteries, over the aortic arch and on to the posterior surface of the left lung. The right crosses the right subclavian artery and then passes behind the superior vena cava to the posterior surface of the right lung. It has meningeal, auricular, pharyngeal and laryngeal branches, and is the main parasympathetic supply to the thoracic and abdominal viscera.

ACCESSORY NERVE (XI)

The nucleus is in the medulla, and the nerve passes forwards and laterally through the jugular foramen, having been joined by fibres from the spinal nucleus (C1–5). These *accessory* fibres join the vagus, and pass to the larynx and pharynx. The spinal part is motor to the sternomastoid and trapezius muscles.

HYPOGLOSSAL NERVE (XII)

The nucleus lies in the medulla, and the nerve leaves the skull through the anterior condylar foramen. It passes over the hyoid bone and then turns medially to supply the muscles of the tongue.

Applied Anatomy

These last four nerves are in such close proximity that they are frequently involved together. Individual lesions do occur, however.

      (a) *IX*. Loss of special and ordinary sensation to posterior third of tongue and soft palate. Test for anaesthesia in the tonsillar fossa.

      (b) *X*. Paralysis of levator palati or vocal cord.

      (c) *XI*. Weakness of sternomastoid, and weakness and wasting of upper fibres of trapezius.

      (d) *XII*. Deviation of tongue to the affected side on protrusion.

In lower motor neurone lesions the tongue is fibrillating and wasted, in upper motor neurone lesions small and stiff.

The X, XI, and XII nuclei are involved in *bulbar* and *pseudobulbar palsies*. The *foramen magnum syndrome* results from *platybasia*; the neck is usually short, and there is a combination of upper motor neurone disease and paralysis of the lower cranial nerves; the IX, X, and XI nerves may be affected in the *jugular foramen syndrome*, from nasopharyngeal tumours or meningiomas, and the IX, X, XI, and XII nerves from *glomus jugulare tumours*, though VII and VIII are also involved frequently and at an early stage.

SPEECH

This involves the selection of words and their production. Production depends upon the integrity of the nerves and muscles concerned with speech; their disorder is termed *dysarthria*, their complete failure *anarthria*. The selection of words depends upon the proper function of large parts of the cerebral cortex, but is possible only if the so-called speech centre is intact. This lies in the dominant hemisphere, and consists of the posterior and inferior parts of the second and third frontal gyri and the adjacent part of the temporal lobe. *Dysphasia* and *aphasia* are the terms respectively applied to difficulty in word selection or its failure. Two forms may be recognised; *expressive aphasia*, in which the word is well known to the subject, but cannot be presented for production, and *receptive aphasia*, in which the word cannot be understood. Expressive aphasia is usually associated with lesions in the anterior part of the hemisphere and receptive aphasia with more posteriorly placed lesions.

THE MOTOR SYSTEM

Anatomy

The Pyramidal Tract. It arises from the precentral gyrus. The fibres converge on the internal capsule and pass down in the cerebral peduncle. It descends through the mid-brain to the pons, where it is divided but not interrupted by the transverse pontine fibres. Some fibres cross the midline in the mid-brain and the pons and serve as upper motor neurones for the motor cranial nerve nuclei. The main bundle comes to lie anteriorly in the brain stem and finally in the pyramid which gives the tract its name. The tract crosses the midline in the lower part of the medulla, decussating with the fibres from the other side (*decussation of pyramids*). A few fibres do not cross, but pass down to the cord anteriorly and lying close to the mid-line. The main pyramidal tract eventually lies in the lateral part of the white matter of the cord and gives upper motor neurone supply to the anterior horn cells.

Stimulation of the motor area in the brain causes discrete contralateral movements, and its extirpation contralateral paralysis. Somatic representation in the cortex is very regular and remains so throughout the length of the pyramidal tract.

Applied Anatomy

Congenital abnormalities of the tract or its injury early in life may be associated with contralateral reduced growth and weakness. Vigorous movements of the unaffected limbs may cause small imitative unwanted movements on the affected side; unwanted movements may also occur at rest. *Acquired* disease of the tract causes contralateral hemiparesis. Abrupt lesions of the tract initially cause flaccid contralateral paresis. At first both plantar responses are extensor. Coma or stupor is the rule; if the dominant hemisphere is affected then aphasia is also present. After some days or a week or two the typical signs of a spastic upper motor neurone (UMN) lesion emerge.

Signs of UMN Lesion

In lesions of gradual onset these may be present from the start. The changes which may be found lie in alterations in tone, power, and the skin and tendon reflexes. Wasting is not apparent except in long-standing hemiplegia with disuse atrophy of muscles, and co-ordination is only disturbed because of weakness and stiffness of the limb.

The Face

The eyes are rarely affected. There may be weakness of the muscles of mastication, detected by deviation of the jaw on opening and weakness in keeping it open. The face is usually affected; there is spastic weakness, particularly of the lower half. The soft palate may rise asymmetrically, deviating from the affected side, and the vocal cord may be paralysed. Weakness of the trapezius is revealed on shrugging the shoulder against resistance, and of the sternomastoid by weakness in turning the head away from the affected side. Spastic weakness of the tongue causes deviation to the affected side on protrusion.

The Limbs

(a) *Spasticity*. There is increase in tone in all the muscles on the affected side, most easily detected in the stronger muscles. It is such that there is initially increasing resistance to stretching, changing suddenly to rapid diminution. This action has been likened to the opening of a clasp knife. But it is this distribution of increased tone rather than its special nature which is important in the recognition of UMN disease.

(b) *Power*. All muscles are weak on the affected side, but there is uneven distribution of weakness, so that in the upper limbs flexors are stronger than extensors, and in the lower limbs extensors are stronger than flexors. In the arm the weaker muscles are the intrinsic muscles of the hand, the shoulder abductors and the extensors of the elbow, wrist and fingers. In the leg, the weaker muscles are the flexors and abductors of the hip, the flexors of the knee, and the dorsiflexors and evertors of the ankle. The hemiplegic posture results from the counterplay of the strong and weak muscles.

(c) *Skin Reflexes*. The abdominal and cremasteric reflexes are abolished or reduced on the affected side, and the plantar response is extensor. In severe hemiplegias this response may be provoked from a wide area of the affected limb. As severity decreases in degree so the sensitive area shrinks and finally only the posterior third of the lateral aspect of the sole of the foot is receptive. To be effective the stimulus may have to be noxious for example by scratching on the outer aspect of the heel with a 'yale key'. Normally this is followed by flexion of the toes, particularly the great toe, at the metatarsophalangeal joints. To be certainly positive biphasic extension and flexion of the first metatarsophalangeal joint should always follow appropriate stimulation.

Signs of hemiplegia may be minimal. They are always reduced, and may be abolished, by rest in bed. In any case either weakness, hypertonia, or deranged skin reflexes may predominate. Flexor plantar responses do not exclude an upper motor neurone lesion.

THE NEUROMUSCULAR JUNCTION

Physiology

The arrival of a nerve impulse at a neuromuscular junction causes the release of acetylcholine. This stimulates a sensitive muscle area (the motor end plate) and initiates a contraction of the muscle bundle. An enzyme (cholinesterase) rapidly destroys acetylcholine, and so permits the muscle to repolarise.

Applied Physiology

Transmission may be deranged in various ways. Procaine and botulinus toxin inhibit the secretion of acetylcholine; physostigmine (eserine), neostigmine, and a number of other drugs (some now used widely as insecticides) destroy cholinesterase, and so perpetuate the actions, both central (muscarine) and peripheral (nicotine) of acetylcholine. The sensitivity of the motor end plate may be reduced either specifically, as for example by Indian arrow poison (curare), or similar substances (gallamine, mephenesin), or as part of a general muscle disorder, for example lead poisoning or potassium deficiency or excess. Inhibition at the neuromuscular junction is believed to be the basis of myasthenia gravis (p. 301).

THE SENSORY SYSTEM

Anatomy

The skin is protected by a superficial and a deep network of sensory end organs. Each organ is supplied by at least two nerve fibres. Not all parts of the skin are equally sensitive. Relatively insensitive areas exist, for example over the medial and lateral condyles of the ankle, and over the elbows. Especially sensitive areas exist over the pads of the fingers and round the lips. The forehead is less sensitive than the rest of the face, and the back of the trunk less so than the front.

Non-medullated fibres conduct all modalities of sensation and pass back in bundles (sensory nerves) to the posterior horns of the spinal cord. Here they divide, and fibres carrying position sense, vibration, and light touch pass into the posterior columns without relaying; those carrying pain and temperature sensation relay in the posterior horn. The relay fibres then cross the midline, and pass upwards in the lateral spinothalamic tracts.

The sacral fibres enter first, and therefore occupy the most medial position in the posterior column and the most superficial in the spinothalamic tract. Conversely the cervical fibres are most lateral in the posterior columns and deepest in the spinothalamic tract.

The spinothalamic tract passes upwards through the brain stem lying superficially (lateral lemniscus) and ends in the (optic) thalamus. The posterior columns end in the gracile and cuneate nuclei in the lower medulla. Some fibres pass to the cerebellum but the main relay crosses the midline in the medulla, decussating with the fibres from the other side (decussation of the fillets). Having crossed the midline these sensory fibres lie deep to the lateral lemniscus, and pass up to the thalamus through the brain stem (medial lemniscus). In the pons they are joined by fibres from the sensory nucleus of V, bearing light touch, pressure, and postural sense from the face (quinto-thalamic tract). The trigeminal ganglion lies in the cavum trigeminale, closely related to the petrous part of the temporal bone. Its peripheral neurones conduct sensation from the face, and its central fibres pass back to three sensory nuclei in the brain stem; the lowest, receiving pain and temperature fibres from the forehead, extends as far down as the upper cervical cord (about C2). The principal nucleus lies in the pons, and it is from this that the quinto-thalamic tract takes chief origin.

Appreciation of crude sensation takes place at the level of the thalamus, but more complex sensations are relayed to the cortex. Sensation is represented in the post-central gyrus in much the same way that the motor cortex is arranged. Besides this direct representation there is an associative area (superior and inferior parietal lobules) lying behind the post-central gyrus concerned with the appreciation of spatial relationships.

Disturbance of sensation may be of two kinds. It may be reduced or absent, or abnormal sensations may be experienced. Neither decreased sensation nor any kind of added sensation alone is of localising value. It is the distribution of sensory change, and the modalities affected, together with associated signs which allow anatomical identification of lesions. Similarly, no kinds of paraesthesiae are specific, although feelings of constriction of limbs or trunk are very commonly associated with posterior column lesions.

Examination of the Sensory System

Each modality of sensation must be individually tested. First an area believed to have normal sensation must be selected, and stimuli first applied here, so that the patient is in no doubt of what he *should* feel. With each modality comparison must be made between the area being tested, the same area on the other side of the body, and the known normal area.

> (a) Pain is tested with a sharp needle or pin. Initially several pricks should be made rapidly over an area of about 1 sq. cm. In this way the possibility of touching an area of apparent anaesthesia between sensory end-organs is obviated. It is important to ask the patient: 'Did it sting as a pinprick

should?', not simply: 'Can you feel this?', for pin prick may be appreciated as a touch where pain sense is impaired but light touch is intact (syringomyelia, p. 297). When this has been done the pin should be firmly pressed to one point, and the patient asked to comment on the sensation. It should be felt as a pinpoint of pain. It may be that the threshold of pain is raised, but when it *is* appreciated the sensation is like a small ring of pain, often with a burning quality, rather than a pinpoint.

This is diagnostic of a partial lesion of pain pathways, but gives no information of the level at which it is affected.

(b) Temperature may be quickly tested with a cold object, such as the blade of a tuning-fork, but if impairment is discovered then careful testing with two test tubes, one filled with cold and one with hot water is necessary.

(c) Light touch can be tested by touching lightly with the finger-tip or with a piece of cotton-wool or the corner of a hand-kerchief. It is important to touch cleanly, and not to rub the skin; this induces tickle, which is conducted by pain pathways.

(d) Position sense should be tested by moving first small and then larger joints and asking the patient to idei ify the direction of movement without looking.

(e) Vibration should be tested with a tuning fork (128 c.p.s.). The handle should be firmly pressed to bony prominences, and appreciation on the two sides compared.

Abnormal sensations (paraesthesiae) are variously described as tingling, pins and needles, burning, coldness, sense of water running over the skin, formication (ants crawling on skin), gripping, and 'compression of a limb'. They imply nothing but disturbance of paths of sensation, and considered alone give no indication at what level disturbance has occurred.

Clinical Interpretation of Sensory Disturbance

(a) Peripheral Neuritis. This causes a disturbance of motor, reflex, and sensory functions, usually of about equal degree. Rarely it is almost entirely sensory, even more rarely only motor. It exists in two forms, a *polyneuritis* affecting all nerves to about equal degree, and *mono-neuritis multiplex*, in which two or more nerves are affected, others being completely spared.

(b) Posterior root lesions (*tabes dorsalis*) cause a widespread disturbance of all modalities of sensation. Degeneration occurs in the posterior columns as fibres pass into them directly; the crossing fibres are relayed, so that no degeneration occurs in the spinothalamic tracts.

(c) Posterior horn lesions (*syringomyelia*) catch the crossing fibres, but spare those passing directly to the posterior columns; hence pain and temperature sense are lost, but light touch preserved. Connecting neurones are also involved, so that the tendon reflexes are interrupted.

(d) Space-occupying lesions of the cord itself involve the spinothalamic tracts from within. Hence cervical and thoracic symptoms appear early, and the more superficial sacral fibres are not immediately involved (sacral sparing).

(e) Extramedullary space-occupying lesions may compress the whole cord and primarily cause upper motor neurone lesions. Later there may be root pains, involvement of long sensory tracts, and lower motor neurone signs at the level of the lesion. The circulation of cerebrospinal fluid (C.S.F.) may be obstructed (*Froin syndrome*, p. 292).

Occasionally extramedullary compression involves predominantly one half of the cord (*Brown-Séquard syndrome*), so that the posterior columns, pyramidal tracts, and spinothalamic tracts are involved on one side of the cord. This causes signs of an upper motor neurone lesion, with loss of position, vibration sense and light touch on the same side as the compression but contralateral loss of pain and temperature sensation.

(f) In the brain stem the disease can be localised by the involvement of adjacent structures. The lateral lemniscus lies superficially and the medial lemniscus deeply throughout their course. Because of this compressing lesions tend to affect contralateral pain and temperature appreciation, whereas intrinsic lesions involve the medial lemniscus and cause contralateral disturbance of position and vibration sense.

(g) Disturbances at the level of the thalamus are rare. Incomplete lesions produce contralateral sensory disturbances. Abnormal sensation, for example burning or stinging may be experienced, and the threshold to pain is increased. Once appreciated, however, there is overreaction to painful stimuli.

(h) The sensory cortex subserves all forms of discriminative sensation. Its functions have been listed as follows (modified from Gordon Holmes).

(1) It relates incoming experiences to previous sensations, and allows the recognition of similarities and differences.

(2) It allows awareness of the postural relations of separate parts of the body.

(3) It locates the sites of stimuli to the body's surface, and enables distinction to be made between one and two simultaneous contacts.

(4) It allows the recognition of the shape, size, weight, texture, and consistency of objects.

(5) It enables the attention to be focused on any given part of the body.

(6) It controls the response of subcortical centres to stimuli.

THE CEREBELLUM

Balance and Co-ordination of Movement

Co-ordination depends upon the smooth contraction of certain muscle groups (agonists) and the equally smooth relaxation of their opposers (antagonists). It is the lateral lobes of the cerebellum which are chiefly concerned in this. The function of the central lobe (vermis) of the cerebellum is to maintain balance; lesions of this lobe cause an inability to stand or to walk.

For the correct maintenance of balance, posture, and co-ordination there must be no proprioceptive defect, no weakness, and muscle tone must be normal. Only when these functions have been shown to be intact should abnormalities be certainly attributed to the cerebellum.

Disease of the lateral lobe of the cerebellum and its connections produces ipselateral derangement of movement. No abnormality is detected when the subject is completely at rest.

The inco-ordination of cerebellar disease results in a *terminal action tremor*. That is to say it occurs only with movement and is worse at the end of movement. It may be detected in various groups of muscles.

(1) The eye; it causes nystagmus on lateral and/or upward gaze.
(2) Speech becomes jerky and abnormally accentuated (scanning speech).
(3) Gait is reeling, usually towards the side of the lesion.
(4) There is loss of muscle fixation, so that if the hand and arm are held extended an abnormal posture results. Added to this there is apparent hypotonia in affected limbs. Because of this the reflexes may be reduced.

Applied Anatomy

The cerebellum is vulnerable to backward spread from infective middle ear disease, which may cause cerebellar abscess. It is very frequently affected by disseminated sclerosis, usually in the superior cerebellar peduncle. Space-occupying lesions of the posterior fossa rapidly cause forward displacement of the brain stem, with obstruction of the flow of cerebrospinal fluid and internal hydrocephalus. In effect, the whole ventricular system is made to behave like a rapidly expanding cerebral tumour; consequently severe headache, papilloedema, and vomiting appear early in the course of quite small space-occupying lesions in the cerebellum.

Occasionally evidence of an upper motor neurone lesion and a cerebellar lesion occur in the same side of the body. This can be caused by one lesion in the mid-brain, catching the descending pyramidal tract before it has crossed, and the tract from the superior cerebellar peduncle to the red nucleus after it has crossed.

THE BASAL GANGLIA AND EXTRAPYRAMIDAL SYSTEM

These are a group of large nuclei situated in the white matter of the cortex just below and lateral to the anterior horns of the lateral ventricles. The corpus striatum (striped body) is divided by the descending pyramidal tract into the caudate ('tail like') and lentiform ('lens shaped') nuclei; these same fibres later separate the lentiform from the thalamic nuclei The lentiform nucleus is seen to consist of two opposing structures, causing a medial pale and lateral darker appearance. The medial pale structure is spherical, and known as the globus pallidus (pale globe), or pallidum; the lateral darker part the putamen (shell).

In the lower vertebrates the corpus striatum is represented only by the pallidum, and for this reason is known as the palaeostriatum (old striped body); in reptiles and birds (and above) the putamen and caudate nuclei appear (neostriatum). The palaeostriatum develops from the between brain; the neostriatum develops from the same embryonic structure as the cortex. In many species the neostriatum is not separated, and in man the putamen and caudate nucleus are continuous anteriorly. The structures are histologically different, in that the palaestriatum is composed of large cells and is rich in medullated fibres, whereas the neostriatum contains smaller cells and has few nerve fibres. The red nucleus is situated high in the mid-brain. It is in two parts; a large upper two thirds containing small cells, and developing at the same time as the cerebellar hemispheres and the expansion of the cortex, and a lower third containing large cells and derived from the 'tween' brain.

The substantia nigra is a group of heavily pigmented multipolar nerve cells, situated high in the mid-brain. The subthalamic nucleus lies close to the midline and below the thalamus.

It appears that these nuclei are the remnants of an ancient motor system; the path of the 'palaeo' system may have been—thalamus—cortex—pallidum—lower third of red nucleus—rubrospinal tract. The path of the 'neo' system is the same, with the modifying effect of the putamen, substantia nigra, and subthalamic nuclei. Besides these pathways must be mentioned many fibres connecting the nuclei to each other, and two efferent tracts, the fasciculus lenticularis and the ansa lenticularis which pass from the globus pallidus to the medial nucleus of the thalamus, short circuiting, as it were, the cortex.

Disease of the basal ganglia cause disorders of muscle tone and movement.

(a) There is a general increase in muscle tone. This hypertonus does not vary during flexion and extension of a joint (c.f. UMN lesions), but joints in the same limb may be affected to unequal degree. Commonly the earliest and most severely affected joints are the neck, shoulder, wrist, and ankle.

The same derangement of tone may be accompanied by tremor; in contradistinction to that caused by cerebellar disease, it is present at rest and often momentarily abolished by movement. It is rhythmic, occurring 5–6 times each second. Sometimes the superimposition of tremor on rigidity causes an apparent jerkiness when the limb is passively flexed (cogwheel rigidity).

The change in tone causes great slowness of execution of voluntary movements. In addition, automatic movements such as blinking, swallowing, and arm swinging are absent or reduced and expressional facial movements much attenuated.

In acute chorea the reverse is true. There is marked hypotonia, automatic movements are increased, and facial expressions exaggerated.

(b) Unwanted movements. In some diseases unwanted movements may occur. These may be caused by the random muscular contractions seen in *chorea* (p. 133), or be of a more violent and flinging nature, as in *hemiballismus*. Slowly changing disorders of tone may cause writhing sinuous movements of limbs (*athetosis*); this may occur with chronic basal ganglia disease in young people. Unwanted movements of another kind are seen in acute chorea; additional movements may occur in either limbs, the face or trunk, when voluntary movements are being executed.

Applied Anatomy

With the exception of the nucleus subthalamicus it is usually impossible to localise disease to one or another nucleus. Commonly they are all affected to greater or lesser degree. It may be said, however, that certain diseases affect chiefly the neostriatum and others the palaeostriatum. Good examples of the former are *hepato-lenticular degeneration* (p. 433; caudate and putamen), *Huntington's chorea*, (p. 300; caudate) and *chronic progressive (senile) chorea* (caudate and putamen); in contrast, the chief changes in the idiopathic form of *Parkinson's disease* (p. 298) are seen in the globus pallidus.

The Cerebro-spinal Fluid

The cerebro-spinal fluid is secreted by the choroid plexuses of the ventricles. That formed in the lateral ventricles passes to the third ventricle through the foramen of Monro. Fluid in the third ventricle passes to the fourth ventricle through the aqueduct of Sylvius, and then to the subarachnoid space through two lateral apertures, the foramina of Luschka and a central foramin of Magendie. It is confined between the pia and arachnoid membranes, and bathes the surface of the brain and spinal cord. It is absorbed into the intracranial venous sinuses.

Many diseases of the nervous system are associated with changes in the pressure or composition of the cerebro-spinal fluid. Specimens for examination may be obtained by lumbar puncture. Normal values are as follows:

    (i) Pressure—60–180 mm. of fluid.
    (ii) Protein—20–40 mg./100 ml.
    (iii) Glucose—50–80 mg./100 ml.
    (iv) Chloride—720–750 mg./100 ml. (as NaCl).
    (v) Cells—2–3 lymphocytes/cu.mm.

Obstruction to the flow of cerebro-spinal fluid is common as a result of subtentorial space-occupying lesions, which obstruct the Sylvian aqueduct by distortion. This causes dilatation of the whole ventricular system, with very rapid rise in the cerebro-spinal fluid pressure.

The Colloidal Gold Reaction (Lange)

The protein content of the fluid consists of albumin and globulin fractions. If the globulin concentration is increased then precipitation occurs on incubation with a colloidal solution of gold. Qualitative and quantitative abnormalities may be detected by mixing CSF with serial dilutions of colloidal gold, ten in all. Characteristic patterns of precipitation are seen in a number of diseases: precipitation in the first dilutions suggests general paresis of the insane (GPI), of the middle dilutions syphilis other than GPI and in the highest dilutions some form of meningitis.

DISORDERS OF THE CENTRAL NERVOUS SYSTEM

EPILEPSY

Epilepsy, the falling sickness, has been recognised and described since earliest times. At first thought to be a general disease, it was Hippocrates who first ascribed it to a disorder of the brain. It was not until 1878 that Hughlings Jackson, as a result of clinical observations, concluded that its basis was a paroxysmal discharge in the brain. This was confirmed in 1929 by Berger who made graphic records of the brain's electrical activity, the electroencephalograph (E.E.G.), and showed that the attacks coincided with the occurrence and spread of an electrical discharge. Recently (1960) Lennox and Lennox have described epilepsy as 'a recurrent disturbance in the chemico-electrical activity of the brain, which manifests itself in a symptom-complex of which impairment of consciousness, perturbation of the autonomic nervous system, convulsive movements, sensory abnormalities, or psychic disturbances are the essential components'.

The aetiology is complex and obscure. Heredity is generally regarded as an important factor since a family history of epilepsy in first or second degree relatives is obtained in about 30 per cent of patients, whatever the nature of their attack. In all epileptics there are predisposing and precipitating causes, though only in some are these causes demonstrable. In addition to the constitutional factor *predisposing causes* include prenatal disorders, birth injuries and neonatal disturbances as well as the more easily recognisable traumatic, inflammatory, neoplastic, or vascular lesions of the brain; the known *precipitating causes* include exhaustion and psychological stress and, more rarely, overhydration, acute anoxia of the brain, hypoglycaemia and hypocalcaemia.

In view of the possible social consequences to the patient of a diagnosis of epilepsy, there is much to be said for avoiding this label when convulsions complicate a pre-existing disorder; thus, a patient who faints from postural hypotension or cardiac arrhythmia and then has a fit as a result of cerebral ischaemia has 'syncope with convulsions' rather than epilepsy.

Clinical Features. Epileptic attacks may take the form of any type of recurrent disturbance of feeling, behaviour, or consciousness which is of primarily cerebral origin, so that their clinical varieties are legion. They may be divided into two groups, *general* epilepsy and *focal* epilepsy. All forms, however, have certain common characteristics.

(i) *They are paroxysmal*, that is to say that the attacks occur from time to time.

(ii) *They are of sudden onset*, as the word ictus, a blow, implies.

(iii) *They are of brief duration;* although attacks may be recurrent, they are individually brief, usually lasting only some minutes.

(iv) *They usually occur for no apparent reason;* although they may be associated with functional or structural changes in the brain, these changes are present and usually unchanged before and after the attack. It is usually impossible to discover exactly why any individual attack occurred.

General epilepsy may be major or minor (*grand mal* or *petit mal.*) Both these forms of general epilepsy (sometimes called central epilepsy) depend in part on a disturbance in the structures of the upper brain stem which are concerned with maintaining the alert or conscious state and each has a characteristic pattern in the EEG.

Grand Mal. In the classical major fit there is a regular sequence of stages, though frequently one or more of these stages are absent. Sometimes the convulsion is heralded by a transient *aura*, which may take a motor, sensory, or psychic form and indicates the site of electrical discharge, but usually the first event is the *tonic stage*, at the onset of which consciousness is lost. The patient falls to the ground, and as all his muscles are in a state of rigid spasm he falls heavily and frequently injures himself. The tonic stage lasts about a minute and as respiration is in abeyance during this time the patient becomes cyanosed. After this comes the *clonic stage*: a series of convulsive movements occurs not only in the trunk and limbs but also in the jaw and tongue so that saliva may be lathered into a 'foam' or the tongue may be badly bitten. The bladder is sometimes evacuated during the clonic stage, which may last for two or three minutes. After this the patient remains in *coma*, usually for only a few minutes but sometimes for some hours; if examined at this stage he is found to have absent corneal and tendon reflexes and extensor plantar responses. On recovering consciousness he usually complains of severe *headache*. After the attack some patients pass into a state of *post-epileptic automatism*, in which they may commit involuntarily anti-social or criminal acts which bring them into the hands of the police.

Petit Mal. These attacks never arise from lesions acquired later than the neonatal period; seen therefore mainly in children, their occurrence in an adult places him in the so-called 'idiopathic' group. They consist simply of a brief interruption of consciousness, in which the patient stops what he is doing or saying for a few seconds and then carries on, or perhaps falls to the ground and immediately picks himself up again.

Focal epilepsy. This term is used to include other ictal manifestations. The basis of such events is a *focal discharge*, and the clinical nature of the attack depends upon its site and intensity, and the patient's innate resistance to its spread, which may be of varying degree.

The attack may include movements, or any change of sensation, simple or complex. It may be so slight as almost to pass unnoticed, or so severe as to end in a general convulsion. It may be followed by a period of confusion and headache.

Brief mention may be made of *temporal lobe epilepsy* (psychomotor epilepsy), the focus of which appears to lie in the anterior part of the temporal lobe. These attacks take many forms in which organised movements, sensations, and emotions occur. Common examples are the déjà vu phenomenon, a feeling of intense familiarity, or feelings of remoteness and unreality, or of pleasure, or hallucinations of smell or taste, accompanied by pallor and sweating and often a feeling of fear. There may be convulsive movements of the limbs or smacking of the lips.

Status Epilepticus. When a series of major epileptic seizures occurs without intervening recovery of consciousness the patient is said to be in status epilepticus, a very dangerous condition which unless promptly and energetically treated may lead to death from exhaustion or hyperpyrexia. Petit mal status also occurs and gives rise to prolonged disorientation.

Diagnosis of Epilepsy. As doctors rarely have the opportunity of seeing patients in an attack, and as there are no helpful physical signs to be found between the attacks apart occasionally from scars of old injuries on the head or tongue, the diagnosis nearly always depends on a carefully taken history. Eyewitness accounts of the attacks should always be sought. On this evidence the diagnosis of grand mal and petit mal can usually be made without difficulty. Focal attacks are often more difficult to recognise as epileptic; helpful points are that they tend to recur in the same patient under the same circumstances, they have a very sudden onset and usually a brief duration.

Whatever the nature of the attack, it is important to remember that epilepsy is a symptom, and the doctor's prime duty is to discover *why* it has occurred. For this reason a careful family history, and a history of previous suspicious episodes must be sought, and a *full* clinical examination of the nervous system made including auscultation over the neck and orbits. All patients should have an E.E.G. and skull radiographs to attempt to demonstrate any focal lesion. However, electrical abnormalities are found in only a proportion of patients with epilepsy. A normal E.E.G. does not exclude epilepsy. Fits may be the only manifestation of early cerebral syphilis, and so the Wasserman and Kahn tests must always be made on the blood, and if there is still reason for doubt, on the C.S.F. too.

Management of Epilepsy. When a patient presents with a recent history of epileptic fits the first question to be answered is whether he has an underlying potentially curable organic lesion. The older the patient when the seizures start the more often can an organic lesion be demonstrated; on the other hand, even in the higher age groups it is only a very small percentage of patients with epilepsy intensively investigated who are found to have a treatable organic lesion. On balance, therefore, it is wrong to perform unpleasant and occasionally harmful procedures such as encephalography, ventriculography, and arteriography except in patients in whom there is some special indication. In general, investigation should be limited to examination of the blood and urine, radiography of the chest and skull, which helps to exclude secondary tumours, and an E.E.G.; if the latter does not show evidence of a local spike focus or of the slow waves which suggest structural disorder of the brain, the patient should be kept under clinical observation, but not investigated further at this stage.

Even if a discoverable cause is removed the epilepsy will not necessarily by this means alone come under control. Patients with epilepsy must be allowed and encouraged to lead as normal a life as possible. Children should stay at school and adults may need help to find useful employment. The life of a patient with epilepsy should be well regulated, and hunger, fatigue, and emotional crises should be avoided as far as possible.

Anticonvulsant Drugs

The decision as to which drug should be used depends on the nature of the attack. For petit mal ethosuximide 250 mg. 4–6 times daily is the drug of choice. It is more effective and less toxic than troxidone and other drugs of the dione series.

In *grand mal* and *temporal lobe epilepsy* a combination of phenobarbitone 30 mg. and phenytoin sodium 100 mg. two or three times a day is usually most effective, but phenytoin may be given alone or may be used in combination with primidone 250 mg. four to six times a day. Primidone may also be given alone but should not be used in combination with phenobarbitone because this may lead to excessive drowsiness. If these drugs alone or together fail to bring the epilepsy under reasonable control then pheneturide (Benuride) may be tried in doses of 200 mg. 3–6 times a day or sulthiame (Ospolot) 200 mg. b.d. or t.d.s. may be tried.

Treatment should be continued until the patient has been free of attacks for at least three and preferably five years and if there are no side effects there is no reason why mild treatment should not be continued indefinitely even if the attacks are under control.

Surgical Treatment. In certain cases of temporal lobe epilepsy when the attacks are difficult to control, amputation of the temporal pole has brought complete relief in about 50 per cent of patients and partial relief in others. Some cases of infantile hemiplegia and of Sturge-Weber syndrome have similarly benefited from hemispherectomy.

Status Epilepticus

Urgent treatment is required, the mortality in inadequately treated patients being as high as 30 per cent. The drug of choice is diazepam 10 mg. by slow intravenous injection and this may be repeated as necessary until control is achieved. If it is ineffective other drugs which may be used are inhalation anaesthetics, intramuscular paraldehyde (10 ml.) intravenous anaesthetics (thiopentone sodium 0·5 g.) or intravenous or intramuscular injection of phenobarbitone (180 mg.). Repeated treatments may be necessary, and careful attention to the patient's airway and if necessary treatment of secondary respiratory infection is essential.

HERPES ZOSTER (SHINGLES)

This common disease is characterised by inflammatory changes which are usually confined to one posterior root ganglion, though rarely they may involve the spinal cord. The causative virus is either identical with or closely related to the virus of chicken-pox, since it is quite common for the healthy contacts of patients with either disease to develop the other. The appearance of shingles often seems to be precipitated by injury or by some other pathological process such as spinal metastases from carcinoma or Hodgkin's disease, or other infections such as meningitis.

Clinical Features. The first symptom is usually severe pain in the distribution of the affected root or roots, often accompanied by swelling of local lymph nodes and followed a few days later by erythema and a vesicular eruption in the appropriate dermatome. At this stage there is often intense irritation as well as pain. The vesicles usually dry up into crusts in a week or so, though if the lesions become secondarily infected they may last much longer and eventually leave permanent scarring of the skin. Special mention may be made of zoster infection in the following special sites:

(1) *Gasserian herpes* involving the first (ophthalmic) division is always serious, since it may lead to blindness either from corneal scarring following ulceration or from a panophthalmitis.

(2) *Geniculate herpes* (The Ramsay Hunt syndrome). This presents with pain in the throat or ear, followed by a vesicular eruption on the pinna, external auditory meatus or fauces and a facial palsy of lower motor neurone type.

(3) *Zoster myelitis* is rare. It may present as a Brown-Séquard syndrome (p. 291) or as a complete transverse lesion of the cord. Recovery within a few weeks is the rule.

Post-herpetic neuralgia is a very troublesome sequela which occurs particularly in elderly patients; the pain may be so severe and persistent as to induce suicidal depression.

Treatment. There is no specific treatment. To prevent secondary infection of the skin lesions they should be kept clean and dry or covered with collodion and in ophthalmic herpes atropine drops and antibiotic drops should be instilled into the eyes. Analgesics must be given to relieve the pain, but drugs of addiction should be avoided since the neuralgia may be very chronic. Claims of dramatic relief following injections of pituitrin

½–1 ml. or cyanocobalamin 1,000 μg., or oral corticosteroid therapy have been made, but their value remains doubtful. Post-herpetic neuralgia is sometimes improved by radiotherapy to the affected ganglia or by repeated applications of an electrical vibrator over the painful area.

MIGRAINE

The essential feature of migraine is a paroxysmal headache. This may be confined to one or other side of the head or may be generalised. The headache may be preceded by an 'aura' which can take the form of some visual disturbance, such as dazzles, fortification spectra or even visual loss which is usually hemianopic. There may be, separately or in addition, some numbness and tingling of face and arms and, more rarely, dysphasia. These symptoms last for some 15–30 minutes and as they pass off the headache develops. The headache lasts on an average some 12–14 hours but may be of shorter and occasionally of longer duration, sometimes lasting several days. At its height it may be accompanied by vomiting and while the headache lasts the patient suffering a severe attack prefers to lie quietly in a darkened room, refusing all nourishment but sipping water. Its frequency is very variable but most people liable to migraine have attacks every few weeks or months.

Pathology

The patho-physiology of migraine is thought to be an initial constriction of vessels which causes the 'aura' and a later dilatation, mostly of branches of the external carotid artery, which causes the headache. The cause is unknown but there is often a family history, the attacks are often related to some emotional disturbance and are sometimes precipitated by eating certain foods, for example chocolate and oranges. Most migrainous subjects are of obsessional temperament and it is typical for attacks to occur during the period of relaxation which follows a spell of intense over-activity; thus 'weekend migraine' is very common. Attacks also frequently occur premenstrually.

Migraine usually starts in the second decade and tends to diminish in frequency in later life.

In a patient liable to migraine an increase in frequency of the attacks is likely to be due to:

(a) anxiety and overwork,
(b) the contraceptive pill,
(c) vascular hypertension,
(d) the menopause,
(e) an underlying structural lesion such as as an angioma or cerebral tumour.

Treatment. This falls into three parts:

(1) The patient must be told, after appropriate steps have been taken, if necessary, that the condition although distressing is not medically serious.

(2) Regular sedation should be given in the form of phenobarbitone or amylobarbitone. This is, in itself, sometimes enough to bring about a considerable decrease in the number of attacks and even to abolish them.

A more specific prophylactic is methysergide (Deseril) a serotonin antagonist which can be given in doses of 3–6 mg. daily. Toxic effects such as skin rashes, disequilibrium and angina are common and it may rarely give rise to retroperitoneal and other fibroses. It should be used only in intractable migraine. Clonidine hydrochloride (Dixarit) 0.025 mg. b.d. is less toxic and is said to reduce attacks by some 60 per cent.

(3) Attacks are best treated by ergotamine tartrate and the important point is to introduce this substance into the body as early in an attack as possible. For this reason tablets are often disappointing in their effect and an injection of ergotamine tartrate 0·25 or 0·5 mg. may be necessary. This the patient should learn to inject himself, so as to avoid delay. Alternatively a suppository containing ergotamine tartrate 2 mg. may be inserted.

MIGRAINOUS NEURALGIA

This variety of paroxysmal headache differs from migraine in that the bouts are of greater frequency and shorter duration.

The headache is sharply localised to one or other supra-orbital region but may spread into the temple, eye, or cheek. Typically it wakens the patient from sleep every night an hour or two after he has gone to bed and is very intense. It lasts from 30–90 minutes and may be accompanied by watering of the eye and blocking of the nose on that side. There may be a partial ptosis and a smaller pupil on the affected side.

Such a headache may also occur irregularly, not necessarily at night or every day and sometimes two or three times within 24 hours. A bout of such headaches usually lasts for several weeks, when there is spontaneous remission. There is, however, a tendency for the headache to recur, usually after an interval of many months and even years, sometimes with a seasonal incidence. It is commoner in men and may occur at any time in adult life, possibly afflicting more often those who are ambitious, hard-working, and conscientious.

Its cause is unknown.

Treatment. Ergotamine tartrate 0·25 or 0·5 mg. must be given by subcutaneous injection or by suppository (2 mg.) prophylactically. If the attacks are occurring exclusively at night the drug is given at bed-time and if, as usually happens, the attacks are prevented, the dose must be withheld every seventh day to see whether the bout has remitted.

If the attacks are irregular or more frequent it will be necessary to give such medication two or three times in 24 hours to make sure of controlling the headache. At the same time the patient may benefit from regular sedation with amylobarbitone. As excessive administration of ergotamine may lead to peripheral gangrene, patients must be warned not to take more than three doses in 24 hours.

CEREBRAL VASCULAR DISEASE

Percutaneous arteriography has added greatly to our knowledge of diseases and disorders of the cerebral blood vessels. It has given more accurate evidence in many cases of the source of intracranial haemorrhage and it has demonstrated that cerebral infarction or ischaemia does not necessarily depend on occlusion, either by embolus or thrombosis, of the cerebral vessels themselves. It has also demonstrated that the heart is not the only source of cerebral embolus. Moreover the arteriographic findings have led to the more routine examination of the carotid and vertebral vessels as well as the cerebral vessels at autopsy, and pathologists now concentrate their attention more on the vascular lesion than on the haemorrhage or infarct.

Intracranial Haemorrhage

This may be *extradural*
subdural
intracerebral
subarachnoid.

Extradural Haemorrhage

This arises as a result of head injury; the source of haemorrhage is usually a ruptured middle meningeal artery. This rupture often underlies a linear fracture of the skull vault at the point where the fracture crosses one of the meningeal arteries.

Clinical Features. The most characteristic story is of head injury with loss of senses and with fairly rapid recovery of consciousness. After a so-called 'lucid interval' a gradually increasing coma supervenes with progressive hemiplegia, fixed dilated pupils, and death unless treatment is prompt.

It is important to remember that there may be no 'lucid interval' and that the initial injury may be of such severity that consciousness is not regained before the effects of the extradural haemorrhage supervene.

Thus in any case of head injury it is not so important to keep close watch on the pulse and blood pressure as it is to observe constantly the *level of consciousness*—that is, the nature and strength of the stimulus required to rouse the patient. If coma is deepening, even though the patient has never been fully conscious, extradural haemorrhage must be suspected. It is useless to wait for the development of hemiplegia and fixed dilated pupils before making the diagnosis because it is then probably too late for effective treatment. In addition to deepening coma the presence of an extradural haemorrhage may be suspected by the discovery of a skull fracture and its presence may be demonstrated, if necessary, by carotid arteriography, when the cerebral vessels will be seen to be displaced inwards by the clot.

The *treatment* is surgical by trephining the skull and evacuating the clot.

Subdural Haemorrhage

The name given to a collection of blood in the subdural space is usually subdural haematoma.

This occurs mostly in elderly patients (and in infancy) and usually as the result of trauma, but this may be quite slight and a history of injury may be lacking. The blood comes from veins and oozes into the subdural space.

Clinical Features. The symptoms start some weeks later with headache and periods of drowsiness and coma. These may be quite brief at first and may be followed by normal alertness, or the drowsiness may fluctuate in severity. For reasons which are not completely understood this tends to be a progressive lesion even after the haemorrhage has ceased and gradually more persistent coma develops. This may be accompanied by signs of hemiparesis and possibly aphasia, due to compression of the brain. Sometimes the compression may be transmitted to the brain stem so that ptosis and ocular palsies develop. Papilloedema and epilepsy are rare.

Diagnosis. The history of head injury, even trivial, must suggest the diagnosis of subdural haematoma in any elderly person with headache and coma, especially with hemiparesis or brain-stem signs. Arteriography may show that the cerebral vessels are displaced inwards by the haematoma intervening clot. It is important to remember that the clot may be bilateral.

The *treatment* is surgical evacuation of the clot.

INTRACEREBRAL AND SUBARACHNOID HAEMORRHAGE

The distinction between these is by no means always clear-cut in that a haemorrhage arising primarily in the cerebral substance may leak into the subarachnoid space and a primarily subarachnoid haemorrhage may plough into the brain. There is some advantage, therefore, in referring to them as *spontaneous intracranial haemorrhage* to distinguish them from the varieties of traumatic haemorrhage already discussed.

Haemorrhage arising in the *subarachnoid* space gives rise to headache which may be so abrupt in onset as to make the patient think he has been struck and there may be rapid loss of senses. Coma may be the first manifestation. The development may be more gradual with a general feeling of ill-ease in the head, gradually increasing suboccipital headache, neck stiffness, and perhaps vomiting. If the onset is accompanied by loss of senses these symptoms and signs will be present when consciousness returns and are likely to persist for some days. If they are slight they are apt to be passed off as fibrositis of the neck or, sometimes, as sunstroke.

In addition there may be mental confusion, aphasia, visual field defect, sub-hyaloid haemorrhage, hemiparesis, with or without sensory loss and auscultation of the skull may reveal a bruit.

The *diagnosis* of subarachnoid haemorrhage is made by lumbar puncture. The important finding is of *xanthochromia*, which is present in 100 per cent of cases after 24 hours; this is the only certain way of distinguishing between subarachnoid haemorrhage and bleeding caused by the lumbar puncture.

A haemorrhage primarily *intracerebral* may produce symptoms of equally sudden onset with loss of senses, and signs depending on the situation of the haemorrhage. This may be not only in the cerebral hemisphere but also in the cerebellum or brain stem. Symptoms may, however, develop more gradually so as to suggest a rapidly expanding lesion and the C.S.F. may contain no blood in as many as 25 per cent of the cases but, when this is so, there is often some xanthochromia or increase of protein or cells. At other times a haemorrhage produces such slight and transient symptoms and signs that its true nature is not suspected.

In practice, by far the most common clinical syndrome is a hemiplegia from a lesion affecting the contralateral internal capsule—a *stroke*.

Strokes may be of slow or sudden onset. If slow, then the underlying lesion is most likely to be thrombotic; if rapid, embolic or haemorrhagic. They are of all degrees of severity. The worst cause immediate loss of consciousness, with bilateral flaccid palsy; the classical signs of UMN lesions (p. 258) develop only after an interval of some hours or days. The least severe present as only the slightest weakness of a limb, usually described as heaviness in the arm and/or stiffness in the leg, with mild headache and a little confusion. If the dominant hemisphere is affected some aphasia may be present. Other signs and symptoms depend upon the involvement of surrounding structures.

Diagnosis. The diagnosis of spontaneous intracranial haemorrhage can usually be made, but this is no longer precise enough. It is important now to try and discover the source of the haemorrhage. This is likely to be:

    (1) a *diseased blood vessel*, with or without vascular hypertension,
    (2) a *ruptured aneurysm*,
    (3) a *leaking angioma*.

(1) Haemorrhage from a diseased blood vessel is likely to occur in elderly patients and in the presence of hypertension which is possibly related to the development of disease in the vessel.

(2) and (3) are likely to be the source in younger patients and in the absence of hypertension. Since both of these, and especially angiomas, can present in other ways in addition to providing a source of haemorrhage, it is opportune to consider briefly their clinical features.

Cerebral Aneurysm

Cerebral aneurysms, which are usually congenital but sometimes develop as the result of atheroma, tend to occur in and around the circle of Willis, the commonest sites being on the internal carotid artery at the origin of the posterior communicating artery, on the anterior communicating artery and at the first bifurcation of the middle cerebral artery. They provide by far the commonest source of primarily subarachnoid haemorrhage and such a haemorrhage is usually the first manifestation of a cerebral aneurysm.

An aneurysm of the internal carotid artery at the origin of the posterior communicating artery may, however, produce frontal headache and an isolated third nerve palsy.

Aneurysm of the internal carotid artery in the cavernous sinus may produce an ophthalmoplegia with sensory loss in the distribution of the trigeminal nerve. If such an aneurysm ruptures it produces a caroticocavernous fistula, with pulsating exophthalmos and a bruit.

Aneurysm in the suprasellar region may cause optic nerve or chiasmal compression with visual loss and optic atrophy.

Cerebral Angioma

This is a congenital arteriovenous malformation which can give rise to symptoms at an early age, but does so most frequently in the second and third decades. It may present with:

> haemorrhage,
> epilepsy,
> headache,
> progressive hemiparesis,

or, which is of more diagnostic help, with a combination of two or more of these symptoms. Recurring haemorrhage in a young person, is in itself suggestive of angioma; and haemorrhage occurring in a person with focal epilepsy or with headache, which resembles migraine but has a constant pattern, is also suggestive.

A bruit is sometimes heard for a few days after haemorrhage from an aneurysm, possibly to be attributed to vascular spasm, but this seldom persists. The commonest cause of a persistent bruit in a young person is a cerebral angioma and its discovery will thus be of significance if the symptoms are otherwise suggestive.

Investigation of Spontaneous Intracranial Haemorrhage

Whatever the clinical assessment of the likely source of haemorrhage it is desirable, in patients in whom the haemorrhage is not likely to prove rapidly fatal, to proceed to arteriography to try and visualise the source of haemorrhage and its site.

The signs will naturally determine whether the carotid tree, on one or other side, or the basilar tree is to be investigated but if there are no signs other than those of meningeal irritation or if the signs are inconclusive, carotid arteriograms should be done first. If these are normal it is important to remember that aneurysms and angiomas also occur in the posterior fossa and that a haematoma without an obvious source can be present in the cerebellum.

Treatment. If no source of the haemorrhage is discovered, treatment is traditionally by rest, good nursing, and such medical measures as will help to keep the patient alive while recovery is taking place; but even so the mortality is about 50 per cent. The possibility now arises, however, that some patients with an intracerebral haematoma may be helped by having the clot removed. This is particularly the case where there seems to be progression of signs, where coma has not been too profound or too prolonged and when the haematoma is relatively superficial.

An aneurysm may be treated surgically by direct attack, if that is possible, so that its neck may be clipped, or it may be packed around with muscle. Another method which is particularly indicated in carotid aneurysms is to tie the common carotid artery in the neck and thus reduce the thrust on the aneurysmal sac.

Some angiomas, depending on their size and situation, can be excised. This is the treatment of choice, but occasionally it may be helpful to tie off the entering arteries. Irradiation is of doubtful value.

CEREBRAL ISCHAEMIA

Apart from haemorrhage causing destruction of brain tissue directly and possibly causing more remote effects by surrounding oedema and compression, cerebral function can be disturbed by ischaemia.

The classical examples of this are where cerebral vessels are occluded by thrombosis or embolus, resulting in infarction, but more recently it has become clear that disease of the internal carotid and vertebral arteries and, indeed, of even more proximal arteries can give rise to clinical pictures indistinguishable from those which have been called cerebral thrombosis. It is no longer possible to think of cerebral ischaemia except in relation to the whole carotido-vertebral system and its cerebral branches.

The classical *source of embolus* is from the heart in the presence of either atrial fibrillation, myocardial infarction with mural thrombus, or bacterial endocarditis. Equally important now is atherosclerosis of the aorta and carotid or vertebral arteries from which mural thrombus or atheromatous material may arise. Rarer causes of embolism are fat, tumour cells, or air.

What actually happens after occlusion by thrombosis or embolism of a cerebral vessel depends on the collateral circulation; the number of anastomotic channels available will determine the size of a given infarct or whether it will occur at all. Upon the size and situation of the infarct will depend the neurological signs.

The diagnosis between thrombosis and embolism is not so important as the diagnosis of each from haemorrhage; the onset of symptoms from embolism is the most sudden and consciousness is not usually lost.

It is now well recognised that infarction can occur without occlusion and an important advance in the understanding of atherosclerotic vascular disease is the recognition of recurrent cerebral ischaemic attacks, usually to be attributed to emboli.

Internal Carotid Artery Disease

The syndrome of the internal carotid artery with ipselateral blindness and contralateral hemiplegia has long been known but it is really carotid arteriography, by demonstrating internal carotid artery occlusion or stenosis, that has led to the recognition of these recurrent attacks. They may occur at any age from the second decade onwards but they are increasingly frequent in older people.

Clinical Features. The episodes are brief, often occurring with great frequency, usually of the same pattern and representing some focal disorder of brain function. The symptoms are characteristically transient monocular blindness with contralateral paresis, paraesthesiae and dysphasia, occurring separately or together, possibly with confusion or other impairment of intellectual function. These symptoms may be followed in time by permanent cerebral damage, possibly extensive and of abrupt onset. In less obvious cases, in which cerebral infarction appears to be the correct clinical diagnosis, the possibility of internal carotid occlusion or stenosis deserves consideration whether the lesion is a large one causing profound hemiplegia or is causing focal symptoms only; ipsilateral Horner's syndrome may be present.

Vertebro-basilar Disease

Similar brief episodes may occur when these arteries are diseased and may be distinguished by impaired vision amounting sometimes to blindness, diplopia, vertigo, dysarthria, tingling around the lips and of the tongue, ataxia, and hemiparesis or tetraparesis.

Treatment of Cerebral Ischaemia

There is no really effective treatment of an established infarct but there may be a possibility of preventing further embolic infarcts. This treatment may be *medical or surgical.*

Medical

A patient with rheumatic or arteriosclerotic heart disease may be helped by the prolonged use of anticoagulants. The same may be so if the embolus arises from the great vessels.

If, however, a cerebral vascular episode is not obviously embolic, there is no way of distinguishing with certainty between haemorrhage and thrombosis, even by examination of the C.S.F. for blood, arteriography, and air-encephalography. Even though, therefore, anticoagulants might be of use in thrombosis they are unsafe.

In the recurrent cerebral ischaemic attacks, which often herald an oncoming stroke, anticoagulants may diminish the frequency of the attacks and delay or prevent the stroke.

Surgical

When the internal carotid artery in the neck is shown to be occluded, operation is rarely indicated and only if the occlusion is known to be recent. If the internal carotid artery is stenosed at its origin an endarterectomy can be performed thus increasing the total blood supply to the brain, the likelihood being that other vessels are similarly involved, and also removing a potential source of emboli. Operations on the vertebral arteries and on the vessels arising from the aortic arch are technically more difficult but are proving increasingly possible particularly in relation to the 'subclavian steal' syndrome when the subclavian artery is narrow or occluded proximal to the origin of the vertebral artery.

Diffuse Cerebral Atherosclerosis

Sometimes the effect of atheroma of the cerebral vessels is such that no obvious stroke occurs but a series of minor episodes gradually lead to a picture of intellectual impairment, into which the patient often has insight; emotional lability, bladder disturbance, and a shuffling gait—*le marche a petit pas*—are other typical features. Sometimes dysarthria and dysphagia develop and complete the picture of *pseudo-bulbar palsy*, so called because the symptoms are the same as those in progressive bulbar palsy, but are due to an upper and not a lower motor neurone lesion. Features of Parkinsonism may also appear.

VENOUS SINUS THROMBOSIS

This occurs as the result of trauma or infection. Infection from the middle ear or mastoid causes lateral sinus thrombosis and that from the face or nasal sinuses may cause cavernous sinus thrombosis or thrombosis of the superior sagittal sinus. Cerebral abscess may be a sequel.

Lateral Sinus Thrombosis

The symptoms are fever, headache and vomiting, and papilloedema may be present. Focal neurological signs are rare.

Cavernous Sinus Thrombosis

The symptoms are pain in and around the eye with proptosis and chemosis. There may be external ophthalmoplegia and papilloedema may develop.

Superior Sagittal Sinus Thrombosis

This is less common but infection may spread from the nasal sinuses and may then pass to the cortical veins giving rise to focal epilepsy and focal neurological signs.

Treatment. This is of the original infection, if present, and as a result of more effective treatment inrecent years by sulphonamides and antibiotics these complications are now relatively rare and are more amenable to treatment when they occur.

INFECTIONS

Acute Pyogenic Meningitis

It results either from primary infection of the meninges and cerebrospinal fluid (CSF), or less commonly by the extension of infection from the middle ear or skull sinuses, or from a cerebral abscess.

The onset is usually acute and is characterised by fever, headache, and vomiting, with the development of a stiff neck and backache. Stupor or coma may follow. Convulsions are rare in adults. *Examination* confirms the neck stiffness and there may be a positive Kernig's sign. Other neurological signs are not found in the early stages.

The diagnosis can be confirmed by lumbar puncture, which reveals a purulent fluid containing several thousand polymorphs, increased protein, greatly decreased sugar and an organism which is likely to be meningococcus, staphylococcus, streptococcus, pneumococcus, or haemophilus influenzae. In meningococcal meningitis morbilliform rashes and petechiae often appear, but this purpuric tendency is rare in other types of meningitis.

Treatment. The principles of treatment are to try to obtain a therapeutic concentration of a suitable antibiotic in the CSF as rapidly as possible. Because of the relatively slow diffusibility of some antibiotics into the fluid, it is usual to combine them with a chemotherapeutic agent which can pass rapidly into the CSF, for example sulphadiazine. In pyogenic meningitis suspected of being other than meningococcal, intrathecal administration of the antibiotic may be necessary. Some useful therapeutic combinations are shown in the Table.

Prognosis and sequelae depend upon the duration of the illness before treatment is begun, and the sensitivity of the infecting agent to the available antibiotics. Most patients do well, and death or serious sequelae occur in less than 10 per cent of cases. These include cranial nerve palsy, focal cerebral lesions, epilepsy, dementia, and hydrocephalus.

Tuberculous Meningitis

It is always secondary to tuberculosis elsewhere in the body, although this may not be manifest. It may occur at any age, most commonly in children and young adults. It is of insidious onset, and usually encephalitis is the striking early feature: this causes confusion, and ultimately stupor or coma. Epileptic fits may occur. Less commonly meningitic signs predominate. Tubercles in the choroid membrane are the only specific finding on clinical examination, but signs elsewhere may suggest tuberculosis.

Diagnosis is confirmed by examination of the CSF. The pressure is increased, and the fluid either clear or opalescent. There are usually 10–50 polymorphs and 50–500 lymphocytes per cu. mm., and the protein is raised. The chloride level falls late in the disease, and is useless in early diagnosis. Expert examination always reveals the tubercle bacillus, usually on direct microscopy, but always on animal inoculation.

Treatment consists of isoniazid (10 mg. per kg. body weight daily), streptomycin (1–2 g. I.M. daily), and para-aminosalicylic acid (100 mg. per kg. daily). After six weeks, isoniazid and P.A.S. alone may be used, and should be continued for 12–18 months (p. 227).

The disease was always fatal before the advent of specific chemotherapy, but with modern treatment the mortality is about 10 per cent. In general, prognosis improves with age and is most serious in infants and young people.

Treatment of Bacterial Meningitis

Infecting Organism	Therapeutic agent	Route of administration			
		Oral*	I.M.	I.V.	I.T.
N. meningitides	sulphadiazine	1·5	1–2·0	1·0	never
Str. pneumoniae	benzylpenicillin and	–	–	4·0 M	–
	sulphadiazine	1·5	1–2·0	1·0	never
H. influenzae	chloramphenicol	50 mg./kg./24hr			–
	and ampicillin	–	–	1·0	–
Esch. coli	ampicillin or ⎱	0·5	0·25	0·25	10–40 mg
	streptomycin ⎰	never	1·0 daily	never	25–100 mg
	and sulphadiazine	1·5	1–2	1·0	never
Ps. pyocyanea	streptomycin or	never	1·0 daily	never	25–100 mg
	colomycin	never	0·75–1 M units	0·25– 0·5 M units	20–100,000 units daily
Staph. aureus	methicillin or ⎱	1·0	1·0	1·0	10 mg
	cloxacillin ⎰	0·5	0·25	0·5	10 mg
	and sulphadiazine	1·5	1–2·0	1·0	never
Purulent fluid, no organisms	benzylpenicillin	–	1·0 M	0·5 M	20,000 units
	sulphadiazine	1·5	1·20	1·0	never
	ampicillin	0·5	0·25	0·25	10–20 mg

I.M. = intramuscularly   I.V. = intravenously
I.T. = intrathecally daily   M = 1,000,000 units

* All doses in grammes unless otherwise indicated. All should be given 4–6 hourly, depending on the clinical condition. Treatment should be continued for 5–10 days; intrathecal treatment until the CSF is sterile.

Virus Meningitis

Presents acutely with predominately meningitic signs and symptoms (p. 279). Usually there is no clue to the infecting agent on clinical examination, although sometimes there may be evidence of an existing virus infection, for example the rash of herpes or the salivary gland swelling of mumps. The diagnosis again depends on examination of the CSF: the pressure is raised, and the fluid is either clear or opalescent. On microscopy lymphocytes are seen, usually between 100 and 1,000 per cu. mm.

Differential diagnosis is from tuberculous meningitis: usually the abruptness of onset, the predominance of symptoms and signs of meningitis over those of encephalitis, the larger number of cells in the fluid, and absence of tubercle bacilli serve to make distinction possible.

Many viruses are capable of affecting the nervous system, but some of the commoner ones are poliomyelitis (below), herpes zoster (p. 270), and lymphocytic choriomeningitis; secondary affection may occur in herpes simplex, mumps (p. 504) and with Coxsackie and Echo viruses (p. 507).

No specific **treatment** is available for virus infections at present, but the prognosis in most cases is good. Sequelae similar to those of acute meningitis (p. 280) occasionally occur.

Poliomyelitis

This is a virus infection which is thought to gain access to the body through the nasopharynx or the alimentary tract. After an incubation period varying from 7 to 14 days, there is first a generalised bodily reaction and then invasion of the nervous system. This is confined to the grey matter, and particularly the anterior horn of the spinal cord and the motor nuclei of the brain stem.

Clinical Features. The prodromal symptoms are fever, malaise, headache, and vomiting and after three or four days, during which they sometimes remit, further symptoms referable to the central nervous system develop. These are increased headache, spinal pains, and paraesthesiae, often localised, and pains in the limbs. There is stiffness of the neck and rigidity of the whole spinal column, usually with drowsiness or irritability. In some patients recovery then occurs but in others this so-called *preparalytic stage* is followed by the appearance of *paralysis*. This usually develops rapidly but may advance for 3 to 5 days. As it develops the fever subsides. The extent and degree of the paralysis are extremely variable, but the legs are involved more often than the arms, and the arms more often than the trunk. In about 15 per cent of patients there is involvement of cranial nuclei and muscles of the face, pharynx, larynx, and tongue may be paralysed. Respiratory paralysis may result either from involvement of the diaphragm and intercostal muscles or by involvement of the respiratory centre in the medulla. Retention of urine sometimes occurs. Reflexes may be abolished. There is no sensory loss.

The *spinal fluid* may be under increased pressure and shows pleocytosis; in the very early stages polymorphs predominate, but later lymphocytes. The protein content may be increased and this may rise further during the first month if paralysis is widespread. The sugar and chloride levels are normal.

Diagnosis. In the preparalytic stage it is from pyogenic and tuberculous meningitis and the history and spinal fluid findings are of help. The appearance of muscular fasciculation is also a sign of great value at this stage. The distinction from other forms of virus meningitis depends upon virus studies or the isolation of the poliomyelitis virus from the faeces.

In the paralytic stage, when there is a lower motor neurone paralysis with muscle tenderness, acute polyneuritis may be suspected. However, poliomyelitis is likely to be asymmetrical, and there is no sensory loss.

Prophylaxis: Poliomyelitis is now prevented by giving 3 drops of live attenuated polio virus to children at 6 months, 7 months, 8 months and $4\frac{1}{2}$ years.

Treatment. In the *preparalytic stage* rest is essential, for there is good evidence that exertion increases the likelihood of paralysis.

If *paralysis* does develop, gentle but frequent passive movements to the weak limbs are given and if pain is troublesome hot packs applied to the muscles give relief. A sedative such as amylobarbitone (15 mg. t.d.s.) is helpful.

During the acute stage of paralysis rigid splinting is to be avoided but a cradle, foot-rest and pillows should be used to prevent shortening of the paralysed muscles. Treatment is directed towards the avoidance of all unnecessary muscle activity and the prevention of painful spasm and contractures.

In the rehabilitation of the patient after the acute stage is over, early and vigorous activity is indicated.

If there are signs of *respiratory failure* the patient must be transferred to a hospital where mechanical artificial respiration can be given.

Cases with early difficulty in swallowing and speaking due to *bulbar involvement* resemble those with respiratory paralysis and the distinction is of great importance because the treatment is different; artificial respiration may be disastrous. Those patients who are unable to prevent secretions in the pharynx from being sucked into the lungs with inspiration must be nursed semi-prone with the foot of the bed raised and must be turned from side to side every two hours.

If respiratory paralysis occurs in bulbar poliomyelitis then either postural drainage must be carried out in a respirator or a tracheostomy must be done and the patient's respiration maintained by intermittent positive pressure.

NEUROSYPHILIS

Syphilis attacks the nervous system either by a meningo-vascular process or by involving the parenchyma; the latter gives rise to tabes dorsalis or general paralysis of the insane or sometimes to a mixture of the two.

Only about 10 per cent of patients with syphilis later develop neurological manifestations, although a higher proportion have asymptomatic involvement in the early stages, characterised only by abnormalities in the C.S.F. What then happens and why only some patients develop clinical neurosyphilis are not known. Symptoms do not appear for some years after primary infection except in the rare cases of acute meningo-vascular syphilis.

Meningo-vascular Syphilis

The lesion is an endarteritis with perivascular inflammation, which is the reaction of the mesoblastic tissues to the spirochaete and its toxins. This proceeds to gumma formation, and the meningeal involvement may be focal or diffuse. The *focal form* is rare and the resulting gumma behaves like any other expanding lesion. In the *diffuse form* the symptoms are headache, often with mental confusion and possibly epilepsy, and there may be papilloedema and neck stiffness. Cranial nerve palsies may develop, the oculo-motor nerves and those in the cerebello-pontine angle being most commonly involved. Optic atrophy may also occur. In a few cases there may be hemiparesis or aphasia, usually transient.

The C.S.F. is abnormal, showing a moderate increase of protein and cells, mainly lymphocytes, and positive serological reactions for syphilis (e.g. Wassermann reaction).

Treatment is by intramuscular injections of penicillin, 1 million units daily to a total of 12–15 million.

Myelitis

A spinal form of meningo-vascular syphilis may lead to a complete or partial transverse myelitis of rapid onset resulting in a variable degree of paraplegia, sensory loss, and sphincter disturbance. This occurs most commonly in the thoracic cord.

A more chronic form of meningo-myelitis usually involves the cervical portion of the cord (*cervical pachymeningitis*) and leads to wasting of the small muscles of the hand and spastic paraplegia. In this respect it resembles motor neurone disease, but the arm reflexes are usually depressed and there may be cutaneous sensory loss.

Tabes Dorsalis

This condition is not so called because the dorsal columns of the cord are involved; the name, which goes back to Hippocrates, was applied first to paraplegia associated with wasting of the back and only later, quite by coincidence, selected to describe a disease in which the posterior columns of the cord were found to be shrunken and, later, demyelinated.

Tabes tends to occur ten years or more after the primary infection and affects males more often than females. Pathologically there is thought to be a lesion of the posterior roots which starts in the lumbo-sacral region of the cord and may extend as far as the cervical cord. Rarely the affection may begin in the cervical cord (cervical tabes). The effect of the lesion is to cause wasting of the posterior columns and demyelination of the fibres passing up the posterior columns; the equally severe involvement of pain fibres is not followed by demyelination because of their relay, as they enter the cord, before crossing to the opposite side.

Clinical Features. 'Lightning pains' are common and characteristic. They are irregularly occurring, sharp, momentary stabs of pain, which tend to involve one spot while the bout lasts and this spot is typically in one or other thigh, calf or ankle. It is rare for two or more spots to be involved at the same time. The pain is variously described as being like a needle or a knife plunged into the leg, but more helpful than any description is the patient's almost invariable tendency to illustrate the sudden, stabbing nature of the pain by gesture. The area where the pain has most recently struck may remain tender for a time. The bouts occur irregularly and tend to be provoked by damp weather.

Other early symptoms may be of *sphincter disturbance*, sometimes bed-wetting due to retention with overflow; *impotence*; *visual disturbances*; or *ataxia*. The unsteadiness is more noticeable in the dark when the patient is deprived of visual aid to guide his steps. Later the ataxia may become more prominent, leading to the characteristic *stamping gait*. Gastric and other *tabetic crises* may occur and *trophic lesions* such as arthropathies and perforating ulcer may develop.

On examination, the pupils are usually small, irregular in outline, fixed to light but contracting on convergence (*Argyll-Robertson pupils*). The knee and ankle jerks are absent and possibly the triceps jerks. Characteristically there is cutaneous analgesia below the knees, over the trunk to the level of T4 and down the inner arm. Deep pain in the calves and Achilles tendons is absent. There is loss of postural sense and vibration sense of variable degree in the legs. There may be ptosis and primary optic atrophy with peripheral constriction of the visual fields, though visual acuity may still be normal.

Trophic changes involve not only the hip, knee, ankle, or small joints of the feet but also the spine (*Charcot's joints*). These joints are grossly disorganised, nearly always painless and unusually mobile considering the amount of destruction present. Arthropathy of the spine may cause painless root lesions and in this way there may develop wasting and weakness of radicular distribution. Otherwise the power in tabes is normal, the apparent paraplegia being due to loss of position sense in the legs.

The C.S.F. in tabes may contain excess cells and protein, a positive Wassermann reaction and an abnormal Lange reaction. It is not always abnormal in all these respects and may sometimes be completely normal.

Specific treatment is by intramuscular injections of penicillin 1 million units daily to a total of 12–15 million units. This will arrest the disease but is unlikely to alter the clinical picture greatly, although lightning pains are sometimes relieved, at least temporarily. Symptomatic treatment may be required for bladder disturbance, especially if the urine is infected. Although considerable disability may result from ataxia, blindness, and arthropathies, the disease is self-limiting and death usually occurs only as a result of urinary infection. The ataxia may be improved by re-educative exercises. Arthropathies may require surgery to promote stability by arthrodesis. Perforating ulcers should have any necrotic bone removed from their base and should be treated by rest. Care should be taken to prevent further trauma.

The C.S.F. should be re-examined after six months to confirm that there is improvement, indicated by a decrease in protein and fewer cells. Although the C.S.F. is likely to become normal eventually, a persistently positive Wassermann reaction is not in itself an indication for further treatment.

General Paralysis of the Insane

This is a chronic spirochaetal meningo-encephalitis, the spirochaetes being in the brain; exactly how they produce the pathological changes is not yet fully understood. These changes comprise thickening of the meninges, atrophy of the convolutions, especially of the anterior two thirds of the brain, with compensatory hydrocephalus and granular ependymitis. Microscopically there is an inflammatory meningeal reaction with peri-vascular infiltration of lymphocytes and plasma cells. Nerve cells degen-erate and iron pigment is deposited.

Clinical Features. The onset is usually insidious, occurring ten years or more after the primary infection. Males are more commonly affected than females.

The early symptoms are those of *dementia* and *personality change*. There may be loss of memory and of judgement, carelessness with regard to spending money and neglect of cleanliness and of general appearance. The personality change is by no means always towards ideas of grandeur and the patient may be depressed or hypochondriacal. Gradually there is complete disintegration of intellect and of personality.

Epilepsy may be an early symptom and may, indeed, be the first mani-festation of the disease at a time when there is nothing to suggest its true nature.

On examination, the physical signs which accompany the dementia are a *slurring dysarthria*, often with an aphasic element so that words are not only incorrectly articulated but wrongly uttered with transposition of syllables; *tremors* of the hands, lips, and tongue; and *spastic weakness* of the legs with brisk reflexes and possibly extensor plantar responses. *Optic atrophy* and Argyll-Robertson pupils (p. 251) may also be present.

The C.S.F. is likely to show increase of protein and cells and a paretic Lange (5555544433) and the Wassermann reaction is always positive. It is usually also positive in the blood, but not so constantly; a negative Wassermann reaction in the blood cannot be taken to exclude general paralysis. If such a diagnosis seems possible the C.S.F. *must* be examined.

Treatment. Untreated general paralysis is fatal within two years or so of its onset and it was this that helped to distinguish it, at the beginning of the nineteenth century, from other forms of insanity. With the intro-duction of malaria therapy in the 1920's a cure was achieved in about 30 per cent of patients and arrest in a similar number. For a time this was combined with penicillin, but the latter is now generally regarded as an adequate treatment by itself. Intramuscular injections of 1 million units daily are given to a total of 12–15 million units.

If the diagnosis is made early the *prognosis* is good, with the possibility of return to normal mental function. The disease can usually be arrested and, when remission is not complete, a proportion of patients can still return to a useful life.

The C.S.F. should be re-examined after six months to ensure that there has been a satisfactory response to treatment, the important feature at this stage being a decrease of protein and cells.

Syphilitic Optic Atrophy

This may occur as an isolated manifestation of neuro-syphilis or it may accompany other clinical symptoms, either meningo-vascular or parenchymatous. The optic discs are dead white but visual acuity may be normal to a late stage, when blindness may develop quite rapidly, central vision being eventually involved in a process of gradually increasing peripheral constriction.

The C.S.F. may be abnormal, but treatment with penicillin is often ineffective in relieving the blindness or preventing its advance to involve an eye still normal at the time of treatment. In these circumstances malaria therapy is still sometimes recommended, but its value is doubtful and its administration not entirely without risk to life. It is also a most unpleasant experience for the patient.

INTRACRANIAL TUMOUR

Under this heading it is convenient to include all expanding lesions inside the skull, abscesses and haematomas as well as neoplasms. Angiomas are excluded since they are congenital arteriovenous malformations and rarely behave as expanding lesions in the absence of haemorrhage.

In adults the common neoplasms are gliomas which are infiltrative tumours, the *meningioma*, an essentially benign tumour, and *metastatic tumours*, usually from carcinoma of the lung or breast. *Neuromas*, usually of the eighth nerve, and *pituitary tumours* are also quite common.

In children, in whom the tumours are usually found in the posterior fossa, the commonest are *medullo-blastoma* and *astrocytoma*, either of the cerebellum or the pons.

Clinical Features. Although the combination of headache, vomiting, and papilloedema is the most characteristic presentation of a cerebral tumour, it is by no means the commonest and the possibility of a tumour may arise when none of these is present. The only indication may be some progressive defect of function, either physical or mental. Thus there may be progressive deafness, visual loss, hemiplegia, and disturbance of speech or its secondary derivatives (reading, calculation, etc.); or progressive personality change or intellectual impairment.

Headache is, however, often a feature. It is usually intermittent, often localised or lateralised, present on waking for a few hours and aggravated, or even precipitated, by coughing and straining. Although often accompanied by increased intracranial pressure it is not due to this but to a distortion or displacement of pain-sensitive structures, which are the dural sinuses, large arteries and sensory nerves. This displacement may also cause obstruction to the C.S.F. pathways and produce *papilloedema*.

Associated *vomiting* is less frequent than headache, but if present also often occurs on waking and may lead to some relief of the headache. Rarely vomiting may occur alone, usually with tumours in the posterior fossa; the probable mechanism is direct involvement of the vomiting centre.

Other symptoms which suggest the possibility of tumour are *epilepsy*, especially if of late onset, and *vertigo*, either of which may occur as an isolated symptom and precede for some time signs of an expanding lesion, in the case of epilepsy possibly for several years. If the epilepsy is focal it may localise the lesion, but if the discharge arises in the temporal lobe area it does not always lateralise it. There is, however, nothing in the pattern of the epileptic attack to indicate for certain the presence of an underlying lesion or to suggest that such a lesion is a tumour.

Mental Symptoms. These may at first consist of no more than tiredness, apathy, or lack of energy, but may proceed to personality change, intellectual impairment and gross retardation, often with incontinence.

Signs. Signs which support the suspicion of cerebral tumour are:

(1) *Papilloedema*

This occurs with obstruction of C.S.F. pathways and is more likely, therefore, with tumours involving the third ventricle, aqueduct, fourth ventricle, and its roof foramina. It is therefore more common with tumours of the posterior fossa and may not be present at all in patients with even large tumours involving the cerebral hemispheres. It must also be remembered that papilloedema occurs in other conditions, such as lateral sinus thrombosis and so-called benign intracranial hypertension; the latter occurs almost exclusively in women, sometimes in association with pregnancy, and may follow mild trauma though often the aetiology is unknown. Papilloedema must also be distinguished from retrobulbar neuritis accompanied by swelling of the disc. The distinction may not be possible simply from ophthalmoscopic appearance; but retrobulbar neuritis is associated with severe loss of visual acuity, which is not an early symptom of papilloedema.

(2) *Focal Neurological Signs*

If these are present, they serve to localise the tumour and may, if this localisation is characteristic, suggest its likely nature. Thus a tumour in the cerebello-pontine angles giving rise to progressive deafness, facial weakness and numbness, and ipselateral ataxia is likely to be an acoustic neuroma. A para-sagittal tumour may be a meningioma, as may be one compressing the olfactory nerve in the olfactory groove and causing anosmia. A tumour causing bitemporal field defects thereby indicates its presence in the region of the pituitary fossa and may be a pituitary adenoma, a craniopharyngioma or a meningioma. General examination of the patient, especially of the lungs or breasts, may suggest the possibility of a metastatic growth, as may the past history of a carcinoma anywhere in the body. A source of infection, either in the ear, the nasal sinuses, or the chest, suggests the possibility of abscess; and this is a common lesion too in patients with cyanotic congenital heart disease.

Special Investigations. It is always necessary to proceed to further investigation so that the presence of a tumour can be verified, its nature determined and appropriate treatment given.

(1) *Radiography*

Radiographs of the skull may show:

Erosion of the posterior clinoid processes, suggesting raised intracranial pressure; of the internal auditory meatus, as in acoustic neuroma; of the skull base in the region of the petrous apex and foramen ovale, as in nasopharyngeal carcinoma extending into the skull.

Expansion of the sella turcica (ballooning) as in chromophobe adenoma or its *destruction* from without as in para-sellar tumours.

Hyperostosis at the sites of election of meningioma, the vault, sphenoid wings, and olfactory grooves.

They may also show lateral *shift of a calcified pineal*, confirming the presence of an expanding lesion, or its downward shift, suggesting the presence of internal hydrocephalus, possibly secondary to tumour.

They may show *abnormal calcification*, which occurs in many tumours, but especially in slow-growing gliomas and in about half the craniopharyngiomas.

If a cerebral tumour is suspected radiographs of the chest must be always taken to exclude or reveal the presence of a bronchial carcinoma.

(2) *Echo-encephalography*

When X-rays of the skull are normal, when there is no abnormal calcifications and when the pineal is not calcified, echo-encephalography can be done to determine the position of the midline structures.

(3) *Electro-encephalography (E.E.G.)*

This may indicate an area of disturbed cerebral function; but a single record cannot distinguish between a vascular and a neoplastic process nor can the E.E.G. distinguish with certainty between a benign and a malignant tumour. The E.E.G. in cerebral abscess contains characteristically slow focal activity. A tumour in the posterior fossa may give rise to bilateral E.E.G. disturbances and the E.E.G. may thus help to distinguish between a posterior fossa and a cerebral hemisphere tumour.

(4) *Brain scan*

This is done using Technetium 99^m, which may be taken up by various abnormal intracranial structures, including neoplasms, abscesses, haematomas and infarcts.

(5) *Lumbar Puncture*

This may be dangerous in the presence of papilloedema and is not likely to add any information of value in cases where there is little doubt about the presence of an expanding intracranial lesion. It may, however, show increased intracranial pressure (normal is up to 180 mm. of fluid) when there is no other evidence of this and it may also show an increased protein content in the C.S.F., especially in acoustic neuroma and basal meningioma.

There may be a pleocytosis, especially in cases of malignant tumours impinging on the ventricular system and it has recently been demonstrated that actual tumour cells may be identified in the C.S.F. In cerebral abscess the C.S.F. usually shows a pleocytosis, about 100 cells and mostly lymphocytic, and increased protein.

If these investigations seem to confirm the suspicion of tumour, then further neuro-radiological investigations may be done. These are:

> cerebral angiography,
> air encephalography,
> ventriculography.

Cerebral Angiography

This involves the injection of a radio-opaque dye into a carotid or vertebral artery. Injection into a carotid artery is particularly indicated if the cerebral lesion is lateralised and if there is some possibility of there being a vascular basis to the symptoms, cerebral angioma and internal carotid artery disease in particular sometimes mimicking a cerebral tumour. Angiography does not always localise an expanding lesion with certainty, especially if it is in the parietal region, but may do so accurately if there is a pathological circulation, as there not infrequently is with very malignant gliomas and metastatic growths.

Vertebral angiography is less frequently indicated but serves a similar purpose.

Air Encephalography

This is the name given to the filling of the ventricular system and the cerebral subarachnoid space with air which is injected either by lumbar or cisternal (cisterna magna) puncture.

The air in the ventricles is less opaque than the surrounding brain and the site, size, and shape of the ventricular system can thus be determined and the presence of any extracerebral, intracerebral, or intraventricular expanding lesion can be demonstrated. Likewise it may be shown that the lesion is, in fact, one of cerebral atrophy.

Ventriculography

Air encephalography is best avoided in the presence of papilloedema or if there is no reasonable doubt about the presence of a tumour. In such cases the air can be introduced through a brain needle into the lateral ventricle through a posterior parietal burr-hole. In certain cases *myodil* may be introduced by this route if it is desired to demonstrate, for example, stenosis of the Sylvian aqueduct.

Treatment. At this stage the presence of a cerebral tumour may have been confirmed and if so its nature must be verified because this will determine the treatment. If investigations so far have been in favour of finding a benign rather than an infiltrating tumour, then a craniotomy should be performed. Craniotomy may also be done even if complete removal of the tumour is impossible if a substantial measure of relief can be anticipated from decompression, or if this is considered the safest or most effective way to verify the nature of a tumour.

If craniotomy is not done then a needle biopsy may provide the necessary verification and may confirm that the tumour is inoperable or may, on the other hand, suggest that it is operable. Exploration with a needle will also be used to find an abscess cavity, to aspirate the pus, and to instil the appropriate antibiotic.

When surgical removal of a tumour is impossible or incomplete irradiation may be considered. If given in association with dexamethazone to control oedema immediate and short term results are often gratifying but the long term results are usually disappointing. This should not contraindicate the use of radiotherapy unless the patient fails to make an initially favourable response to dexamethazone.

SPINAL CORD COMPRESSION

One of the most important clinical syndromes from the diagnostic point of view is that of gradual compression of the spinal cord.

Symptoms. It may occur at any age from a variety of causes and the earliest symptom may be *pain*. This pain is intermittent and precipitated or aggravated by coughing, straining, movement, jolting, and jarring. It is radicular in distribution and thus, depending on the situation of the lesion, passes down the arm or leg or is of girdle distribution round the trunk.

Following pain the next symptom from a lesion within the cervical or thoracic spine is a tendency to drag the legs on account of spasticity, especially on exertion. Progressive weakness, sensory loss, and sphincter disturbance gradually develop. A lesion within the lumbar spine causes a flaccid weakness.

Signs. The signs depend on the *level* of cord compression; it is the demonstration of a motor, sensory, or reflex *level* which leads to the diagnosis of a focal lesion of the spinal cord.

There are wasting and weakness of lower motor type at the level of compression, and pyramidal weakness below it. *Reflexes* may be depressed at the level of the lesion and increased below it, with extensor plantar responses. The level of pain and temperature impairment may fall below the level of the lesion in early compression, on account of the lamination of the spinothalamic tract, but this will rise as the compression increases. The demonstration of a partial *Brown-Séquard syndrome* (i.e. pyramidal and posterior column signs more prominent on one side and pain and temperature loss more prominent on the other) confirm that the lesion is of the cord.

Compression of the conus and cauda equina cause early sphincter disturbance and impotence. A flaccid paralysis of the legs then develops, with wasting and fasciculation of the affected muscles, and sensory loss to all modalities over the lower lumbar and sacral dermatomes.

Once the suspected level of the lesion is discovered the spine must be carefully examined, especially at that level, for signs of a gibbus, other deformity, or tenderness.

Investigations

Radiological

Radiography of the spine may reveal vertebral destruction or erosion or the changes of spondylosis; the latter is a particularly common cause of cord compression in the cervical region. Radiographs may also show changes of Paget's disease or of Pott's disease. A chest radiograph must be taken, since spinal metastases commonly arise from a bronchial carcinoma.

Lumbar Puncture

This is a very valuable investigation not only so that the C.S.F. may be examined but in order to do the *Queckenstedt* test to investigate the possibility of a block in the spinal subarachnoid space. This is performed by pressing on the jugular veins in the neck; if there is a free rise and fall of fluid in the manometer, there is no block. If there is no rise on jugular compression it is then necessary to press on the abdomen. If this produces a rise and fall of fluid in the manometer and further compression of the jugular veins again produces no response, then a block has been demonstrated in the spinal subarachnoid space, which confirms the suspicion of cord compression. A rise of fluid in the manometer on jugular compression, but no fall, indicates a partial block from which the same conclusion may be drawn. If there is a block the protein content of the C.S.F. is likely to be increased (*Froin syndrome*). If the puncture is above the level of a cauda equina compression, manometry will be normal but the protein may be increased, especially if the lesion is a neurofibroma.

Differential Diagnosis. A lesion causing focal compression of the spinal cord must be distinguished from other lesions which have a spastic paraplegia as part of the clinical picture. These are:

(1) *syringomyelia,* in which the arm reflexes are lost and there is dissociated cutaneous sensory loss,

(2) *syphilitic meningo-myelitis,* in which there may be other evidence of syphilis such as pupillary abnormalities and in which the C.S.F. shows appropriate changes,

(3) *disseminated sclerosis,* in which there is evidence of multiple lesions,

(4) *motor neurone disease,* in which there are no sensory symptoms or signs and no sphincter disturbance,

(5) *subacute combined degeneration* of the cord due to B_{12} deficiency, in which there are gastric achylia, possibly a macrocytic anaemia and megaloblastic marrow and a significantly lowered serum B_{12} (normal 150–800 pg.)

(6) On rare occasions a spastic paraplegia is caused by a *para-sagittal cerebral tumour* involving the leg areas.

Myelography

If focal compression of the cord remains a possibility, myelography must be done in order to demonstrate conclusively a compressing lesion and its exact situation, not only in the spinal column but with regard to whether it is outside the cord (*extramedullary*) or inside the cord (*intra-medullary*). Myelography involves the injection of a radio-opaque dye, such as Ethiodan, either by the lumbar or cisternal (cisterna magna) route and by appropriate tilting the dye can be followed through the entire extent of the spinal subarachnoid space. In this way any filling defect in the sub-arachnoid space or any displacement of the spinal cord can be seen on screening and can then be recorded on film.

The films may show some compression of the cord *from without*, the cause of which might be:

(1) primary tumour—meningioma or neurofibroma,
(2) secondary carcinoma,
(3) cervical spondylosis,
(4) extradural abscess,
(5) Hodgkin's disease.
(6) myeloma,
(7) Pott's disease,
(8) Paget's disease.

There may be *expansion of the cord*, suggesting an intramedullary lesion which may be syringomyelia or a tumour such as glioma or ependymoma.

Treatment. Before treatment is embarked upon, surgical exploration may be necessary to verify the nature of a compressing lesion. If a menin-gioma or neurofibroma is found it is removed. Cervical spondylosis is best treated, in the first place, by immobilisation in a collar, but laminectomy and decompression may be indicated later. A soft, single disc protrusion in a young person may be removed and an anterior inter-body fusion car-ried out. Pott's disease is treated by chemotherapy and Paget's disease, which usually causes compression in the upper thoracic region, may be helped by decompression. Intramedullary tumours, extramedullary carci-nomas, and other deposits may respond to radiotherapy.

MOTOR NEURONE DISEASE

This is the name usually given to a condition, of unknown aetiology, in which there is progressive degeneration of the anterior horn cells, the motor nuclei in the medulla and the upper motor neurones in the spinal cord, brain stem, and to some extent in the cerebral hemispheres. The condition affects men about twice as often as women. It is rare under twenty and the greatest incidence is in the fifth and sixth decades.

Although the degeneration observed pathologically is not strictly confined to motor pathways, there are never any sensory symptoms, apart from occasional painful cramps in the muscles about to become involved. Nor are there any sensory signs or sphincter disturbance.

Clinical Features. There are three patterns of clinical presentation:

> progressive bulbar palsy,
> progressive muscular atrophy,
> amyotrophic lateral sclerosis.

Either of the first two may appear alone for many months, but the second and third often appear together as amyotrophic lateral sclerosis (i.e. muscle wasting, usually of the arms, with pyramidal involvement, usually of the legs) to which picture features of progressive bulbar palsy are sometimes added.

Progressive Bulbar Palsy

Slowly progressive wasting and weakness develop in the musculature of the tongue, palate, and pharynx, secondary to degeneration of the motor nuclei in the medulla, causing *dysarthria* and *dysphagia*. The most important sign is a *wasted fibrillating tongue*.

Progressive Muscular Atrophy (PMA)

This usually starts with wasting and weakness of the small muscles of the hands, not necessarily symmetrical, as a result of degeneration of anterior horn cells. The wasting tends to spread proximally and fasciculation may be widespread. Far less often the wasting and weakness start in the muscles of the feet and legs. In the absence of associated upper motor neurone involvement the reflexes are depressed in proportion to the degree of wasting.

Amyotrophic Lateral Sclerosis

With degeneration of the upper motor neurone spastic weakness develops, with increased reflexes and extensor plantar responses. The clinical picture at any one time will depend on the extent to which the upper and lower motor neurones are involved in the spinal cord.

With involvement of the upper motor neurone in the brain stem and above, the picture of 'pseudo-bulbar palsy' develops, either on its own, in which case the symptoms are dysarthria and dysphagia but due to a spastic rather than an atrophic weakness, or there may be a combination of both upper and lower motor neurone signs. With the development of pseudo-bulbar palsy there is emotional lability and the jaw-jerk is increased.

Treatment. No treatment is known which will influence the course of this condition, which is a progressive one. If the picture remains one of progressive muscular atrophy the prognosis is rather better than when the upper motor neurone is involved, when the expectation of life is about three years after the diagnosis has been established. With progressive bulbar palsy the outlook is similar; death results from inanition and pulmonary infection.

PERONEAL MUSCULAR ATROPHY (Charcot-Marie-Tooth)

This is a familial condition of unknown cause. There is atrophy of the anterior horn cells and posterior columns and associated interstitial neuritis of the peroneal nerves.

It presents as muscular wasting, starting in the feet and rising steadily over the years to the junction of the middle and lower thirds of the thigh. The small muscles of the hand and the distal third of the forearm may waste similarly. Despite extreme wasting power is remarkably preserved and active life for many years is the rule. All modalities of sensation are affected over the wasted muscles.

Only symptomatic treatment is possible but life expectancy is little reduced.

OCCUPATIONAL CRAMPS

This is an uncommon group of disorders affecting the muscles of the hand when engaging in vocational repetitive movements. The classical example is *writer's cramp*, but others such as seamstress's or telegraphist's cramp have been described. With increasing use of mechanical appliances they have become less common.

Characteristically the muscles are only affected when performing the particular task, for example writing. Initially there is pain in the muscles followed by cramps, eventually necessitating the cessation of the activity. No abnormality is found on examination. The only effective treatment is the complete avoidance of the painful activity for 6 to 9 months; symptomatic relief from cramp may be obtained with aspirin (300 mg.); splinting the hand and wrist is sometimes helpful.

Nothing is certainly known of the cause of the condition, but it is thought that psychological factors are important. The chief differential diagnosis is from Parkinson's disease, which may present with cramps in the hand and micrographia.

SPASMODIC TORTICOLLIS

This is an uncommon condition. It occurs only in adults, and affects the sexes equally. Outbreaks have been described following epidemics of encephalitis and rarely it is associated with Parkinson's disease. In 1959 the condition was induced in monkeys by lesions in the cephalic part of the reticular formation, the occiput turning towards the side of the lesion.

It may begin abruptly or gradually and consists of irregular spasms of the muscles supporting the head, notably of one sternomastoid. The head is irregularly displaced; usually it is rotated, occasionally flexed. It may be so slight as almost to pass unnoticed, or be so severe as to handicap the patient completely. As it persists it is associated with hypertrophy of the affected muscles and usually with derangement of the cervical spine.

Treatment consists of exercises to the neck with the object of stretching the affected muscles fully. This may be combined with amylobarbitone sodium 15 mg. t.d.s. Other drugs sometimes of use are promethazine (50 mg. t.d.s.), chlorpromazine (100 mg. t.d.s.), meprobamate (400 mg. t.d.s.) or reserpine (0·25 mg. t.d.s.). Alternatively, surgical division of the accessory nerve and upper anterior cervical roots may bring relief.

NEUROFIBROMATOSIS

This condition is usually manifest between twenty and forty and affects the sexes equally. It consists of hyperplasia of the fibrous connective tissue supporting the nerves. It occurs in a number of clinical forms.

(a) *Multiple neurofibromata* (von Recklinghausen's disease)

Multiple tumours arise from cutaneous nerves, and project as lumps, some pedunculated, all over the body. There are also patches of melanotic pigmentation of the skin and often congenital spinal deformities, for example spina bifida or spondylolisthesis. There is no curative treatment, but large tumours may be excised.

(b) *Individual neurofibromata*

These may arise from any nerve, and cause no symptoms unless the nerve passes through a constriction at the site of the tumour. Examples are:

(1) The *radial* as it pierces the lateral intermuscular septum, the *median* as it passes behind the tendonous bridge joining the origins of the flexor digitorum sublimis, and the deep branch of the *ulnar* nerve as it passes into the hand.

(2) Neurofibromata may arise on the *spinal nerve roots*, so that part of the tumour is within the spinal canal and part is in the thorax or abdomen. These so-called 'dumb-bell' tumours are occasionally discovered on chest radiography, but usually present with spinal-cord compression (p. 291).

(3) *Auditory* or (less commonly) *trigeminal nerve* tumours. They arise in the cerebello-pontine angle. They are insidious, and usually present as gradually increasing deafness and tinnitus. Vertigo may occur. This is followed by impairment of sensation of the forehead and cornea (V) sometimes complicated by corneal ulceration, and ipselateral facial weakness. Large tumours may cause ipselateral signs of cerebellar derangement (p. 263).

These tumours are all associated with raised C.S.F. protein (about 80–120 mg./100 ml.), and with expansion of the internal auditory meatus when visualised radiologically.

Treatment of all these conditions is surgical, the results depending upon the extent of the disease at the time of intervention. Rarely the tumours may undergo sarcomatous change.

(c) Rarely there is diffuse overgrowth of all the nervous supportive tissue, so as to cause hypertrophic chronic peripheral neuritis.

SYRINGOMYELIA AND SYRINGOBULBIA

Syringomyelia is a cystic degeneration of the grey matter of the spinal cord, until recently of unknown cause. There is now good evidence that in some patients, and possibly quite a large number, the primary lesion is a developmental or acquired anomaly in the region of the foramen magnum which obstructs the flow of C.S.F. from the foramina in the roof of the 4th ventricle. C.S.F. is thus forced into the central canal causing first a hydro-myelia and then rupture of the ependyma permits fluid to seep into the central grey matter. Symptoms do not usually appear until early adult life or later and men are more frequently affected.

Clinical Features. The early involvement of grey matter interrupting the crossing pain and temperature fibres and the reflex arc, determines the cardinal signs of syringomyelia which are:

(1) *dissociated cutaneous sensory loss,* with loss of pain and tem-perature sensation and preservation of touch, vibration, and position sense.

(2) *loss of reflexes.*

The process usually starts in the cervical enlargement so that the dis-sociated sensory loss appears over a forequarter and the arm reflexes are lost.

The *symptoms* which are likely to bring the patient under observation are:

pain in the arm,
wasting of small hand muscles,
spastic weakness of the legs.

These are features which are present in a number of conditions and *on examination* the important additional diagnostic findings will be absent reflexes and dissociated sensory loss, which may not be present over the whole forequarter and may not even be present anywhere in the arm but be confined to upper cervical dermatomes. Fasciculation, rather coarse, may be present over the arms and chest and there may be a scoliosis. Arthropathy (Charcot joints) may be present in the cervical spine and, more rarely, in the shoulder and elbow joints.

Treatment. Radiotherapy to the affected part of the cord is thought to be helpful in some cases, especially in relieving pain. In other patients operation to restore a normal circulation of C.S.F. and decompress the expanded cord is now the treatment of choice.

Syringobulbia

Cavitation may occur in the medulla and does so usually in association with syringomyelia, but sometimes alone. The cavity has a fairly constant situation, in the postero-lateral part of the tegmentum, and involves, unilaterally or bilaterally,

(a) vestibular pathways,
(b) the descending root of the trigeminal nerve,
(c) sympathetic and taste pathways,
(d) the nucleus ambiguus,
(e) the emerging fibres of the hypoglossal nerve.

The *presenting symptoms*, which are sometimes of quite acute onset, are thus *vertigo, pain,* or *sensory loss* over the face or *hoarseness*. The *signs* are *nystagmus*, usually rotary, *dissociated sensory loss* over the face (not with a peripheral nerve distribution), *loss of taste, Horner's syndrome, vocal cord paralysis*, and a *wasted tongue*.

The condition may be slowly progressive, but may arrest and remain stationary for many years.

BASAL GANGLIA SYNDROMES

Parkinsonism

Paralysis agitans, first described by Parkinson in 1817 and later named Parkinson's disease by Charcot, is characterised by a combination in varying degree of rigidity, tremor and bradykinesia (slowness of movement) that cannot be totally accounted for by rigidity. Rigidity is the most constant feature and sometimes appears alone.

There may be a genetic factor in some 25% of cases. An imbalance between the transmitter substances acetylcholine and dopamine in the striatum is now postulated and drugs which either inhibit the former (atropine and other solanaceous alkaloids) or increase the latter (*l*-dopa) give benefit in certain cases.

Clinical Features. *Rigidity*. The effect of the rigidity is to interfere with the normal play of facial expression; with speech, so that the patient mumbles in a monotonous voice; and with posture and movement. Due to the rigidity of the neck and trunk muscles, the posture becomes stooped and there is disturbance of gait, so that starting to walk is often difficult and thereafter the patient has a tendency 'to walk at a running pace'. When walking, one or both arms may hang immobile by the side.

The patient often complains of weakness of an arm not, as he says, for picking up large things like a bucket of coal, but for picking up small things, and there is inability to perform fine finger movements. The writing becomes smaller and illegible.

Tremor. The characteristic feature of the tremor is that it is present at rest and may be momentarily inhibited by using the arm. The tremor usually starts in a hand or arm and may then involve the leg. It may remain unilateral or then involve the other side. The lower jaw may also become tremulous. Tremor stops during sleep.

In the absence of the characteristic tremor, the most important finding is *rigidity*, a resistance to passive movement at a joint throughout the full range of movement at that joint. Rigidity is found early in neck muscles, in the shoulder, wrist, and at the ankle, and may later become generalised. The small hand muscles are often *weak*, in addition to showing poverty of movement, but there is no other significant weakness and no reflex change or sensory loss. The **glabellar tap** is an interesting physical sign: blinking in response to tapping the root of the nose ceases in normal adults after a few taps, but in parkinsonian patients it persists indefinitely.

Pathology

Paralysis agitans in the classical form is a systemic degeneration affecting a neuronal system whose nodal point is the substantia nigra. It usually develops in late middle age. About 100 years after Parkinson's description it became clear that a similar picture could be associated with encephalitis lethargica, coming on either at the time of the acute illness or later, the substantia nigra and its connections being the seat of an inflammatory rather than a degenerative change. More recently it has been recognised that certain features of Parkinsonism are associated with cerebral arteriosclerosis. There are, however, some distinguishing features.

Post-encephalitic Parkinsonism

In this the rigidity and tremor are identical but there may be added features which serve to distinguish it such as oculo-gyric crises, spasms of neck muscles, dribbling, a greasy skin, and behaviour disorders. The onset is nearly always before the age of forty.

Arteriosclerotic Parkinsonism

This is more easily distinguished and is commonly associated with hypertension or other evidence of vascular disorder, with dementia, pyramidal signs, sphincter disturbance, and a more shuffling gait. Tremor is less prominent than rigidity. This is a disease of old age.

Parkinsonism due to drugs

Parkinsonism may be a side effect of drugs of the phenothiazine group (e.g. chlorpromazine) or of the butyrophenane group (e.g. haloperidol). These drugs can also cause oculo-gyric crises, previously seen only in post-encephalitic parkinsonism.

Treatment

Medical. Tincture of stramonium and related drugs of the solanaceous group were for long the treatment of choice in the Parkinsonian syndrome.

Then a series of synthetic drugs of the same nature was developed of which benzhexol (artane) is a useful representative. It may be given in tablets containing 2 mg. or 5 mg. up to a total of 12–18 mg. daily; it sometimes causes mental upset as a side effect. Another useful preparation is orphenadrine (Disipal) 50–100 mg. t.d.s.

More recently, following observations that dopamine was depleted in the basal ganglia of patients with Parkinsonism, dihydroxyphenylalanine (*l*-dopa), the precursor of dopamine which does not cross the blood-brain barrier, has proved effective in the treatment of about two thirds of the patients with Parkinsonism. The response is usually greater than that to the anticholinergic drugs already mentioned and bradykinesia is relieved more than rigidity and tremor. An initial dose of 250 mg. t.d.s. is gradually increased by increments of 250 mg. every three days or so and it seems that a total daily dose of between 2 g and 8 g will produce a satisfactory response. Side-effects are nausea, anorexia, hypotension and involuntary movements usually starting in the face. Psychiatric disturbances also occur.

Amantadine (Symmetrel) may also be tried in doses of 100 mg. daily for a week and 100 mg. twice daily thereafter.

Surgical. Recently operation has been helpful in suitable patients. The operation is a stereotactic one in which a destructive lesion is made in the globus pallidus or anterior thalamus. It is especially indicated in unilateral involvement in patients under sixty in whom there is no evidence of cerebral atherosclerosis. Tremor and rigidity are relieved more than bradykinesia and possibly operation plus *l*-dopa will prove to be the most effective treatment.

HUNTINGTON'S CHOREA

This is an adult, hereditary, progressive chorea, with dominant inheritance, affecting the sexes equally and occurring in the third or fourth decade.

The early *symptoms* are usually involuntary movements of a fidgety and jerky character, accompanied by grimacing. As the condition progresses the arms become clumsy, the gait unsteady and signs of dementia appear, with personality change and memory and intellectual impairment.

There is no treatment and the condition usually ends in death in about fifteen years. The chorciform movements may respond to tatrabenazine (Nitoman) 75–300 mg. daily.

FRIEDREICH'S ATAXIA

This is the commonest member of a group of heredo-familial degenerative disorders.

Pathology. Degeneration is seen in the posterior columns, less marked in the lateral columns and cerebellum, and sometimes affects the optic nerves.

Clinical Features. The onset is in the first or second decade and the first symptom is unsteadiness of the gait followed later by clumsiness of the hands. Dysarthria develops and weakness is added to the ataxia. On examination nystagmus is present, there is intention tremor of the arms, pyramidal weakness of the legs with absent knee and ankle jerks and extensor plantar responses. There is impairment of postural and vibration sense. There may be optic atrophy. Pes cavus and scoliosis are characteristic and the E.C.G. may show cardiac arrhythmia.

The condition tends to be slowly progressive and no treatment is known which will arrest its course.

MYASTHENIA GRAVIS

This is a disease characterised by abnormal fatigue of striated muscle and rapid recovery after rest. The pathology is still far from clear, but there seems to be a biochemical defect associated with abnormal behaviour of acetylcholine at the myoneural junction. The symptoms can be present in the new-born child of a mother with myasthenia gravis, and will be transient. They can come on at any age and affect the sexes about equally; the highest incidence occurs in the second and third decades and in this age group women are more commonly affected.

Clinical Features. Fatigue may occur in any muscle or muscle group but most commonly involved are those in which weakness gives rise to diplopia, dysphagia, dysarthria, and difficulty in chewing. Muscles of the trunk and limbs are involved first in about 30 per cent of the cases. Affected muscles tire quickly on exercise, for example dysarthria develops in the course of conversation or difficulty in chewing in the middle of a meal; and all symptoms tend to become worse by the end of the day and to be relieved to some extent by next morning. The disease also shows complete remissions.

Myasthenia can occur as a *symptom* in carcinomatous neuropathy and in thyrotoxicosis.

Signs. On examination there is no wasting or fasciculation and there may or may not be permanent weakness. The most important feature to demonstrate is pathological fatigue. This may be done by asking the patient to look up without blinking for a prolonged period, during which time ptosis may develop, or by asking him to raise his arm above his head thirty or forty times, a movement he may find more and more difficult to perform. In both instances power will return to normal after a few seconds' rest. There is never any reflex change or sensory loss.

Diagnosis. If the diagnosis is in doubt and weakness is present, a diagnostic test may be carried out by giving an intramuscular injection of neostigmine 2 mg. or 2·5 mg., with atropine 1·0 mg. to prevent abdominal colic. Increase in power is quite striking after 20 to 30 minutes in the patient with myasthenia gravis, but a slight improvement, particularly if only subjective, has no significance.

Treatment. This is, in the first place, by tablets of neostigmine bromide (15 mg.); one or two tablets should be taken as often as is necessary to maintain normal power. Alternatively tablets of the longer-acting pyridostigmine (60 mg.) may be given in the same way.

If the weakness is severe, especially of the muscles of swallowing, an intramuscular injection of neostigmine 2 mg. may be necessary first thing in the morning and before meals.

Thymectomy is of undoubted benefit in some cases and is indicated if the response to medical treatment is unsatisfactory. It seems to be of especial benefit if the total history is short. It does not replace treatment by neostigmine, which is afterwards usually required in smaller doses.

Operation is not indicated in the first place for a thymoma, whose presence may be discovered by an abnormal mediastinal shadow on radiography; but surgery may be considered after irradiation.

DEMYELINATING DISEASES

Demyelination in the central nervous system occurs in response to various pathological processes, but under this heading will be considered only diseases in which it is possibly the primary lesion.

Disseminated Sclerosis

The commonest of these conditions is disseminated sclerosis. Patches of demyelination occur at different times and in different places throughout the central nervous system, giving rise to the 'plaques' which in their final stage form grey, translucent scars in the white matter.

The *cause* of this condition is unknown. Some still regard it as an infection, others as an allergic reaction of the nervous system or the result of a metabolic upset or deficiency disorder. The disease is more common in temperate climates and about 60 per cent of patients have their first manifestation between the ages of twenty and forty, the onset being rare below the age of fifteen or over fifty. In this country it is half as common again in women as in men. Although intercurrent infection is likely to cause at least transient deterioration, there is no clear evidence that this or trauma can precipitate the disease and the risk of operation or pregnancy in producing a relapse is no longer considered a serious one. Although there is no evidence that pregnancy influences the long-term course of disseminated sclerosis, extra care may be helpful during the puerperium.

Clinical Features. Disseminated sclerosis is essentially pleomorphic and many symptoms and signs may appear singly or together; it is the *evidence of multiple lesions* on which the diagnosis ultimately rests. Unilateral *retro-bulbar neuritis* is often an early feature, the vision in one eye becoming misty, possibly with a central scotoma, or absent. Movement of the eye may be painful and there may be swelling of the optic disc. Vision usually returns to normal, but the disc subsequently shows abnormal pallor.

There may be *weakness* of one or both legs, sometimes with a sensory level indicating a transverse lesion of the cord. Sometimes there is defect or *loss of postural sense* in one or other arm giving rise to a useless arm. There may be *numbness* or *tingling* in the hands or feet, which may also be painful. There may be *vertigo, diplopia*, sphincter disturbance, usually causing increased frequency or *urgency* but sometimes retention, or impotence. *Tremor* and *dysarthria* may develop

In the early stages there may be complete remission of symptoms which may last for many years, but with recurrent episodes remissions are likely to be less complete and increasing permanent disability usually develops, ending in paralysis of the legs, often with painful flexor spasms, ataxia of the arms due to tremor or postural loss, and urinary infection. In many patients, however, the disorder remains fortunately mild and interferes little with ordinary life. Occasionally, and more often when the disease is of late onset, it may be steadily progressive from the first.

Diagnosis. The diagnosis depends on (1) the *demonstration* of multiple lesions, by means of symptoms and signs and (2) the *exclusion* of a focal lesion either in the brain or in the spinal cord, such as spinal tumour or cervical spondylosis, system disorders, e.g. subacute combined degeneration of the cord or Friedreich's ataxia. In doubtful cases the C.S.F. may contain changes of diagnostic help, especially a paretic Lange in the presence of normal protein, indicating a relative increase of gamma globulin. The W.R. is negative.

Treatment. There is no specific treatment which is known for certain to influence the course of the disease. Arsenic, pyrotherapy, low fat diet, intrathecal injection of P.P.D. and many others have been tried without obvious success in a disease in which spontaneous remissions make the assessment of any specific remedy difficult. Corticotrophin has, however, been shown to be helpful in the treatment of retrobulbar neuritis and in hastening recovery in other acute episodes of disseminated sclerosis; it should be given by daily injections for about a month. There are also many opportunities for symptomatic treatment which must not be ignored. A pill containing ext. belladonnae sicc. 30 mg. may relieve sphincter disturbance; chlorpromazine 50 mg. t.d.s. may relieve vertigo; and patients sometimes feel the benefit of weekly, or more frequent, injections of cyanocobalamin 1,000 µg. When the patient's mobility is affected rehabilitation by physiotherapy is important. In the later stages good nursing will help the prevention of bed-sores.

Neuromyelitis Optica

This is a closely related disease in which there is demyelination in the optic nerves and in the spinal cord, where it may be limited to a few segments or be diffuse.

The cause is unknown but it may develop at an earlier age than disseminated sclerosis. The *clinical picture* is that of bilateral retro-bulbar neuritis occurring simultaneously or consecutively, followed by a transverse myelitis which causes a spastic paraplegia or quadriplegia with sensory involvement and sphincter disturbance.

Except in its most typical form the clinical picture is indistinguishable from disseminated sclerosis, unless it develops at an earlier age.

Recovery may be complete or practically so, but relapse does sometimes occur leading to symptoms and signs characteristic of disseminated sclerosis.

Treatment. Corticotrophin is given and the management is as for disseminated sclerosis.

Diffuse Sclerosis

This term includes a number of conditions whose chief feature is a widespread demyelination in the cerebral hemispheres. They usually occur early in life and both sporadic and familial types occur. They are progressive, usually rapidly, and are not necessarily symmetrical. They are characterised clinically by epilepsy, dementia, visual disturbance, and diplegia.

DISORDERS OF THE PERIPHERAL NERVOUS SYSTEM

Root Lesions

Radiculitis has been shown in recent years to be the cause of some disorders formerly referred to as neuritis (e.g. the interstitial neuritis causing sciatica); it arises usually from disorders of the spine. Of these the commonest are lesions of the intervertebral disc, which usually occur where the spine is most mobile, that is in the cervical and lumbar regions. The lesions are produced either by trauma or by degeneration and lead to a protrusion or osteophytic overgrowth (spondylosis) which may be either central or lateral. A central protrusion causes cord or cauda equina compression (p. 291); it is lateral protrusion which is considered here. A single root is usually involved, the symptoms naturally depending on the situation of the lesion.

Cervical Spondylosis

The early symptom is pain which may at first be confined to the neck but later passes down the arm. The pain is intermittent, aggravated by coughing, straining, exertion, and jarring and is distributed according to the *myotome*; that is, it appears in muscles predominantly supplied by the root involved. At the periphery tingling may occur in the fingers in accordance with the *dermatome*. The pain is often most troublesome at night.

Thus in a C6 root lesion pain passes down the outer arm and may cause tingling in the thumb and index finger; in a C7 root lesion pain passes down the posterior aspect of the arm and forearm and may cause tingling in the index and middle finger; in a C8 root lesion pain passes down the inner arm and forearm and may cause tingling of the ring and little fingers.

Signs. Neck movements are usually restricted. Weakness and fasciculation of the muscles supplied by the root involved sometimes develop. In the case of a C6 root these are predominantly biceps, brachioradialis, and the radial extensor of the wrist, and the biceps and 'supinator' jerks are depressed or absent. In the case of a C7 root the triceps, the ulnar extensor of the wrist, finger extensors, and lower pectoral muscles are affected and the triceps jerk is depressed or absent. In the case of a C8 root the finger flexors are the muscles involved and the finger jerk, if originally present, may be absent. Significant sensory loss is rarely found. Other roots are less commonly affected and involvement of more than one root at a time is unusual.

Diagnosis. The fact that cervical spondylosis is the commonest cause of a root lesion must not lead to the neglect of other possible causes, especially primary spinal tumours and metastatic deposits.

Radiographs of the cervical spine may show narrowing of the appropriate disc space and osteophytic encroachment on the intervertebral foramina.

Treatment. In the first place, if the severity of the pain warrants it, this should be rest in bed with the arm supported on pillows in the most comfortable position. Analgesics will be required for a few days and the rest should be continued for some days after the pain has subsided. Manipulation is sometimes successful but possibly dangerous. If permanent relief is not achieved in a few weeks, the wearing of a cervical spine support for 3 to 6 months is often helpful. The condition tends to recur.

Lumbar Spondylosis

As in the neck, root lesions in the lumbar spine are usually attributable to spondylosis; the roots most commonly involved are L5 and S1, somewhat less commonly L4. The prominent symptom is pain which has the usual intermittent character of root pain and is precipitated by coughing, straining, jolting, and so on and is distributed in accordance with the *myotome*, with paraesthesiae at the periphery in the *dermatome*. Thus in an L4 root lesion there is pain in the anterior thigh passing down into the inner leg; in an L5 root lesion there is pain passing down the outer thigh into the outer leg; in an S1 root lesion there is pain passing down the back of the thigh into the calf. Muscle cramps, especially in the calf, sometimes develop.

Signs. With involvement of the lower lumbar and first sacral roots there is likely to be limitation of straight leg raising and there may be a scoliosis determined by spasm of the erector spinae muscles on the side of the lesion.

These may be the only abnormal signs, but weakness, wasting, and fasciculation are sometimes present; in an L4 lesion these are found in the quadriceps, and the knee jerk may be depressed or absent. In an L5 lesion the earliest and sometimes the only weakness is in the extensor hallucis longus and there is no associated reflex change. In an S1 root lesion weakness is of plantar flexion and the ankle jerk is depressed or absent. The jerks may disappear in the absence of weakness; there is seldom any significant sensory loss.

Radiographs may show appropriate changes in the lumbar spine, but they are often normal. Their main importance is in helping to rule out more serious lesions such as metastatic carcinoma.

Diagnosis. The possibility of other lesions causing radiculitis must be considered, especially primary tumours of the cauda equina and metastatic deposits. In these cases the condition is progressive, and if there is any doubt about the diagnosis lumbar puncture and myelography should be done.

Treatment. The condition varies in severity and tends to come in attacks which are sometimes fairly mild and pass off without any particular treatment. If severe, treatment in the first place should be complete rest, the patient being flat but not necessarily on the back. Bed-boards or placing the mattress on the floor, are sometimes helpful. At first analgesics may be necessary, but rest should be continued for some time after the pain has subsided and may have to be continued for 4 to 6 weeks. Thereafter gradual rehabilitation is necessary. Some advocate traction, epidural injection or manipulation and in resistant cases a plaster jacket or other lumbar support may be helpful. Operation has not proved sufficiently successful to make it the treatment of choice and should not be considered until other methods have failed to produce relief of pain. It is not likely to influence any residual weakness in the abscence of pain.

The patient who has once had radiculitis from lumbar spondylosis (sciatica) should be advised against heavy lifting with the back flexed, though recurrence may take place without any apparent precipitation.

CERVICAL RIB SYNDROME

A rib arising from the seventh cervical vertebra may produce no symptoms or signs. Sometimes, however, it may produce clinical features which are likely to be predominantly either vascular or neurological.

The vascular symptoms are usually due to vascular occlusion from embolus arising from a mural thrombus which has formed in the subclavian artery distal to its narrowing as it passes over the cervical rib. The patient complains of pain in the forearm which has the character of ischaemic muscle pain, spreading sometimes to involve the whole arm. This pain develops especially with use and is relieved by rest. In addition the hand is cold and becomes blue when dependent.

The neurological symptoms are caused by involvement of the lower cord of the brachial plexus, formed by the C8 and T1 roots. There is pain down the inner arm and forearm with tingling of the ring and little fingers. This pain develops with the arm in use, especially with lifting and carrying. The patient may also complain of a weakness of the grip and of a tendency to drop things.

Signs. There is weakness and possibly wasting of the finger flexors and of the small muscles of the hand. There may be slight cutaneous sensory impairment over the inner forearm, corresponding palm, and little and ring fingers. A rib may be palpable in the supraclavicular fossa.

Radiographs may show a cervical rib and one giving rise to symptoms should be removed surgically.

NEURITIS

This is the term usually applied to disorder of a peripheral nerve from whatever cause. The cause is, however, rarely inflammatory and commonest is some form of trauma. There will be considered here the clinical features which develop when the function of certain nerves is disordered by pressure.

Radial Nerve

The radial nerve is compressed typically when the arm is hung over a chair in a drunken stupor (drunkard's palsy), but it is exposed to compression in other ways as it winds round the radial groove on the humerus.

The muscles which are thus paralysed are the brachio-radialis, the extensors of the wrist and fingers and the long abductor of the thumb. There may be a small area of cutaneous sensory loss over the first dorsal interosseous.

Ulnar Nerve

The ulnar nerve may be injured by pressure in bed, when the development of symptoms and signs is likely to be rapid; but the onset is usually more insidious and occurs in association with previous damage around the elbow in the region of the medial epicondyle, or when the ulnar groove is unusually shallow and the nerve unduly exposed, or when the nerve tends to slip out of the groove with flexion of the elbow. When there is no obvious abnormality at the elbow joint, as is sometimes the case, it has been suggested that the nerve may be compressed where it passes into the forearm between the heads of flexor carpi ulnaris.

Pain is not a feature of this compression and the earliest symptoms are numbness of the little finger and corresponding palm and inability to *adduct* the little finger so that it tends to be caught when the hand is put in a pocket or into a glove. Later, weakness progresses to involve all the interossei and wasting of these muscles appears. The numbness becomes more intense and may be found by the patient to involve the ulnar aspect of the ring finger.

Signs. There will be a variable degree of wasting and weakness of the interossei, but the bulk of the abductor pollicis brevis and its power will be normal. The function of this muscle is to abduct the thumb at right angles to the palm and the muscle bulk can be palpated alongside the first metacarpal bone. Sensory loss of variable degree will be confined to the little finger and the inner half of the ring finger. Arthritic changes may be found at the elbow, or the groove may be shallow and the nerve tend to dislocate.

Treatment. Treatment is surgical, the nerve being transplanted from the ulnar groove, if there is evidence of disorder there, to the anterior aspect of the elbow. If the elbow seems normal the nerve may be decompressed as it passes between the heads of the flexor carpi ulnaris.

Median Nerve

Compression of the median nerve in the carpal tunnel has long been known to cause wasting of the muscles of the thenar eminence, with paralysis of abduction and opposition of the thumb, and cutaneous sensory loss over the thumb, index, middle, and radial half of the ring finger. This florid picture is, however, comparatively rare.

More recently it has been shown that milder forms of compression are responsible for acroparaesthesiae in the hand even when signs are slight or absent. This is now usually referred to as the *carpal tunnel syndrome,* which is common.

It occurs mostly in women, appearing usually for no apparent reason although, as will be seen, its development is related to use of the hands. In men there is usually a discoverable cause as, for example, arthritis of the wrist following injury, ganglion of the wrist joint, acromegaly or myxoedema. These causes do, of course, operate also in women, in whom pregnancy may be an additional precipitating factor.

The early symptoms are intermittent, usually nocturnal tingling of the fingers, usually of one hand and usually the hand the patient uses most. This tingling may spare the little finger and is sometimes most prominent in the *ring and middle* fingers. It wakens the patient, who may drop the arm out of the bed, sit up, and rub it or get up and swing it until sensation is restored.

This may happen more than once in the night. The tingling may be accompanied by pain in the hand, at the elbow or more rarely in the shoulder. The symptoms tend to be worse during a night which follows a strenuous day with the hands as, for example, doing the family washing.

As the condition progresses the patient has not only troubled nights but finds that on waking in the morning at the ordinary time the fingers feel swollen and are numb. This passes off in about twenty minutes but while present causes disability such as difficulty in doing up buttons.

Later, symptoms occur during the day. They are brought on especially by gripping, as in various forms of housework, and knitting or even holding a newspaper is sometimes enough to precipitate uncomfortable numbness so that the activity must be stopped. The tingling is sometimes painful and may be permanent.

Finally, abnormal signs may appear. They may be quite slight, and consist of weakness of the abductor pollicis brevis with cutaneous sensory impairment within the distribution of the median nerve. Sometimes there is *over-reaction* to pin-prick rather than hypoalgesia.

Diagnosis. This is rarely difficult when the history is typical and when abnormal signs, however slight, are present. Symptoms of this nature have for long been thought to arise from *cervical ribs or related anomalies,* but the neurological picture bears no resemblance to this and even if a cervical rib is discovered it can only be relevant in so far as it impedes the circulation through the subclavian artery and thus facilitates ischaemia at the wrist. *Cervical spondylosis* is also sometimes held to account for the symptoms; in this connection the not infrequent finding of tingling involving predominantly the middle and ring fingers is helpful, for this is not a radicular distribution. In general the tingling is too widespread for cervical spondylosis, which does not cause early-morning numbness.

Treatment. The early symptoms can be relieved by resting the hands and patients have often noticed this when on holiday or on coming into hospital. This is, however, rarely a practicable solution ard other methods of relief must be found. Weight reduction may be of value. If the symptoms are purely nocturnal, splinting the wrist in the position of slight dorsiflexion at bed-time often ensures an untroubled night but seldom leads to permanent relief. Symptoms which are troublesome both by day and by night may be relieved by injection of hydrocortisone at the wrist, but although this can lead to permanent relief the incidence of relapse is high. With troublesome symptoms and especially when abnormal signs are present, *operation* is indicated and this is undoubtedly the most immediate and most effective method of producing lasting relief. The operation is one of decompression by division of the flexor retinaculum at the wrist. In assessing the results of this operation, which is very successful in the vast majority of patients in whom the diagnosis has been correctly made, it is important to realise that the immediate effect of the operation will be to relieve only the symptoms which are *intermittent*. Any tingling which is constant and any weakness or sensory loss may be improved immediately but, depending on its severity, will take some time to recover. If the weakness and wasting of the abductor pollicis brevis are profound then complete recovery may not take place for many months.

In myxoedema treatment of the primary condition will in most cases relieve the symptoms.

Lateral Cutaneous Nerve of Thigh

This nerve is compressed as it passes from the pelvis under the lateral aspect of the inguinal ligament where it may become involved in the origin of the sartorius muscle. This compression may give rise to numbness over the lateral aspect of the thigh and to pain. Hence the name *meralgia paraesthetica*. The pain and numbness develop usually in men in middle life and sometimes as a result of weight increase.

This pain develops typically on exertion and may be severe enough to halt the patient so that this is a cause of intermittent claudication (intermittent limping) and thus may resemble the symptoms caused by ischaemia in the leg. The pain is relieved by rest but may return with further exertion.

On examination sensory loss may be demonstrated over a somewhat variable area on the lateral aspect of the thigh corresponding to the whole or part of the distribution of the lateral cutaneous nerve.

Treatment. Weight reduction may be sufficient to relieve the symptoms but decompression of the nerve may be necessary.

Lateral Popliteal Nerve

Owing to its superficial course as it winds round the neck of the fibula, this nerve is particularly subject to pressure, for example from splints. The effect of this is to cause a flaccid foot drop with paralysis of eversion of the foot and of dorsiflexion of the foot and toes. There may be cutaneous sensory impairement over the lateral aspect of the leg and the dorsum of the foot.

Mononeuritis Multiplex

Lesions of nerves so far considered may be termed mononeuritis in the sense that only a single nerve, whether mixed or purely sensory, has been involved. In these cases the only pathological process considered has been one of compression but there are certain conditions, not due to pressure, in which there may be involvement of two or more nerves but still something less than a polyneuritis; this clinical picture is referred to as a *mononeuritis multiplex*, that is the involvement of several peripheral nerves by the same pathological process. The conditions which may give rise to this picture are:

> alcoholic poisoning,
> diabetes mellitus,
> polyarteritis nodosa,
> leprosy.

All these conditions, with the possible exception of leprosy, may at other times give rise to a true polyneuritis.

Polyneuritis

The most characteristic feature of polyneuritis is its symmetry; there is symmetrical motor, reflex, and sensory change. Tachycardia is common.

The effect of polyneuritis is usually to cause peripheral symptoms and signs, but the essential lesion may well be central. Although there are some well-recognised causes of polyneuritis, many cases remain obscure.

Symptoms. The early symptoms are usually persistent tingling and numbness of the hands and feet accompanied by peripheral weakness. They come on at varying rates and the speed of development is helpful in the diagnosis of the cause.

Signs. The signs of a polyneuritis are weakness, usually more marked peripherally, reflex loss, and cutaneous sensory disturbance, also peripheral.

Diagnosis. The clinical diagnosis of polyneuritis is not difficult but the discovery of the cause often is; and even when the cause seems established the mechanism whereby a polyneuritis occurs is difficult to understand. In some cases the vasi nervorum are affected, as for example, in *polyarteritis nodosa* and possibly *diabetes mellitus*, or as a result of some toxic effect or metabolic disturbance.

Toxic effects are produced by *heavy metals, chemical substances* used in industry, agriculture and the home, and *certain drugs*, for example isoniazid. Metabolic disturbances which may give rise to polyneuritis include *dietary and vitamin deficiency, infection, carcinoma, pernicious anaemia, amyloid disease,* and *porphyria.*

Acute Infective Polyneuritis

This is usually of rapid development, the onset often being associated with an upper respiratory infection and accompanied by fever. There is initially peripheral tingling, soon followed by weakness which may spread rapidly to involve *proximal muscles* and sometimes those of respiration, which is a danger to life. There is sometimes facial weakness and this is occasionally bilateral. The tendon reflexes are lost. Peripheral sensory loss may be severe but is often quite slight. The spinal fluid usually shows considerable increase in protein, up to 300 mg./100 ml. or more, but without cellular increase. This dissociation which is referred to as the *Guillain-Barré syndrome* is not, however, specific to this condition and may be found in diphtheritic, diabetic, and other forms of polyneuritis.

Treatment. Steroid therapy may be of value in the early stages but otherwise there is no specific treatment. Recovery is likely to be slow and is occasionally incomplete. The prognosis is good if death from respiratory failure can be prevented. It is therefore essential to have the patient removed to where a respirator is available if there should be any question of involvement of muscles of respiration.

Subacute and Chronic Polyneuritis

In these forms the diagnosis of polyneuritis is usually clear enough and a search must be made for the cause. Palpation of peripheral nerves may reveal hypertrophy and suggest the possibility of hypertrophic interstitial neuritis, amyloid or leprosy, but there is a tendency for nerves to hypertrophy in any long-standing chronic polyneuritis.

In *alcoholic polyneuritis* the calves are exquisitely tender and a pyruvate tolerance test shows impaired pyruvate metabolism, the cause of this neuritis probably being thiamine deficiency.

The polyneuritis may be accompanied by the syndrome of confusion, disorientation, memory loss, and a tendency to confabulation described by *Korsakoff*, or by the encephalopathy described by *Wernicke*; this is characterised by vertigo, nystagmus, ocular palsies, ataxia, and stupor. These features are likewise due to thiamine deficiency and treatment is by large doses of the vitamin intravenously.

In *lead neuritis* the extensor muscles of the wrist and fingers are almost exclusively involved and sensory symptoms and signs are rare. Other evidence of lead poisoning is not always present and a history of exposure must be sought. The diagnosis can be established by a provocative dose of calcium versenate and the demonstration of excess excretion of lead in the urine. If this is positive treatment is by means of calcium versenate.

In *diabetic polyneuritis* the symptoms are predominantly sensory and are usually confined to the legs, which may be painful. Arthropathy and perforating ulcer may develop in the feet. The diagnosis rests on the finding of diabetes mellitus which will require appropriate and energetic treatment with insulin.

In polyneuritis associated with *porphyria* (p. 430), there may be in addition abdominal pain and mental disturbance. Excess excretion of porphyrins may be found in the urine.

CARCINOMATOUS NEUROPATHY

This includes a group of neurological syndromes which appear in patients with a carcinoma, usually in the lung and far less frequently in the ovary or elsewhere. The neuropathy does not depend on the presence of metastases and the mechanism of its causation is unknown.

The neuropathy may appear before the carcinoma is discovered, may be present at the time the carcinoma is diagnosed or may appear later. Its appearance, its nature, and its extent bear no relation to the size of the carcinoma. It runs a variable course, sometimes undergoing partial spontaneous remission and is not greatly influenced by removal of the growth.

Syndromes so far recognised include polyneuritis, often predominantly sensory; neuro-myopathic pictures, with muscle wasting and weakness which is often variable and may include features of myasthenia gravis, even the response to neostigmine (p. 302); syndromes depending on cerebellar degeneration; and a clinical picture resembling subacute combined degeneration of the cord. Sometimes two or more of these clinical pictures are combined and the very fact that they are so bizarre may suggest the diagnosis.

DEFICIENCY STATES

Deficiency of thiamine causes *beriberi* which is characterised by polyneuritis sometimes with associated oedema, which may be due to associated cardiac failure. Such deficiency in temperate zones is usually due to failure of absorption associated with persistent vomiting or gastro-intestinal disease. This may be the basis of so-called alcoholic polyneuritis. Treatment is by the intravenous administration of thiamine.

Deficiency of other members of the vitamin B complex in addition to thiamine give rise to *pellagra*, which is characterised by gastrointestinal disturbance, skin eruptions, and mental change. These features are thought to be due to a deficiency of nicotinic acid and treatment is by intravenous administration of this together with thiamine.

Deficiency of cyanocobalamin (vitamin B_{12}) may give rise to:

    (1) *anaemia,*
    (2) *peripheral neuritis,*
    (3) *subacute combined degeneration of the cord,*
    (4) *dementia,*
    (5) *optic atrophy.*

The anaemia is discussed elsewhere (p. 469) and is nearly always present when the neurological symptoms develop; occasionally they occur when there is no abnormality of the circulating blood or even the bone marrow. Histamine fast achlorhydria is always present, however. In doubtful cases the diagnosis may depend on the estimation of the serum cyanocobalamin and the demonstration of its deficiency.

Subacute Combined Degeneration of the Cord

This condition, so called because of the combined involvement of the posterior and lateral columns (postero-lateral sclerosis), usually starts in the fifth or sixth decade and affects the sexes equally. The early symptoms are tingling in the hands and feet followed by increasing numbness, especially of the legs, with the development of ataxia and finally of weakness.

On examination the legs are usually flaccid and weak and the knee and ankle jerks are absent. The plantar responses are extensor and there is impairment of touch and vibration sense, often well marked in the legs and less in the arms.

The diagnosis is not difficult when there is a macrocytic anaemia and a megaloblastic bone marrow, but sometimes these are not present when gastric achlorhydria is. The diagnosis then rests between this, disseminated sclerosis of the late spinal type, and cervical spondylosis, both of which can equally give rise to a postero-lateral sclerosis. They may be distinguished by estimation of the serum vitamin B_{12} level.

Treatment. This is by injection of cyanocobalamin 1,000 μg. intramuscularly at first every second day but gradually less frequently so that eventually a maintenance dose may be given once a month; it must be continued for life.

Dementia

Mental symptoms are sometimes present in subacute combined degeneration of the cord, but may appear alone. It is important to remember the possibility of B_{12} deficiency in any case of dementia for which there is not already a satisfactory explanation, especially as it responds well to treatment with vitamin B_{12} if the diagnosis is established early.

Optic atrophy is an uncommon but very serious complication of B_{12} deficiency. It is treated in the same way as subacute combined degeneration of the spinal cord, but significant recovery is unusual.

TRIGEMINAL NEURALGIA

This is a pain in the face of unknown cause, usually severe and of a stabbing, lancinating, shooting character. The typical features are:

(1) The pain is confined to the distribution of the trigeminal nerve, involving first either the maxillary or the mandibular

division and much more rarely the ophthalmic division. The pain may then spread to involve two or all divisions. It is occasionally bilateral, usually consecutively.

(2) The pain is paroxysmal, a bout of pain lasting for as little as a few seconds but not usually for more than 15 to 20 minutes.

(3) The pain is precipitated by touching the face, as in blowing the nose or in washing, or by facial movement as in talking, laughing, eating, and so on.

Such a pain usually occurs for the first time between the ages of fifty and seventy, and more often in women. Typically the first attack lasts for a few weeks and is followed by a complete remission. The pain returns after months or years and as time passes the periods of remission become shorter and the periods of pain become longer. There may, however, be no lasting remission at any time, although the pain remains paroxysmal throughout and never becomes constant.

Signs. There are no abnormal signs in the absence of any previous attempts at treatment. Patients with a similar or even indistinguishable pain who show abnormal signs may have a neoplasm, such as an acoustic neuroma, an angioma in the posterior fossa, or disseminated sclerosis. In the latter disease there is about a 2 per cent incidence of trigeminal neuralgia, but on the other hand between 5 per cent and 10 per cent of patients with trigeminal neuralgia will be suffering from disseminated sclerosis; the neuralgia in these cases being sometimes bilateral, and the treatment is the same as in the cases where no cause is discovered.

Treatment. Trigeminal neuralgia can always be relieved by numbing the face and abolishing the sensory impulses which precipitate the pain. Such numbness may, however, cause discomfort and should only be produced when the patient is likely to find it preferable to the pain. Fortunately the fact that the early attacks are likely to be brief and to remit for months or even years makes delay practicable. The early attacks are best treated with analgesics. The most effective drug is *Tegretol* which is really an anti-convulsant. Treatment should be started with 100 mg. t.d.s. and may be increased to 200 mg. q.i.d. Relief is obtained in about 75 per cent of patients and is usually apparent within 48 hours. Side effects include dizziness and skin rashes. In the end more definitive treatment may be undertaken. In elderly patients in whom the pain is confined to the mandibular division this branch can be injected peripherally with alcohol. This will abolish the pain, but the nerve will regenerate and function will return. Fortunately, however, the pain does not always return with the return of function and relief may be long lasting.

If the pain is more widespread the injection must be made into the Gasserian ganglion, thus destroying the nerve cells, or an intracranial operation must be performed to divide the sensory root. Numbness after these procedures, successfully performed, is permanent and relief of pain complete. Certain dysaesthesiae sometimes develop over the face and cause some distress, but if the procedure is properly timed the vast majority of patients will be grateful for the relief of pain.

When the whole of the face is numbed patients must wear glasses with a sidepiece to protect the insensitive cornea and guard against ulceration.

FURTHER READING

Brain's *Clinical Neurology*, 3rd ed., edited by R. G. Bannister, Oxford University Press, London, 1969.

Holmes, G. *Introduction to Clinical Neurology*, 3rd ed., revised by Brian Matthews, Livingstone, Edinburgh, 1969.

Merritt, H. H. *Textbook of Neurology*, 4th ed. Kimpton, London, 1968.

CHAPTER SEVEN

DISEASES OF MUSCLE

EPIDEMIC MYALGIA (Bornholm disease)

This is an acute epidemic myalgia, thought to be of virus origin. The onset is acute and the intercostal muscles are most frequently affected. Pain is severe and respiration is shallow, rapid, and painful. A pleural rub may be heard, and affected muscles are tender. Low-grade fever is the rule, and there may be a lymphocytosis in the blood. The disease lasts 7 to 10 days and no serious complications or deaths have been reported. Treatment is symptomatic.

WASTING OF MUSCLES

Introduction. This may result as a secondary phenomenon from disuse, or because the blood or nerve supply is impaired. It may be caused by malnutrition and it occurs in old age. It may, however, present as a primary disorder of muscle or one in which muscle is chiefly involved.

Widespread weakness and wasting of muscle is an uncommon but not rare clinical phenomenon at all ages. In the past there has been much confusion in its diagnosis, and many cases still remain mysterious. Interest in recent years has served to clarify some of the clinical syndromes and increasing use of the electromyograph (E.M.G.) and histological examination of biopsy specimens has given greater precision to some diagnoses. For descriptive purposes it is convenient to separate cases of muscle wasting occurring in infancy from those first noticed in childhood or adult life. Those diseases confined to infancy will not be discussed.

THE MYOPATHIES

They are genetically determined, and are thought to represent inborn errors of muscle metabolism. Onset is usually in childhood or early adult life. Wasting is symmetrical and progress is slowly but inexorably downhill. Remissions do not occur. Similar cases frequently occur in the same family.

Clinical Features. The chief complaint is of gradually increasing weakness in the affected muscles. There are no sensory changes nor any systemic disturbance, and the only pain in the condition is from joints deprived of adequate muscular support. The disease begins proximally, and posture is usually disturbed, causing a marked lumbar lordosis. The muscles are always weak and wasted; fasciculation never occurs. Some fibres may be replaced by fat, giving the muscle an unduly bulky appearance which contrasts strangely with the weakness (*pseudohypertrophy*).

Certain groups of muscles are commonly affected, and give rise to well-recognised clinical syndromes. These patterns of disease are frequently known by the names of those who first described them; it is important to realise that minor variations are the rule and that the descriptive titles given to the diseases are at best generalisations.

(1) **Pseudohypertrophic muscular dystrophy** (Duchenne, Erb.)
Affects principally the shoulder and hip girdles, later the calves. The muscles commonly affected by pseudohypertrophy are the deltoids, glutei, and gastrocnemius; these last cause the characteristic waddling gait.

(2) **Facio-scapulo-humeral dystrophy** (Landouzy-Dejerine)
Begins in the face, and spreads centrifugally to involve the upper limb girdle and arms. No pseudohypertrophy.

(3) **Arm and shoulder** (Erb)
Occurs between the ages of fifteen and thirty, starts in the biceps, triceps, and deltoids.

(4) **'Distal Myopathy'** (Gowers)
This is a rarity. Most cases so described are in fact suffering from cervical spondylosis (p. 304) or dystrophia myotonica (*vide infra*). A true distal myopathy starting in the hands and spreading centripetally does occur. It is not uncommon in Scandinavia, but extremely rare in this country.

Course and Prognosis. All these conditions progress inexorably to the patient's death in 5 to 25 years. This is usually from intercurrent infection, frequently respiratory following inhalation of food or saliva. The sphincters are never affected.

No treatment influences the disease.

DYSTROPHIA MYOTONICA

Introduction

This is an hereditary disease, with onset usually in the early thirties. It is believed to represent an as yet unidentified error of metabolism.

Clinical Features. (a) *Symptoms.* Early complaints are of *weakness*, usually first manifest as difficulty in swallowing, nasal voice, and weakness of the hands. To this may be added slowness, difficulty in relinquishing grip, and stiffness, from *myotonia*.

(b) *Signs.* Weakness is manifest in the facial muscles, those of deglutition and particularly the sternomastoids, which may be greatly wasted or absent. The neck extensors, in contrast, are never affected. The hands are weak. Affected muscles may show sustained contraction on direct percussion.

Associated features are baldness, chiefly vertical, cataracts, testicular atrophy, and dementia. There is an infrequent association with diabetes mellitus. Goitres, sometimes toxic, may occur. Psychopathic behaviour is common.

Special Investigations

E.M.G. shows the typical picture of myotonia.

Treatment is with quinine sulphate (300 mg. t.d.s.). Prognosis is bad. The condition proceeds inexorably to death in the early forties. Anaesthetics, particularly when muscle relaxing drugs are given, are particularly hazardous.

POLYMYOSITIS

Introduction

Polymyositis is more important than the myopathies, because of its relative frequency, difficulty in diagnosis and particularly because of the prospect of effective treatment. It may be caused by a number of disease processes. It occurs equally in males and females, and although it can begin at any age it is commonest between thirty and sixty.

It may be seen in association with carcinoma of the bronchus, some collagen disorders (systemic lupus erythematosus, dermatomyositis, polyarteritis nodosa), sarcoidosis, during treatment with fluorine-containing steroids, or with Cushing's syndrome. In many cases no cause can be discovered, but when one is found it is most frequently *carcinoma of the bronchus*.

Clinical Features. It is patchy in distribution and erratic in its course. It may progress rapidly for a few months, then remit or even regress a little. It frequently affects the nuchal extensor muscles, so that the head hangs forward. No muscle is immune, including the ocular muscles, and sometimes ptosis is the first evidence of the disease. Occasionally the heart is affected. Fever, malaise, tachycardia, and pain on muscular contraction may all sometimes occur. Severe Raynaud's phenomenon is a common accompaniment.

Special Investigations. E.M.G. and muscle biopsy show typical features and enable the diagnosis to be made with certainty in a high proportion of cases. The E.S.R. may be raised, and there may be a polymorphonuclear leucocytosis in the blood.

Differential Diagnosis

This is chiefly from myopathy, and certain helpful features are tabulated.

	Myopathy	*Myositis*
(1) Family history	Usually present	None
(2) Age of onset	Usually before 35	Usually after 35
(3) Course	Relentless; no remissions	Erratic; remissions common
(4) Pattern of affection	Symmetrical	Patchy
(5) Extensor nuchal muscles	Spared	Affected
(6) Systemic disturbance	None	May be marked
(7) Raynaud's phenomenon	Rare	Common

Treatment is with steroids (prednisolone 5–25 mg. t.d.s.) and physiotherapy. *Prognosis* depends upon the cause, but in general the course is gradually downhill over 5 to 10 years, although long remissions are possible.

LESS COMMON CAUSES OF WEAKNESS AND WASTING OF MUSCLE

Thyrotoxic Myopathy

May occur either in association with thyrotoxicosis or myxoedema, or occasionally in euthyroid states. Eye signs of thyrotoxicosis are commonly absent. Muscular changes may precede any change of thyroid function. The effects are usually confined to the proximal muscle groups, and are worse in the legs. Hyperthyroidism may be revealed by laboratory investigation (p. 440) at this stage, and the full clinical picture is usually apparent within a few months. The muscles show typical E.M.G. changes.

Diabetic Myopathy

Occurs chiefly in middle-aged mild diabetics. It begins with pains in the thighs and legs, and goes on to moderately severe weakness and wasting of the buttocks and thighs. E.M.G. suggests denervation, but no sensory changes are found. The protein is raised in the cerebrospinal fluid and both E.M.G. and histology suggest that the disease is primarily an affection of anterior horn cells.

Lead Myopathy

Is rare in this country. It is commoner in men than women, and results most frequently from inhaling volatilised lead. It affects the arms more than the legs, and usually begins in the extensors of the fingers and wrists. Sensory changes are very rare. Frequently there is a history of industrial exposure, and often of abdominal cramps, without diarrhoea ('the dangles, with dry colic'). There may be a lead line on the gum, or a blue anal ring. Anaemia is common, and the red cells may contain punctate basiphilic granules. Collection of urine after giving chelating agents shows an excess of lead excretion (p. 565).

FURTHER READING

Walton, J. N. (Editor), *Disorders of Voluntary Muscle*, 2nd edition, Churchill, London, 1969.

CHAPTER EIGHT

DISEASES ASSOCIATED WITH DISORDERED IMMUNITY

Introduction

It is now realised that a number of diseases are associated with disordered immunity and in particular the mechanism of hypersensitivity and concept of auto-immune disease and immune-complex disease have gained wider recognition.

In this chapter the first part is devoted to a general summary of the immune reaction and its relationship to clinical medicine. In the rest of the chapter a description is given of certain diseases of connective tissue in which there is evidence of disordered immunity. This group includes systemic lupus erythematosus, rheumatoid arthritis, polyarteritis nodosa and dermatomyositis. Other diseases such as asthma, acute nephritis, some forms of the nephrotic syndrome, haemolytic anaemias, ulcerative colitis and a variety of skin rashes are associated with disordered immunity and are considered under the appropriate systems.

IMMUNOLOGICAL REACTIONS IN CLINICAL MEDICINE

Immunology has its roots in the observation that persons surviving certain infectious diseases seldom suffer from the same disease again. Apart from conferring specific resistance to various pathogens, it is now realised the immune system plays a fundamental role in other biological reactions of great clinical importance; the nature of these is outlined in this section.

Nature of the Immune Response

(i) *Immunoglobulin Production.* The immune response is initiated by foreign antigens, usually associated with pathogenic organisms or their products. Antigenic compounds may be complex proteins or carbohydrates of large molecular size. Many antigens which initiate a specific antibody response can be observed to undergo phagocytosis by tissue macrophages (p. 321). These cells do not synthesise antibody but appear to participate in the immune response by concentrating antigen and passing it to adjacent lymphocytes. The latter cells, which are derived from precursors in bone marrow, are widely distributed in lymph nodes, spleen, marrow and lymphoid tissues of the lung and gastro-intestinal tract. After antigenic stin ul .tion they divide and differentiate into plasma cells which contain and secrete antibody molecules.

Serum antibodies are confined to the γ-globulin fraction and are referred

IMMUNE RESPONSE

Schematic representation of the immune response.

to as immunoglobulins (Ig). They are large proteins containing 2 heavy and 2 light polypeptide chains. The different classes of immunoglobulin (IgG, IgA, IgM, IgD, IgE—see below) are distinguished by the structure of

PROPERTIES OF HUMAN IMMUNOGLOBULINS

	IgG	IgA	IgM	IgD	IgE
Structural					
Molecular weight	150,000	160,000 (serum) 370,000 (secretory)	900,000	170,000	200,000
Heavy chain classes	γ	a	μ	d	e
Light chain types	$\varkappa, \lambda$	$\varkappa, \lambda$	$\varkappa, \lambda$	$\varkappa, \lambda$	$\varkappa, \lambda$
Carbohydrate (%)	2·9	7·5	11·8	11·3	10·7
Biological					
Serum concentration (mg./100ml.)	800–1700	140–400	50–200	0·3–40	0·01–0·04
Antibody activity	+	+	+	+	+
C fixation	+	0	+	0	0
Placental transfer	+	0	0	0	0
Seromucous secretion	0	+	0		+
Tissue sensitisation	0	0	0	0	+
Combination rheumatoid factor	+	0	0		
Attachment to macrophages	+	0	+		

their heavy chains. Each Ig chain is made up of repeating units of about 70 amino acids enclosed by a disulphide bond. This arrangement is of interest since antibodies have evolved to perform two distinct functions which are separately localised in the molecule.

(a) Each antibody combines with a specific antigen. Every individual can probably make at least 10^5 antibodies with different specificities. The portions of the molecule which interact with antigen are called combining

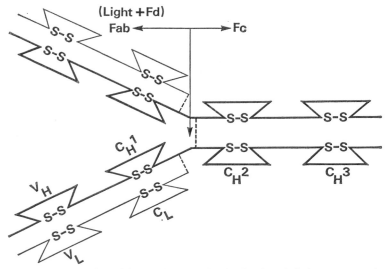

Schematic representation of the antibody molecule showing 4-chain structure, site of cleavage by the enzyme papain (arrowed) and distribution of repeating units bounded by intra-chain disulphide bonds. The units labelled V_H and V_L contain the antigen binding sites while the C_H and C_L-units carry sites for other activities such as complement fixation and membrane attachment.

sites and there are two on each 4 chain molecule. These sites are generated by the interaction of the N-terminal units (V_H and V_L) of heavy and light chains, which show great variability of structure and are different in antibodies of distinct specificities. The V regions are common to all classes of immunoglobulins so that antibodies of a given specificity may be distributed in all the major Ig classes.

(b) Antibodies also carry out various effector functions which are consequent upon interaction with complement or with specific cells or membranes of the body. These effector sites are in C regions of the antibody molecule and given sites are present on some immunoglobulin classes but absent from others, e.g. only IgG and IgM have sites for complement fixation and only IgE has a site for attachment to mast cells, which is the basis for sensitisation of autologous tissues. These differences between the immunoglobulin classes account for the remarkable diversity of biological reactions mediated by serum antibody.

(ii) *Cell-mediated Immunity.* In addition to the immunoglobulin response outlined above, antigenic stimulation frequently leads to the production of cells resembling small lymphocytes but carrying specific combining sites on their surface. These lymphocytes are derived from cells originating in bone marrow, but modified in some way by passage through the thymus gland (p. 321). Their surface receptors appear to have a structure related to that of the serum immunoglobulins, but the chemical identity of the two kinds of antibody has not been established. Cell-mediated immune responses are directed predominantly against intracellular pathogens and organised tissues. Sensitised lymphocytes after combination with antigen can exert a cytotoxic effect by producing factors which activate macrophages.

(iii) *Immunological Paralysis.* Cells of the immunological system can respond in two alternative ways to the presence of antigen. On the one hand, antigenic stimulation, as outlined above, may induce the cycle of cell proliferation and differentiation which culminates in humoral or cell-mediated immunity. On the other hand, antigen may lead to specific immunological paralysis; this is not merely a failure to produce specific antibody, but is characterised by long-lasting loss of the capacity to synthesise antibodies specific for the paralysing antigen. Injection of antigens during foetal life tends to induce specific paralysis rather than antibody production, but specific paralysis can also be induced in adults by using the appropriate antigen dose or by modifying the physical character of the antigen. The mechanisms which determine whether an antigen will induce specific paralysis rather than antibody production are not fully understood. In some instances, the removal from antigen preparations of aggregated material liable to phagocytosis converts an immunising protein antigen into one inducing specific paralysis. This suggests that, at least in these instances, the immune response is initiated by antigen which has been modified by passage through macrophages while specific paralysis follows the direct interaction of antigen with lymphocytes.

Disorders of Antibody Production

Clinical disorders may be associated with either diminished or increased antibody production. The most severe forms of antibody deficiency affect both cell-mediated and humoral immunity, but in other syndromes only one of these immune responses may be affected while the other remains intact (p. 324).

An excessive production of Ig leading to a diffuse increase of gamma-globulin detected on electrophoresis of serum is seen in many clinical disorders (p. 324) and results from proliferation of many different clones of lymphoid cells. The proliferation of a single clone, on the other hand, leads to production of monoclonal Ig which is homogeneous on electrophoresis and belongs to a single Ig class. This occurs in multiple myelomatosis and macroglobulinaemia, in association with various lymphomata and unrelated neoplasms and also, quite commonly, as an 'idiopathic' condition without detectable underlying pathology.

DISORDERS OF ANTIBODY PRODUCTION

1. Deficient Production

   (i) *Reduced cell-mediated and Ig responses*
       Alymphyocytic agammaglobulinaemia
       Agammaglobulinaemia with Thymoma

   (ii) *Reduced Ig response only*
        Transient hypogammaglobulinaemia of infancy
        Infantile agammaglobulinaemia
        Acquired agammaglobulinaemia

   (iii) *Reduced cell-mediated response only*
         Thymic aplasia

2. Excessive Production

   (i) *Diffuse hypergammaglobulinaemia*
       Chronic infections
       Granulomata
       Hepatic Disease
       'Connective tissue' Disease

   (ii) *'Monoclonal' Ig production*
        Multiple Myelomatosis (IgG, IgA, IgD, or IgE)
        Macroglobulinaemia (IgM)
        Lymphoma
        Unrelated neoplasm
        Idiopathic 'gammopathy'

Reactions Mediated by Immunoglobulin

Humoral antibodies are of fundamental clinical importance, not only in regard to protective immunity, but also in a wide range of pathological states involving either immediate hypersensitivity reactions, auto-antibody formation or reactions to circulating immune complexes.

(1) *Protective Immunity.* Immune reactions involve the primary interaction of antibody with the pathogen or its toxic products. Only in rare instances, however, e.g. some forms of viral immunity and toxin neutralisation, does this primary interaction constitute an effective immune response. Immunity is usually dependent on subsequent reactions of the bound antibody either with complement which leads to cell lysis, e.g. of Gram-negative bacteria, or with the surface of macrophages which promotes phagocytosis of the pathogen, e.g. pneumococci. It follows that protective immunity in systemic infections is mainly dependent upon IgG and IgM antibodies since only these can fix complement and attach to macrophages. IgA is the predominant antibody of seromucous secretions and fulfils an important protective role at the epithelial surface of pulmonary and gastrointestinal tracts. Although IgA does not fix complement, it can act synergistically with lysozyme, present in seromucous secretions, to cause bacterial lysis.

Whether the immune response to infection is clinically effective or not depends mainly upon the serological character of the pathogen and its distribution in the body (p. 325). Lasting immunity occurs with organisms of uniform antigenicity widely distributed in the circulation, e.g. pertussis infection. Recurrent infections may be caused by serological

IMMUNE RESPONSE TO VARIOUS INFECTIONS

Clinical Immunity	Serology	Distribution of Pathogen	INFECTIONS			
			Bacterial	Rickettsial	Viral	Protozoal
Lasting	Uniform	Systemic	Pertussis	Q-fever	Measles, Mumps, Rubella, Small-pox, Yellow-fever, Chicken-pox	
Strain-specific	Varied	Systemic or Localised	Streptococcal, Staphylococcal, Pneumococcal	Typhus	Polio, Common-cold, Influenza	Trypanosomiasis
Poor	Uniform or Varied	Localised	Brucella		Common-cold, Influenza, Trachoma, Gonorrhoea	Malaria
Ineffective			Tetanus		Herpes	

variants of the original infecting pathogen, e.g. pneumococcal infections, or occur after localised infections which evoke a feeble immune response, e.g. diphtheria. Immunity may be totally ineffective where the organisms persists in modified form, e.g. the herpes virus as DNA or where the lethal dose of a toxic product, e.g. tetanus toxin, is less than the immunising dose.

(2) *Anaphylactic (Type I reactions)*. These reactions which include general and localised forms of anaphylaxis depend upon an immune response fundamentally similar to that responsible for protective immunity. There has long been speculation regarding the underlying mechanisms responsible for such dramatically divergent reactions. It is now established that immediate hypersensitivity is mediated by one class of immunoglobulin, IgE (below) and atopic individuals tend to produce this antibody in res-

TYPES OF ALLERGIC REACTION

	Anaphylactic Type I	Cytotoxic Type II	Immune-complex Type III	Cell-mediated Type IV
Clinical examples	anaphylaxis	Acquired haemolytic anaemia	serum sickness	tuberculin sensitivity
Examples of Antigens	penicillin	red cell iso-antigens	foreign serum	tuberculoprotein
Antibody	IgE	IgG or IgM	IgG or IgM	—
Passive transfer	serum	serum	serum	lymphocytes
Skin reaction	'immediate' (15 minutes)	—	'immediate' (4–8 hours)	'delayed' (24–48 hours)

ponse to antigenic stimulation. The serum concentration of IgE is very low (p. 321) and most of this antibody is attached to tissue mast cells which are then said to be sensitised. On subsequent exposure, the antigen (allergen) reacts with tissue bound IgE and as a result the sensitised mast cells undergo degranulation, liberating various pharmacologically active compounds which cause the characteristic allergic symptoms (below). Desensi-

MECHANISM OF HYPERSENSITIVITY

Fig. 3.   Mechanism of local and generalised anaphylaxis. Antigenic stimulation of a susceptible subject leads to synthesis of IgE antibody which becomes attached to mast cells. A subsequent exposure to the same antigen leads to its combination with cell-bound IgE and consequent degranulation of mast cells and discharge of pharmacologically active compounds which cause anaphylaxis.

tisation of atopic individuals can sometimes be achieved by injecting very small doses of the allergen. This stimulates the production of IgG antibody and on subsequent, natural exposure the allergen combines mainly with the predominant IgG (blocking) antibody so that reactions due to combination with IgE are prevented below. It is apparent that the biological conse-

Desensitisation of an atopic subject by injecting small amounts of the allergen may induce the formation of IgG antibody. By combining with the allergen after natural exposure the IgG acts as a 'blocking' antibody and prevents combination with IgE on sensitised mast cells.

quences of antibody reactions depend fundamentally upon the relative proportion of the reacting Ig classes.

(3) *Auto-antibodies* (*Cytotoxic Type II reaction*). The remarkable ability of the immunological system to distinguish 'self' from 'non-self' is thought to depend upon the development during foetal life of specific paralysis to auto-antigens. The appearance of auto-antibodies could, therefore, result from changes in the structure of auto-antigens (e.g. by drugs or infectious agents), entry into the circulation of antigens normally shielded from the immune system (e.g. spermatozoa, lens protein or thyroglobulin), the presence of cross-reacting heteroantigens (e.g. group A streptococci, which have antigens also present in human heart tissue) or mutation of lymphoid cells. Viral infections which cause viral antigens to be deposited on cell surfaces may also induce antibody formation against the infected tissues (e.g. as probably occurs in post-measles encephalitis).

Auto-antibodies are being found in association with an increasing number of pathological states (p. 328). In many instances their presence is of diagnostic value, but several facts throw doubt upon the role of most of these antibodies in the *initiation* of pathological lesions. Many auto-antibodies occur in only a proportion of patients with the particular clinical syndrome and conversely, specific auto-antibodies are often found in the absence of the relevant disease. In addition, their presence or level may show little correlation with the clinical state and auto-immune lesions are not usually induced by passive transfer of auto-antibodies. Long-acting thyroid stimulator (LATS) is an exception to this statement since thyrotoxicosis may occur in new-born offspring of thyrotoxic mothers who have

PROPERTIES OF SOME COMMON AUTOANTIBODIES

Disease	Antibody	Antigen	Test	Positive in
Rheumatoid arthritis	Rheumatoid factor (IgM)	Altered γ-globulin	Rose-Waaler Latex-particle } agglutination	Rheumatoid arthritis 70%. S.L.E. 20%. Normal 5%. Sjogren's syndrome 75%.
Systemic lupus erythematosus	L.E. factor (IgG, IgA or IgM)	Deoxyribonucleohistose (nuclear protein)	L. E. cell phenomenon or immunofluorescence	S. L. E. 90%. Rheumatoid arthritis 50%. Sjogren's syndrome 75%.
Thyroiditis	IgG or IgM	Thyroglobulin Thyroid microsomes	Precipitin reaction or Agglutination C^1 fixation	Hashimoto's disease 100%. Thyrotoxicosis, Ca thyroid, non-toxic goitre 60%. Normal females 15%. Pernicious anaemia 40%.
Thyrotoxicosis	LATS (IgG)		Release of labelled hormone from thyroid	Thyrotoxicosis 60%.
Acquired haemolytic anaemia	IgG (non-agglutinating)	rH	Indirect haemagglutination (Coombs test)	AHA 80%.
Pernicious anaemia		Intrinsic factor Parietal cell	Binding of Radioactive Vit.^{n} B_{12} Immunofluorescence	Pernicious anaemia 50%. Thyroiditis 30%.

circulating LATS. This observation strongly supports the idea that some forms of thyrotoxicosis are caused by an autoimmune reaction involving a serum IgG antibody.

(4) *Immune Complex (Type III reaction)*. Antigen-antibody complexes present in the circulation may form micro-precipitates in small blood vessels, fix complement and lead to accumulation of polymorphonuclear leucocytes, vascular occlusion and perivascular inflammation. Such lesions may occur in individuals injected with large doses of penicillin or horse serum (e.g. during passive immunisation for diphtheria or tetanus) who form antibodies which combine with the circulating antigen. The resulting syndrome, which is known as serum sickness, is characterised by glomerulonephritis, myocarditis, joint effusions, urticaria and pyrexia. Certain forms of pulmonary alveolitis which follow inhalation of fungal antigens, e.g. farmer's lung, also represent a reaction to circulating immune complexes, There is at present considerable interest in the possibility that various forms of renal disease, arthritis and periarteritis of obscure etiology are caused by a similar immune mechanism.

(5) *Cell-mediated Immunity (Type IV reaction)*. Sensitised lymphocytes of thymic origin are involved especially in immunological reactions against organised tissues carrying foreign antigens. Such antibodies are therefore primarily responsible for rejection of foreign grafts, immunological responses to tumours and possibly for certain autoimmune reactions. Cell-mediated immunity probably also plays an important role in specific resistance to intra-cellular infections including tuberculosis, leishmaniasis, leprosy and some viral infections, and may be responsible for many of the papular and vesicular rashes which accompany common infectious diseases. The presence of cell-mediated immunity is indicated by the delayed hypersensitivity response, i.e. an inflammatory lesion appearing 24 hours after intradermal challenge with the antigen and characterised by local infiltration of the tissue with round cells.

The importance of cell-mediated immunity in suppressing tumour growth has been demonstrated in vitro and is also indicated by the unusual frequency of neoplasms in association with lymphoid deficiency or administration of anti-lymphocytic serum. Immune reactions can only occur against cells carrying altered or foreign antigens such as those found in viral or chemically induced tumours. Such responses have been demonstrated particularly in Burkitt's lymphoma, nasopharyngeal carcinoma, osteogenic sarcoma and carcinoma of the colon and bladder. The frequent failure of the immune system to prevent growth and spread of tumours in the body may be attributed to poor antigenicity of the neoplasm or immunological deficiency. In addition, serum antibody which cannot destroy organised tumour tissue may block the action of the potentially effective cell-mediated immune response and so enhance the growth of the tumour. As in the case of immediate hypersensitivity discussed above, the relative proportions of different tumour antibodies are of prime importance in determining their final biological effects.

SYSTEMIC LUPUS ERYTHEMATOSUS

Introduction

This is a disease almost confined (90 per cent) to young women (aged 30–50). Rarely it is familial, and generally patients have enjoyed good health before its onset. Systemic lupus is associated with complex disorders of immunity and it is not known which is the primary disturbance. It is protean in its manifestations, but most cases show fever, weight loss, and leucopenia. Among the disorders of immunity, certain symptoms occur:

(a) There is undue sensitivity of the immune system with the production of autoantibodies (see p. 327) against erythrocytes and platelets, and in particular the production of the antinuclear factor, an IgG immunoglobulin with an affinity for the nuclei of the patient's own cells and especially the nuclei of the leucocytes. The nuclear material from the damaged leucocytes is responsible for the LE (Hargreaves) cell phenomena.

(b) There is also evidence for circulating immune complexes in the blood (see p. 329) which may be responsible for the vascular lesion found in lupus.

Clinical Features

(a) *Arthritis and Myalgia*. It may present with all the clinical features of rheumatoid arthritis (p. 336), or with a migratory arthritis resembling rheumatic fever. Myalgic pains and tenderness are common.

(b) *Pleurisy and Pneumonia*. Starts with acute pleurisy, sometimes with effusion, often bilateral. With this there may be a true pneumonitis, causing symptoms of pneumonia. Secondary infection is common and can be very misleading. Leucopenia throughout is the rule.

(c) *Proteinuria and Nephrotic Syndrome*. Proteinuria is the commonest single finding in SLE, occurring in 80 per cent of cases. It may be gross, and a classical nephrotic syndrome (p. 388) may develop. Hypertension is common, and death in uraemia may result.

(d) *Pericarditis, Myocarditis, and Endocarditis*. Acute pericarditis may be the first evidence of the disease. Loud and persistent friction rubs are common, and there may be effusion. The heart muscle itself can be affected causing tachycardia and dilatation of the heart. The valves too may be damaged (*Libman-Sacs endocarditis*) on both sides of the heart, with typical murmurs resulting. Congestive cardiac failure may supervene.

(e) *Blood Dyscrasias and Splenomegaly*. Normocytic normochromic anaemia is the rule, but there may be coincident iron deficiency with hypochromia. Acute haemolytic anaemia occasionally occurs, and there may be thrombocytopenia. The spleen is frequently enlarged, usually not very greatly.

(f) *Skin*. Skin rashes are not uncommon in SLE, but are not necessary for the diagnosis. It is unusual for discoid lupus to disseminate, although it may do so. The rash is typically of butterfly-wing distribution, over the nose and cheeks; the area is purplish red, raised and slightly indurated. Classical findings are blocking of follicular openings with horny plugs, and the presence of telangiectases. Almost any type of rash can occur, however, and no area of the body is immune.

(g) *Hepatitis.* Hepatomegaly is found in about 30 per cent of cases, and sometimes a syndrome resembling acute viral hepatitis (p. 83) occurs. More commonly the disease is ingravescent, progressing to chronic hepatitis which is frequently complicated by arthritis.

(h) *Nervous System.* This is usually spared, but epileptic fits may occur. Rarely there is peripheral neuritis or focal neurological signs and symptoms, probably resulting from arterial changes. In acute SLE there may be retinal changes, consisting of soft white patches (cytoid bodies) distributed along the arteries or veins, and sometimes mild papilloedema.

Special Investigations. The criterion of diagnosis is the presence of the so called Hargreaves cell (L. E. cell). Essentially this is the demonstration of the ingestion of dead nuclear material by intact white cells, usually polymorphs, under the influence of a factor present in the serum. The cell may be found in the peripheral blood, or more frequently the bone marrow. A specific *antinuclear serum factor* can be demonstrated in the gamma-globulin fraction of the serum proteins.

Treatment. General measures include bed rest, good diet, analgesics, and the management of the arthritis (p. 337). *Steroids* are most effective in controlling symptoms, although they do not necessarily prolong life. Large doses may be required. Occasionally *immunosuppressive drugs* (azothioprine or cyclophesphamide) may be useful but carry definite risks. *Chloroquine* in doses of 0·2–0·4 g. daily has been used but is frequently disappointing.

Prognosis. Prognosis must be guarded. There is much to commend the division of the cases into benign and malignant (Hill), in the same way as hypertension. Benign cases may progress very slowly for many years, but once the malignant phase begins, and particularly once there is marked renal involvement, the outlook is bad, patients usually only surviving a year or two.

POLYARTERITIS NODOSA (PAN)

Introduction

Polyarteritis nodosa is believed to be due to the formation of an antigen-antibody-complement complex (see p. 329). This may occur in the arterial wall causing a vasculitis, or it may be formed in the blood and deposited in the vessel wall.

The cases are best grouped into those with preceding lung involvement (30–40 per cent) and those without it (50–60 per cent). Some defy classification. In both groups there are striking constitutional effects, including loss of weight, fever, tachycardia, raised E.S.R., increased gamma-globulin levels, sometimes increased alpha 2 globulin, leucocytosis with eosinophilia (extreme if there is lung involvement), and anaemia, usually normochromic normocytic.

Clinical Features

(a) *With Lung Involvement.* The disease may start at any age, and has equal incidence in both sexes. A respiratory illness always precedes the other evidences of PAN, sometimes (25 per cent) by many years. Its features are asthma, chronic bronchitis, and recurrent pneumonia. There is no family history of asthma, and there is usually a high (albeit intermittent) eosinophilia (1,500–50,000 per cu. mm.). Radiography of the chest may show anything from transient symptomless shadows to chronic abscesses.

These symptoms are associated with a tendency to granulomatous lesions of the nose *Wegner's granuloma*, and there may be superficial ulceration throughout the gastrointestinal tract, especially in the mouth. Other evidences of visceral granulomatoses may be found, but these are not marked.

(b) *Without Lung Involvement.* This type occurs twice as commonly in men as in women, and increases with longevity. The incidence is maximum in the seventh decade.

(c) *Additional Features.*

(1) *Gastrointestinal involvement* occurs in 80 per cent of patients. Usual complaints are of poorly localised abdominal pain. The liver and spleen may be palpable, and shallow ulcers may occur in the gastrointestinal tract and sometimes bleed severely. About 10 per cent of cases present as an acute colitis, and may progress in a way similar to ulcerative colitis (p. 78).

(2) *Cardiac Involvement.* The coronary vessels are involved in about half the cases, and may give rise to typical symptoms (p. 153). The heart muscle may be affected causing tachycardia and dilatation.

(3) *Nervous Involvement.* Peripheral neuritis is common (35 per cent) and it may take the form of mononeuritis multiplex (p. 310). Focal lesions in the nervous system are less common, but do occur. They are caused by affection of cerebral vessels.

(4) *Renal involvement* occurs in over 50 per cent of cases. It causes proteinuria with microscopic haematuria, and granular and hyaline casts. A specific glomerulitis has been described, and death from malignant hypertension or uraemia may result.

(5) *Arthritis and Arthralgia.* A typical rheumatoid type of arthritis may occur; less frequently there is an atypical

arthralgic illness resembling rheumatic fever. Muscle pain and tenderness are common, and the pectoral muscles are frequently affected.

Special Investigations

The combination of leucocytosis, eosinophilia, and high E.S.R., should lead one to suspect the diagnosis. It can be proved by microscopy of biopsy material, either from a superficial lesion or from the pectoral muscle.

Treatment. Is general and specific, as for SLE (p. 331).

Prognosis must be guarded. Ninety per cent of patients are dead within five years of onset. Those without lung involvement survive a little longer than those with pulmonary disease.

DERMATOMYOSITIS AND SCLERODERMA

Introduction

It is probable that these two clinical syndromes represent extremes of the same pathological process. Points in favour of their unity are the identical distribution of the skin changes in both, and the presence of muscular weakness, Raynaud's phenomenon and calcinosis. They may present at any stage. Dermatomyositis occurs equally in either sex but scleroderma is commoner in women. They are much more rare than SLE or PAN, and the general manifestations of connective tissue diseases previously discussed may occur in both.

Clinical Features

(a) *Dermatomyositis* may present in acute or chronic forms. The diagnostic triad is of non-suppurative polymyositis, dermatitis, and oedema. Many types of skin reaction have been recorded in the acute form but there is usually a generalised erythematous macular rash, whereas in the chronic form cutaneous telangiectases with periorbital oedema and heliotrope discoloration of the eyelids is common. All transitional forms between these rashes and the appearances of scleroderma have been recorded; calcinosis may occur. Muscular weakness is the rule, sometimes with tenderness and pain on use of muscles, including isometric contraction. Ultimately fibrosis occurs and contractures may result. The heart muscle may be affected causing a myocarditis with disproportionate tachycardia.

Special Investigations. The plasma levels of creatine phosphokinase (CPK and aldolase are greatly elevated in the acute phase of the disease. Typical patterns are seen on electromyography, and muscle biopsy may be diagnostic.

Prognosis in acute dermatomyositis is bad. In about half the recorded cases death results, either from myocarditis or bronchopneumonia from involvement of the intercostal muscles. Less acute forms may merge imperceptibly into the picture of scleroderma, but the lungs and alimentary tract are always spared.

(b) *Scleroderma*

In this condition the skin becomes hard and rigid, initially thickened from fibrosis, later atrophic and shiny, with telangiectases. It exists in two forms, local and systemic. *The local form* (morphoea) is confined to the trunk, and the lesions vary in size from a centimeter in diameter or less to great sheets encasing the whole trunk. The local form is not associated with systemic upsets, and does not usually change to the generalised form.

The commonest of the *systemic syndromes* is progressive symmetrical scleroderma with sclerodactylia (acrosclerosis). It begins insidiously with stiffness of the hand, later progressing to complete rigidity and joint fixation. The earliest sign is a disappearance of the wrinkles over the extensor surfaces of the knuckles. Later the hand seems to be encased in a hard, shiny glove, like a marble statue. Bone and joint destruction may be severe. Similarly the face may be affected, and very gradually the ability to open the mouth widely is lost and mobility of expression is impaired. The skin appears shiny, often pigmented, and with multiple telangiectases. Calcinosis in the hands is common, and severe Raynaud's phenomenon is frequent. In the *Thibierge-Weissenbach syndrome* these changes are accompanied by sclerodermatous involvement of the oesophagus and dense pulmonary infiltration. Dysphagia and dyspnoea are common complaints. Other parts of the alimentary tract and other organs, notably the heart and kidney, may be involved.

Prognosis is bad, both for life and health. Death may result from intercurrent infection, cardiac failure, or uraemia.

Treatment with steroids (p. 572) should be started as soon as the diagnosis is made but frequently fails to halt the progress of the disease.

GIANT-CELL ARTERITIS (Temporal arteritis)

Introduction

This is not proved as a collagen disease, but is believed to represent an auto-immune reaction. It occurs in the elderly, being excessively rare before fifty-five. Commoner in women than in men, it presents local and general features.

Clinical Features

(a) *General.* Malaise, fever, weight loss, anorexia, aches, and pains in muscles (p. 335), peripheral polyarthritis, and osteoporosis frequently precede local changes.

(b) *Local changes* are produced by acute inflammation of the arteries. All arteries, including the coronary vessels, may be affected, but particularly those of the scalp and brain, hence the older name of temporal arteritis.

The commonest arteries to be affected are those of the *scalp*, particularly the temporals. There is a persistent dull, throbbing headache and the skin overlying the vessels is inflamed. The scalp is tender locally, and arterial pulsation is absent. In extreme cases, where several vessels are affected, there may be necrosis of the scalp. *Intracranial vessels* may be involved. Their narrowing causes turbulence in the blood flowing through them, so that loud murmurs may be heard through the skull over them. The *eye* is commonly affected, and blindness from retinal arterial disease is frequent. Personality changes from impairment of the blood supply to the frontal lobes are the rule, and a curious indifference to the disease marks its early stages. Later depression is common. No vessel is safe from attack and focal neurological signs may occur.

Special Investigations. The E.S.R. is always raised, and usually over 50 mm./hr. (Westergren). Leucocytosis is the rule, and the gamma-globulin levels may be raised in the plasma. Microscopy of biopsied vessels is diagnostic. They show an acute inflammatory change; the chief feature of the lesion is the presence of giant cells, though this is not a specific finding, as they may be seen in other arterial diseases. However, their profusion is such that they may reasonably give title to the disease.

Treatment is with steroids (p. 572). *Prognosis* is fairly good provided treatment is started before serious complications have occurred. The eye lesions are little influenced by treatment, and terminal mental changes are common.

POLYMYALGIA RHEUMATICA

This is a disease of the elderly, who present with pain and stiffness of the limbs, particularly the arms, local tenderness of muscle, and malaise. Fever is usual, and the E.S.R. raised. Some patients subsequently develop an arteritis and biopsy of the temporal artery is justified to diagnose this complication which can lead to retinal artery thrombosis unless vigorously treated with steroids (p. 572). Treatment with small doses of steroids is usually very effective, and most patients can be weaned from the drug after a year or so.

SJØGREN'S SYNDROME

This uncommon disease is almost confined to middle-aged women. It is characterised by progressive dryness of the eyes, nose, mouth, larynx, and vagina, which is produced by atrophy of the lachrymal, salivary, and mucus glands. The patients usually present with complaints of grittiness or soreness of the eyes, sometimes with dryness of the mouth. On examination the dryness is apparent, and the lachrymal and salivary glands may be enlarged. In the later stages hyperaemia of the conjunctiva and filiamentary keratitis may be seen. Polyarthritis of the rheumatoid type, and splenomegaly are occasionally found. The Latex and Rose Waaler tests are positive in 75 per cent of the patients. Treatment is unsatisfactory. Local application to the eye of methyl cellulose drops may relieve symptoms, and steroids may be tried systemically. Prognosis is generally bad.

RETROPERITONEAL FIBROSIS

A rare disorder of unknown aetiology, although in a number of patients it appears to be associated with the use of *methysergide* in treating migraine. The fibrosis extends over the posterior abdominal wall, frequently involving the ureters and producing an obstructive nephropathy. It may also obstruct the inferior vena cava or aorta. Rarely the fibrosis extends upwards into the mediastinum.

Clinical Features include general malaise, slight fever, low back or abdominal pain and a variety of urinary symptoms, polyuria, chronic renal failure and sometimes anuria.

Intravenously pyelography may show a deviation medially of the ureters. The urine may contain leucocytes or red cells and the E.S.R. is frequently considerably raised.

Treatment. There is no specific treatment, but the various forms of obstruction caused by fibrosis may be relieved surgically.

RHEUMATOID ARTHRITIS (RA)

Introduction

Women are affected three times as frequently as men, and the usual age of onset is between twenty-five and fifty-five (mean forty years in both sexes). There is a slight (5–10 per cent) familial tendency, and the disease is essentially one of temperate climates. Dramatic remissions may be observed during pregnancy or jaundice. There is a striking racial incidence; it is virtually unknown in Negroes and Eskimoes.

The most obvious disorder of immunity in rheumatoid arthritis is the presence in the serum of most patients of the 'rheumatoid factor'. This is an IgM globulin which will react with human IgG antigen provided that antigen is aggregated or fixed to particles (latex balls or red cells). Evidence suggests however that the rheumatoid factor does not cause rheumatoid arthritis but develops as a consequence of the disease. It seems most probable that rheumatoid arthritis is initiated by circulating immune complexes (see p. 329), but the cause is still unknown.

Clinical Features. (1) There is usually a *prodromal illness* lasting weeks or months, in which fatigue, malaise, weight loss, sweating (particularly of the palms and soles), tachycardia and pains and stiffness in the limbs are common. There is low-grade fever, and the E.S.R. is raised. There may be leucocytosis.

(2) *Arthritis.* The prodromal illness is followed by the appearance of arthritis. This is essentially a peripheral polyarthritis. It usually begins in the metacarpo-phalangeal or interphalangeal joints of the hands, less commonly the feet, and spreads proximally to involve the wrists and elbows, or ankles and knees. Shoulders and hips may be affected, but this is

uncommon. The spine is rarely involved. Less commonly only one joint is affected, usually of middle size, and the disease may remain 'fixed' there for months or years.

Affected joints are tender, swollen, and hot, and movement is painful. Muscles moving the joints waste, and in advanced cases dislocation may occur. The appearance of the hands, with swollen joints, wasted muscles, sometimes dislocated fingers, and ulnar deviation is very characteristic. Radiography shows loss of joint space, soft tissue swelling, and rarefaction of bone, sometimes with small cyst formation.

(3) *Associated Features.* Commonest of these is the appearance of chronically swollen bursae. Less frequently subcutaneous nodules may be felt, or ganglia appear in tendons, especially those round the wrist. There is widespread wasting of all connective tissue elements, including the blood, which may show normochromic normocytic anaemia and leucopenia. Circulatory disturbances are common; the hands and feet are cold and blue, with anomalous sweating. In some cases there is generalised lymphadenopathy with splenomegaly and skin pigmentation (Felty's syndrome). A similar condition occurs in children (Still's Disease), with the added features of calcification of the cornea and cataract formation.

Special Investigations. There is no specific laboratory test for rheumatoid arthritis. Over half the cases possess a serum factor which agglutinates sensitised sheeps' red cells or latex balls, but this may also occur in systemic lupus erythematosis or scleroderma. Diagnosis must be based upon a clinical assessment and the exclusion of other polyarthritic syndromes (*vide infra* p. 338).

Treatment. This is general, local, and specific. Of the *general* measures, none is more important than rest, both physical and mental. Initially there should be a period of bed rest, and if necessary sedation. Sleep must be insured with analgesics and hypnotics. Diet should be varied and plentiful, if necessary with a vitamin supplement. Iron deficiency should be corrected if it exists; otherwise anaemia must be treated by transfusion.

Local Treatment. In the acute phase the arthritic joints should be immobilised, preferably with light detachable plaster of Paris or plastic splints. Much relief may be found from warmth. Two perils must be avoided in this period. The first is joint fixation, to be averted by full passive movement of the affected joints at least twice daily, and the second muscle wasting. It is a counsel of perfection to aim at avoidance of wasting above and below an acutely affected joint, but it may be minimised by insisting on isometric contractions of surrounding muscles at least twelve times every hour. In the subacute phase splints may be retained for part of the day, but as soon as pain permits active voluntary movement should be encouraged. In both the acute and subacute stages much improvement may result from the local injection of 50–100 mg. of hydrocortisone into the affected joint.

In the chronic phase orthopaedic and manipulative procedures including synevectomy may be of value.

Specific Measures

(a) *Salicylates* are both analgesic and in large doses anti-inflammatory. Soluble aspirin in doses of 4–6 g. every 24 hours is usually satisfactory but should not be used in those with peptic ulcers.

(b) Other anti-inflammatory analgesics are used. *Indomethacin* 25 mg. daily increasing to 25 mg. three times daily or as a 100 mg. suppository at night is most generally useful, although it may cause headaches and rarely mental disturbance. *Phenylbutazone* in doses of 100 mg. three times daily reduced to the minimum necessary is very effective but produce gastric bleeding, blood dyscrasias, rashes and water retention.

(c) *Steroid hormones* are effective in relieving the symptoms Unfortunately their withdrawal is usually followed by relapse, and their long continued use attended by many side effects (p. 572). They are best given in short courses with gold.

(d) *Gold.* Interest has been revived in gold salts since the Empire Rheumatism Council's trial of 1961 showed benefit from a combination of IM gold injections and short courses of steroids. Toxic effects include skin rashes, blood dyscrasias and renal damage. Of these, skin rashes are by far the commonest. They can be minimised by avoiding gold in psoriatics, or other rheumatics with skin rashes. A test dose (10 mg.) should be given first, and the total dosage should not exceed 1 g., divided into 20 injections of 50 mg. each. Before each injection an inquiry for irritation at the site of the previous injection should be made, and if there was itching no more gold should be given for three months. The urine should be tested for protein before each injection, and frequent observations should be made on the haemoglobin level, and white count.

(e) *Chloroquine* and its derivatives are also sometimes useful; their longterm prescription may lead to liver damage, retinal degeneration and corneal opacities. Weekly inquiry should be made for visual disturbance; the earliest sign of retinal damage is the appearance of halos round light objects. Gastrointestinal upsets, skin rashes and depigmentation of the hair may also occur.

Prognosis. Prognosis should be extremely guarded initially until the rate of progress of the disease has been assessed. In general it may be said that patients whose symptoms start very early or very late in life do worst, and those in middle life fare best.

Other Conditions in which Peripheral Polyarthritis may Occur

Arthritis indistinguishable from RA may occur with SLE, PAN (p. 331), or scleroderma. It may complicate achalasia of the cardia (p. 65), Crohn's disease (p. 77), or chronic brucellosis (p. 509). Sometimes it is the only evidence of ankylosing spondylitis, and it may appear with sarcoidosis (p. 233). Rarely gout (p. 427) takes a polyarthritic course. Psoriasis occurs with polyarthritis sufficiently often to warrant a separate descriptive title, *psoriasis arthropathica*; the nails are always pitted by the psoriasis, and there is a marked tendency to bone resorption and consequent severe deformity. If destruction is extreme the condition is known as *arthritis mutilans*. This may also occur in uncomplicated RA.

Chronic infection, particularly chronic gonorrhoea affecting the prostate or salpinx, may cause a polyarthritis, and the unwary may be trapped by hypertrophic pulmonary osteo-arthropathy (p. 208), usually associated with clubbing of the finger-nails, or by the generalised form of osteo-arthritis (*vide infra*).

ANKYLOSING SPONDYLITIS (AS)

Introduction

This is a disease which is ten times as frequent in men as in women. It starts usually between fifteen and thirty-five years. It has a moderately strong tendency to be familial, and has been ascribed to a dominant gene with about 70 per cent penetrance in males and about 10 per cent in females. Persons poisoned with *cryolite* (sodium and aluminium fluoride) and those living in areas where there is a very high concentration of fluorine in the local water develop bone changes clinically indistinguishable from AS.

Clinical Features. (a) *Symptoms*. Clinically the commonest initial complaint is of low back pain, usually wakening the patient from his sleep in the early morning. This is associated with general stiffness of the spine. Other presenting complaints are frequent. Iritis (20 per cent) may precede all other symptoms for months or years. Non-specific urethritis occurs frequently at some time in the illness, and may present. In about 10 per cent of cases the first symptoms are from peripheral joints, usually feet, ankles, or knees. There may be tenderness of the heels, over the symphysis pubis, the greater trochanters, the ischial tuberosities, the iliac crest, or the sterno-manubrial joint. With these goes a general disturbance of health, low fever, malaise, lack of energy, and loss of weight.

(b) *Signs*. On examination the patients are usually rather tall, pale, and slender. There is a tendency to sweating, especially of the palms and soles. The normal lumbar lordosis is lost and mobility, particularly of the lumbar spine, is reduced. The respiratory excursion is poor, usually less than 2 inches. There may be pain on 'springing' the sacro-iliac joints, which may be tender on pressure. Other tender points may be found as described.

(c) *Associated Features*. The heart may be involved, and if it is the aortic valve is most commonly affected. The usual lesion found is aortic incompetence. Abdominal hernias, usually indirect inguinal, are found in up to 25 per cent of patients.

The E.S.R. is always very high in the active stage of the disease, and there may be normochromic normocytic anaemia. *Diagnosis* usually depends upon the radiographic demonstration of lesions in the sacroiliac joints. Stereoscopic views may be necessary for adequate visualisation. The earliest changes are widening of the joints with blurring of the margins; this is followed by sclerosis of the adjacent sacrum and ilium, and eventually by destruction of the joint space. The condition must be differentiated from *condensans ilii*, a benign affection of young women sparing the sacrum, and *tuberculosis*, which is usually unilateral. The spine too may be affected, and eventually all the vertebrae become joined by bridges of bone, the so-called 'bamboo' spine.

Ultimately the whole skeleton may be locked, warranting the first description (Connor, 1695) of 'An extraordinary humane skeleton, whose vertebrae, the ribs, and several bones down to the os sacrum, were all firmly united into one solid bone, without joynting or cartilage'.

Treatment. In the early stages physiotherapy may be given in an attempt to reduce ankylosis and deformity. Posture is important, and rest on a hard level bed during treatment must be insisted upon. If aspirin 0·5g. every four or six hours fails to give adequate relief from pain, phenylbutazone 50 mg. three times daily often proves very effective but its administration must be carefully supervised as it may aggravate or induce peptic ulceration and occasionally causes serious blood dyscrasias. Radiotherapy to the affected joints will sometimes arrest or retard the condition, but its use is followed by an increased incidence of leukaemia. Corticosteroids may give great symptomatic relief, but should only be given for acute exacerbations which cannot be controlled by other measures.

REITER'S SYNDROME

This is almost confined to men and may occur at any age after puberty, and consists of the association of urethritis, conjunctivitis, and arthritis, usually in that order, and sometimes accompanied by visceral manifestations. Its incidence varies between 1 and 3 per cent of all new cases of urethritis in different reported series.

Clinical Features

(1) *The urethritis* follows sexual intercourse after an interval of about 1–4 weeks. It is non-bacterial, and often associated with some balanitis. It is not influenced by antibiotics. (2) *Conjunctivitis* is bilateral and follows 1–3 weeks after the urethritis. It is sometimes accompanied by uveitis, and rarely keratitis. Usually it is mild, and lasts about a week or ten days. (3) *The arthritis* follows within a week or two of the conjunctivitis. It is usually a subacute polyarthritis of the small- and middle-sized joints; occasionally it is confined to one large joint. It is the most persistent of the triad, and may last 2 or 3 months. (4) There are signs of a *general infection*, with fever, malaise, and raised E.S.R. Skin rashes, and ulceration of the mucous membranes are common, and there may be involvement of muscle and tendon. Plantar fasciitis is common, and may progress to the formation of a calcaneal spur.

The disease is usually mild and self limiting, but relapses are common, and chronic affection possible, particularly if there is associated chronic prostatitis. Treatment of the urethritis is with tetracycline 25 mg. four times daily for a week, although response is variable.

Pain may be controlled by salicyclates although in severe and persistent disease phenylbutazone or steroids both systemic or local may be required.

FURTHER READING

Copeman, W. S. C., *Textbook of the Rheumatic Diseases*, 4th edition. Livingstone, Edinburgh, 1969.

Dixon, A. St. J., *Progress in Clinical Rheumatology*. J. & A. Churchill, London, 1965.

Humphrey, J. H. and White, R. G., *Immunology for Students of Medicine*, 3rd edition. Blackwell Scientific Publications, Oxford, 1970.

Samter, M., *Immunological Diseases*, 2nd edition. Little Brown & Co., Boston, 1971.

Roitt, I., *Essential Immunology*. Blackwell Scientific Publications, Oxford, 1971.

CHAPTER NINE

DISEASES OF CALCIUM METABOLISM
AND BONE

INTRODUCTION

Bone

As Fourman has stated bone consists of connective tissue made rigid by the orderly deposition of mineral. The connective tissue of bone consists of collagen fibres lying in a polysaccharide ground substance. In this connective tissue framework are deposited crystalline bone salts which consist of calcium, phosphate and carbonate; the proportion of these ions may vary but dahlite (Ca CO_3 . $2Ca_3$ $(PO_4)_2$) is probably the commonest combination. In addition to calcium bone contains about one third of the total body sodium.

Calcification depends on the concentration of calcium and phosphate at the bone face and on other variables such as pH. The exact mechanism is not known but it is clear that phosphatase plays a part, perhaps by raising the local concentration of phosphate; a rise in plasma alkaline phosphatase therefore indicates an increased rate of breakdown and renewal of bone. Recently a hormone *calcitonin* has been described. It is secreted by the thyroid, parathyroid and thymus and causes deposition of calcium and phosphate in bone. Its clinical significance is not known.

Vitamin D is probably not directly concerned with calcification of bone but its general effect on calcium metabolism is such (p. 345) that when it is deficient the osteoid tissue of growing bone fails to calcify. The salts of bone are not metabolically inactive; rapid exchange can occur between the minerals in bone and those in the tissue fluids. Furthermore bone is not a static structure but is constantly being remodelled by a process of breakdown and renewal. Osteoclasts are concerned with bone resorption and osteoblasts with calcification.

Metabolism of Calcium

Calcium is absorbed from the small intestine. The average daily diet contains about 1–2 g. of calcium and of this about 100–200 mg. is absorbed, the exact amount being regulated by the needs of the body. In health about 100–200 mg. are excreted daily in the urine. Most of the body calcium is in bone. This is undergoing continuous absorption and excretion with a turnover of about 400 mg. daily and here again calcium release equals calcium uptake.

If the calcium in the diet is increased, balance is maintained largely by a decrease in absorption and urinary excretion rises little. Conversely, if the diet is deficient in calcium, absorption is increased and urinary excretion decreases. Vitamin D is essential for the absorption of calcium from the gut and if it is deficient calcium loss exceeds intake with subsequent decalcification of bones. Excessive urinary loss, however, is balanced by an increase in uptake and decalcification is unusual.

The plasma normally contains between 9·0–10·5 mg. of calcium per 100 ml. A little over half of this is ionised, most of the remainder is bound to protein (chiefly albumen) and a small fraction is diffusible but unionised. The ionised fraction plays the most important part in the clinical states hypo- and hyper-calcaemia, although its concentration is rarely measured. Because of the binding to calcium to protein, total calcium levels are influenced by plasma protein concentration and corrections may be required. The binding of calcium and plasma albumen is also affected by pH; acidosis decreases protein-binding and thus increases the ionised fraction. The level of plasma calcium is controlled by the *parathyroid* glands. A fall in plasma calcium increases parathormone secretion and vice versa. The actions of parathormone are:

(1) To mobilise calcium from bone and thus increase the plasma calcium concentration.

(2) To increase the renal excretion of phosphate and thus to lower plasma phosphate concentration.

The non-protein-bound calcium and phosphate pass freely through the glomerulus. About 95 per cent of the filtered calcium is reabsorbed, probably by the distal tubule. The urinary excretion of calcium is only slightly dependent on dietary intake. In health it should not exceed 300 mg./24 hrs. Phosphate is both reabsorbed and excreted by the renal tubules. In addition small amounts of calcium are excreted by the intestine.

HYPOCALCAEMIA

Introduction

The commonest cause of a sustained fall in plasma calcium is parathyroid hormone deficiency, for under normal circumstances any lowering of plasma calcium leads to increased secretion of parathormone with mobilisation of calcium from bone and return of the blood level to normal. Hypocalcaemia also occurs rarely in vitamin D or calcium deficiency (i.e. steatorrhoea, rickets or during lactation) or in renal osteodystrophy.

Long-standing hypocalcaemia produces striking structural changes in the body. Reduction in the level of ionised calcium in the blood causes increased neuromuscular excitability, and the clinical syndrome of tetany. This usually appears when the total plasma calcium level has fallen to about 7·0 mg./100 ml. It is also seen in alkalosis where, although the total plasma calcium concentration is normal, the ionised fraction is reduced. It is probable too that magnesium and potassium can play a part in the genesis of tetany.

Clinical Features of Tetany

Symptoms

> (1) Paraesthesiae in lips, nose and fingers.
> (2) Spontaneous muscle cramps.
> (3) Epileptic fits.
> (4) Laryngeal spasm in children.
> (5) Rarely arteriolar spasm, with pallor and raised blood pressure.
> (6) Psychoses may develop.

Signs

The diagnostic point is the demonstration of increased neuromuscular excitability. *Chvostek's sign* is elicited by tapping over the facial nerve as it emerges from the parotid gland beneath the zygoma. A hemi-facial twitch constitutes a positive response. Minor contractions confined to the angle of the lips should be ignored. The combination of twitching of the eyelids and the lips is usually significant but for certainty there should be movement of the whole side of the face. *Trousseau's sign* consists in the application of a sphygmomanometer cuff to the arm and raising the pressure to above the patients systolic blood pressure for three minutes, by which time the hands should have adopted the classical 'main d'accoucheur' position—wrist and metacarpophalangeal joints flexed and fingers extended. Severe cases may show *Schultze's sign*; the tongue is protruded over a spatula held transversely to the mouth, and sharply percussed, when a transient dimpling is seen.

Signs of Long-standing Hypocalcaemia

Long-standing hypocalcaemia is associated with striking ectodermal defects. There may be coincident tetany.

> (1) Dry, scaly skin.
> (2) Loss of eyelashes, sparse eyebrows, patchy alopecia and scanty axillary, and pubic hair.
> (3) Wrinkling and brittleness of nails.
> (4) If present before they are fully formed, hypoplasia or aplasia of teeth.
> (5) Changes in nervous system; cataracts are common and so is calcification in the basal ganglia and dentate nuclei. Papilloedema occurs rarely.

Differential Diagnosis of Hypocalcaemia and Tetany.

(1) *Alkalosis* usually results from hyperventilation; this is commonly hysterical but may be an epileptic phenomenon. It produces a fall in the

concentration of ionised calcium in the plasma, partly by raising the pH of the blood and partly by increasing the level of plasma citrate which combines with free calcium. Hyperventilation produces transient attacks of tetany. A history of overbreathing is diagnostic but subjects vary considerably in the amount of hyperventilation required to produce tetany. Typical findings in the blood are a reduced pCO_2, with a normal or slightly reduced bicarbonate and a normal total calcium concentration. *Treatment* consists of re-breathing from a paper bag.

Tetany may also occur with alkalosis due to acid loss from prolonged vomiting or gastric aspiration or rarely after ingestion of too much alkali.

(2) *Hypoparathyroidism* is usually the result of too radical thyroidectomy (secondary hypoparathyroidism). Transient tetany may develop soon after operation and in a few patients symptoms persist. In others the onset of symptoms may be delayed for several years. Occasionally the parathyroids are absent or non-functioning (primary hypoparathyroidism).

Clinical Features. The typical findings in parathormone deficiency are due to hypocalcaemia. They consist of tetany and sometimes epilepsy combined with widespread ectodermal defects (see above). Patients with primary hypoparathyroidism frequently develop chronic monilia infection of the skin. The plasma calcium level is low and the phosphate is high. The 24 hour urinary calcium output is usually low.

Pseudohypoparathyroidism is a rare condition in which the parathyroid functions normally but the tissues are incompletely responsive to parathormone. In addition to showing the features of hypocalcaemia these patients are short of stature and have thickset bodies, round faces, and short hands and fingers.

(3) *Osteomalacia and Rickets*. In these disorders (p. 348) there is a decrease in calcium absorption. However, a lowered plasma calcium level is unusual, presumably because the parathyroid glands maintain it at a normal level by mobilising calcium from bone, although the evidence for this is scanty. Occasionally, however, hypocalcaemia with attendant symptoms is found.

(4) *Chronic renal failure* may be complicated by disorders of calcium metabolism including hypocalcaemia (p. 375).

(5) Occasionally patients are seen with recurrent tetany where there is no apparent biochemical abnormality.

Treatment of Hypocalcaemia

(1) *Tetany* can be abolished by injecting calcium gluconate (10 ml. of a 10 per cent solution) slowly intravenously.

(2) The diet should be of adequate calorie value and have a high protein and calcium content. This latter is achieved by giving calcium lactate 5·0–10·0 g. daily.

(3) Patients with hypoparathyroidism are best treated with vitamin D (50,000–200,000 units daily) by mouth. This increases calcium and phosphate absorption from the gut.

The dose is best controlled by estimation of plasma calcium and phosphorous levels.

HYPERCALCAEMIA

Hypercalcaemia may result either from increased calcium absorption (vitamin D poisoning or milk poisoning) or from increased calcium mobilisation from bone as in hyperparathyroidism, sarcoidosis or primary bone disease.

Clinical Features. Several systems are affected by hypercalcaemia.

(a) *Kidneys.* Hypercalcaemia interferes with reabsorption of water by the renal tubules producing polyuria and causing thirst. Eventually calcium may be deposited in the renal tubules producing nephrocalcinosis and renal stones.

(b) *Voluntary muscle.* There is decreased neuromuscular excitability, which may lead to general muscular weakness.

(c) *Gastro-intestinal tract.* Decreased excitability also affects smooth muscle causing constipation. Anorexia and vomiting are also common.

(d) Patients with hypercalcaemia may feel generally ill and depressed.

(e) *Deposits of calcium* may occur in the conjunctivae and around joints as well as in the kidney.

(f) If bone is affected by the primary disease there may be pain and weakness perhaps with fractures.

(g) Severe hypercalcaemia produces confusion, coma, anuria and death. Such symptoms develop at a blood level between 16–20 mg./100 ml.

Differential Diagnosis of Hypercalcaemia

(1) Primary Hyperparathyroidism

Usually results from one or more parathyroid adenomas; less commonly all four glands show diffuse hypertrophy. Carcinoma of the parathyroids is rare, but these tumours are always hormone-secreting. About 70 per cent of the patients are women. The disease exists in two clinical forms, with and without involvement of bone. Whether these represent two distinct fundamental disorders is not known but it seems more probable that bone changes are merely due to more severe disease, the basic cause of both types being overproduction of parathormone (p. 343).

Clinical Features

(a) *Without bone disease* (80%); presents with symptoms of hypercalcaemia (see above) or of renal stones. About 10 per cent of patients with recurrent renal stones have hyperparathyroidism and it must be emphasised that renal stones may be the only signs of the disorder. If hypercalcaemia persists over long periods there is progressive renal destruction with stones and finally fibrosis with renal failure. There is an association between hyperparathyroidism and duodenal ulcer.

(b) *With bone disease* (20%); this may be either generalised, with skeletal pain, waddling gait, loss of height, pseudoclubbing and bony tenderness; or localised, when tender bony lumps occur. These are the *"brown tumours"* of hyperparathyroidism; they contain osteoclasis, but unlike the osteoclasiomas they are not locally malignant. They usually arise in the jaw or tibia, though no bone is immune. These localised and generalised forms of skeletal involvement are not mutually exclusive.

Special Investigations

Biochemistry

(1) In primary hyperparathyroidism the plasma calcium level is usually persistently above normal, though occasionally it may be only intermittently raised so that several estimations are advisable if the condition is suspected clinically. Changes in the plasma protein concentration affect the level of bound calcium and thus of total calcium and a correction for these fluctuations may have to be made. It is important to avoid prolonged compression of the arm when taking blood as this may concentrate plasma protein and thus give falsely high figures for calcium. Hypercalcaemia due to hyperparathyroidism can be distinguished from that due to other causes by giving cortisone 100 mg. daily for ten days. In hyperparathyroidism the plasma level of calcium is unchanged; in other conditions it is reduced. The daily urinary excretion of calcium is nearly always increased. The plasma phosphate level may be reduced but this is not constant particularly when there is concomitant renal damage. The plasma alkaline phosphatase level is usually raised if there is involvement of bone.

Radiology. Early radiological changes occur in the phalanges which show subperiosteal and phalangeal tuft erosion and the laminae dura surrounding the roots of the teeth disappear. Later changes consist of fuzziness of trabeculae and in long-standing cases widespread patchy erosions and cystic changes occur with bowing and sometimes fractures of pelvis and long bones. "Brown tumours" may be present. Calcification appears in soft tissues.

Treatment. The treatment of primary hyperparathyroidism is surgical and prognosis is good provided renal damage is not too extensive.

Secondary Hyperparathyroidism with hypertrophy of the parathyroid glands occurs secondary to chronic renal failure (see renal osteodystrophy) and with long-standing steatorrhoea. In secondary hyperparathyroidism the plasma calcium level is only very rarely higher than normal.

(2) **Sarcoidosis** (p. 233). About 20 per cent of patients have raised serum calcium level; this bears no relationship to increase in plasma globulin or to involvement of bones. It appears to be due to an increased absorption of calcium. It is accompanied by hypercalcuria which may lead to nephrocalcinosis or stone formation.

(3) **Myelomatosis.** The bone changes and raised plasma and urinary calcium levels closely resemble those of hyperparathyroidism. Bence Jones proteinuria and abnormal plasma proteins are strongly in favour of myelomatosis. Marrow biopsy is diagnostic.

(4) **Carcinomatosis.** With or without osteolytic secondary deposits, may be associated with hypercalcaemia. The reason is obscure but there may be some substance produced by the tumour which releases calcium from bone.

(5) **Paget's Disease of Bone** (p. 352). If these patients are immobilised, e.g. in a plaster spica for a fractured femur or kept in bed for a long period, the plasma calcium (otherwise normal) may rise to very high levels.

(6) Overdosage with **Vitamin D** or undue sensitivity to its actions cause hypercalcaemia.

(7) **Milk Alkali Syndrome.** Patients with peptic ulcers who have taken very large quantities of milk and alkalis may develop hypercalcaemia, hypercalcuria and tissue calcification.

HYPERCALCIURIA

Hypercalciuria is important because it may lead to nephrocalcinosis and renal stone formation. The main causes are:

(1) Hypercalcaemia (see above).

(2) Increased absorption of calcium as in vitamin D excess or sarcoidosis.

(3) Increased bone breakdown as in immobilisation and Paget's disease.

(4) Renal tubular disorders.

(5) Idiopathic hypercalciuria.

Idiopathic hypercalciuria is now believed to be a disorder of calcium absorption. On a low calcium diet absorption and excretion are normal, but as the amount of calcium in the diet is increased so a larger fraction than normal is absorbed and the urinary calcium rises often to figures of 400–800 mg. Ca excreted in 24 hours.

Hypercalciuria can thus be controlled by a low calcium diet but this may prove irksome. Calcium absorption can also be decreased by giving sodium cellulose phosphate (1·0 g. three times daily with meals).

RICKETS AND OSTEOMALACIA

In adults the syndrome is known as osteomalacia, in children as rickets, and both are due to vitamin D deficiency. A similar syndrome may occur in chronic renal failure (renal osteodystrophy) and in certain disorders of the renal tubules; these are considered below.

Vitamin D is obtained from the diet and is also formed by the action of sunlight on sterols in the skin. Coloured people living in Britain are therefore particularly susceptible if their diet is deficient in the vitamin. In coeliac disease and steatorrhoea, deficiency is due to poor absorption.

Lack of vitamin D leads to decreased absorption of calcium from the gut. This is associated with a fall in extracellular calcium concentration and it is believed (although the evidence is incomplete) that this in turn stimulates the production of parathormone. The plasma calcium is thus usually kept at normal levels, but there is an increased urinary excretion of phosphorous and the plasma phosphorous concentration is lowered. The calcification of osteoid depends in part on the solubility product of calcium and phosphorous $(Ca)^3 \times (P)^2$ in the plasma and tissue fluids. When this is decreased as in vitamin D deficiency there is a failure to calcify *osteoid*. In rickets the main changes are seen where new bone is being formed from the epiphyseal cartilage. In the adult there is no new bone formation at the epiphysis but remodelling of bone continues throughout life and in osteomalacia too there is a failure to calcify new bone.

Clinical Features

Rickets. The earliest clinical symptoms are tiredness and muscular weakness. There is bone pain and pain on movement. Dentition is delayed and the teeth may be deformed and quickly become carious. Swelling and tenderness of the distal ends of the radius and ulna are common, and so is the rickety rosary (costochrondral swellings). Frontal and parietal bossing of the skull occurs and occipito-parietal flattening may result from the softness of the skull (craniotabes).

If the child can stand or walk, bowing of the legs may result from weight bearing, and kyphoscoliosis may appear.

Radiographs show widening and decreased density of the line of calcification next to the metaphysis, with irregularity and concavity of the metaphysis itself. In severe cases there may be rarefaction with deformities in the shaft of the bone.

Osteomalacia. Early symptoms are fatigue, stiffness and skeletal pains followed by muscular weakness and hyporeflexia. The gait is waddling and there is marked adductor spasm. Costochondral swelling is common, and there is striking spinal curvature and the pelvic outlet is narrowed. Pathological fractures may appear in the pelvis and long bones, and may be exquisitely painful. Occasionally the plasma calcium level is low enough to produce tetany.

Radiology. Pseudo-fractures (Milkman, Looser) are the most frequent defect. These are lines of increased translucency running in from the surface of the bone, commonly found in the upper ends of the humerus and femur and in the pubic rami. They are strips of decalcification occurring in relationship to arteries or in areas of stress. In severe cases the bones show generalised decalcification with deformity and fractures.

The biochemical changes are similar in rickets and osteomalacia.

Treatment. Depends on the cause. For simple dietary deficiency, vitamin D 0·05 mg. (2,000 units) or liq calciferol (BP) 1·0 ml. (3,000 units), with calcium lactate 10·0 g. daily, are sufficient. In steatorrhoea doses of vitamin D up to 50,000 units daily by mouth may be required, or 20,000 units can be injected weekly. Treatment should be continued until healing occurs and a watch kept for vitamin D poisoning. In steatorrhoea a gluten-free diet will frequently decrease the oral vitamin D requirements.

Vitamin D Resistant Rickets. This small group have the symptoms of rickets but do not respond to small doses of vitamin D. The onset is usually late and there may be a family history. They are associated with disorders of renal tubular function.

(a) *Phosphaturic rickets* is probably due to a failure of the renal tubules to reabsorb phosphorous. The plasma calcium concentration is normal and the phosphate low. The bony lesions respond to large doses of vitamin D (100,000–500,000 units daily) and a supply of phosphorous in the form of sodium phosphates should be added to the diet.

(b) *Renal tubular acidosis* (p. 385) and *Fanconi's syndrome* (p. 385) may both be associated with rickets.

RENAL OSTEODYSTROPHY

Renal or uraemic osteodystrophy is a disease of calcium metabolism associated with chronic renal failure. The bones show a number of changes including an increase in osteoid at the metaphysis, with fibrous replacement and new bone formation elsewhere. In the blood there are a normal or lowered calcium level, a normal or raised phosphorous level and frequently evidence of acidosis. The blood urea is always raised.

The cause of these changes is not fully understood. There is good evidence of resistance to the action of vitamin D leading to decreased absorption of calcium from the gut and failure to calcify osteoid. In addition there is often increased parathyroid activity (*secondary hyperparathyroidism*) with enlargement of the glands and typical changes in the bone (see below). Rarely the parathyroids become autonomous causing hypercalcaemia (*tertiary hyperparathyroidism*).

Clinical Features. In children dwarfism with bone deformities similar to those found in rickets are the most prominent features. In adults the symptoms of chronic renal failure usually overshadow the bone lesions although bone pain and fractures occasionally occur. The other feature is metastatic calcification which is occasionally palpable but is more frequently seen in radiographs. The radiological changes in the bones are complex and may be divided into:

(1) Changes similar to rickets (p. 348).

(2) Changes similar to hyperparathyroidism, with subperiosteal absorption of bone often most marked in the phalanges.

(3) Patchy osteosclerosis most marked in the skull. The vertebrae

may show alternating bands of sclerosis and decalcification producing the 'rugger jersey' spine.

(4) Metastatic calcification may be widespread, both muscles and particularly blood vessels being affected.

Treatment. Bone symptoms can be relieved by giving vitamin D in large doses (100,000–200,000 units daily) with calcium gluconate 5·0 g. b.d. The dose of vitamin D should be controlled by blood calcium estimations.

If metastatic calcification is a problem and the blood phosphate level is raised, phosphate absorption can be decreased by giving aluminium hydroxide orally.

OSTEOPOROSIS

This may be defined as an atrophy of bone; although the volume of the bone remains the same, its content of bone tissue decreases. It affects both bone matrix and calcium and is most evident in the axial skeleton.

Aetiology

(1) *Idiopathic (Senile) Osteoporosis* is a common disorder. Atrophy of the skeleton is part of the general process of ageing, and starts at about the age of twenty. In certain people atrophy progresses fast enough to produce symptoms which usually appear in late life. This occurs more commonly in women than in men. It has been suggested that oestrogen or androgen deficiency may be partially responsible for the condition, or that the patient may have been in mild negative calcium balance for a long period, but the cause is not really known.

(2) In *Cushing's syndrome* and *steroid administration* a negative nitrogen balance and failure to form bone matrix are important.

(3) *Hyperthyroidism* and *acromegaly* may be complicated by osteoporosis and are associated with increase loss of calcium in the urine.

(4) *Immobilisation* leads to osteoporosis and increased excretion of calcium in the urine, sometimes complicated by stone formation.

(5) In *intestinal malabsorption* osteoporosis may co-exist with osteomalacia.

(6) *Rheumatoid arthritis* is frequently associated with osteoporosis especially in those treated with steroids.

Clinical Features. The disease may be symptomless, or there may be pains in the back, round the trunk, or down the limbs. They are made worse by jarring or flexing the spine, but rarely have the characteristics of root pain. Sudden severe back pain suggests the collapse of a vertebra. On examination, the spine is shortened so that height is lost and the distance from the ground to the iliac spine exceeds that from the iliac spine to the crown. Gross kyphosis is the rule and may decrease the vital capacity, but compression of the spinal cord is almost unknown. The consequent buckling of the trunk causes a characteristic transverse skin crease across the upper abdomen above the umbilicus. The infolded skin is keratinised, emphasising that the changes are of long standing. Radiographs show rarefaction of the spine and biconcave (cod fish) vertebrae. No typical biochemical changes are recognised.

Treatment consists of mobilising the patient and the administration of hormones and calcium. Women may be given ethinyl oestradiol 0·1 mg. daily. In men nor-androstenolone (Durabolin) 25 mg. intra-muscularly once weekly or nor-ethandrolone (Nilevar) 10 mg. three times daily are satisfactory. A reasonably high protein diet and calcium 1·0 g. daily (calcium Sandoz three tablets daily is a useful preparation) are necessary to replace deficiencies. Relief of pain often occurs within a month or so, though it is rare for radiological improvement ever to be seen.

PAGET'S DISEASE OF BONE (Osteitis Deformans)

Paget's disease usually affects a number of bones to greater or lesser degree, but some bones are completely spared. This is in distinction from osteomalacia and osteoporosis where the whole skeleton is affected, albeit unequally. Sometimes Paget's disease affects just one bone, particularly the tibia, femur, a clavicle, or a vertebra. It is rare before forty and affects men more than women in the proportion of 3:2. Occasionally it is familial. No disorder of metabolism has been identified, nor is there any indication that it is an inflammatory process. Two clues to its cause are the association with Hashimoto's disease and the occurrence of a similar disease in horses fed on a diet low in calcium and high in phosphorus (*big head disease*). It is said to be rare in oriental countries, where the phosphorus content of the diet is low.

The bones in order of affection are the sacrum, pelvis, spinal column (from below upwards), femur, tibia, skull, fibula, clavicle, humerus, rib. The hands and feet are almost always spared. Clearly the distribution is to some extent governed by stress and strain; the part of the skull which is particularly affected is at the sites of origin of the temporal muscles.

Clinical Features. The earliest symptom is pain, usually in the lower back, and often worse at night. Headaches are common, and there may be an unpleasant feeling of hotness from circulatory derangements. Deafness, often of nerve type, is common and the patient may have noticed increase in the size of his head. The picture may be complicated by platybasia (p. 256), and pathological fractures are common.

Examination of advanced cases shows enlargement of the head, kyphosis, shortening of the spine and bowing of the long bones, especially in the legs. The bones are highly vascular and act as an arteriovenous shunt. This causes tachycardia, wide pulse pressure with a collapsing pulse, and dilatation of the heart. The limbs and extremities are hot, and often a murmur can be heard over affected bones. *Congestive cardiac failure* of 'high output' type may supervene. In the earliest cases these signs are absent, but there is limitation of hip movement, especially rotation, by pain.

The *serum alkaline phosphatase* level is always raised, often to great heights (50–150 K.A. units/100 ml.). No other biochemical abnormality is found in the blood unless the patient is immobilised, when the serum calcium level rises. The changes in the bones are essentially the result of increased resorption, and are characterised by cystic fibrosis, in this respect resembling hyperparathyroidism. Radiography shows a typical picture; there is increase in total diameter of affected bones, with thickening and broadening of the cortex, and abnormal architecture of the cortex and cancellous bone. In some cases only the proximal part of a long bone is affected, and the area immediately beyond its distal extent is rarefied (*osteoporosis circumscripta*). The disease spreads distally, progressing about 1 cm. every two years.

Complications are frequent. *Pathological fractures* are common, and generally heal well. *Deafness*, either from auditory nerve compression or otosclerosis, is ultimately the rule, and the optic nerve too may be compressed, causing *blindness*. Vertebrae may collapse and cause *spinal cord compression* and the effects of platybasia (p. 256) may be extreme. As more bone is involved so the tendency to *cardiac failure* increases. It is claimed that both hypertension and atheroma are more common than usual in Paget's disease. But the most serious (and least common) complication is the occurrence of *sarcomatous change* in the affected bone.

No effective treatment is available; pain is sometimes relieved by steroids or radiotherapy.

OSTEOPETROSIS (Albers-Schönberg's disease)

The outstanding feature is a great increase in bone density so that radiographically they warrant the description of 'marble bones'. It exists in three forms foetal, juvenile and adult. The foetal form may be diagnosed radiographically *in utero*, and death always occurs shortly after birth. It is sporadic, whereas the juvenile and adult forms are familial and have Mendelian recessive characters.

Clinical Features. The *juvenile form* is severe, and death before puberty is the rule. Effects are produced by increase in size of bones, so as either to compress nerves (auditory, optic) or to encroach on the medullary cavity and to interfere with blood formation. This causes anaemia initially, later leuco-erythroblastic anaemia, ultimately marrow aplasia. Attempts at extramedullary haematopoiesis cause hepato-splenomegaly and generalised lymphadenopathy. *In adults* the disease is relatively benign. About one third of all cases sustain pathological fractures which heal badly; otherwise there are no symptoms or signs, and the diagnosis is made by chance radiography.

There is no special change in blood chemistry, but radiography shows a typically symmetrical increase in bone density. Characteristic appearances in individual bones are described, e.g. 'celery stick' in long bones, 'sandwich' vertebrae, and 'bone within bone' in the carpal and tarsal bones.

CONGENITAL ABNORMALITIES OF BONE

(a) **Osteopsathyrosis** (Osteogenesis imperfecta) exists in two forms, intrauterine and infantile. The intrauterine form causes multiple fractures in utero and death either before or shortly after birth. The infantile form presents as pathological bone fragility, resulting in frequent fractures. The bone changes are probably evidence of defective osteoblastic activity; other abnormalities are blue sclerotics and a tendency to dislocation of the joints, evidence of a more widespread mesenchymal disorder. Those who survive to early adult life almost all develop deafness from otosclerosis.

Clinically these children are pathetically deformed from frequent fractures, and the skull becomes egg-shaped. The appearance is reminiscent of Humpty Dumpty.

(b) **Achondroplasia.** This disease appears in foetal life, and is hereditary. In most instances the pattern of occurrence is of Mendelian dominance, but sometimes recessive characters appear. There is defective ossification of bones formed in cartilage. For this reason the skull vault and spinal bones are normal, but the arms and legs are abnormally short, like those of a dachshund.

These are the typical circus dwarfs. The average height is about 4 feet; the trunk is normal but the arms and legs are short and the head misshapen. The vault appears large and the face is small with a sunken bridge to the nose. Musculature is well developed, and the hands rather small; the fingers are almost equal in length.

Many achondroplastics are stillborn, or die soon after birth. In those who survive the expectation of life is normal. No treatment is useful.

TYPICAL BIOCHEMICAL CHANGES IN SOME METABOLIC BONE DISEASES

	Plasma Ca	Plasma PO_4	Plasma HCO_3	Blood Urea	Alkaline Phosphatase	Urine Ca
	(mg./ 100 ml.)	(mg./ 100 ml.)	(mEq./ litre)	(mg./ 100 ml.)	(K.A. units)	(mg./ 24 hrs.)
Normal	9–10.5	3–4	24–28	20–35	5–13	120–240
Rickets or Osteomalacia	7–10	1–3	Normal	Normal	5–50	10–100
Osteoporosis	Normal	Normal	Normal	Normal	Normal	Normal
Primary Hyper-parathyroidism	11–17*	1–4*	Normal*	Normal*	10–100†	250–800
Renal Osteodystrophy (Secondary Hyperparathyroidism)	6–10	4–15	Decreased	Raised	10–100	50–150

* If renal failure occurs these figures approximate to those of renal osteodystrophy.
† Usually raised if there is bone involvement.

MARFAN'S SYNDROME

Marfan's Syndrome is a hereditary disorder of connective tissue. There is no particular sex incidence and it can appear in incomplete forms.

The main manifestations are:

1. *Skeleton.* The bones are elongated and thin and the span exceeds the height. The palate is high arched and the hands show arachnodactyly.

2. *Cardio-vascular System.* There is necrosis of the elastic tissue of the aortic wall leading to aneurysm formation, dissecting aneurysm or aortic incompetence, sometimes with superimposed bacterial endocarditis.

3. *The lens of the eye* may be dislocated.

4. *The urine* may show increased excretion of hydroxyproline a constituent of collagen.

There is no treatment.

FURTHER READING

Fourman, P. and Royer, P., *Calcium Metabolism and Bone.* 2nd edition, Blackwell, Oxford, 1968.

CHAPTER TEN

DISEASES OF THE KIDNEY

Introduction

The kidney has two main functions:

(1) The excretion of the end products of metabolism and of foreign substances and their metabolites. These include such substances as urea, uric acid and creatinine and a large number of drugs or their breakdown products.

(2) The maintenance of the tissue fluids at a constant composition. The kidney is concerned not only with the concentration of various substances in the tissue fluids, but also helps to maintain the pH and volume of the latter within physiological limits.

There is a continual tendency for the composition of the tissue fluids to change. This results from wide variation in the intake of fluid and electrolytes and from the changes in the rate of metabolism which occur from hour to hour, resulting in uneven production of the end products of metabolism. The kidney must respond to these changes by excreting varying quantities of fluids and electrolytes; and as many of the end products of metabolism are acid it is continuously excreting hydrogen ions.

THE STRUCTURE OF THE KIDNEY

The functional unit of the kidney is the *nephron*. This consists of a glomerular tuft, situated in the cortex, and a tubule. The tuft leads into the proximal convoluted tubule which in turn leads to the loop of Henle which dips into the medulla, turns back on itself and ends in the distal convoluted tubule, which drains into a collecting tubule. There are about one million nephrons in each kidney.

The *blood supply* to the glomerulus is directly from the renal artery. Efferent vessels leaving the glomerular tuft form a capillary network around the convoluted tubules, ending in a branch of the renal vein.

The cells lining the convoluted tubules and part of the ascending limb of the loop of Henle are columnar epithelium whereas those lining the rest of the loop are much flatter.

RENAL FUNCTION

THE GLOMERULUS

The glomeruli receive blood almost direct from the renal arteries at a considerable pressure. It seems probable that glomerular filtration is a passive process and that glomerular fluid is an ultrafiltrate, the formation of which depends on the balance between the capillary hydrostatic pressure forcing water and solutes through the glomerular membrane and the osmotic pressure of the plasma proteins keeping it within the vessel. Provided that the concentration of plasma proteins is constant, the rate of glomerular filtration depends therefore on the intraglomerular pressure and stresses the need for an adequate blood pressure and flow to maintain glomerular filtration.

The *glomerular filtrate* contains water with glucose, sodium, chloride, potassium, urea, uric acid, creatinine, and a number of other substances. It contains a little protein, which is reabsorbed in the proximal tubule. The volume of the glomerular filtrate is enormous, probably about 180 litres/24 hours.

The *glomerular filtration rate* (G.F.R.) can be measured. This is done by giving a substance which passes freely through the glomerular membrane and is not reabsorbed by the renal tubules. The rate of excretion of this substance is therefore the same as its rate of filtration.

TUBULAR FUNCTION

The tubules selectively reabsorb the various constituents of the glomerular filtrate so as to maintain the composition of the body fluids constant and at the same time allow the excess of electrolytes, products of metabolism, and water to pass to the collecting tubules and be excreted as urine.

The table shows the approximate composition of the glomerular filtrate and urine in 24 hours.

Substance	Amount in glomerular filtrate	Amount excreted in the urine
Sodium	600 g.	6 g.
Potassium	35 g.	2 g.
Calcium	5 g.	0·2 g.
Glucose	200 g.	—
Urea	60 g.	35 g.
Water	180 litres	1·5 l.

(After Robinson)

Reabsorption of Water

(a) *Diuresis*. About 85 per cent of the water filtered by the glomerulus is reabsorbed by the proximal tubule. It is believed that this is a passive process and follows the active reabsorption of sodium. The remaining water, greatly diminished in volume but with the concentration of sodium unaltered, then passes to the distal tubules and collecting ducts where further reabsorption occurs. This distal reabsorption is under control of the antidiuretic hormone (A.D.H.) from the posterior pituitary. Osmo-receptors in the paraventricular and supra-optic nuclei respond to changes in plasma osmolarity. Dilution of the plasma decreases the release of A.D.H. so that less water is reabsorbed in the distal tubules and collecting ducts and diuresis results.

When an osmotic diuretic is given reabsorption by the proximal tubule is decreased and the volume arriving at the distal tubule is so great that only a fraction can be reabsorbed. This is why in chronic renal failure there is a failure to concentrate urine. The increased amount of filtered urea which is not reabsorbed acts as an osmotic diuretic.

(b) *Urine Concentration.* When the osmolarity of the plasma increases, there is an increased release of A.D.H. which leads to concentration of the urine. The mechanism of this action has now been clarified. The loops of Henle as they dip into the renal medulla act as a *counter current multiplier*; sodium passes across from the ascending to the descending limbs so that as the urine descends into the loops it becomes more and more concentrated and as it ascends it becomes more dilute. The osmotic concentration which develops in the lowest part of the loops is reflected in the interstitial tissue of the medulla and renal papillae.

The action of A.D.H. is to render the cells lining the collecting ducts more permeable to water, so that when urine passes down these ducts and through the area of high osmotic concentration in the renal papillae, water is absorbed from the ducts and the urine becomes concentrated.

Reabsorption of Sodium and Excretion of Acid

Under normal conditions about 80 per cent of sodium reabsorption occurs in the proximal tubule, largely in association with chloride and with an osmotically equivalent volume of water. The remainder occurs in the ascending limb of the loop of Henle and in the distal tubule.

Sodium reabsorption is adjusted so that the total body sodium remains constant. One of the important controlling mechanisms is the hormone *aldosterone* which is secreted by the adrenal cortex. Aldererone causes increased tubular reabsorption of sodium and excretion of potassium and is produced in response to a fall in blood volume or a decrease in renal blood flow.

Some substances are actively absorbed from the tubules; they are some-times called *high threshold substances* and include sodium, potassium, calcium, and glucose. Other substances are only slightly absorbed by the passive process of back diffusion; these are known as *low threshold substances* and include urea.

A number of substances can be actively secreted by the renal tubules, for example hydrogen ions and potassium. Certain foreign substances can also be excreted by the renal tubules including diodone, para-aminohippuric acid, and penicillin. The first two are sometimes used to measure the renal plasma flow.

The metabolic processes of the body lead to the production of various acids. The chief one is carbonic acid, the end result of oxidization of foodstuffs, and this is eliminated in the form of its anhydride carbon dioxide, which is excreted through the lungs. The other important acid products of

Tubular Mechanism for Excretion of Acid and Conservation of Sodium

metabolism are phosphoric and sulphuric acids. The excess hydrogen ions of these acids are absorbed by the buffer systems of the blood, mainly the sodium bicarbonate system, with the release of CO_2 which is excreted by the lungs.

One of the chief functions of the kidney is to excrete these excess hydrogen ions and conserve sodium, which is the principal cation of the extra-cellular fluid. This is done in the renal tubules by the replacement of the sodium ions which have been filtered through the glomeruli by hydrogen ions from the cells of the tubules.

Because the kidney cannot produce a urine of below pH 4·5 it is necessary to reduce the number of free hydrogen ions in the urine. This is done in three ways:

(1) In an acid urine hydrogen ions combine with ammonia:

$$NH_3 + H^+ \rightarrow NH^+_4$$

(2) The buffer systems of the urine (largely phosphate) absorb hydrogen ions without producing too great a change in pH of the urine.

(3) Hydrogen ions combine with bicarbonate ($V. I$).

These mechanisms are important for without them the kidney could only excrete a small amount of acid (i.e. hydrogen ions); moreover, the exchange of hydrogen ions and sodium would be curtailed, with resulting loss of sodium (as may occur in chronic renal failure).

Excretion of Bicarbonate

When hydrogen ions are excreted into the renal tubules they combine with bicarbonate:

$$H^+ + HCO_3^- \rightleftharpoons H_2CO_3 \rightleftharpoons H_2O + CO_2$$

The carbon dioxide thus produced diffuses back into the tubular cells to reform bicarbonate. This is the most probable method of bicarbonate reabsorption, although it is possible that bicarbonate ions are absorbed as such.

If, however, plasma bicarbonate is raised, less hydrogen ions are exchanged for sodium and this results in the excess bicarbonate being excreted and the urine becoming alkaline.

Excretion of Potassium

It appears probable that all the filtered potassium is absorbed by the proximal tubules and that further potassium is excreted by the distal

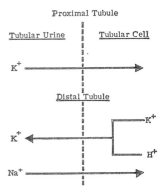

Tubular Mechanism for Excretion of Potassium

tubules. The pathway of tubular potassium excretion competes with that for hydrogen ion excretion, so that increased hydrogen ion excretion decreases potassium excretion and vice versa. Potassium is also exchanged for sodium by the renal tubules, so that if little sodium is available potassium excretion is decreased. Finally certain drugs, particularly chlorothiazide and the adrenal steroids, increase renal excretion of potassium.

HORMONES PRODUCED BY THE KIDNEY

Renin is an enzyme which splits off a polypeptide *angiotensin* from plasma protein. Angiotensin is important in the control of blood pressure and blood volume. It has a direct constricting action on the arterioles and also promotes salt and water rentention by stimulating the release of *aldosterone* by the renal cortex.

Erythropoietin stimulates the production of erythrocytes. Overproduction may be responsible for the polycythaemia seen in some patients with renal tumours.

THE URINE

Volume. The volume of urine passed in 24 hours in health usually lies between 400 and 3,000 ml. The urinary output of normal people is modified by fluid intake and by loss of fluid in sweat and the stools.

Appearance. The colour of normal urine varies from deep yellow to almost colourless. The colour is due to the presence of urochrome.

Specific Gravity. The specific gravity can be roughly estimated by a hydrometer. In health it varies between 1002 and 1032. The specific gravity of urine depends on the weight of substance in solution. Generally speaking a high specific gravity indicates that the kidney is capable of concentrating the urine, but glucose in the urine can cause a high specific gravity even when the kidney is concentrating poorly.

Proteinuria. Protein in the urine, provided that there is no lesion of the urinary tract, indicates that excess protein has leaked from the blood to the urine across the glomerular membrane. Being the smallest molecule, albumen leaks the most easily, but if the glomerular leak is severe all fractions of the plasma proteins may appear in the urine. Proteinuria is found in almost every variety of renal disease and generally speaking its presence is evidence of disease of the renal parenchyma. The amount of protein in the urine is no indication of the severity of the renal damage and it is a common experience to find only a small amount of protein in the urine of some patients with advanced renal disease (notably advanced pyelonephritis). However routine methods of detecting protein (such as 'Albustix') have become so sensitive that a faint trace (30–40 mg./litre) may be found in the urine of many apparently healthy patients. If there is no suspicion of renal disease on other grounds this finding should be disregarded.

In patients with significant proteinuria who are otherwise symptom free it is important to avoid over-investigation, but it is necessary to exclude treatable lesions and form an idea of the seriousness of the underlying disease and of the prognosis. The first step is to decide whether the proteinuria is intermittent or persistent.

Intermittent proteinuria. In some patients proteinuria is intermittent and may be related to posture, exercise and other factors. It may occur in a wide variety of renal diseases but in young people is frequently due to

orthostatic proteinuria. In this condition protein is found in the urine secreted when the subject is up and about, but is absent from urine secreted when he is recumbent. Urine passed on rising therefore contains no protein.

It is believed to be due to kinking of the inferior vena cava as it passes behind the liver, which occurs only in the upright posture. The rise in pressure in the inferior vena cava is transmitted to the renal veins and causes proteinuria. The condition is harmless and is unrelated to renal disease. However, before orthostatic proteinuria is diagnosed renal disease must be excluded and investigations should include renal function tests, examination of the urinary deposit and an intravenous pyelogram.

Persistent proteinuria is most commonly due to glomerulonephritis either with minimal glomerular change or to changes of the proliferative or membraneous type. It may also be due to pyelonephritis or surgical renal disease. If no abnormality is found on clinical examination and renal function studies and the pyelogram are normal and the urine contains no red cells, the patient should be observed. Provided there is no deterioration in renal function over a year or two further investigation such as renal biopsy is unnecessary and the prognosis is usually good. The presence of hypertension, impaired renal function or red cells in the urine suggests progressive renal disease and carries a much worse prognosis.

Cells in the Urine. These are best examined in a fresh unspun sample of urine. The number of cells are counted in a Fuchs-Rosenthal chamber and urine should not normally contain more than one red cell and fifteen white cells per cubic millimetre.

Haematuria. Blood in the urine may arise from the kidney or from the renal tract. If it arises from the kidney it is intimately mixed with the urine; if from the lower renal tract it may appear only at certain phases of micturition. Large amounts of blood in the urine are obvious; smaller amounts give it a smoky appearance and minimal haematuria can only be detected by centrifuging the urine and examining the deposit under the microscope for red cells. Haematuria must be distinguished from haemoglobinuria and various drugs which may colour the urine red, notably phenindione.

Important causes of haematuria are:

From the Kidney	*From the renal tract*
Acute nephritis	Papilloma of the bladder
Infarct of the kidney	Acute pyelitis or cystitis
Subacute bacterial endocarditis	Carcinoma of the renal tract
Hypernephroma	Prostatic hypertrophy
Overdosage with anticoagulant	Tuberculosis of the renal tract
drugs	Renal stone
Bleeding diseases	
Injury to the kidney	

Pus in the Urine. Pyuria may be severe enough to cloud the urine and may also impart a 'fishy' odour to it. Often it is only found after microscopical examination of the centrifuged deposit. It may occur in any infective condition of the urinary tract.

Casts in the Urine. Casts are composed of Tamm Horsfall protein, a normal constituent of urine which has solidified in the renal tubules. If they contain cells, either epithelial cells from the renal tubules or leucocytes or red cells, they are called *cellular casts*. If these cells have undergone cloudy swelling the casts are called *granular casts*. Casts which do not contain cells are called *hyaline casts*.

A few hyaline casts are often found in the urine of normal people. Cellular and granular casts in excess are found only in renal disease.

USUAL URINE ABNORMALITIES IN RENAL DISEASE

Disease	Appearance	Volume	Specific Gravity	Protein	Deposit
Acute Nephritis	Smoky or red	Decreased	High	Present	Red cells and casts
Nephrotic syndrome	Normal or pale	Normal	Normal range at first, low and fixed later	Present in large amounts	Casts
Chronic renal failure	Pale	Increased	Low and fixed	Trace	Casts and few red cells
Essential Hypertension	Normal	Normal or increased	Normal range or low and fixed	0 to small amounts	Normal or excess casts
Acute renal infection	Cloudy 'fishy' odour	Often decreased	Normal range unless previous renal damage	Present	Pus cells and bacteria

RENAL FUNCTION TESTS

Renal function resolves itself broadly speaking into filtration and reabsorption. A number of tests have been devised which assess one or other of these aspects of renal function. It must be realised that renal function tests merely indicate the degree of impairment of one aspect of renal function; they rarely indicate the nature of the underlying disease. Moreover, they are relatively insensitive and there may be considerable renal damage before these tests show evidence of impaired renal function.

The Blood Urea and Blood Creatinine

The blood urea should always be estimated in patients with suspected renal disease. Although it is a rough-and-ready test of renal function it is simple to perform and often gives as much information as more elaborate investigations.

The normal blood urea level lies between 15–40 mg. per 100 ml. Elevation indicates considerable interference with glomerular function; this may be due to primary renal disease, or be secondary to a failure of the renal circulation. It should also be remembered that in the face of diminished glomerular function the blood urea can be lowered by a low protein diet. Unfortunately, although the estimation of the blood urea level is easy it is not a very sensitive test of glomerular function; on a normal protein intake glomerular filtration must be reduced by about 30 per cent before there is any rise in blood urea level. Blood creatinine levels can be used in the same way (Normal range 0·7–1·5 mg./100 ml.).

TESTS OF GLOMERULAR FILTRATION RATE (G.F.R.)

The G.F.R. can be measured by giving a substance which is completely filtered by the glomerulus and is neither absorbed nor excreted by the tubules. Such a substance is the polysaccharide inulin. Under these circumstances the excretion of inulin in the urine (in mg./min.) divided by the plasma level of inulin (in mg./ml.) gives the number of ml. of plasma filtered per minute. The general calculation is given by the formula:

$$\text{G.F.R./per min.} = \frac{\text{Urine vol. per min.} \times \text{Urine concentration of inulin}}{\text{Plasma concentration of inulin}}$$

In practice inulin clearance studies are rather complicated to perform so that urea or creatinine (two substances which occur naturally in the blood) are often used.

Urea Clearance Test

The urea clearance is defined as the number of ml. of blood completely cleared of urea per minute. This figure may be obtained by estimating the amount of urea excreted through the kidneys each minute and dividing it by the blood urea level. Some urea is reabsorbed by the renal tubules but provided the urine flow is kept above 2 ml./ minute, the urea clearance bears a constant relationship to the glomerular filtration rate (i.e. urea clearance = $\frac{2}{3}$ glomerular filtration).

The test is performed on the fasting patient. Before the test he drinks 1 pint of water in order to keep the urine flow above 2 ml./per minute. The bladder is emptied before the experiment and at the end of one and two hours. Blood is taken for the estimation of urea level in the middle of the test.

The urea clearance is given by the fraction

$$\frac{\text{Urine volume per minute} \times \text{Urine urea concentration}}{\text{Blood urea concentration}}$$

Under these conditions the normal urea clearance is about 75 ml. per minute and the patient's urea clearance is usually expressed as a percentage of this figure. Levels which are below 70 per cent of normal are usually considered to show impaired renal function.

Creatinine Clearance Tests

The rate of clearance of creatinine from the blood almost exactly parallels glomerular filtration although in man there is slight tubular excretion of creatinine. If however there is a massive proteinuria the creatinine clearance may give an erroneously high figure for glomerular filtration. Creatinine clearance is estimated in a similar fashion to urea clearance, but as the blood creatinine levels are very constant a 24-hour collection of urine can be used. Generally speaking, creatinine clearance provides the most practical method of measuring G.F.R.

Single Shot Clearance

A substance such as Cr^{51} EDTA which is not metabolised and is excreted only by glomerular filtration is injected intravenously. The rate of its disappearance from the blood which is measured by timed blood samples is proportional to the glomerular filtration.

TESTS OF TUBULAR FUNCTION

Concentration Test

The most widely used test for tubular function is that which measures the ability of the tubules to produce a concentrated urine, although as will be seen, this may depend on other factors than function of the tubules.

Method 1. This depends on stimulating the production of A.D.H. by dehydration. The patient is allowed to take nothing by mouth after his midday meal. He empties his bladder again next morning at 7.0 a.m., 8.0 a.m. and 9.0 a.m. (still fasting) and if renal function is normal, the specific gravity of one of these samples will be 1025 (900 m. Osm./litre).

Method 2. The discomforts of dehydration can be avoided by injecting 5 units of pitressin tannate in oil in the morning. Urine samples are taken over the next 24 hours. The specific gravity of one specimen should exceed 1020. Excessive fluid intake should be avoided during this period.

Patients with many forms of renal disease are unable to concentrate the urine which is then found to have fixed specific gravity (about 1010).

The inability to concentrate, which is easily shown by the concentration test, may be due to severe damage to the tubular cells so that these are unable to respond to the circulating ADH; more often it is due to an osmotic diuresis produced by a decreased number of nephrons each trying to excrete an increased load of soluble substances such as urea.

The Ability to Produce an Acid Urine

This is an important aspect of tubular function, for if the kidney cannot secrete an acid urine it is failing in one of its most important functions, the excretion of the acid products of metabolism.

A simple test of the kidney's ability to produce an acid urine is by giving ammonium chloride by mouth in a dose of 0·1 g. per kilo body weight. The urine should then become acid (pH 5·3 or less) within five hours. Failure to produce an acid urine under these circumstances indicates a derangement of tubular function.

In chronic renal failure even with a systemic acidosis, the kidney can still usually produce an acid urine but in various tubular disorders particularly renal tubular acidosis, it cannot produce a pH of less than 6·0.

ACUTE RENAL FAILURE

Acute renal failure is a serious condition with a mortality of about 30 per cent. The exact cause is not known but factors certainly implicated are:

(1) Sustained hypotension from haemorrhage, shock etc. leading to inadequate perfusion of the kidneys.

(2) Free circulating haemoglobin—usually from mismatched transfusions.

(3) Extensive tissue damage.

(4) Concealed accidental haemorrhage.

(5) Septicaemia—particularly with E. coli and staphylococci.

(6) Renal disease—this includes acute glomerular nephritis, renal tract infection and obstruction from various causes including sulphonamide overdosage.

Clinical Features. In the first (*oliguric*) stage of acute renal failure the urinary output drops below 700 ml./24 hours (30 ml./hour). During this period urea and potassium released from cell breakdown accumulate with ever rising plasma levels. The failure to excrete hydrogen ions causes an acidosis with a fall in plasma bicarbonate. The patient becomes sleepy and stuporose, nausea and vomiting are frequent. The chief danger is cardiac arrest due to hyperkalaemia.

In the oliguric stage, *acute renal failure must be distinguished from acute retention of urine and other forms of mechanical obstruction of the urinary tract.* Simple dehydration can be excluded by measuring the S.G. and urea content of the urine. In acute renal failure the S.G. is around 1010 and the urea content less than 600 mg./100 ml. In dehydration the S.G. is above 1015 and the urea content above 2·0 g./100m l.

If there is doubt whether acute renal failure is incipient rather than fully developed it is justifiable to give mannitol 100 ml. of a 12·5% solution intravenously. In incipient renal failure this may cause a diuresis and prevent complete renal shut down from developing.

Occasionally acute may be superimposed on chronic renal failure. This can frequently be diagnosed by straight radiography or tomography of the abdomen, which will show the outline of the contracted kidneys.

The *oliguric* phase usually lasts from one to twenty-one days and is followed by a *diuretic* phase. The urinary output rises sharply until the patient is passing huge volumes of dilute urine which is largely glomerular filtrate as the renal tubules are not yet working. The danger now is excess loss of water, sodium and potassium. Slowly the urine volume and composition return to normal as tubular function recovers.

Throughout both phases many patients have a bleeding tendency and all are highly susceptible to intercurrent infection.

Treatment: is aimed at keeping the patient alive until spontaneous recovery of renal function occurs.

Proper management requires frequent measurement of the fluid and electrolyte state of the patient.

To prevent infection, barrier precautions should be observed and the patient given benzylpenicillin 500,000 units daily; large doses are unnecessary as the drug is hardly excreted.

(a) In the *oliguric phase*, fluid and electrolyte loss should be replaced but overhydration must be avoided. It is important also to supply sufficient calories so that tissue breakdown is minimised and the release of urea and potassium is kept to a minimum. To achieve this:

(1) At least 1500 calories should be given every day. This can be achieved by giving Hycal (Beechams) orally, which is a high strength glucose solution containing 425 calories per bottle (175 ml.). Just sufficient of this solution should be given to replace fluid loss in the tears, breath, and sweat; this is about 500 ml. in an adult and may be increased to 1,000 ml. if the patient is feverish and sweating. If the kidneys are secreting any urine the amount of glucose solution may be further increased by the volume of urine passed in the previous 24 hours. Foods containing no protein or potassium can be given if tolerated. Patients who cannot tolerate this regime, usually because vomiting is severe, may be given fluid as a 30% fructose solution intravenously through a polythene catheter every 24 hours. If liver function is disturbed, a 30% glucose solution should be used. This is rather liable to lead to venous thrombosis and it is therefore necessary to place the tip of the catheter in the right atrium, or if a peripheral vein is used 500 units of heparin and 5·0 mg. hydrocortisone should be added to each bottle to prevent clotting. If vomiting is troublesome it can often be controlled by chlorpromazine 50 mg. intramuscularly. Should electrolytes deficiencies develop due to vomiting, they must be corrected.

(2) Tissue breakdown should be minimised by giving an anabolic steroid (norethandrolone 25 mg. I.M. weekly).

(3) If plasma potassium levels continue to rise they can temporarily be controlled by adding 25 units of insulin to each bottle of 30 per cent dextrose and by giving resonium A 15 g. three times daily by mouth, if the patient can take it.

With this regime most patients can be maintained until diuresis occurs.

Dialysis is required if:

(a) Clinical condition deteriorates, with drowsiness, twitching etc.

(b) Blood urea rises above 200 mg. particularly if it is rising rapidly (more than 50 mg./100 ml. in 24 hours).

(c) Plasma potassium rises above 7·5 m.Eq./litre.

(d) Plasma bicarbonate falls below 15 m.Eq./litre.

(b) In the *diuretic* phase, which may develop very quickly, the aim of treatment is to replace the large amounts of water, sodium and potassium which are lost in the urine.

NEPHRITIS

Classification

Nephritis may be defined as bilateral, non-suppurative diffuse disease of the kidneys. It has a large number of causes, of which each generation produces its own classification, some based on morbid anatomical findings and some on clinical features. No classification has been entirely satisfactory. Nephritis presents at the bedside as a number of syndromes each with several causes. It is proposed here to describe three syndromes:

Acute nephritis.
Nephrotic syndrome.
Chronic renal failure.

Not every patient will fit neatly into one of these three groups and many intermediate types will be encountered. Nevertheless, most cases can be so classified.

ACUTE NEPHRITIS

The syndrome of acute nephritis usually presents as oedema which affects the face as much as the rest of the body, a decreased output of urine which contains blood and albumen, and usually some rise in blood pressure.

The causes of acute nephritis are:

(1) Acute glomerulonephritis (Type I nephritis).
(2) Polyarteritis nodosa.
(3) Anaphalactoid purpura.
(4) Radiation to the kidneys.

Much the most common is *acute glomerulonephritis*, which is probably an allergic reaction to a previous streptococcal infection and is due to an antigen-antibody complex in the blood which damages the glomerular membrane.

ACUTE GLOMERULONEPHRITIS

Pathology. Macroscopically, the kidneys appear hyperaemic. On micro-scopy the glomeruli show inflammatory changes with increased numbers and swelling of the capsular cells, and sometimes polymorph infiltration. In a proportion of cases the tubular cells show some damage.

Many of the clinical features can be explained by the morbid anatomical findings. The widespread damage to the glomeruli is responsible for blood and protein leaking into the urine. The oedema is probably due to a marked reabsorption of salt and water by the relatively undamaged tubular cells and partially to a concomitant widespread capillary damage.

Clinical Features. Acute glomerulonephritis occurs most commonly in children and adolescents. There is usually a history of a streptococcal throat infection one to three weeks previously. The onset is fairly sudden with malaise, shivering, and fever and some patients complain of a pain in the loins or abdomen. Vomiting in children is common.

Examination shows oedema, particularly around the eyes and giving the face a characteristically puffy appearance. The blood pressure is usually moderately raised, the pressure in the neck veins is often elevated, and auscultation of the lungs often reveals fine râles from oedema. *The urine* is decreased in volume during the early stages of the disease; it is of high specific gravity and contains protein and red cells. The amount of blood is usually sufficient to produce a smoky appearance in an acid urine. The E.S.R. is raised. The blood urea, provided there is no previous renal dam-age, may be within normal limits; frequently, however, it is raised.

About 85–95 per cent of children with acute nephritis make a complete and permanent recovery. A diuresis occurs after a few days, following which the temperature settles, the oedema subsides, the blood pressure falls and the blood and protein disappear from the urine. Proteinuria is generally the last of the abnormal signs to go and may take several months or even a year or more to disappear completely. In the remaining 10 per cent or so of patients the disease takes one of two courses:

(1) In a few patients the symptoms and signs persist with increas-ing evidence of renal failure and death occurs, usually within a year, from uraemia and hypertension. In this group early epithelial crescent formation is common.

(2) A further small group of patients develop complete anuria, this is a very serious complication and most of them die unless treated with dialysis.

(3) Some patients apparently make a good recovery, but con-tinue to pass albumen in the urine and although they may feel perfectly well for many months or even years they even-tually develop either the nephrotic syndrome or chronic renal failure.

In adults the development of persistent renal damage is more common.

Observations. The following observations should be made on a patient with acute nephritis:

(1) Daily urine volumes.
(2) Temperature and pulse chart.
(3) Daily examination of the urine and measurement of its protein content.
(4) Daily blood pressure.
(5) Weekly E.S.R.
(6) Weekly Addis counts, if available.

Treatment is designed to maintain water and electrolyte balance and to provide adequate calories until spontaneous recovery of renal function occurs. In the early stages the patient is kept in bed but is usually allowed up when his general condition improves even if there are still red cells and protein in the urine. There is no evidence that prolonged bed rest improves the prognosis.

The diet should contain at least 1000 calories, largely in the form of carbohydrate and fat to prevent endogenous protein breakdown, but only 20–30 g. of protein daily. It is also important to restrict the salt intake as the retention of salt is in part responsible for the oedema and raised blood pressure. Such a diet consists of bread and butter (salt free), jam, honey, cereals, and fruit. Potatoes baked in their jackets or mashed with salt-free butter are a good source of calories. The most useful fluids are barley water, fruit drinks containing glucose, or weak tea with very little milk. At the beginning of treatment fluids should be restricted to 750 ml. in 24 hours; as the urinary output increases the fluid intake is increased. The usual method of calculation is 500 ml. plus a volume equal to the amount of urine passed in the previous twenty-four hours.

On this regime a diuresis usually develops within a few days; when this occurs the patient's diet may be increased to include vegetables, milk, eggs, cheese, fish, and meat.

Procaine penicillin 600,000 units daily should be given for a few days at the beginning of treatment to clear streptococci from the throat. Otherwise there is· no evidence that any drug influences the course of acute glomerular nephritis.

Complications include fits and cardiac failure. Fits can be controlled by giving diazepam 2·5–10·0 mg. intravenously and cardiac failure is treated along the usual lines (see p. 111).

Convalescence. As the clinical state improves the patient should make a gradual return to full activity. Proteinuria may persist for up to a year and there is nothing to be gained by prolonging convalescence until it has entirely disappeared. A gradual return to full activity should be made. On returning to normal life, chills and throat infections should be avoided as much as possible and streptococcal throat infections must be treated vigorously with antibiotics if they occur. Wholesale removal of tonsils should not be practised, but if they are grossly diseased they should be taken out at a later date. Many physicians now believe that phenoxymethyl penicillin 250 mg. daily by mouth should be given for several years to prevent streptococcal throat infection and thus diminish the chance of further attacks of nephritis.

RECURRENT HAEMATURIA

Recurrent haematuria is a syndrome in which haematuria occurs at the height of the infection and not after the lapse of some days as in patients with the more serious acute diffuse nephritis. Most patients give a long history of repeated attacks of haematuria without oedema and without developing any evidence of impaired renal function or hypertension. Treatment should be directed to treating the infection and the patient should be kept in bed until the urine returns to normal. Prognosis should be guarded.

THE NEPHROTIC SYNDROME

The nephrotic syndrome is characterised by heavy proteinuria, low plasma proteins and oedema. There are a number of causes of this state:

(1) Subacute glomerulonephritis. This accounts for a little over half the cases of nephrotic syndrome in the adult. The disorder is of unknown cause. It most commonly arises de novo, but sometimes follows an episode of acute glomerulonephritis. It has also been called nephrotic nephritis or Type II nephritis.

(2) Diabetic nephropathy.

(3) Systemic lupus erythematosus.

(4) Amyloid disease.

(5) Thrombosis of renal veins or inferior vena cava.

(6) Poisoning by mercury, troxidone or other substances.

Pathology of the Nephrotic Syndrome. The nephrotic syndrome is the result of excessive loss of plasma proteins in the urine. This is due to glomerular damage of differing aetiology. The smaller albumen molecules pass more easily through the damaged glomerular membrane than the larger globulin molecules and there is therefore a disproportionately large loss of albumen. With increasing glomerular disease the leak of the larger-molecular-weight proteins increases and it is possible to measure the profile of the protein leak by measuring the clearance of protein of differing molecular weights. The fall in plasma proteins, particularly albumen, leads to a low plasma osmotic pressure and diffusion of fluid into the tissue spaces, forming oedema and causing a fall in blood volume. It seems probable that the fall in blood volume stimulates the release from the adrenal cortex of excess aldosterone which in turn is responsible for the retention of more salt and water. The loss of gamma globulin which contains the circulating antibodies makes patients with this condition highly susceptible to intercurrent infections. In the early stages this protein leak may be the only disorder of renal function, but if the disease progresses there is obliteration of the nephrons and picture of chronic renal failure develops.

The nature of the glomerular lesion varies. In glomerulonephritis three types of change may be found:

(1) *Minimal change.* In this type little abnormality can be seen in the glomerulus on light microscopy. It accounts for 80% of childhood nephrotics but is rare in adults. Patients with minimal change usually respond well to steroids; if these are ineffective or produce excessive cushingoid changes a cytotoxic immunosuppressive agent may be tried.

(2) *Proliferative changes* may vary from minor glomerular fibrosis to rapid proliferation with crescent formation. The prognosis is thus variable; a few may respond to steroids or cytotoxics. This form is more common in adults.

(3) *Membranous change.* The wall of the glomerular capillary is thickened by deposition of antibody and complement. The course is usually gradually downhill and it is unaffected by treatment. Membranous changes are confined to adults.

The other causes of the nephrotic syndrome usually produce characteristic changes in the glomerulus (p. 387). Difficulties may arise however. Disseminated lupus erythematosus may produce lesions in the glomeruli which are indistinguishable from membranous or proliferative glomerular nephritis. Thrombosis of the renal vein, where presumably mechanical factors are responsible for the glomerular lesion, may resemble membranous glomerular nephritis, as does mercury poisoning, which may also cause changes in the proximal renal tubules.

Clinical Features. The onset of the nephrotic syndrome is usually insidious. The appearance of oedema is preceded by a period of proteinuria; when the plasma albumen drop below a critical level (2·0 g./100 ml.) oedema begins to appear. At first this may be confined to the ankles and be fleeting, but as the disease progresses it extends until finally it may affect the whole body, so that the face is pale and puffy, the legs show particularly severe distention and fluid may accumulate also in the peritoneal cavity, the pleural cavities and the pericardium. In the early stages of the disease, the blood pressure is not usually raised and the blood urea level may be normal or even low. The urine contains large amounts of protein, usually more than 5·0 g. in 24 hours; in addition it may contain red cells, the persistence of which usually indicates a severe lesion and a poor prognosis. The serum cholesterol level is high, the reason for this not being clear.

The *course* of the disease is variable and depends to some degree on the underlying cause. The oedema may persist, often fluctuating in severity for weeks, months, or even years. Ultimately, in the majority of patients renal failure develops. The blood pressure and blood urea levels begin to rise, the proteinuria and oedema often diminish at this stage and death ultimately ensues from renal failure. Before the introduction of antibiotics many of these patients died of intercurrent infection, but such infections can now usually be controlled.

Bowman's capsule

Bowman's space

Normal glomerulus

Basement membrane

Endothelial cell

Membranous
glomerulo-nephritis

Severe proliferative
glomerulo-nephritis
with crescent

It must be realised that the determination of the cause of the nephrotic syndrome may be difficult, but it is important from the point of view of prognosis and treatment. Frequently the precise diagnosis can be established only by renal biopsy.

Treatment. When the cause of the nephrotic syndrome has been determined it is occasionally possible to remove or treat that cause, for example drug-induced renal damage or amyloid disease. In most patients, however, the only treatment possible is that of the renal disease itself.

Treatment of the nephrotic syndrome is aimed at reducing proteinuria and oedema, restoring the plasma proteins to normal and combating intercurrent infection as it arises. In the majority of adult cases all these objectives cannot be achieved, but temporary remission of symptoms is usually possible.

The main methods of treatment are:

(1) *Bed Rest.* Bed rest is advisable if the patient is grossly oedematous but probably does not influence the course of the disease, so when the oedema lessens the patient should be allowed up.

(2) *Diet.* The chief cause of the oedema is the loss of plasma proteins and the retention of sodium. A diet with a high protein and low salt content should be prescribed. It must be realised, however, that the speed of replacement of plasma protein is limited by the liver's ability to manufacture proteins from amino acids. The absorption of salt can be further restricted by the use of ion exchange resins. A resin 25 per cent in the potassium and 75 per cent in the ammonia phase is suitable in a dose of 15 g. three or four times daily by mouth. If this method is used a careful watch must be kept on the blood electrolytes as potassium deficiency may develop.

(3) *Steroid Treatment.* Most patients with the nephrotic syndrome should be given a trial of steroid treatment. Prednisolone is better than cortisone, as it has less sodium-retaining properties. When treatment is successful there is a progressive decrease in proteinuria with diuresis and disappearance of oedema. The mode of action of steroids is not known, but presumably they alter the characteristics of the glomerular membrane. 24-hour protein excretion must be estimated when assessing the effect of treatment, as the protein content of isolated samples may be misleading.

There are many schemes of dosage and the most suitable has not yet been settled. In children aged ten years and upwards, 60 mg. of prednisolone are given daily for 14 days. The dose is then reduced by 10 mg. every five days, until a daily dose of 10 mg. is reached. If the urine is now protein-free this dose is continued for three months and then tailed off. If proteinuria persists the dose is adjusted and may be continued for longer periods.

In adults steroids are not so effective and it is usual to start with 40 mg. of prednisolone daily and modify subsequent dosage according to the response.

(4) In patients failing to respond to steroids a remission may be obtained with *immuno-suppressive drugs*. These drugs are toxic to the lymphocyte series of cells, and may therefore decrease antibody formation. Azathioprine (150 mg. daily) or cyclophosphamide 2–5 mg./kg. daily reducing when the white count falls are most commonly used, and great care is required as too high a dosage will cause bone marrow depression. There is some evidence that cyclophosphamide is the more effective.

(5) *Diuretics* are used as symptomatic treatment for the nephrotic syndrome. Frusemide (p. 114) is particularly useful, especially if there is some reduction in the G.F.R. Spironolactone may be given in addition to frusemide to inhibit the effect of excessive aldosterone secretion.

(6) *Infection*. Any intercurrent infection must be treated with an adequate antibiotic.

(7) *Mechanical drainage*. Mechanical drainage is occasionally required; tapping of the chest or paracentesis of the abdomen should be performed if large accumulations of fluid embarrass respiration or cause discomfort. Similarly, if all else fails, multiple punctures of the legs performed under strict aseptic precautions, will allow drainage of fluid from the legs.

The *prognosis* of the nephrotic syndrome is variable. In about 60 per cent of children and a considerably smaller proportion of adults, steroid treatment produces a complete remission. Whether this represents a total cure is not yet known. Steroid treatment is most successful in the group with no histological renal lesion, or with minimal proliferative changes. In those with marked proliferative or membranous changes steroids may improve symptoms and decrease proteinuria, but they do not usually produce more than a transient or incomplete remission and probably do not alter the course of the disease.

CHRONIC RENAL FAILURE

Chronic renal failure may be the end result of a number of widely differing diseases of the kidney. It occurs when the damage to the kidney is such that it is unable to carry out its functions properly. It is by definition of gradual onset. In the early stages it may be asymptomatic and can only be diagnosed by investigation. If the disease of the kidney is progressive, symptoms will sooner or later appear. The clinical picture produced by advanced chronic renal failure is often called *uraemia*. Some of the symptoms of uraemia can be related to underlying biochemical abnormalities consequent on renal failure; other symptoms are as yet without adequate explanation. The clinical picture of fully developed uraemia may vary somewhat as one or other biochemical abnormality predominates, but generally speaking it is remarkably consistent.

Renal Function in Chronic Renal Failure

In chronic renal failure there is a considerable decrease in the number of functioning nephrons and thus in the glomerular filtration rate. Those nephrons which remain appear to function normally so that disturbances of function are probably due to overloading of the remaining nephrons, rather than to any abnormality of the nephrons themselves. However, sometimes there is evidence of specific tubular defects. The result is a loss of flexibility of renal function.

(1) **Urea Retention.** The excretion of urea depends on the GFR; when this drops to about 30 per cent of normal, retention of urea occurs. The raised concentration of urea in the plasma increases the concentration of urea in the filtered fraction and by this means an adequate excretion is maintained.

(2) **Polyuria and Hyposthenuria.** The passing of large volumes of urine of a specific gravity around 1010 (300 mOs/litre) is characteristic of chronic renal failure, this is associated with the loss of the normal diurnal rhythm of urine production so that nocturia is a common feature. This is largely an osmotic diuresis due to the increased filtered load of urea, although occasionally (particularly in pyelonephritis) damage to the tubular concentrating mechanism is contributory.

(3) **Acidosis.** Acidosis is a common feature of chronic renal failure. With the falling GFR, there is a decreased filtration of H+ ions. In addition, although the kidneys are still capable of secreting an acid urine, there is a reduced production of ammonia and a reduced excretion of phosphate which are not therefore available to combine with H+ ions (p. 359), so that total acid elimination is diminished. Also the tubules are less efficient at reabsorbing bicarbonate.

(4) **Electrolyte Loss.** The long-continued osmotic diuresis interferes with distal tubular function resulting in some increased loss of sodium and potassium in the urine, but severe electrolyte depletion is unusual. Rarely sodium loss may be considerable, perhaps due to some local lesion of the renal tubules, and leads to 'salt losing' nephritis. In the very late stages of renal failure, particularly if there is oliguria, retention of sodium and more particularly of potassium may occur.

(5) **Calcium.** The disorders of calcium metabolism are considered on page 350.

(6) **Anaemia.** The anaemia of chronic renal failure may be due to a failure of production of erythropoietin by the damaged kidneys, though other factors are probably involved.

The Early Clinical Features of Chronic Renal Failure

The onset of renal failure is usually insidious. Symptoms may be minimal, but may include some polyuria, nocturia, and perhaps some loss of energy. On examination the blood pressure is usually raised and the urine contains a little protein together with a few red cells and granular casts. The blood urea level is a little raised, but in the early stages of renal failure this can often be restored to normal by a diet low in protein. This stage may persist for a considerable period, sometimes years, before the classical terminal picture develops and it is in this stage that judicious management of diet, fluid intake, and electrolyte balance can keep the patient in moderately good health.

The Terminal Clinical Features of Chronic Renal Failure

For convenience these may be considered systematically:

Central Nervous System. The patient is at first tired and listless and as the disease progresses, he becomes drowsy and may finally lapse into coma. Muscular twitching and sometimes epileptiform convulsions may occur.

The biochemical abnormality underlying the symptoms arising in the nervous system is not clear, but it seems probable that they are due to an upset in balance of the blood electrolytes. The muscular twitching can sometimes be relieved by intravenous calcium salts.

Alimentary System. The tongue is dry and coated with a dirty brown fur, the breath has an uriniferous smell and hiccoughs, nausea, and vomiting are often distressing symptoms. Sometimes bleeding from the gastro-intestinal tract occurs leading to haematemesis or bloodstained diarrhoea. These symptoms are caused by the excretion of urea into the gut, where it breaks down and releases ammonia. This is highly irritant.

Respiratory System and Acid Base Balance. Acidosis causes a typical gasping form of respiration known as Kussmaul breathing; Cheyne-Stokes respiration may also occur in the terminal stages.

Pulmonary oedema may occur. Pulmonary infection is not uncommon and may be due to unusual bacteria such as E. coli or to fungi.

Cardiovascular System. Hypertension is frequently found in association with chronic renal failure and is probably due to sodium and water retention and perhaps to a disturbance of the renin/angiotensin system (see p. 361). It may produce no symptoms, but more commonly the vascular system is severely affected. This is most easily seen in the retinae which show:

(1) Papilloedema.
(2) Soft exudates which often take the form of a star at the macula. They are caused by oedema of the retina.
(3) Haemorrhages into the retina.
(4) Thickening of the arteries with variations in calibre and tortuosity, increased light reflex, and nipping at the arteriovenous crossings.

Pericarditis frequently appears in the late stages of renal failure. It may cause chest pain and usually a loud rub. Effusions are uncommon. The cause is unknown.

A small proportion of patients die from heart failure or cerebrovascular accidents, although the majority die of renal failure itself.

Skin. The skin is dry and becomes yellowish or brownish in colour and since the sweat glands excrete urea or other substances normally excreted by the kidney, pruritus is common. Occasionally there is so much urea in the sweat that it crystallises on the skin to give a 'urea frost'.

Blood. Microcytic normochromic anaemia which is resistant to iron treatment is very common in uraemia. It can only be relieved by blood transfusion.

The Skeleton. A small proportion of cases of chronic renal failure show widespread decalcification which is sometimes called renal rickets (p. 350).

The Urine. The urine volume per 24 hours is increased and there is nocturia. It is usually of fixed specific gravity (between 1010 and 1012) and contains protein, although often in quite small amounts. Microscopy shows increased numbers of red cells and granular casts.

Causes of Chronic Renal Failure

In patients with chronic renal failure the possible causes should be considered, although often an exact diagnosis is not possible. The most important are:

(1) Chronic glomerulonephritis.
(2) Chronic pyelonephritis.
(3) Malignant hypertension.
(4) Polyarteritis nodosa.
(5) Disseminated lupus erythematosus.
(6) Polycystic kidney.
(7) Renal tuberculosis.
(8) Multiple or recurrent renal stones.
(9) Prostatic obstruction.
(10) Diabetic nephropathy.
(11) Amyloid disease.
(12) Myelomatosis
(13) Chronic analgesic abuse.

CHRONIC GLOMERULONEPHRITIS

Clinical Features. Chronic glomerulonephritis may follow an attack of acute or subacute glomerulonephritis or it may occur without any history of renal disease. It may develop immediately after the attack of acute glomerulonephritis, or there may be a latent period of many years in which albuminuria is the only symptom of the underlying and progressive renal damage.

Sooner or later the symptoms of uraemia develop, often complicated by severe hypertension. When this occurs the progress is usually steadily downhill and most patients are dead within two years. Complications which reduce the renal blood flow, for example gastrointestinal haemorrhage, diarrhoea, or vomiting, cause rapid deterioration in the patient's condition and may prove fatal.

Treatment of Chronic Renal Failure. There is unfortunately no way of preventing the progress of renal damage in most patients with chronic renal failure. All that can be done is to help the kidney to function as well as possible under the circumstances. Patients can frequently be kept alive and in moderately good health for years. The important points in management are:

(a) *Fluid intake* should be at least 3·0 litres daily. In chronic renal failure the excretion of urea and other waste products is proportional to the urinary flow, so a high urine output is essential. These patients can very easily become dehydrated, with a sharp deterioration in renal function. Provided fluid is given by mouth overhydration is not likely; if vomiting is troublesome and fluids are given intravenously, care is necessary.

(b) Severe *dietary restrictions* are irksome and it is doubtful if they are useful. When the blood urea rises above 100 mg./100 ml. the daily intake of protein should be reduced to 40 g. and the diet should be largely composed of carbohydrates and fat, producing 2,000 calories. As failure becomes more severe the protein intake may be reduced to 20 g. daily, or the Giovenetti diet may be used. This diet provides the minimal necessary quantity of first class protein. The continued osmotic diuresis may cause salt deficiency, and this can be prevented by taking salt in cooking and with meals. The fall in plasma pH and bicarbonate can to some extent be controlled by sodium bicarbonate 5·0 g. daily orally. For the treatment of disturbed calcium metabolism see page 350.

(c) The *anaemia* of renal failure does not respond to haematinics and should be treated with blood transfusion. It is usually fruitless to try and maintain a normal P.C.V. by repeated transfusions and many of these patients get along very well with a P.C.V. of 25 per cent or even lower.

(d) If the *hypertension* which accompanies the renal failure is very severe and in the malignant phase, it will accelerate the progression of the renal damage. Provided this damage has not progressed too far (i.e. a blood urea of under 100 mg./100 ml. may be taken as a rough guide) it is worth while trying to lower the blood pressure to safer levels by means of drugs (p. 127).

(e) Sometimes these patients appear to be in a terminal state as a result of renal circulatory failure from dehydration. They should be rehydrated with 5 per cent dextrose or if there is concomitant sodium deficiency 0·16 M sodium lactate should be used as it will also help to correct the acidosis. Thereafter the patient should be treated as for acute renal failure (p. 366).

(f) Eventually a stage is reached at which only symptomatic treatment can be given. Chlorpromazine often prevents the nausea and vomiting and morphine may relieve discomfort and alleviate anxiety and fears.

(g) *Maintenance Haemodialysis and Renal Transplant.* When the glomerular filtration rate falls below about 3 ml./minute terminal renal failure has been reached and the patient will die. It is now possible to maintain such patients in fair health by haemodialysis.

The patient is given a permanent arterio-venous shunt or fistula and through this is attached to a dialysis machine for about twelve to fourteen hours two or three times a week. The choice of patients for such treatment is not always easy, as a certain amount of mental resiliance is required, and they should not be suffering from any progressive systemic disease outside the kidneys. Hypertension however is no bar and is often considerably improved after dialysis has been started.

Renal transplant with either a cadaver or live donor kidney offers another method of rescuing patients with terminal renal failure, and if successful enables them to lead a more normal life than on dialysis.

URINARY TRACT INFECTION

Three clinical syndromes of urinary tract infection will be described:
    (1) Acute lower urinary tract infection.
    (2) Acute pyelonephritis.
    (3) Chronic pyelonephritis.

The relationship between these three syndromes is not yet defined. There is little doubt that infection of the lower urinary tract can be followed by an acute pyelonephritis; in fact many authorities do not distinguish between upper and lower urinary infection. How often an attack of acute pyelonephritis fails to clear up and is followed by latent infection finally terminating in the scarred and contracted kidney of chronic pyelonephritis is not known. The problem is further bedevilled by the difficulty in diagnosing chronic pyelonephritis, which in fact may be discovered only as postmortem. It is however apparent that recurrent renal infection in childhood is an important cause of the contracted, scarred kidneys of chronic pyelonephritis found in adult life. Childhood pyelonephritis is often associated with reflux of urine from the bladder on micturition and it interferes with the growth of the kidneys so that they never reach full size. Recurrent infection in children should therefore always be taken seriously.

The Significance of Bacilluria. E. coli is the common infecting organism; others include staphylococcus aureus, proteus vulgaris (frequently associated with stones), pseudomonas pyocyaneus and streptococcus faecalis.

The culture of a *fresh* specimen of urine (a mid-stream or catch specimen is satisfactory) is essential in the investigation of urinary tract infection. The work of Kass has shown that the urine of normal individuals does not contain more than 10,000 organisms per ml. of urine. In urinary tract infection, even if it is latent, it is usual to find more than 100,000 organisms/ml.

Acute Infections

Acute Lower Urinary Tract Infection

This is a disease of women. The short female urethra allows infection to spread from the perineum to the posterior urethra and the trigone of the bladder. The urethral glands may become chronically infected and the disease become recurrent.

Clinical Features. This is a very common disease. It may be precipitated by minor trauma such as sexual intercourse (honeymoon cystitis) or complicate such conditions as prolapse. The symptoms are frequency and dysuria; general symptoms are not common. The condition frequently settles in a few days. The main dangers are:

(1) The infection may become recurrent.

(2) During the acute attack there may be reflux of urine from the bladder up the ureters causing an ascending infection and acute pyelonephritis.

Culture of the urine may show the infecting organism but is quite often sterile.

Acute Pyelonephritis

The term pyelonephritis is used to emphasise that with inflammation of the ureters and renal pelvis there may also be infection of the renal parenchyma; this is important because in patients who have a long history of recurrent or chronic infection, the kidneys may become so damaged that hypertension and renal failure eventually develop (see chronic pyelonephritis).

Acute pyelonephritis may follow lower urinary tract infection (see above). Sometimes it is blood-borne, particularly in staphylococcal infections. Urinary stasis also predisposes to infection which is frequently seen therefore in *pregnancy*, in men with *bladder neck obstruction* due to prostatic enlargement and in patients with *neurological disorders* which interfere with the emptying of the bladder.

In children, bladder neck obstruction may be combined with reflux of urine into the ureters on micturition, probably due to some congenital defect. This can be demonstrated radiologically by a micturating cystogram; its recognition is important since early surgical correction may prevent progressive renal damage. Infection may also complicate *renal stones* and *neoplasms* with the renal tract. Finally it seems likely that other forms of parenchymal renal disease such as glomerulonephritis may predispose to bacterial infection.

In men pyelonephritis is nearly always secondary to some abnormality in the urinary tract.

Clinical Features. The onset is usually sudden, although there may be a short history of lower urinary tract infection. Symptoms include fever, shivering and rigors, general malaise, aching in one or both loins and sometimes in the suprapubic region, frequency and dysuria. On examination there is usually tenderness over one or both kidneys. There is a leucocytosis and a large number of pus cells are found in the urine.

Treatment of Acute Infection

(a) *Acute lower urinary tract infection* usually responds to a ten day course of sulphonamide (see p. 383). Recurrent attacks may be troublesome and may lead to pyelonephritis. They require a full urological investigation to exclude a local cause and often cystoscopy and urethral dilatation may in itself lead to improvement. It must be admitted however that in spite of investigation and treatment many women suffer from recurrent attacks and few come to serious harm.

(b) *Acute pyelonephritis.* The patient is nursed in bed and given a fluid intake of at least three litres a day. A urine sample should be sent for culture and to determine sensitivity of the organism to antibiotics. Since the usual E. coli infection is found only in an acid urine, an alkaline mixture containing 3·0 g. each of sodium citrate and sodium bicarbonate is given two-hourly until the urine becomes alkaline and then in reduced dose to keep it alkaline. In addition, treatment is started with a sulphonamide (see p. 383). On this regime, symptoms and signs should usually subside within a few days; if they have not, a sulphonamide-resistant organism is probably responsible and the result of the initial urinary culture will reveal its nature. The sensitivity tests now show the most suitable antibiotic to use.

It is very important to eradicate infection from the kidney and the initial course of treatment which should last two weeks is best followed by a further two weeks' treatment with another antibiotic to which the infecting organism is sensitive (usually tetracycline or ampicillin). The urine should be cultured one month after apparent cure to ensure that there is no persistent bacilluris.

Children, who are particularly liable to develop persistent infection and all patients with recurrent chronic infection require a complete urological investigation, long-term treatment with antibiotics over several months and prolonged follow-up.

Renal Infection in Pregnancy

Routine urine tests show that about 5% of pregnant women have a significant bacteruria (more than 100,000 organisms per ml.), although they may be symptomless at the time, and these patients are particularly liable to develop clinical infection later in pregnancy. About 2–3% of all pregnant women develop clinical renal tract infection. This is believed to be due to dilatation of the ureters and interference with urinary flow by the foetus. Urinary infection appears to be associated with an increased incidence of toxaemia and foetal abnormality.

Clinical infection should be treated (see above) and a sulphonamide or ampicillin is usually satisfactory. Patients with asymptomatic bacteriuria should be given a week's course of antibiotic treatment and thereafter be observed throughout the pregnancy. A few patients whose kidneys have already been damaged by previous infection may require treatment throughout pregnancy. Sulphadimidine 0·5 g. t.d.s. is usually satisfactory (provided the organism is sensitive). However, sulphonamides must be stopped four days before delivery as they interfere with binding of bile pigments by the infant's plasma proteins, and thus increase the risk of kernicterus.

Chronic Pyelonephritis

Chronic pyelonephritis is probably the commonest cause of chronic renal failure in this country but its pathogenesis is still something of a mystery. One or both kidneys may be affected. In the terminal stages the kidneys are contracted and irregularly scarred. There are areas of round cell infiltration most marked in the medulla with periglomerular fibrosis. Most patients

Drug	Dose	Comment
Sulphamethizole	100–200 mg. q.i.d.	Very soluble in urine. Forced fluids not required.
Sulphadimidine	2·0 g. start 1·0 g. 6 hourly	High fluid intake.
Septrin–Bactrim	1 tab. b.d.	Very effective.
Nalidixic Acid	1·0 g. q.i.d.	Wide antibacterial range. Side effects— photosensitivity and neurological disorders.
Nitrofurantoin	100 mg. t.d.s.	Sterilises urine but may not eradicate parenchymal infection. May cause neuropathy if given to patients in renal failure and should be avoided in pregnancy.
Tetracycline	250 mg. q.i.d.	Generally useful—wide range. Must not be used in renal failure as it raises the blood urea or in pregnancy or young children as it discolours teeth.
Ampicillin	250 mg. q.i.d.	Expensive but effective against many strains of E. coli and proteus.
Penicillin		Useful in staphylococcal and some strains of proteus infection.
Cephalexin	250 mg. q.i.d.	Useful in renal failure in reduced dosage.
Streptomycin	1·5 g. daily I.M.	Rapid resistance so short course. Best in alkaline urine. Toxic effects liable with renal failure.
Colistin	50,000 units per kilo body weight daily	Useful in pyocyaneus infection.

give a history of recurrent or chronic bacterial infection, often extending back to childhood and women will have suffered exacerbations of symptoms in pregnancy. In others there is no such history and even *post-mortem* it may be impossible to culture bacteria from the kidney. Whether such cases are due to a latent infection or to some other cause is not known. The consumption of large amounts of phenacetin over long periods has been implicated as a cause of pyelonephritis-like changes in the kidney (p. 388) as is also gout and some rare hereditary nephritides.

Chronic pyelonephritis may complicate renal stones and structural abnormalities of the renal tract.

Clinical Features. Chronic pyelonephritis may present as a chronic or recurrent infection with fever, shivering attacks, aching in the loins and perhaps some frequency. It is then easy to diagnose.

Sometimes, however, it presents as chronic renal failure (see p. 375) with no history of infection, and may be difficult to distinguish from other causes of this syndrome. Renal failure may be preceded by a symptomless proteinuria of many years duration.

Features suggesting chronic pyelonephritis:

(1) The presence of pathogenic organisms in the urine (see bacilluria above).

(2) The presence of increased number of white cells in the urine, which also contains protein. In pyelonephritis the injection of prednisolone 40 mg. i.v. will sometimes provoke a rise in white cell excretion in the urine for some hours after injection and this can be used as a diagnostic test.

(3) As chronic pyelonephritis attacks mainly the renal medulla, abnormalities of tubular function are more prominent than in chronic glomerulonephritis. Inability to concentrate the urine appears early and some patients lose excessive amounts of sodium through the kidney.

(4) Straight radiography may show irregularity in the outline of the kidneys due to coarse scarring, and they may be unequal in size. The cortex may be thinned and the calyces may show clubbing.

The diagnosis may be confirmed by renal biopsy which may give a positive bacteriological culture or precipitate a flood of organisms into the urine. It will also show the typical histological features.

All patients with suspected chronic pyelonephritis should have an intravenous pyelogram and usually cystoscopy and micturating cystogram or retrograde pyelogram to exclude any structural disorder which requires surgical treatment.

Treatment. If an infecting organism is identified, its sensitivity to all relevant antibiotics should be determined. Eradication of infection usually requires treatment for months. It is reasonable to start with six months' continuous treatment, changing the antibiotics every fortnight, during which time the urine should become sterile and free of excess leucocytes. Thereafter the urine must be cultured at regular intervals and treatment instituted as required. In renal failure the dose of antibiotic must be halved and streptomycin should not be used. Results of treatment are often disappointing and relapses frequent.

If a patient with chronic pyelonephritis develops renal failure he should be treated as already described (p. 378). The following points however should be remembered:

(1) Renal failure in these patients may be precipitated by an acute exacerbation of renal infection and antibiotic treatment may induce a remission.

(2) Patients with chronic pyelonephritis are particularly prone to electrolyte disturbance, correction of which may produce considerable improvement in renal function.

DISORDERS OF TUBULAR FUNCTION

A small number of patients will be encountered who appear to have disorders of tubular function without much evidence of glomerular disease. In many of these patients the disorder is congenital but in others it is the result of various forms of renal disease, particularly chronic pyelonephritis. These disorders may be simple or multiple and may affect nearly every aspect of tubular function. Two such disorders are considered here:

Fanconi's Syndrome

Fanconi's syndrome is a familial disorder in which there is a failure of reabsorption of phosphate, amino acids and sugar by the proximal renal tubules resulting in the appearance of these substances in the urine. In addition the renal tubules are so deranged that the kidney cannot produce an acid urine.

Clinical Features. The syndrome usually presents in childhood with polyuria, thirst, and stunting from renal rickets. Ultimately chronic renal failure develops.

Renal Tubular Acidosis

In this condition there is a failure of the tubule to produce an acid urine (below pH 6·0). This results in an excessive secretion of bicarbonate, which is replaced in the plasma by chloride ions, leading to hyperchloraemic acidosis. This condition is often complicated by excessive calcium loss in the urine and calcification of the kidneys (nephrocalcinosis).

Clinical Features. (1) *In infants* renal tubular acidosis is characterised by failure to thrive, dehydration, and vomiting. The urine is never more than slightly acid. If the child survives, renal function tends to become normal and the disease does not progress into adult life.

(2) *In adults* the main symptoms are osteomalacia of the skeleton and calcification of the kidney which may ultimately lead to chronic renal failure. Sometimes in addition there are symptoms of potassium deficiency.

Treatment is to try and correct the acidosis by giving citrates and to replace the calcium deficiency if present.

RENAL LESIONS IN SYSTEMIC DISEASE

The Kidney in Hypertension

Although hypertension causes some changes in the renal arterioles, this is not usually enough to interfere seriously with renal function and renal failure occurs very rarely in essential hypertension. In the small group of hypertensives in whom there is a very high diastolic blood pressure associated with marked arteriolar changes and papilloedema, often called malignant hypertension, severe renal damage can, however, rapidly develop. The arterioles become thickened and the afferent arterioles of the glomerulus undergo hyaline necrosis with subsequent ischaemic lesions of the glomerulus.

Clinical Features of Malignant Hypertension. In addition to the usual symptoms of severe hypertension (p. 124), the patient develops evidence of renal damage: albumen, casts, and red cells appear in the urine and the blood urea rises.

Treatment. The blood pressure must be reduced (p.127) before severe and irreversible damage to the kidney is produced. There is some evidence that if the blood pressure is lowered early enough some of the renal changes which have already occurred may be reversible.

UNILATERAL RENAL DISEASE AND HYPERTENSION

The experiments of Goldblatt showed that ischaemia of one kidney in the dog produced hypertension, and a small proportion of patients with hypertension have demonstrable unilateral renal disease. Hitherto, however, removal of the abnormal kidney, although occasonally dramatically successful, has seldom cured the hypertension.

The unilateral renal disease may be pyelonephritis, hydronephrosis, or stenosis of the renal artery. This last type exactly mimics Goldblatt's experiment and it is in this group that nephrectomy or relief of the stenosis should be successful, for it is renal ischaemia which is important in producing hypertension. The problem is to separate this small group from the large number of patients with hypertension from other causes.

Clinical Features. Suspicion should be aroused if the patient is young (under 40) with severe hypertension of rapid onset and with a negative family history. Physical examination is unhelpful except that a murmur may be heard over the affected renal artery.

Pyelography may show the renal shadow to be smaller on the affected side, and the dye may be more concentrated by the ischaemic kidney and thus produce a denser shadow.

I-131 hippuran is handled by the kidney in the same way as P.A.H. It can be injected intravenously and its uptake and excretion monitored by counters over the kidneys. In renal ischaemia and other forms of renal disease inequality of the traces is found. It is, therefore, a useful screening test.

If these investigations reveal unilateral renal disease which might be ischaemic the next step is to confirm the presence of stenosis by aortography which outlines the renal arterial tree. Even the presence of a stenosis, however, does not necessarily imply that the kidney is ischaemic. *Divided renal function studies*, for which under standard conditions the urine is collected from each kidney separately are rarely required.

When the kidney is ischaemic the pattern of tubular function changes. Essentially the tubules reabsorb more of the filtered load of water and proportionally even more of sodium. This means that the urine from the ischaemic kidney is:

(a) Decreased in volume.
(b) Higher in P.A.H. concentration.
(c) Lower in sodium concentration, and
(d) The inulin and P.A.H. clearances are often decreased on the ischaemic side (but this is not characteristic of ischaemia and may occur with any type of renal damage).

Treatment. The correct management is very difficult, for no test shows without doubt which patient will derive benefit from operation. If there is unequivocal evidence of unilateral renal artery stenosis and the other kidney is normal there is about a 50 per cent chance of relieving the hypertension by nephrectomy or by some plastic operation on the stenosed renal artery. If there is doubt it is usually better to lower the blood pressure with drugs. In general the present trend is to be more conservative with these patients.

Diabetes Mellitus

Albuminuria is common in patients with diabetes. Sometimes in addition there may be other evidence of renal involvement such as a nephrotic syndrome or chronic renal failure. It is only recently that the various renal diseases associated with diabetes have been classified. They are:

(1) *Pyelonephritis.* This is probably the commonest lesion and accounts for the majority of diabetics who develop chronic renal failure.
(2) *Glomerular lesions.* There are two types:

(a) The Kimmelstiel-Wilson lesion, which is characterised by nodules of eosinophilic material in the glomerular tuft and is almost entirely confined to diabetics.
(b) A generalised thickening with sclerosis of the basement membrane of the glomerular capillary. This change may be found in other types of renal disease.
The relationship between these changes and clinical evidence of renal disease is not clear but it would seem that the nodular lesions are not necessarily associated with clinical renal disease, which correlates much more closely with the generalised sclerosis.
(3) *Arterial changes.* The smaller arteries of the kidney may show thickening and sclerosis.

Treatment is directed to controlling the diabetes as well as possible, although it is not certain whether this prevents the development of renal disease. It is very important to recognise chronic pyelonephritis, as in this group it may be possible to control the infection with antibiotics and thus halt or slow down the progress of the disease.

Subacute Bacterial Endocarditis (p. 162)

The presence of red cells in the urine is a very useful diagnostic test for subacute bacterial endocarditis. The kidney may show diffuse changes indistinguishable from acute glomerulonephritis or patchy lesions which affect only part of the glomerular tuft. It is believed that both these lesions are due to an allergic response. Chronic renal failure may ensue if the infection is not controlled.

Rarely larger emboli may cause frank renal infarcts.

Amyloid Disease (p. 432)

Amyloid disease is usually secondary to chronic sepsis or rheumatoid arthritis. It usually produces a nephrotic syndrome and now that more accurate diagnosis is available by means of renal biopsy it does not appear to be as rare as was formerly considered.

The presence of amyloid within the body can usually be confirmed by rectal biopsy or by the *Congo red test*. This depends essentially on rapid absorption by amyloid of the dye, which disappears from the circulation after intravenous injection more quickly than normal.

Systemic Lupus Erythematosus (p. 330)

A renal lesion is an important feature of S.L.E. and about 40 per cent of those with renal involvement develop a nephrotic syndrome terminating in chronic renal failure. Rarely it presents as a progressive acute nephritis. The glomerular lesions are variable and include basement membrane thickening (wire loop appearance) and cell proliferation indistinguishable from glomerulonephritis. Diagnosis therefore may depend on evidence of lupus elsewhere. The disease is usually rapidly progressive in spite of treatment with steroids, although in a few patients the downhill course is prolonged over many years.

Polyarteritis Nodosa (p. 331)

The arteritis frequently affects the kidney producing glomerulitis and small areas of infarction. The patient presents with acute nephritis and recurrent bouts of haematuria are a prominent feature. Occasionally the nephrotic syndrome or chronic renal failure may occur.

Anaphylactoid Purpura

A small number of patients with anaphylactoid purpura have haematuria and proteinuria. Oedema is rare but disappearance of the proteinuria is characteristically rather slow, although complete recovery is usual.

Analgesic Nephropathy

The prolonged use of analgesics is associated with the development of renal damage, the usual pathological picture being that of renal fibrosis with papillary necrosis and sometimes even detachment of the papillae. It seems that phenacetin is the most important analgesic involved. However, analgesics are quite often given as mixtures and it is difficult to completely exonerate other mild analgesics such as aspirin and paracetamol.

Clinical Features. The patient may present with chronic renal failure, hypertension, recurrent renal infection or haematuria. Straight X-ray may show calcification of the papillae which may outline the papilla if they are lying free in the renal pelvis. Pyelography may show small irregular kidneys similar to chronic pyelonephritis. The dye may show detachment of the papillae and may outline the spaces found by the disappearance of the pyramids.

Treatment. There is no specific treatment, but if the analgesic is stopped renal function should not deteriorate further and may actually improve.

NORMAL VALUES

Plasma Concentrations

Bicarbonate	25–29 m.Eq./litre
Potassium	4–5·5 m.Eq./litre
Sodium	138–145 m.Eq /litre
Creatinine	0·7–1·5 mg./100 ml.
Urea	20–40 mg./100 ml.

24 hour Urine Output

Calcium	50–250 mg.
Potassium ⎫	Depends on intake
Sodium ⎬	Usually 50–200 m.Eq.
Urea	10–30 g.

Renal Function (corrected to 1·73 sq. m. surface area)

Renal plasma flow	approx. 600 ml./min.
Glomerular filtration rate	approx. 112 ml./min.
Urea clearance	approx. 75 ml./min.
(urine flow > 2 ml./min.)	

Maximum concentrating capacity—up to SG 1020–1032

(800–1,200 m. osmoles/litre)

FURTHER READING

Merrill, J. P. *The Treatment of Renal Failure.* 2nd Ed. Grune & Stratton, New York, 1965.

Wardener, H. F. de, *The Kidney.* 3rd Ed. J. and A. Churchill, London, 1968.

Pitts, R. F. *Physiology of the Kidney and Body Fluids.* 2nd edition, Year Book Medical Publishers Inc., Chicago, 1968.

Black, D. A. K., Edited by, *Renal Disease.* 3rd edition. Blackwell Scientific Publications, Oxford, 1971.

Cameron, J. S., and Russell, A. M. E., *Nephrology for Nurses*, William Heinemann, London, 1970.

CHAPTER ELEVEN

DISORDERS OF WATER AND MINERAL METABOLISM AND OF ACID/ BASE BALANCE

Introduction

A normal man with a body weight of 70 kg. contains about 42 litres of water. The proportion of the body which is accounted for by water varies with sex and age.

Adult man: 60 per cent of weight is water

Adult woman: 50 per cent of weight is water

Infant: 65 per cent of weight is water

Fat, which contains no water, also influences these figures and in very obese subjects the proportion of body weight due to water may be significantly lower.

In considering disturbances of water and electrolyte balance the body water is divided into the intra and extracellular spaces or compartments. The intracellular space contains about 70 per cent and the extracellular space about 30 per cent of the body water.

The extracellular space can be further subdivided into the intravascular space and the interstitial fluid. Ions and water pass freely between these compartments and although the capillaries are largely impermeable to protein so that the concentration of protein is much higher in the plasma than in the interstitial fluid, the interstitial and plasma spaces may be regarded as a single compartment.

The most important ions are:

		Plasma (mEq./litre)	Intracellular Fluid (mEq./litre)
Cations	Na	136–142	11
	K	4·0–5·5	164
	Ca	5·0	2
	Mg	2·0	2·8
Anions	Cl	95–105	0
	HCO_3	25–28	10
	HPO_4	2	110
	SO_4	1	18
	Protein	16	66
	Organic Acids	6	5

Extracellular Osmolality 285 mOs./litre.

The intra and extracellular spaces are separated by the cell membrane which is freely permeable to water but in health is largely impermeable to sodium and potassium. In health the cell water and the extracellular fluid are isoosmotic.

It can be seen that the main extracellular cation is sodium and the main intracellular cation is potassium. The maintenance of the high concentration gradient of these ions across the cell membrane is dependent on energy-producing metabolic activity within the cell.

Changes in the concentration of these ions in either the intra or extracellular spaces result in the passage of water from the low concentration to the high concentration space until the osmolalities of the two spaces are again equal. The shift of water results in the shrinkage and expansion of the respective spaces.

In general, therefore, it can be stated that provided there is adequate hydration the amount of sodium in the body determines the volume of the extracellular fluid and the amount of potassium in the body the volume of the intracellular fluid.

CLINICAL DISORDERS

The diagnosis of clinical disorders of salt and water metabolism requires an awareness of the circumstances in which these disorders may occur; if these are remembered diagnosis is not usually difficult. However, it is usually much harder to assess the extent of the disorder.

The management of these conditions is made more precise by daily measurement of intake and output of water and electrolytes and estimation of plasma levels of electrolytes. The main measurements required are careful records of the volume and electrolyte content of oral and intravenous fluids, the levels of sodium, potassium, bicarbonate and chloride in the plasma, and the volume of urine passed in each 24 hours. In more complicated disorders measurements of sodium and potassium concentrations in the urine may be necessary. In special cases the volume and electrolyte content of other excreta (vomit, aspirate and faeces) may be needed. Regular weighing is a most useful guide to net fluid balance.

Losses which may be expected are given below:—

Aspirate ⎫ Vomit ⎰	Water, H^+ K^+ Na^+
Fistulae	Water Na^+ K^+ HCO^-_3
Diarrhoea	Water Na^+ K^+
Osmotic diuresis (as in uncontrolled diabetes)	Water Na^+ K^+

Some assessment of renal function is very useful and measurement of blood urea is usually sufficient for this purpose. Good renal function is a great help in returning the patient to normal fluid balance provided ions and water are supplied in adequate quantities. The problem is much harder when renal function is impaired.

Disorders of water and electrolyte balance.

If intake and output records are available from the start of the patient's illness the nature and degree of the disorder of electrolyte and water balance can easily be calculated. However, for most patients records are either incomplete or non-existent. Diagnosis must usually be made on clinical grounds and confirmed by plasma concentrations of electrolytes, although as will be seen below these may only give a very rough idea of the extent of the disorder. There are now methods of measuring the total body sodium and potassium, but they are not generally available for routine use and are slow and clumsy.

Finally it must be remembered that it is unusual for a single disorder to exist alone. Any change in the total body electrolytes affects the amount of water in the body, and loss of more than one electrolyte occurs frequently. Although for simplicity individual disorders are examined separately, in practice combinations are the rule.

WATER

The volume of body water depends on the amount ingested and the output in the urine; in addition about 500 ml./24 hrs. are lost through the lungs and skin. Diarrhoea or excessive vomiting are also factors in some patients. Healthy kidneys require to excrete at least 700 ml./24 hrs. to get rid of waste products. Many patients do not have healthy kidneys and the urine output may have to be considerably higher to prevent uraemia.

Dehydration. Isolated dehydration is not common in this country and usually results from decreased intake. Comatose or debilitated patients may not be given sufficient water. Excessive loss of water from the intestinal tract or through the kidneys is much more common, but, except in diabetes insipidus, there is a concomitant loss of electrolytes and thus a complicated picture.

In pure water deficiency shrinkage of both the intra and extracellular spaces occurs (see p. 390). The main symptoms are thirst due to a rise in the osmolarity of the extracellular fluid and in severe cases confusion or coma. Signs are not prominent except for a dry mouth. The volume of urine is low and the urine is concentrated. The plasma proteins, sodium and haemoglobin are raised.

Treatment. Water should be given by mouth or intravenously as 5 per cent dextrose solution. The amount required may be difficult to assess, but the plasma sodium level or osmolality may be used as a guide.

Overhydration. This occurs when excessive water intake is combined with failure of water excretion. The common causes are acute renal failure or excessive production of antidiuretic hormone such as occurs in the first forty-eight hours following major surgery. The excess water is distributed evenly through the intra and extracellular spaces. Subcutaneous oedema may be present and pulmonary oedema detected by rales at the lung bases. Clinical features are confusion, convulsions and ultimately coma. The plasma electrolytes and osmolarity are low.

Treatment. In mild cases it is sufficient to restrict water intake. If over-hydration is severe it will be necessary to give hypertonic saline (2N or 5N) to raise the plasma sodium level (and thus osmolality) of the body water. If there is acute renal failure some form of dialysis may be needed to remove excess water.

SODIUM

The freely exchangeable sodium in the body (about 2500 mEq.) is almost entirely confined to the extracellular space. There is in addition a considerable amount of sodium in bone but it is not available for exchange.

In health the amount of exchangeable sodium in the body depends on intake and loss in the urine. Normal kidneys are very effective in regulating excretion to keep the body sodium steady. If there is severe loss or excessive intake, particularly if renal function is temporarily or permanently disturbed, upsets in sodium balance occur.

Sodium Depletion. This can be caused by excessive loss, usually from the *gastrointestinal* tract or through the *kidneys.* Gastrointestinal loss results from vomiting, diarrhoea, and fistulae. Renal loss is usually the result of prolonged diuretic therapy, although it may also occur in uncontrolled diabetes (p. 417) or with renal tubular lesions.

Vomiting causes sodium deficiency, not only from loss in the vomit but also by producing an alkalosis, and thus an obligatory excretion of sodium in an alkaline urine. Decreased intake is not common in this country, but in the tropics excessive sweating plus a low salt intake can be important.

As the sodium concentration (and thus the osmolality) in the extracellular space falls, water is lost both in the urine and into the intracellular space (p. 390) so that the volume of the extracellular space including the blood volume decreases. Finally, this adjustment fails and the sodium concentration in the extracellular space falls. This means that by the time the plasma sodium is significantly reduced, considerable depletion has occurred.

Clinical Features are weakness, vomiting and cramps. The shrinkage of the extracellular space causes hypotension (particularly postural), lax skin and sunken facies. The plasma sodium concentration is reduced with severe depletion but owing to the fall in extracellular volume the plasma sodium concentration under-estimates the extent of sodium deficit.

Treatment. If charts are available, the degree of sodium depletion can be calculated, but this is unusual. There is no ideal way of establishing sodium deficiency which is suitable for routine use. A rough approximation may be obtained by multiplying the number of millequivalents the plasma sodium is below normal by the total body water, i.e.
Deficiency in mEq. Na =

$$140 - \text{observed Na conc.} \times \frac{60 \ (50 \text{ for women})}{100} \times \text{body weight in Kg.}$$

This formula assumes (incorrectly) that sodium is distributed throughout the body water and makes no allowances for the shrinkage in the extracellular space. However, these two errors tend to cancel each other and thus allow an approximate estimation of sodium deficiency.

It is usual to spread the repletion of sodium over 24–48 hrs. It should also be remembered that the day to day loss of sodium may be continuing, and sodium depletion is frequently associated with water depletion so that correction of dehydration may also be required. A patient with severe sodium depletion may easily need as much as 10 litres of water and 1000 mEq. of sodium. Sodium is usually given as N sodium chloride solution, though if the plasma sodium concentration is below 120 mEq/litre, 2N sodium chloride should be used. If sodium depletion is associated with acidosis, due perhaps to uncontrolled diabetes or excessive intestinal loss, $\frac{1}{6}$M sodium lactate can be infused or 100 ml. of 8·4 per cent sodium bicarbonate (1 mEq./ml.) can be added to whatever infusion fluid is used. During the repletion period, continued observation of the clinical and biochemical state of the patient is necessary.

In patients in whom it is suspected that cardiac function is impaired a careful watch must be kept on the jugular venous pressure and the bases of the lungs as over-rapid infusion can precipitate heart failure and pulmonary oedema. A jugular venous pressure line is useful if available.

POTASSIUM

Potassium is the major intracellular cation. It plays an important part in cell membrane activity and in the contraction of muscle. In health the adult male body contains about 3000 mEq. of potassium, the amount being regulated by renal excretion, although the conservation of potassium by the kidneys is not as effective as that of sodium.

Potassium is also excreted into the gut in the bile and intestinal fluid, but is reabsorbed. If, however, there is excessive loss of intestinal fluid, depletion can occur.

The intracellular distribution of potassium makes the measurement of total body potassium very difficult. Unfortunately the plasma potassium concentration, though usually giving some indication of the situation, may be misleading especially as considerable depletion (up to 200 mEq. K) can occur with no fall in the plasma level and without development of symptoms. More accurate methods of measuring total body potassium are available but are not suitable for routine use.

Potassium Depletion. Excessive loss of potassium can occur from the *gastrointestinal tract*, due to vomiting, fistulae, or prolonged diarrhoea. Prolonged use of purgatives is an occasional cause. Severe *renal loss* occurs in prolonged diuresis, usually from the use of diuretic drugs, but also in diabetes mellitus (p. 417) or the recovery phase of acute renal failure. Steroids also cause increased renal potassium loss, and it is a feature of Conn's Syndrome (p. 449).

Loss of potassium from the cell causes a fall in intracellular osmolality, and thus loss of water from the cell. There is some shift of hydrogen and sodium ions into the cell and thus an intracellular acidosis and an extracellular alkalosis. The plasma pH is therefore raised and the raised bicarbonate concentration increased, whereas the urine, which reflects the intracellular pH, will be acid.

Clinical Features are muscle weakness and fatigue, and in severe depletion actual paralysis may occur. The muscle of the intestine may lose tone, causing ileus. Potassium depletion can also damage the cells of the renal tubule producing polyuria and failure of acidifying powers. Potassium depletion sensitises the heart muscle to the effects of digitalis, and may be responsible for the development of overdosage. The plasma potassium is usually low in severe depletion and the ECG shows typical changes (see below).

Treatment. The extent of potassium depletion is impossible to assess and estimations based on plasma levels will usually be misleading. In general it can be said that depletion severe enough to produce symptoms means a deficit of at least 500 mEq. and with severe symptoms it may be considerably higher.

Whenever possible potassium should be given by mouth. Potassium chloride is most satisfactory in doses of 10–15 g. (130–200 mEq.) daily. Prolonged use of potassium chloride sometimes produces intestinal ulceration with stricture formation. Potassium Chloride effervescent tablets (Sancto K), (12 mEq. K and 8 mEq. Cl per tablet, or tablets of 'Slow K' (8 mEq./tablet) which contain potassium chloride in a slow release form, seem to be free from side effects. Satisfactory natural sources of potassium are fresh orange juice (5·0 mEq./100 ml.) and tomato juice (6·0 mEq./100 ml.).

If intravenous replacement is necessary a potassium chloride solution containing 1·5 g. KCl (20 mEq. K) in 10 ml. can be added to 500 ml. of infusion fluid. In general, potassium should not be infused at a greater rate than 1 g. KCl (13 mEq.) in every four hours, and great care is required if renal function is impaired as there may be a sudden swing to hyperkalaemia.

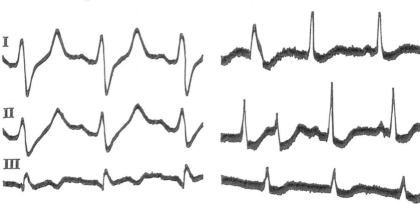

E.C.G. from patient with a raised serum potassium level (9 mE./l.): note wide QRS and tall T waves.

E.C.G. from patient with low serum potassium level (2·7 mE./l.: note extrasystole, wide QRS and S–T depression.

Potassium Excess. The symptoms of potassium excess develop when the extracellular potassium concentration is raised and most commonly occurs when the kidney fails to excrete potassium. This is found in acute renal failure when oliguria is frequently associated with widespread muscle injury, infection and fever, all of which tend to release potassium from the tissues into the extracellular space. In chronic renal failure the kidneys usually excrete potassium normally or even in excess until the terminal stages. In conditions of circulatory failure a combination of low partial pressure of oxygen and reduced renal blood flow leads to migration of potassium from the cell and raised plasma levels. A mild hyperkalaemia may also be seen in Addison's disease, and is due to aldosterone deficiency.

Clinical Features. The main effect is on muscle. The patient becomes increasingly weak and may eventually become paralysed with hypotonic and absent reflexes. The heart's action becomes irregular and heart block and asystole may ensue. The ECG shows typical changes (p. 396). The diagnosis is confirmed by estimating the plasma potassium level, and a concentration of over 7·0 mEq./litre can be dangerous but the rate of rise is also important.

Treatment

(a) *Preventative*
> (1) High calorie diet, low in potassium.
> (2) Ion exchange resin in the sodium phase, Resonium A (Beyer) 15 g. four times daily, by mouth.
> (3) Dialysis.
> (4) If possible correct the underlying cause.

(b) *Emergency*
> (1) Infusion of 30 per cent glucose intravenously with 25 units of insulin per 500 ml.
> (2) 10 ml. of calcium gluconate (10 g./100 ml.) slowly I.V.

ACID/BASE BALANCE

Physiology

The intracellular pH is believed to be about 7·0. The end products of non-nitrogenous metabolism are carbon dioxide and small amounts of organic and inorganic acids. These substances are temporarily buffered by the intracellular buffers but ultimately pass from the cells and are carried in the blood to their sites of elimination (the lungs and the kidneys) with a minimal change in plasma pH. Carbon dioxide being a gas is excreted via the lungs and the organic and inorganic acids are excreted by the kidneys.

Excretion of Carbon Dioxide. On entering the blood carbon dioxide is converted to carbonic acid by the enzyme carbonic anhydrase in the red cells. This reaction is so rapid that dissolved CO_2 may be considered as an effective acid. Measurements are usually given in terms of partial pressure of carbon dioxide (pCO_2) rather than concentration of carbonic acid. Some

90 per cent of the hydrogen ions released by the dissociation of this carbonic acid combine with haemoglobin, thus preventing a large fall in blood pH. In the tissues the release of oxygen from haemoglobin allows the uptake of hydrogen ions by the imidazolyl groups on the haemoglobin molecule.

$$HbO_2 + CO_2 + H_2O \xrightarrow{\text{carbonic anhydrase}} H^+Hb + HCO_3^- + O_2$$

Oxygen in the lungs similarly causes a release of hydrogen ions which combine with bicarbonate with the formation of carbon dioxide which is excreted. In addition some carbon dioxide is carried on the amine groups of haemoglobin and plasma proteins.

$$H^+Hb + O_2 \rightarrow HbO_2 + H_2O + CO_2 \uparrow$$

Maintenance of pH and Excretion of Hydrogen Ions. The stable pH of the blood is preserved by a number of buffer systems. These consist of strong bases which on the addition of hydrogen ions (acid) form weak acids. The bases and weak acids which act as buffers in this context are frequently called buffer bases and buffer acids.

The pH of the blood depends on the ratio buffer base to buffer acid. It can be derived from the equation propounded by Henderson and Hassalbalch in 1908.

$$pH = pK + \log\left(\frac{\text{buffer base}}{\text{buffer acid}}\right)$$

The buffer systems of the blood with their approximate relative buffering capacity are:

% of Total Capacity		*% of Total Capacity*	
HCO_3^-/H_2CO_3	37%	Hb/HbH	34%
HPO_4^{--}/H_2PO_4	5%	Protein/PrH	24%

If hydrogen ions are added to these buffer systems, they combine with the buffer bases to form weak buffer acids. The fall in pH resulting from the addition of acid is therefore minimised.

In the plasma the compensation is almost entirely due to HCO_3/H_2CO_3 system because CO_2 can be excreted immediately.

$$HCO_3^- + H^+ \rightarrow H_2CO_3 \rightarrow H_2O + CO_2 \uparrow$$

and the ratio $\log \dfrac{HCO_3}{H_2CO_3}$ (i.e. pH) maintained at near normal levels.

Similarly if hydrogen ions are removed from the system and the pH rises, buffer acid is changed into buffer base with the release of hydrogen ions and the increase in pH is minimised.

The *total buffer base* is the sum of all the buffers (bicarbonate + protein + Hb + phosphate). If ventilation is normal then the plasma bicarbonate level reflects the total buffer base. If however there is an abnormality of ventilation then this is no longer true. This is because retention or deficit of carbon dioxide (and thus carbonic acid) will influence bicarbonate levels without altering the total buffer base. i.e.

$$\text{i.e.} \quad H_2CO_3 \;\rightarrow\; H^+ + HCO_3^-$$
$$\downarrow$$
$$\text{Buffer base}$$

The hydrogen ion released thus reduces the buffer base, but at the same time bicarbonate is added. The net result being no change in total buffer base, but an increase in bicarbonate. The terms 'base excess' or 'base deficit' are used to indicate abnormalities of total buffer base.

The role of haemoglobin in the excretion of carbon dioxide has already been considered. In addition small amounts of hydrogen ions (about 75 mEq./24 hrs.) are produced as organic and inorganic acids (sulphuric and lactic). They are accommodated in the buffer systems of the blood and excreted in the urine. Provided the influx from the cells equals efflux through the kidneys, the pH of the blood remains constant.

Clinical Applications

Introduction. Acid/base disturbances can be divided into those which are primarily due to disorders of carbon dioxide excretion (respiratory) and those due to inequality of acid or base production or excretion (metabolic or non-respiratory). The symptoms due to acid/base disturbances are ill-defined and are often overshadowed by the primary disease. Once the possibility is recognised the diagnosis is usually not difficult.

Investigation. The bicarbonate buffer system of the blood is usually studied as it is the easiest to measure. Bicarbonate is usually estimated by the autoanalyser or the Van Slyke method using venous blood. Provided that respiratory function is normal this estimation usually gives an adequate approximation of the buffer base situation in the blood. If however there is CO_2 retention it will underestimate the deficiency in base and vice versa, so that where there is a respiratory disorder or where the situation is complicated, it is necessary to measure additionally the plasma pCO_2 or pH. The pCO_2 can be measured by the rebreathing method or by the Astrup method using capillary or arterial blood. Mixed venous blood can also be used but gives a figure about 6 mm. higher than arterial blood. If two of the three variables (pH, pCO_2 or bicarbonate) are known the third can be calculated.

Acid/base disorders are often associated with electrolyte deficiencies, so that the plasma and often urinary concentrations of sodium and potassium should be measured. Estimation of blood urea levels gives an indication of overall renal function.

Normal Values

$$\text{Plasma pH} = 7\cdot35\text{--}7\cdot45$$
$$\text{Plasma bicarbonate} = \;24\text{--}28 \text{ m.Eq./litre}$$
$$pCO_2 = \;36\text{--}42 \text{ mm.Hg.}$$

Disorders of Carbon Dioxide Excretion

1. Impaired Excretion (Respiratory Acidosis)

The carriage of carbon dioxide from the tissues to the lungs is described above. In health ventilation is physiologically maintained so that the partial pressure of carbon dioxide in the alveoli is about 40 mm.Hg., the concentration of dissolved carbon dioxide in arterial blood being that which is in equilibrium with this partial pressure.

If there is inadequate alveolar ventilation, the partial pressure of carbon dioxide rises leading to an increase in the dissolved carbon dioxide (hypercarbia).

This causes a fall in the ratio $\dfrac{HCO_3^-}{pCO_2 \text{ (increased)}}$ and therefore a fall in pH.

The decrease is minimised by the other buffer bases combining with carbon dioxide and being converted to buffer acids with the release of bicarbonate.

$$\text{Buffer base} + CO_2 + H_2O \;\rightarrow\; \text{Buffer acid} + HCO_3^-$$

Following carbon dioxide retention the excess hydrogen ions are excreted by the kidney, producing an acid urine and reabsorption of bicarbonate by the tubules is increased.

Impaired carbon dioxide excretion occurs:

    (1) Most commonly in chronic bronchitis, emphysema and asthma. It may occur acutely in bronchial obstruction with collapse.

    (2) More rarely with depression of respiration in morphia or barbiturate poisoning, or from weakness of the respiratory muscles in poliomyelitis.

Clinical Features. Symptoms usually appear when the pCO_2 rises to 60 mm.Hg. The patient is dyspnoeic and cyanosed (due to the concomitant hypoxia) with a full pulse and warm extremities from peripheral vasodilation. The blood pressure is frequently raised in acute hypercapnia. Further increase in pCO_2 brings about confusion with twitching and finally coma. Papilloedema may develop due to cerebral vasodilation. The treatment is directed towards increasing alveolar ventilation and relieving hypoxia.

2. Excessive Excretion (Respiratory Alkalosis)

This is due to hyperventilation which leads to excessive loss of carbon dioxide and to a rise in the ratio $\dfrac{HCO_3^-}{pCO_2 \text{ (decreased)}}$ and a rise in plasma pH.

This is minimised by the other buffer acids converting to buffer bases with the release of hydrogen ions which combine with bicarbonate.

$$\text{Buffer acid} + HCO_3^- \rightarrow \text{Buffer base} + H_2O + CO_2$$

Renal conservation of hydrogen ions results in an alkaline urine.

Excessive excretion of carbon dioxide is often due to hysterical over-breathing and is a constant feature of salicylate poisoning; rarely it is found in subjects with alveolar block causing hypoxia but not affecting carbon dioxide excretion and it may also complicate various forms of cerebral damage.

Clinical Features are increased neuromuscular excitability with twitching, paraesthiae and tetany. The easiest treatment is to raise the pCO_2 in the alveoli by rebreathing from a bag. In those with cerebral damage careful depression of respiration with morphia is sometimes useful.

Disorders of Hydrogen Ion Excretion

1. Gain of Acid or Loss of Bicarbonate (Metabolic Acidosis)

When the rate of production of hydrogen ions exceeds the rate of excretion either because of increased ingestion of acid substances, undue metabolic production of acids or impaired excretion by the kidneys, the condition of metabolic acidosis develops.

The rise in pH is minimised by the acid combining with buffer bases,

$$\text{Buffer base} + H^+ \rightarrow \text{Buffer acid}$$

resulting in a fall in the ratio $\dfrac{\text{Buffer base}}{\text{Buffer acid}}$.

A similar state can result from the loss of bicarbonate ions.

An excessive influx of acid into the blood can arise from the following causes:

    (a) Ingestion of substances which produce acid, the commonest being ammonium chloride and aspirin.

    (b) Increased production of acid occurs with severe exercise, in uncontrolled diabetes mellitus and sometimes after major surgery.

    (c) Tissue hypoxia as may occur in cardiac arrest leads to rapid production of lactic acid with resulting acidosis.

    (d) In both acute and chronic renal failure the kidneys fail to excrete sufficient acid.

Bicarbonate deficiency follows loss of intestinal secretions due to diarrhoea or fistulae. There is frequently an associated sodium and potassium deficiency. Failure of the renal tubules to reabsorb bicarbonate with subsequent deficiency also occurs with renal tubules acidosis.

Clinical Features are tiredness and weakness with increased respiration, and finally unconsciousness.

Treatment

(1) Relief of the primary cause if possible.

(2) Re-establishment of optimal renal function, i.e. correct dehydration and electrolyte deficiencies.

(3) Restoration of depleted buffer bases by the infusion of 0·16 M sodium lactate or by the addition of 8·5 per cent sodium bicarbonate (approx. 1 mEq./ml.) to whatever infusion is being used. As a rough guide the total base deficiency can be calculated:

25 — Plasma bicarbonate (mEq./litre)

$$\times \ 0\cdot3 \ \text{body weight in Kg.}$$

This will almost certainly underestimate the deficit and further base will be required, the amount depending on the levels of plasma bicarbonate. A watch must be kept for tetany.

2. Loss of Acid or Gain of Bicarbonate (Metabolic Alkalosis)

Gain of bicarbonate is due to its excessive ingestion in the treatment of peptic ulcer. Healthy kidneys can cope with almost unlimited amounts of bicarbonate but if there is renal disease, base excess may develop. Loss of acid is usually due to vomiting or gastric aspiration. Metabolic alkalosis can also complicate potassium deficiency (p. 395).

The rise in pH results in buffer acid being changed to buffer base.

$$\text{Buffer acid} \ \rightarrow \ \text{Buffer base} + H^+$$

and a rise in the ratio $\dfrac{\text{Buffer acid}}{\text{Buffer base}}$.

The kidneys secrete an alkaline urine containing large amounts of sodium and bicarbonate.

Clinical Features include clouding of consciousness and in addition there may be paraesthesiae, tetany and convulsions.

Acid loss from vomiting or aspiration is often coupled with sodium and potassium deficiency. This is due partially to loss in gastric secretion and to increased excretion in the urine.

Treatment. It is usually sufficient to correct dehydration and electrolyte deficiencies and the kidneys will excrete the excess base.

Definitions

Acid. A substance which donates hydrogen ions. Strong acids are those which are highly dissociated in solution, and weak acids are those poorly dissociated in solution.

Base. A substance which accepts hydrogen ions. A strong base accepts hydrogen ions more readily than a weak base. Important physiological bases are bicarbonate, dibasic phosphate and some amino acids.

Buffer Base. A base which takes part in the buffer systems of the body.

Acidosis and Alkalosis. These terms can not be precisely defined. They are generally used to indicate the primary direction of the change of plasma pH, acidosis indicating a fall and alkalosis a rise in pH.

	Partial Pressure CO_2	*Plasma pH*	*Plasma Bicarbonate*
Impaired excretion CO_2 (respiratory acidosis)	Increased	Decreased	Increased
Excessive excretion CO_2 (respiratory alkalosis)	Decreased	Increased	Decreased
etention of acid or loss of base (metabolic acidosis)	Normal or Decreased	Decreased	Decreased
Loss of acid or retention of base (metabolic alkalosis)	Normal	Increased	Increased

Plasma changes in Acid-Base Disorders.

FURTHER READING

J. S. Cameron in *Medical Treatment* (Vol. III). Edited by K. S. Maclean and G.W. Scott, J. & A. Churchill, London, 1970.

Victor Wynn in *The Scientific Bases of Surgery*. Edited by W. T. Irvine. J. & A. Churchill, London, 1965.

CHAPTER TWELVE

DISEASES OF METABOLISM

DISORDERS OF CARBOHYDRATE METABOLISM

Introduction—Metabolism of Carbohydrate

Glucose is absorbed actively from the small intestine, and passes through the portal vein to the liver. Here it is phosphorylated and some is stored as glycogen, some broken down to pyruvate, and some dephosphorylated and passed into the plasma. These changes are effected by enzyme systems. The normal fasting plasma level of glucose is 50–100 mg./ml. Glucose passes freely through the glomerular filter, and is totally reabsorbed by the cells of the proximal tubule. If the plasma glucose level (and hence the level in the glomerular filtrate) is above about 180 mg./100 ml. then the tubule's power of reabsorption is exceeded, and sugar appears in the urine.

Glucose passes from the plasma into the interstitial fluid and then into the cell. Inside the cell it is again phosphorylated, and either stored as glycogen, or broken down to pyruvate and then to CO_2 and water, with consequent release of energy, or converted to fatty acids and ultimately to fat. It has been estimated from tracer studies in animals that of the total glucose which is daily metabolised 67 per cent is oxidised to CO_2 and water, 30 per cent converted to fatty acids, and only 3 per cent stored as glycogen. Sixty-five per cent of this glucose is dietary in origin, 30 per cent arises from gluconeo-genesis, and 3 per cent only from glycogen.

A number of hormones serve to regulate carbohydrate metabolism. Of these the most important is insulin, which is a protein released from the beta cells of the islets of Langerhans in response to a rise in plasma glucose levels.

It circulates both in a free form and bound to the albumen and alpha-2 globulin of the plasma.

The total plasma insulin content in fasting normal subjects is about 1 milli-unit per ml. and this increases after a rise in plasma glucose. In adult diabetics normal levels are often found with a slow rise in response to glucose. Low values are found in young diabetics after prolonged insulin treatment.

The action of insulin varies in different tissues but in general it increases the uptake of glucose and suppresses the release of non-esterified fatty acids by adipose tissue.

Thyroxine is mildly hyperglycaemic in effect, but pituitary and adrenal hormones, and the secretion of the alpha cells in the islets of

Langerhans, glucagon, are all hyperglycaemic. How important the hormones other than insulin are in clinical diabetes is uncertain.

DIABETES MELLITUS
Introduction

Diabetes mellitus occurs in all parts of the world. The age at which the disease is first recognised clinically ranges from early childhood to old age; over 50 per cent of patients are first diagnosed over the age of 50 years. The sex ratio was believed to show a predominance of females over males, but recent surveys suggest that it is 1:1.

It is easiest to consider it as a breakdown of the body's insulin-glucose economy. Thus, certain conditions such as steroid therapy, pregnancy, obesity, etc., may overtax the insulin resources; they may fail in idiopathic diabetes, or with primary pancreatic disease. Since the recognised disease runs in families it has been suggested that predisposition to diabetes is related to a recessive gene of low penetrance. However, there is controversy over this point, and a multifactorial aetiology and inheritance is also possible.

Prevalence

Before World War II, prevalence studies in western countries suggested a rate of 0·7 per cent. An investigation in 1946–7 based on screening by glycosuria in Oxford, Mass., indicated that for every known case there was another unrecognised case, raising the prevalence to 1·99 per cent. Since then many surveys have been carried out, and it appears that the prevalence of diabetes is very low (0·1 per cent or less) in unmechanised primitive societies, rising to high levels (up to 7 per cent in some cases) in under-exercising industrial communities with extended life span.

Pathological Chemistry

Glucose Tolerance Tests. After an 8–12 hour (usually overnight) fast, the true blood sugar in arterial, capillary or venous samples ranges in most subjects from 50–100 mg. per cent; these levels are regarded as normal. A fasting blood sugar over 100 mg. per cent is suggestive of diabetes mellitus and over 130 mg. per cent is now generally accepted as diagnostic. However, in many persons who sooner or later develop complications of diabetes, the fasting blood sugar, which depends on the time since the last meal, may be under 100 mg. per cent. A more reliable indication is obtained with tolerance tests. The oral glucose tolerance test is in widest use. After taking a fasting blood sugar sample, 50 g. (in the U.S.A. 100 g.) of glucose are given in 250 ml. water with noncaloric flavouring to prevent nausea. Further blood samples are then taken at half-hour intervals. The early form of the curve depends on the opening of the pylorus, the intestinal absorption and liver glucose uptake. Patients with rapidly emptying stomachs often show a brisk early peak (steeple or lag curve). At 2 hours, current W.H.O. levels of true blood sugar for the suspicion of diabetes (i.e. needing further study) are 120 mg. per cent for capillary blood and 110 mg. per cent for venous blood, and for the acceptance of the diagnosis of diabetes 140 mg. per cent and 130 mg. per cent respectively.

In all cases where diabetes is diagnosed, the renal threshold for glucose must be determined, as glycosuria is the simplest, and therefore most widely used, method for judging control.

Metabolic Consequences of Failure of Insulin Action

Glycosuria. When insulin is not available the blood glucose level rises. When glucose levels exceed the renal threshold glycosuria results, which may be detected in concentrations as low as 0·1 per cent by glucose-specific tests or as a reducing substance by less sensitive (0·25–2·0 per cent) means, e.g. Benedict's Solution (sensitive to homogentisuric acid and other hexoses) or tablets such as those available commercially as Clinitest.

All the latter less sensitive methods which are semiquantitative are of particular value for following the control of the diabetic *providing always* that the renal threshold is known. Recent surveys indicate that the threshold tends to be lower than 180 mg. per cent among young adults, and higher in elderly subjects. It may fall during pregnancy, and recover after parturition.

Dehydration and Shock. Intense uncontrolled glycosuria can result in an osmotic diuresis of 7–10 litres/day with resulting intense thirst. Unless adequate replacements are given, this polyuria leads to large losses of sodium and potassium.

Ketoacidosis (p. 416). Insulin failure is accompanied by ketoacidosis. This is due to:

(1) Accumulation of ketoacids.
(2) Accumulation of incompletely metabolised carbohydrate, i.e. pyruvic and lactic acid.

In the absence of insulin, adipose tissue releases large quantities of free fatty acids which circulate to the liver where they are burnt to carbon dioxide. When this mechanism becomes overloaded, acetyl co-enzyme A accumulates and becomes condensed to aceto-acetic acid and acetone. These can be burnt by muscle, but if produced in sufficient quantities they accumulate in the blood and appear in the urine and the breath.

The resulting acidosis causes a fall in plasma bicarbonate.

Causes of Diabetes

Clearly, there are many points in the sequence of events between insulin synthesis and release, its clearance and action, and glucose uptake by the various organs, where abnormality or biochemical fault may upset the normal balance and produce the diabetic state.

Pancreatectomy or chronic pancreatitis removes the source of insulin production. With advancing years, protein synthesis is generally slowed down and this also applies to insulin production. It is not surprising therefore that recent studies show a high prevalence of hyperglycaemia (up to 50 per cent) among the elderly. The close correlation between obesity and diabetes indicates that under-exercise and the deposition of adipose tissue lead to a breakdown in the body's insulin-glucose economy despite over-production of insulin by the beta cells.

In young diabetics there seems to be an idiopathic failure of beta cell function. About 80 per cent of all diabetes occurs in elderly obese patients, and nearly all the rest in young thin ones.

Minutes after 50 g of Glucose

The mean glucose tolerance curves in sex and age groups (40–50 subjects per group) in apparently normal people.

The aggravation of hyperglycaemia in Cushing's disease, by steroid therapy and in pregnancy, may be attributed in part to changes in protein metabolism, and in part to alteration of tissue sensitivity to insulin. The association between acromegaly and diabetes and the production of intense ketonuria when growth hormone is given to insulin-dependent diabetics indicates that this hormone, too, increases the body requirement for insulin.

Symptoms and Presentation

Depending largely upon the severity and rapidity of the metabolic decompensation, hyperglycaemic patients may present in four ways, irrespective of the possible precipitating factors.

1. *Acute Onset.* The patient suffers intense polyuria, polydypsia, rapidly loses weight, becomes ketoacidotic and unless treatment is begun usually passes into coma within a few days or weeks. Less frequent symptoms include irritability, vomiting, abdominal pain, muscle cramps and peripheral tingling. This onset is usual (but not universal) among children and adolescent diabetics, but may occur among the elderly.

2. *Gradual Onset.* There is much less intense thirst and polyuria, although nocturia may be noted. The obese may lose 1–2 st. over a period of

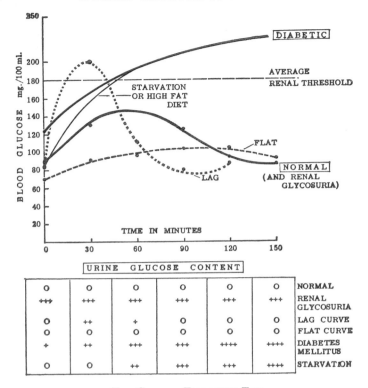

The Glucose Tolerance Test.

months, or may have gained weight lately. Pruritus vulvae or crops or boils may occur; lassitude is common, and middle-aged males may complain of loss of libido, and impotence. This onset is usual in middle life, but may be observed among younger and older patients.

3. *Symptoms of Complications.* Many older people present with symptoms from the complications of diabetes in the eye (cataract, retinitis), peripheral nerves (neuritis), kidneys (nephrotic syndrome), blood vessels (gangrene, intermittent claudication, and coronary artery disease).

4. *Asymptomatic Glycosuria.* Many adult and elderly patients are detected at the stage before symptoms (but not necessarily signs) emerge, as a result of the chance findings of glycosuria at insurance examinations or in routine testing. This glycosuria must be distinguished from other reducing substances (with Clinistix or Testape) and from renal glycosuria by a glucose tolerance test. Because diabetics' health and enjoyment of life may be grossly impaired without the patient recognising any specific diabetic symptoms, early detection and treatment is now being widely advocated and practised.

Signs and Complications

The diabetic patient must be examined thoroughly to establish the diagnosis, to assess the severity of the metabolic decompensation and/or complications, to decide on treatment and to judge progress.

Evidence of glycosuria may be provided by penile irritation or balanitis in men, and the excoriations of pruritus vulvae in women.

(1) *In the Eyes*

    (a) Diabetic retinitis—ophthalmoscopic examination shows earliest a shiny 'wet' retina, then venous engorgement. 'Blot' haemorrhages, actually capillary microaneurysms, have been detected in 95 per cent of hyperglycaemic cases after 15–25 years. More serious disturbances of blood lipids lead to scattered 'hard' waxy exudates. Most serious is proliferative retinitis where delicate new vessels grow forward into the globe. These may cause haziness of the vitreous, haemorrhages, retinal detachment, fibrosis, scarring and loss of vision.

    (b) Diabetic cataracts—in older patients these are associated with generalised clouding of the lens, sometimes with (6–10) radially arranged 'faults'—sharp edged opacities like spokes in a farm wagon wheel.

    (c) Iritis rubeosa—reddening of the iris at the margin of the pupil due to microaneurysms which may lead to glaucoma.

(2) *In the Blood Vessels*

Evidence of impaired circulation to the feet should be carefully sought (cold toes, or foot, atrophic skin, poor hair or nail growth) as gangrene here is severely incapacitating and should be prevented by foot care whenever possible. Particularly significant are small ischaemic areas which seem to be related to the obstruction of endarteries with glycoproteins.

    (a) All peripheral pulses should be palpated: absent ankle pulses may occur with ageing, but are more common among diabetics.

    (b) The main vessels should be auscultated for the occasional bruit, especially the abdominal aorta, renal arteries, iliac and femoral vessels.

    (c) Blood pressure should be measured lying and standing to detect sympathetic neuropathy.

    (d) An electrocardiogram should be recorded.

(3) *In the Nervous System*

    (a) Peripheral neuropathy. Many people over 65 years of age lose one or both ankle jerks and vibration sense over the malleoli, but these may also be signs of early diabetic peripheral neuritis. If bilateral, diabetes should be excluded. Usually confined to the lower limbs, neuropathy is associated with tingling and pain, stocking anaesthesia and, in severe cases, muscle weakness and wasting.

(b) Mononeuritis multiplex (p. 310). A peripheral nerve is suddenly affected, leading to muscle weakness and wasting and an area of anaesthesia.

(c) Radiculitis (rare). This may precede clinical recognition of diabetes. It is associated with pain, tingling or scalding sensations in the segment affected and is frequently self-limiting to about two years.

(d) Amyotrophy.

(e) Pupillary changes and palsies of the extra ocular muscles (rare).

(f) Damage to the autonomic nervous system causing impotence, nocturnal diarrhoea, postural hypotension and loss of sweating over the lower limbs.

(4) *In the Renal Tract* (see page 387)

(5) *In the Skin*

(a) At blood sugar levels over 200 mg. per cent, glucose appears in the sweat. Skin infections, particularly boils and monilial infections of the vulva, are common in diabetics.

(b) Hypercholesterolaemia and hyperlipaemia occasionally lead to the formation of xanthomata in the skin, small hard yellowish nodules up to a few millimetres in diameter.

(c) Insulin may lead to changes in the skin (in 20–30 per cent of cases) either hypertrophy at the site of injection or atrophy, locally or remote from the injection site. These changes are more common in young people, and in adults are much more common in women than in men.

(6) There is an association between tuberculosis and diabetes, and all suspected cases should have a chest radiograph.

The Classification of Diabetes

Diabetes produces a number of clinical pictures. The current W.H.O. recommendations regarding definitions and classifications are as follows:

(1) Recognised onset during growth between ages 0–14 years (*Infantile or Childhood Diabetics*). These patients usually present with severe initial symptoms and rapidly become insulin-dependent.

(2) Recognised onset between 15 and 24 years (*Young Diabetics*). These patients usually have an acute onset of symptoms and most may be expected to become insulin-dependent. However, in the tropics, cases in this age group may resemble the adult cases (see below).

(3) Recognised onset between 25 and 64 years (*Adult Diabetics*). Growth onset, insulin-dependent diabetes may occur up to the age of 22 or 23 years, but between 20 and 35 years such cases merge into the adult-onset cases who are much less insulin-dependent. These patients begin with variable symptoms and may or may not need insulin.

(4) Recognised onset over 65 years of age (*Elderly Diabetics*). These patients frequently present with symptoms of the complications of diabetes and can often be controlled without insulin.

It should be noted that all classifications refer to the age WHEN THE DIABETES WAS RECOGNISED, *not* the current age of the patient.

In addition to these classifications by age, the W.H.O. Committee recognised certain other types of diabetes which were defined as follows:

Juvenile type diabetes. This term should refer to cases of any age group who require insulin and who are prone to attacks of ketosis.

Brittle diabetes. It was recommended that this term be used as little as possible. It refers to juvenile-type cases who prove difficult to stabilise between hyperglycaemia and ketosis on the one hand and hypoglycaemia with symptoms on the other. Genuine brittle diabetics are very uncommon and the brittle state does not necessarily persist.

Insulin-resistant diabetes. This term should be reserved for patients requiring over 200 units insulin daily.

Endocrine diabetes. Cases where the disordered carbohydrate tolerance can be attributed to the endocrinological disease, e.g. Cushing's syndrome.

Treatment of Diabetes Mellitus

Introduction

In the past there have been two schools of thought, those who advocated strict control and those who felt that provided the patient was not hypoglycaemic or ketotic, little needed to be done. Longer experience suggests that only by the most careful control can complications be postponed and life prolonged. Unfortunately even the strictest control by present methods will not prevent complications developing ultimately in some cases; nevertheless the incidence of complications is less and expectation of life is far greater in those diabetics who have always been carefully controlled.

Control may be measured by the urinary glucose provided that the renal threshold is normal and that the renal function is not impaired. It should be checked by blood-sugar estimation every three months. The aim should be to keep the urine as nearly sugar free as possible, and in any case not to allow more than 8 g./24 hrs. of glycosuria. This means that if the patient excretes 1,500 ml. of urine in 24 hours no sample should contain more than ½ per cent (0·5 g./100 ml.) of sugar. Added to this the patient should be 'lean and spry', neither gaining nor losing weight, eating an adequate and enjoyable diet, taking exercise reasonable for his age, free from all diabetic complications, and subject to neither hyperglycaemia nor hypoglycaemia at any time in the 24 hours.

Treatment of Adult and Elderly Diabetics

When a patient is discovered to be a diabetic he should be fully examined clinically, and any complications noted. A chest radiograph should be taken, and the urine tested for sugar, acetone bodies, protein, and casts. A mid-stream specimen of urine should be cultured. Any existing infection should be treated, and a diet suitable to his age and occupation prescribed. If he is obese then weight should be reduced near to ideal levels. The majority, about 80 per cent, of diabetics present with obesity and mild diabetes in the second half of life. They represent the *'elderly'* type of diabetic. Almost all of them can be treated by diet alone provided they will co-operate. It is essential to reduce them to near their ideal weight, and this can only be done by dieting. In effect this means eating less food than the patient requires, so that the body is forced to draw on fat depots as a source of energy. When the weight is reduced to something close to the ideal for the age, height, and sex, then a diet supplying adequate but not excess calories should be prescribed, with limitation of carbohydrate. In general, patients are offered too much to eat. Only the heaviest labourers require more than 3,000 calories daily; most patients need between 1,800 and 2,500 calories, and women rather less than men. Few patients are adequately controlled on diets containing much more than 150 g. carbohydrate in 24 hours. It is important to realise that some diabetics may take up to *four weeks* to respond fully to diet.

Oral Hypoglycaemia Agents

There are many advantages in the use of oral agents for the control of diabetes mellitus. Injections are never welcome at any age, and may be impossible in the aged, handicapped or partially sighted patient. If it could be shown that these preparations were able to control (p. 411) diabetes as effectively as they lower the blood sugar then there would be few reservations about their use. Unfortunately, this is far from certain, indeed recently it has been suggested that the tendency to develop vascular disease may be increased in patients where hyperglycaemia is controlled by tablets and dietary restrictions neglected.

It is therefore wise to restrict the use of oral hypoglycaemia agents to those patients in whom diet manifestly fails despite conscientious effort by the patient and doctor, and whose hyperglycaemia can be controlled by tablets without recourse to insulin. This is a small group of patients, and at present oral hypoglycaemia agents are more widely prescribed. Further observation is required to settle the point.

The precise mode of action of the available preparations is not certainly known. Two chemical groups, the sulfonylureas and the diguanides are used at present. The first are believed to act on the pancreas and to increase the endogenous supply of insulin; the diguanides are thought to act chiefly on muscle, and to increase glucose uptake at the cellular level. Hypoglycaemia may occur with the sulfonylureas, but is rare with the diguanides.

Of the sulfonylureas, tolbutamide and glibenclamide have short actions, and must be given two or three times daily. Chlorpropamide has a long action, and need be given only once daily. Its full effects are not seen for a week. Acetohexamide and tolazamide are intermediate in their time of action. Hypothyroidism and jaundice from biliary stasis have been attributed to these drugs, and certainly they occasionally cause rashes, fever, or flushing after food. The diguanides are of relatively short action, and should be given two or three times daily. Their chief toxic effects are on the gastrointestinal tract, and they may cause anoexia, nausea, vomiting and diarrhoea.

ORAL HYPOGLYCAEMIC COMPOUNDS

Approved name	Proprietary name	Average daily dose (mg.)	Strength of tablets (mg.)	Contraindications
Sulfonylureas:				
Tolbutamide	Rastinon	1,500	500	
Chlorpropamide	Diabinase	250	100, 250	liver disease renal failure
Acetohexamide	Dimelor	1,000	500	
Tolazamide	Tolanase	250	100, 250	
Glibenclamide	Euglucon	15	5	
Diguanides:				
Phenformin	Dibotin	75	25, 50	renal or liver disease
Metformin	Glucophage	1,500	500	renal or liver disease

Treatment of Juvenile Diabetes

All young thin diabetics require both insulin and diet, and need to have these matched to the amount of physical exercise they take daily. Clearly a heavy worker will need more calories and more insulin than a clerk. It follows that for adequate control a regular amount of activity and a regular diet are essential, and certain occupations, such as commercial travelling, or the stage, are unsuitable careers for young diabetics to choose. Variation in diet and activity are a major problem during school years, but with patience and persistence most juvenile diabetics remain reasonably well controlled whilst being educated. In general, these children are not suitable for boarding-schools. A useful general guide is to prescribe not less than 70–80 g. protein per day, not more than 150–200 g. carbohydrate and the balance of calories needed as fat.

Insulin

Insulin is a polypeptide, and if taken by mouth is digested to its constituent amino acids. It must therefore be injected subcutaneously at least once daily. A standard insulin syringe should be used, and needles not smaller than size 19. The site of injection should be varied daily; the from of the thigh, over the deltoid muscles, and the lower abdomen are the most convenient sites for self-inoculation. Repeated use of the same site may lead to hypertrophy or atrophy of the subcutaneous fat locally, and to interference with insulin absorption.

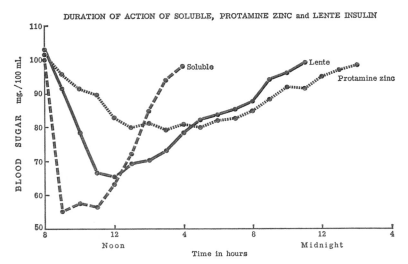

DURATION OF ACTION OF SOLUBLE, PROTAMINE ZINC and LENTE INSULIN

Insulin is prepared from the pancreases of cattle or pigs, or less commonly sheep. Pure crystalline insulin 1 mg. is equivalent to 22·2 international units. A number of different preparations is available.

(a) *Soluble* (Regular, Toronto) *Insulin* (SI) is supplied in concentrations of 20, 40, or 80 units per ml.

(b) *Protamine zinc insulin* (PZI) is supplied as 40 or 80 units per ml.

(c) *Insulin zinc suspension* (IZS) (Danish Insulin) which is prepared either in quick-acting amorphous form (semilente) or the slow-acting crystalline form (ultralente). *Lente insulin* is a mixture of three parts of semilente and seven parts of ultralente. Mixtures of other proportions to suit individual requirements can be made. Other insulins, for example Isophane, Globin and Biphasic, have not found wide usage in the U.K.

The importance of clear prescription of insulin is stressed. The variety, strength, and dose should all be indicated, e.g. ℞ IZS lente (40/c.c.) 20

units subcutaneously each morning. Many emergencies in practice are avoided by this simple expedient.

Most diabetics are controlled on mixtures of SI and PZI. Provided that the injection is given at once and not left to stand both may be drawn into the same syringe and injected as a mixture. Recently more use has been made of insulin zinc suspension. Most diabetics requiring less than 60 units of insulin daily can be easily controlled with lente insulin. Most patients requiring between 60 and 100 units are better managed with a mixture of SI and PZI. Those few patients requiring very large doses of insulin should receive two or more injections of soluble insulin daily.

Controlling Diabetes with Insulin

Assuming a normal renal threshold, the urine may be used as a rough index of control. The patient is told to test the overnight urine, and then after breakfast, lunch, and tea, and immediately before bed, and to record the results. An initial dose of 20 units of SI in the morning just before or just after breakfast and 10 units just before or just after dinner are prescribed, and the effect on the urinary glucose observed. Changes should not be made at less than three-day intervals unless hypoglycaemia occurs. Appropriate adjustments are made until the patient is sugar free and not hypoglycaemic; this is much best done as an outpatient and with the patient at work.

When control appears adequate the patients may be changed to one injection daily of IZS or to a mixture of SI and PZI. It is important to remember that SI can be mixed with PZI, but not with IZS. To effect the change, the total number of units required daily is considered. If it is less than 60, then a straight change to an equivalent dose of IZS may be made (unit for unit). Some slight adjustment of this dose may subsequently be required. Between 60 and 100 units better control is achieved with mixtures of SI and PZI. Four-fifths of the total daily requirements of SI are taken, and a quarter of this given as SI, and three-quarters as PZI. Again, some slight adjustment of dose is likely to be required, always remembering that retard insulins act chiefly at night and are therefore reflected in the morning urine, and that soluble insulin acts by day. Before assuming adequate control a series of blood sugars should be estimated throughout an average day. Although sounding complicated this is a simple method of control and works well in almost all cases.

Once control is achieved the urine need be tested only once daily, but at a different time each day, so that in five days tests are made at all critical times. Hospital attendances can also become infrequent; well-controlled cases should be reviewed quarterly, when blood sugar and urine tests for sugar, ketones, and protein should be taken. Careful records of weight must be kept, and chest radiographs taken annually. Care of the feet should be emphasised, especially in the elderly, and chiropody arranged when necessary.

Complications of Insulin Treatment

(1) Repeated use of the same site for insulin injections may lead to a gross thickening of subcutaneous tissues, chiefly fat, so-called *lipohypertrophy*. In other patients the subcutaneous fat rapidly disappears at the site of injections (*lipoatrophy*). This usually occurs early in insulin treatment, and cannot be avoided by varying the injection site. It is usually self limiting.

(2) *Hypoglycaemia* may result from an insulin overdose; this may be caused by mis-measurement, by unwittingly using insulin of increased strength (40 or 80 instead of 20 units per ml.) or by the too-rapid action of insulin, either from increased physical activity or from failing to take an expected meal. Treatment, see p. 423.

Difficulties in Diabetic Control

Insulin resistance in insulin-requiring diabetics is rare. The diagnosis is usually made either when insulin is incorrectly prescribed (for 'elderly' diabetics) or incorrectly given. The common cause of failure of control if insulin is correctly prescribed and injected are:

(1) *Failure to Diet.* It is difficult to persuade patients with only minor symptoms to accept dietary restriction. Failure to comply is soon revealed by serial observation of body weight. Alcoholics, narcotic addicts, and psychopathic patients are unable to accept restrictions, and suffer accordingly.

(2) *Cryptic Infection.* Pulmonary tuberculosis is the most serious of these, chronic pyelonephritis the commonest. Septic teeth tonsils and adenoids, especially in children, may be important. Cholecystitis should be excluded.

(3) *Marked Variation in Physical Activity.* This applies particularly to schoolchildren, when great ingenuity must be used to balance diet, activity, and insulin. Some adult occupations are too irregular to be suitable.

(4) Genuine *insulin resistance* rarely exists. It occurs when there is failure of absorption of insulin from a too frequently used site at which either severe lipoatrophy or hypertrophy has occurred, when there are antibodies to insulin present in the plasma, and when there are abnormalities of intracellular glucose metabolism which are not wholly corrected by insulin. These cases may present as unstable, or brittle diabetics, who pass easily and rapidly from hypo- to hyperglycaemia and ketosis.

Diabetic Crisis Ketoacidosis

Untreated diabetes eventually leads to coma; but short of coma there is still a medical emergency. The occurrence of glycosuria of 2 per cent or more, with ketonuria and ketonaemia, in a drowsy patient who appears ill should be regarded as a *DIABETIC CRISIS*. It must be appreciated that all degrees of crisis exist; the severity is proportional to the ketosis, not to the level of the blood sugar. In the presence of renal disease, ischaemic or other, urinary ketones are not an adequate index of ketosis. Blood ketones or plasma bicarbonate should be estimated.

Before starting treatment a careful examination must be made to try to discover the initiating cause of the crisis; infection, infarction, trauma, or neglect being the commonest. But treatment is a matter of urgency, and should not be unduly delayed by prolonged search for causes. Two other words of warning. The patients should be disturbed as little as possible; routine nursing procedures may be omitted until the patient is fully conscious. Better a dirty diabetic than a clean corpse. Second, while there is ketosis there will be resistance to the action of insulin. As soon as ketosis begins to subside, sensitivity to the action of insulin increases sharply; it is possible to precipitate hypoglycaemia by too vigorous therapy. The regime detailed below is suitable for a diabetic deeply in coma. It should be discreetly interpreted for minor stages of crisis.

Treatment of Diabetic Crisis. The objects of treatment are first to treat precipitating causes, including infection; second to correct dehydration; third to replace lost minerals; and lastly to re-establish the metabolism of carbohydrate.

(1) *Insulin.* Only soluble insulin should be used. One hundred units should be given at once, one third intravenously, the rest intramuscularly, *not* subcutaneously. If the initial blood sugar level is known the number of units of insulin required may be derived by dividing the blood sugar figure by 10: e.g., if the blood sugar is 1200 mg. % give a total of 120 units of insulin. Three to five hundred units may be needed in 24 hours.

(2) *Replacement Therapy.* Intravenous replacement of lost fluid and cations is essential to prevent circulatory failure and to maintain renal function. Early correction of the metabolic acidosis also renders the tissues much more sensitive to the action of insulin. One litre of 1/6 M. sodium lactate should be given intravenously at the rate of 15–20 ml. per min. This should be followed by 1·0 litre of N-saline unless facilities are available to measure plasma bicarbonate, when either saline or sodium lactate may be used, depending on the degree of acidosis. Once the serum potassium level is known total replacement must be made (p. 396).

(3) *Antibiotics.* One million units of benzyl penicillin should be given intramuscularly at once and daily thereafter for five days.

(4) *Clinical Studies.* When appropriate insulin and antibiotic therapy has been instituted, blood may be withdrawn from the needle inserted for intravenous therapy for chemical analyses. Every effort should be made to obtain this initial sample, and to have full investigation—sugar, ketones, haematocrit, plasma bicarbonate, sodium, potassium, and urea—made of it. These results serve as an invaluable base line. A catheter may be left indwelling in the bladder, and all urine withdrawn hourly and tested for ketones and sugar. Although this predisposes to urinary infection, it is justified by the value of these hourly observations in heralding a sudden swing to hypoglycaemia. Finally, if there has been vomiting a stomach tube may

be passed and the stomach emptied. Gastritis is always present in severe diabetic ketosis, and there may be gastric haemorrhage. Four grams of potassium chloride dissolved in 40–50 ml. of water should be left in the stomach, and if no blood has been withdrawn the tube may be left *in situ* until the patient is able to swallow. An E.C.G. is useful at this stage; it may show evidence of hyper- or hypokalaemia or reveal a myocardial infarct, which may have been the initiating cause of the coma. If the blood pressure falls below 100 mm. Hg. systolic then nor-adrenaline may be added to the intravenous infusion.

Subsequent Treatment. (a) In mild diabetic crisis, where the initial blood sugar does not exceed 500 mg./100 ml. and there is only moderate ketosis, some improvement in blood sugar and ketones will be apparent after two hours. No further insulin should be given at this stage, but the existing infusion should be changed to 5 per cent glucose. If the urine withdrawn from the bladder after three hours still shows 2 g. per cent or more glucose, or if the blood glucose is still over 350 mg. per cent a further 50 units of soluble insulin (in an adult) are given intramuscularly. Further treatment should be governed by two-hourly observations of blood glucose and the patient's clinical condition.

(b) In severe cases, where the initial blood glucose level exceeds 500 mg. per cent and there is marked ketosis and acidosis, much greater insulin resistance is likely. Blood may be withdrawn through the infusion needle every hour (see later), and blood glucose estimated; 50 units of soluble insulin should be given intramuscularly every half hour until there is a fall of the blood glucose level to below 300 mg. per cent. This indicates that glucose (and potassium) are passing into the cells and that carbohydrate is being metabolised; the infusion should at once be changed to 5 per cent dextrose. Now is the time when hypoglycaemia or hypokalaemia are probable. Two-hourly estimations of blood glucose, plasma bicarbonate, and potassium are required. Further insulin requirements should be decided in the light of blood and urinary glucose levels. It must be appreciated that insulin will continue to be required for normal metabolism after the crisis has passed, and should be prescribed as two or more doses of SI daily. If the blood potassium levels or the E.C.G. show evidence of deficiency then a supplement must be added to the infusion (p. 396). In mild cases potassium may be given by mouth, 4 g. potassium chloride in 50–60 ml. water every four hours. As soon as the patient can swallow, good natural sources are fresh orange juice, tomatoes, and Horlicks.

As the crisis lessens clinical examination should be repeated. Undetected infection or silent myocardial infarction must be suspected if the patient fails to respond in four to six hours.

Non-Keto-Acidotic (Hyper-Osmolar) Diabetic Coma

Although this condition was first described in 1886 it is only in recent years that it has been widely reported, and at the time of writing appears increasingly common. The reasons for this change are not apparent.

It occurs in elderly often obese subjects, more frequently females than males, and in the U.K. is commonest in immigrants from the West Indies. It is of insidious onset, and usually presents as disordered consciousness, ranging from mild confusion to deep coma. Focal neurological signs may develop, and epilepsy has been recorded. The outstanding features on clinical examination are deranged consciousness, dehydration (p. 393) and the absence of ketosis.

When the diagnosis is suspected it may be confirmed by measuring the blood sugar level, which is always greatly raised, and the plasma bicarbonate to exclude acidosis. From the serum sodium, potassium, sugar and urea the serum osmolality may be derived from the formula proposed by Jackson and Forman (1968) as follows:

$$\text{Serum Osmolality} = 2(\text{Na}^+ + \text{K}^+) + \frac{\text{sugar}}{18} + \frac{\text{urea}}{6}$$

Results accord well with direct measurements, and in normal subjects values of less than 300 m. Osm./Kg. should be derived. In hyperosmolar coma figures ranging from 300–500 m. Osm./Kg. may be found.

Treatment consists of correcting the dehydration and hyperosmolality intravenously. The repair fluid of choice is 0·5 normal sodium chloride, supplemented by water by mouth or naso-gastric drip. Care must be taken not to provoke pulmonary oedema by too rapid intravenous therapy, and the progress of treatment can be monitored by serial haemotocrit studies. There is no indication for bicarbonate in the absence of acidosis, and hyperglycaemia is corrected with insulin (p. 417).

Prognosis has been variably reported, but with earlier recognition of the condition is improving. Subsequent management of the diabetes (p. 412) is not difficult.

Hyperosmolality of comparable degree also occurs in ketotic diabetic coma, and the outstanding difference in the present group is the absence of ketotis rather than the presence of hyperosmolality. The explanation of the absence of ketosis is not at present known.

Diabetes in Special Circumstances

(a) *Pregnancy*. Diabetic women are less fertile, more prone to miscarry and to toxaemia of pregnancy and hydramnios than their healthy sisters. Their babies are more likely to die *in utero*, to be born grossly overweight, to suffer congenital malformations or to perish shortly before or after birth. Whereas the maternal mortality rate has improved markedly in the last twenty-five years, the foetal mortality in babies born to diabetic mothers remains at about 20 per cent.

Diabetes almost always becomes more severe during pregnancy; indeed, it may be precipitated or unmasked by it. Insulin requirements usually increase sharply for the first trimester, remain steady for the second, and usually increase but occasionally decrease during the third. They decline very sharply after parturition and close observation is necessary to avoid hypoglycaemia. Breast feeding almost always fails, and many obstetricians artificially suppress lactation immediately after birth. Because the power of the cells in the proximal renal tubule to reabsorb glucose is impaired in pregnancy the renal threshold falls, and therefore the urinary glucose is not an adequate index of control and blood glucose levels must be estimated.

Because of the dangers of intra-uterine death, termination of pregnancy either by induction of labour or elective caesarian section is indicated at 36 weeks. Some of the fatalities in the infants can be traced to a hyaline membrane lining the alveoli, a few to hypoglycaemia, but many remain unexplained.

(b) *During Infection.* Insulin requirements increase with infection, and this is true of gastro-enteritis with vomiting and anorexia. The prescribed insulin dose should always be given, and if glycosuria or ketonuria persists it should be increased. Even minor infections in diabetes should be treated seriously.

(c) *During Surgical Operations.* Mild diabetics undergoing short anaesthetics for elective surgery may safely forgo their insulin until they return to the ward. In more severe diabetics, or for prolonged procedures, the usual dose of insulin should be given and an intravenous infusion of 4 per cent dextrose saline set up. When the patient is unconscious estimations of the blood glucose level are made every hour. More insulin or glucose is given appropriately. When severe diabetic ketosis coexists with a surgical emergency, operation should be postponed as long as possible while the treatment for crisis is instituted. In some cases grave risks must be accepted and the time of surgical intervention decided by consultation between physician and surgeon.

DIABETES INSIPIDUS

Introduction. This is a rare disease, characterised by the excretion of a large (10–20 litres/24 hours) urinary volume and consequent great thirst. It is caused either by an absence of antidiuretic hormone from the posterior pituitary gland, or by an inability of the distal renal tubule to respond to its action. Failure of secretion may occur when disease processes affect the region of the pituitary, for example tumours (*c.* 50 per cent), inflammatory disease (*c.* 25 per cent), vascular changes (*c.* 10 per cent), trauma (10 per cent) and Hand-Schüller-Christian disease (*c.* 2–3 per cent).

Clinical Features. The effect of the diuresis is to cause intense thirst, and if fluids are withheld dehydration is rapid, and the signs and symptoms of water deficiency (p. 393), soon appear. The urinary specific gravity is always low, and the urea and chloride levels in the urine reduced. The condition should be suspected in all patients secreting over 4 litres of urine per 24 hours and drinking more than 5 litres per 24 hours. It must be differentiated from diabetes mellitus (glycosuria), terminal renal failure (proteinuria, uraemia) and hysterical over-drinking. Only the last is difficult to separate. Distinction is achieved by showing that intravenous hypertonic saline will temporarily inhibit the diuresis in hysterical patients. It has no effect in diabetes insipidus.

Symptomatic treatment is by means of pitressin, either posterior pituitary powder as snuff, or pitressin tannate (0·5–1·0 ml. daily) intramuscularly or subcutaneously (but never intravenously). A salt-free diet is also useful. Some patients are helped by thiazide diuretics and chlorpropamide is sometimes of value. Cure can only be achieved by treating the cause.

Nephrogenic diabetes insipidus is almost always congenital, very rarely the result of destruction of the distal renal tubule in pyelonephritis. The congenital form is easily recognised by the family history, its early onset, male predominance, and failure to respond to pitressin. Low sodium diets are recommended as treatment, but prognosis is poor.

Inappropriate Secretion of Anti-Diuretic Hormone

In some patients with malignant disease, almost always carcinoma of the bronchus, anti-diuretic hormone may be secreted by the tumour cells and cause water retention with progressive dilution of the plasma electrolytes and urea. This usually presents clinically as a "low sodium syndrome" (page 394). Treatment is by water restriction, aldosterone, and the treatment of the underlying condition.

HYPOGLYCAEMIA

Introduction. Symptoms usually appear when the blood glucose has fallen to between 40 and 50 mg./100 ml. They seem more related to the rate of fall than to the actual level reached, and commonly occur when patients are hungry. Sometimes they can be averted by eating carbohydrate, e.g. chocolate.

Symptoms are of rapid onset and begin with slight unsteadiness, tremulousness, difficulty in concentration, and often headache. They proceed to irrational behaviour, stupor, and coma. Urine may be voided.

Signs. The patient becomes pale, sweats, and the pulse is initially rapid and jerky. When coma is complete the pulse and blood pressure are normal. Severe and prolonged hypoglycaemia may produce irreversible cerebral changes. Epileptic fits may occur and coma may proceed to death.

Causes of Hypoglycaemia

(1) *Insulin overdose*; mismeasured doses, failure to take an expected meal, over-exertion.
(2) *Idiopathic* (functional).
(3) *Liver disease.* Cirrhosis, subacute necrosis.
(4) *Gastrointestinal disease*—post gastrectomy syndrome; steatorrhoea; after alcoholic excess.
(5) *Endocrine.* Hypopituitarism, hypothyroidism, adrenal in-

sufficiency, as a premonitary occurrence in diabetes mellitus, and in insulin-secreting tumours of the pancreas.

(6) *Sarcomas, secondary carcinomatosis.*

(7) Use of *chlorpropamide*, and other *hypoglycaemic drugs,* especially in non-diabetics.

(8) Side-effect of salicylatis, anti-histamines or mono-amine-oxidase inhibitors.

Careful history and clinical examination will make nearly all these conditions sufficiently obvious. Only when it occurs before the onset of diabetes mellitus, when it is idiopathic, or when it is due to an insulin secreting

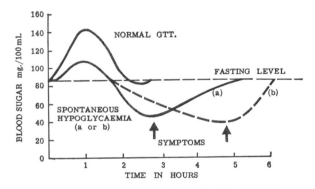

GLUCOSE TOLERANCE TESTS IN NORMAL SUBJECT
AND IN SPONTANEOUS HYPOGLYCAEMIA

tumour is a glucose tolerance curve usually necessary for diagnosis. In diabetes mellitus the curve is typical (p. 408). The last two conditions may be separated by measuring fasting blood-sugar levels hourly for five hours.

REPEATED FASTING BLOOD SUGAR LEVELS
IN SPONTANEOUS HYPOGLYCAEMIA

In idiopathic (functional) hypoglycaemia the blood-glucose levels are normal, and remain so. In the presence of insulin-secreting tumours or other organic causes, the fasting levels are low, and the blood sugar continues to fall through the test.

Treatment. Unless von Gierke's disease is suspected, or the coma has been long-standing or very severe the patients may be revived with adrenalin. A sugar-containing drink—hot sweet tea or sugar in hot water—is prepared, and an injection of 5–10 minims of 1 : 1,000 adrenaline solution subcutaneously is given. This produces a transient hyperglycaemia, with partial recovery of consciousness, during which the sweet drink can be given. Failing this, a stomach tube can be passed and the sweet drink given through this. It is better to give an intravenous injection of 20 ml. of 50 per cent glucose solution.

Subsequent treatment depends on the cause of the hypoglycaemia. If it is due to an insulin-secreting tumour (extremely rare) this should be removed surgically. If due to 'spontaneous hypoglycaemia' then best results are obtained with a high-protein diet and small frequent meals.

DISORDERS OF FAT METABOLISM

OBESITY

This is a serious disease, common in prosperous communities. It results from eating more food than is required. The common cause accounting for over 90 per cent of cases of this hyperphagia is gluttony, but it may also occur in hypothalamic disorders or as a sequel to severe emotional stress. The rate of weight gain is proportional to the extent of dietary excess over requirement; once obesity is established, however, it may be maintained by quite small food intake. Fat can only be removed by eating less food than is required. Actuarial analysis shows that even minor degrees of obesity decrease the expectation of life, and gross fatness severely so. Weight is gained in myxoedema, but is not due to fat.

Obesity may occur at any age; it is most common in the prosperous years of life, and the appearance of the plump matron or city alderman is familiar. Rarely the distribution of fat is unusual. In Cushing's syndrome (p. 449) it affects the head, neck, and shoulders chiefly, and spares the legs; the reverse is true in *lipodystrophia progressiva*. This is most common in women, who show little fat above the waist, but are obese about the buttocks and legs. There is a rare association of obesity with cystic disease of the ovaries (*Stein-Leventhal syndrome*, p. 456). Many fat women have menstrual irregularities which usually remit when ideal weight is achieved.

The appearance of fat is due to hypertrophy of fat-bearing cells. If obesity appears early in life, then the actual number of fat bearing cells may be greatly increased. In some cases local hyperplasia occurs, causing painful fatty lumps in the adipose tissue (Derum's disease). Obesity may occur in children, most frequently the young child of elderly parents. Fat accumulates generally, but is well marked in the mons pubis; this sporran of fat overhanging normal genitalia (where there is no subcutaneous fat) often leads wrongly to a diagnosis of *Froelich's syndrome*, an extremely rare condition.

The effects of obesity are widespread. Extra effort is required for all activity, and extra blood and energy for the metabolism of fat. This increases the demands on the heart and lungs, and excess obesity may itself cause heart failure from restriction of respiratory excursion. The appearance of these grotesquely bloated patients in severe congestive cardiac failure, markedly cyanosed, with polycythaemia rubra, and gross oedema (*Pickwickian syndrome*) is unforgettable. Even minor degrees of obesity may induce failure in an already diseased heart.

Direct mechanical effects of obesity too must be considered. Joints and ligaments suffer from the extra weight that they are called upon to support. Osteoarthritis is common in the knees, and skeletal pains from undue tension in ligaments are the rule. The skin creases are exaggerated, and become keratinised. They are difficult to keep clean, and fungus infection and other skin sepsis is common. Because of the insulating effect of fat it is difficult for the body to lose heat. In spite of profuse sweating discomfort may be acute in hot weather. Added to these are the more mundane difficulties of obtaining appropriate clothes, rising from chairs, and entering and alighting from vehicles.

There also exists a predisposition to certain diseases. Diabetes mellitus (p. 405) is much commoner in the obese, and there is increased tendency to atheroma. Hypertensives are commonly overweight, and the risks of anaesthesia and surgery are greatly increased in the obese.

Treatment. The energy equivalent of adipose tissue is so great that exercise is of little value in treatment. It is calculated that a pound of fat would be lost for every 25 miles run! There is no benefit from hot baths, purgation, or massage. Nor is there any place for thyroid extract, which may cause irreversible exophthalmos. It may be that a few patients are helped a little by diuretics, but undoubtedly the main treatment is simply dietary restriction.

Many suitable diets for the treatment of obesity are available. Mild cases may follow a quite simple diet, merely avoiding fat and carbohydrate in normal meals. This may be reinforced by a day's starvation during the week. Drastic restriction is required in more severe degrees of obesity. The most extreme cases resemble the addiction states, and are best admitted to hospital, and supplied with only 200 calories daily; extra vitamins and iron should be given if this is undertaken. Most patients will tolerate this for 2 to 3 weeks, after which the diet may be increased to 400 cals. daily. After a week or so apparent constipation occurs, from reduced faecal residue. This may be treated with methyl cellulose and liquid paraffin 15·0 ml. at night. The ultimate objects are to restore the patient to his ideal weight, to enable him to conquer his hyperphagia, and to be discharged content to eat a normal diet. These may imply a profound alteration in his way of life; simple psychotherapy and supportive interviews may be necessary for some months.

ATHEROMA

Introduction. Arterial disease as a sequel to atheroma is a major cause of ill health. Deaths attributable to it are increasing exponentially in all civilised countries. There are many features which make it probable that it is of environmental origin. For example, man is the only mammal in which atheroma is significant; it is rarely present at birth, but increases in extent and severity throughout life. It may, however, be modified by endogenous factors. It is rarely severe in healthy women until the menopause; it is more extensive and has more complications in patients with certain maladies, for example diabetes mellitus, familial xanthomatosis, and nephrosis. It results in either abrupt or slow closure of arteries, with consequent deprivation of vital tissues of blood. It is ubiquitous and is a major cause of hospital admissions. It is the underlying cause of angina pectoris, and coronary artery disease, of cerebral vascular disease, intermittent claudication and gangrene, of much atrial fibrillation and retinal disease and most mesenteric thromboses.

Etiology. Of the endogenous factors, a familial history and hyperlipidaemia are the most constant associations. The technique of plasma electrophoresis has led to the easy separation of the protein fractions and subsequent staining for fat has shown where the lipids are bound to protein

TYPE	NORMAL	I	II	III	IV	V
ELECTROPHORETIC LIPOPROTEIN PATTERNS — CHYLOMICRONS origin / BETA LIPOPROTEIN / PRE-BETA LIPOPROTEINS / ALPHA LIPOPROTEIN						
CHOLESTEROL mg/100ml	180–220	+	+	++	NORMAL or LITTLE +	+
TRIGLYCERIDES mg/100 ml	50–150	+++	NORMAL or LITTLE +	+	+	++
GLUCOSE TOLERANCE TEST	NORMAL	NORMAL	NORMAL	40% IMPAIRED	IMPAIRED	IMPAIRED
URIC ACID mg/100 ml	3–7	NORMAL	NORMAL	+	+	+

Plasma electrophoretic patterns, cholesterol, uric acid and triglyceride levels, with glucose tolerance tests in normal and hyperlipidaemic subjects. (after FREDRICKSON)

moieties. Plasma cholesterol and triglyceride levels have also been examined, and from these data a 'lipid profile' of the plasma has been constructed (above). The patterns of lipid carriage so derived point to at least five phenotypes (Fredrickson 1968).

Type I (Exogenous Hypertriglyceridaemia)

This is a rare disease affecting chiefly children, and inherited as an autosomal recessive. In the few adult cases recorded, no relationship with atheroma has been demonstrated. It is characterised by creamy plasma from excess of chylomicrons following about 15 hours after a fatty meal.

Type II (Hyperbeta Lipoproteinaemia)

A common disease of adult life, inherited as a Mendelian dominant character. It is strongly associated with the development of atheroma. In the heterozygotes subcutaneous xanthomata of the elbows, hands, knees and heels may occur. It may occur as a secondary phenomenon to a variety of diseases, for example, myxoedema, nephrosis, myeloma, and liver disorders.

Type III ('Broad Beta Disease').

A disease, occurring chiefly in men aged 20 to 40 years and inherited as an autosomal recessive. It is characterised by the appearance of flat linear deposits of lipids in the subcutaneous tissues, usually of the hands (planar xanthomas), and of lumpy deposits at the elbows, knees, and buttocks (tubo-eruptive zanthomas). It is strongly associated with the early appearance of atheroma.

Type IV (Endogenous Triglyceridaemia)

This is the commonest of the five groups described. It occurs in adult life, but neither its cause nor its inheritance are currently known. It is believed to reflect an imbalance between the endogenous synthesis and removal of glycerides, and is frequently unmasked by obesity. It is often seen in association with other diseases, for example, diabetes mellitus and the nephrotic syndrome. There is a strong association with early atheroma. On examination, lipaemia retinalis, eruptive xanthomata, and hepato-splenomegaly may be found.

Type V (Mixed Hyperlipidaemia)

This is an uncommon lipid pattern seen usually between 10 and 30 years. It is commonly secondary to other diseases, for example, nephrosis, diabetic acidosis, and myxoedema. Clinically it resembles type IV but recurrent bouts of abdominal pain are common. The nature of its inheritance is not yet known nor is its relationship to type IV at all clear. No certain association with early atheroma has been found.

(1) *Prophylactic*

Weight reduction benefits types III, IV and V, and specific dietary restrictions are also of value as follows:

Type I	very low fat
Type II	low fats, and these should be polyunsaturated (i.e. vegetable).
Type III	balanced fat and carbohydrate content
Type IV	low carbohydrate
Type V	low carbohydrate and fat

(2) *Local*

In some cases parts of arteries may be resected and replaced by grafts. This is almost confined to the larger vessels, for example, the carotid and lower aorta or femoral arteries.

(3) *General*

(a) Control of predisposing factors such as heavy smoking, obesity, arterial hypertension, and lethargy.

(b) When symptoms appear, e.g. in coronary heart disease (p. 153) and arterial disease (p. 170).

GOUT

Uric Acid Metabolism

The complex compounds in the cell nucleus consist of a protein to which is joined a large polymer named nucleic acid. This is constructed of a number of nucleotides, each consisting of one molecule each of a base (purine or pyrimidine), a pentose (ribose or desoxyribose) and phosphoric acid. When nucleoprotein is broken down nucleic acid is first split off and then degraded to its constituents, ending as xanthine and finally uric acid. This diffuses from the cell into the plasma, is excreted freely by the renal glomerulus and poorly reabsorbed by the tubules. Some uric acid may be secreted by the distal tubule. The normal blood level is 2–5 mg./100 ml. and 300–600 mg. per 24 hours are excreted in the urine.

It is clear that the blood uric acid may be derived from breakdown of either ingested or endogenous nucleoprotein. It may also be synthesised by the body cells from simple constituents (glycine, glutamine, and ribose phosphate) which are readily available.

Serum levels are raised in primary gout, and in conditions in which there is increased nucleoprotein turnover, for example the leukaemias (particularly myeloid), polycythaemia (primary or secondary), or chronic haemolytic anaemias. It may also be increased in renal disease associated with reduced G.F.R., or from administration of chlorothiazide or its derivatives.

Introduction

Although the clinical syndrome of gout may occur in any of these conditions the relationship to the level of uric acid in the blood is by no means absolute. This and the predilection of the disease for certain specific tissues, and its precipitation and localisation by trauma, all point to there being some as yet undiscovered tissue factor concerned. The mechanism of production of hyperuricaemia in secondary gout is increased nucleoprotein turnover, or rarely renal retention. In primary gout, however, there is some evidence that increased endogenous synthesis may be the underlying cause. Relatives of patients suffering from primary gout may also develop the disease, and a proportion of them show hyperuricaemia without gout. Inheritance is determined by a single dominant gene.

Clinical Features

(1) *Arthritis*. This is usually an acute intermittent monoarthritis. The commonest joint to be affected is the first metatarso-phalangeal, but none is immune. The large joints are only occasionally affected, and a generalised polyarthritis of the rheumatoid type is a rarity. The attacks may be precipitated by overactivity, trauma, or diuresis; frequently no cause can be found. They usually begin at night, are sudden in onset, and are extremely painful. Movement is excruciatingly painful. On examination the joint is red, hot, swollen, glazed, and exquisitely tender. Left untreated the attack develops in an hour or two, and remits over six or seven days. It is frequently followed by desquamation of the overlying skin, with intense itching. The attack is accompanied by malaise and extreme irritability, with fever and leucocytosis.

(2) *Deposits* of crystals of sodium biurate occur in the subcutaneous tissues of the dorsum of the hands, the bursae, particularly the olecranon bursa, the tendons, especially in the forearm, and in the cartilage of the ears, nose, and sometimes eyelids. Typical subcutaneous deposits (tophi) vary in size from peas to pigeons' eggs. The overlying skin is thin and shiny, and the tophus may have ulcerated through and become infected. Sodium biurate is also deposited in the cartilage and juxta-articular bone of the affected joint. Uric acid and (more rarely) xanthine concretions may form in the kidney, either as tubular gravel, or as large pelvic stones.

(3) *Associated Disorders*

(a) Certain acute musculo-skeletal conditions occur more frequently than would be expected by chance in gouty subjects. These include acute tenosynovitis, acute subtendonous bursitis, and acute supraspinatous tendonitis.

(b) Deposit of crystals in the kidney predisposes to infection and chronic pyelonephritis; this may cause hypertension.

(c) There is an occasional association with diabetes mellitus. The structural resemblance of the uric acid molecule to alloxan, a potent beta-cell poison will be recalled.

Diagnosis

(1) The simplest and most certain way is to puncture a tophus with a sterile needle, extract a little of the deposit on the needle point, and examine it microscopically. Typical acicular crystals are seen.

(2) Estimation of the blood uric acid level is usually valuable. It is raised to about 6–7 mg./100 ml. in typical cases.

Treatment

(a) *Acute Episodes*

Acute attacks of gout are best treated with phenylbutazone 100 mg. three times daily until symptoms are relieved. It is unsuitable for long-term administration and should not be used at all in patients with a history of dyspepsia. Colchicine (0·5 mg. two-hourly) may be given, but has the disadvantage of causing diarrhoea. Prednisolone may also be used: an initial dose of 20–30 mg. should be given orally, followed by 10 mg. eight-hourly until symptoms are relieved. Once this is achieved the dose should be reduced progressively, and omitted in two to three days.

Throughout the attack the limb should be supported, and the patient remain at rest. The affected joint may be dressed with lotio plumbi et opii (B.P.), and protected from the weight of bedclothes.

(b) *Management of Chronic Gout*

(1) *Diet.* The chief source of the blood uric acid is endogenous metabolism, and therefore dietary restrictions need be slight. It is wise to avoid high purine foods, and alcoholic excess, and the patient should reduce to his ideal weight. At least five pints of fluid should be drunk daily to minimise stasis and precipitation of urate in the kidney.

(2) *Excretion of uric acid.* A number of substances interfere with the reabsorption of uric acid by the renal tubule. Of these only sulphinpyrazone and probenecid need be considered. It is clear that once the diagnosis of gout is made, treatment to be wholly effective must continue for the rest of the patient's life. For this reason, toxic effects, palatability, and cost of these substances must be considered. To be effective 50–100 mg. sulphinpyrazone four times daily are required, or 0·5 g. of probenecid four times daily. With this treatment acute episodes become less frequent, and eventually cease. Tophi absorb and may be painful, and the process may not be complete for a year or more.

This treatment causes an increased amount of urate in the urine. If there is a history of urate stone formation or if the treatment is not effective then allopurinol may be given. This inhibits the enzyme xanthine oxidase, and so prevents the conversion of xanthine to uric acid. Initially treatment may precipitate acute attacks of gout so that it is wise to start with small doses (50 mg. three times daily) later increasing to 2–400 mg. daily in divided doses.

PSEUDOGOUT

Closely resembles gout. It usually occurs in middle life, and afflicts one or more joints. There is a tendency for the larger joints, particularly the knee, to be affected. The attacks of acute arthritis last days, or a week or two. Occasionally 'pseudotophi' are seen in the ears.

Radiographs show striking calcification in cartilage, and none of the rarefied areas in bone seen in gout. Aspiration of the fluid from an acutely inflamed joint shows crystals of *calcium pyrophosphate,* as opposed to uric acid crystals in a gouty joint.

Treatment is the same as acute gout The disease runs a prolonged course, and joints that are repeatedly affected tend to become osteo-arthritic.

PORPHYRIA

In man, porphyrins are synthesised chiefly in the liver and bone marrow, and the clinical syndromes associated with their disordered metabolism may be divided into the *hepatic* and *erythropoietic* varieties. The initial precursor is glycine, which is changed first to delta-amino-levulinic acid (ALA) and then to porphobilinogen (PBG). This is converted chiefly to uroporphyrin III with a little uroporphyrin I. The uroporphyrin III is further metabolised to protoporphyrin, and finally to haem. It is then available as a protein prosthetic group. In health up to 100 μg./24 hours of porphyrin appears in the urine, of which 60–80 per cent is coproporphyrin I; there is also some uroporphyrin present. The faecal porphyrin amounts to 200–300 μg./24 hours, chiefly coproporphyrin I.

A number of clinical syndromes are associated with disorders of porphyrin metabolism, primary or secondary. The secondary ones are asymptomatic with the exception of lead poisoning, and may occur after poisoning with a large number of substances toxic to the bone marrow. These include phosphorous, arsenic, sedormid, sulphonal, and trional. Lead is the most important, for the occurrence of abdominal colic, constipation, vomiting, and motor polyneuritis makes the differential diagnosis from acute intermittent porphyria a matter of moment. Other evidence of plumbism (p. 565), however, and the occurrence in the urine only of coproporphyrin III, which is colourless, and the absence of porphobilinogen, serve to distinguish it.

Of the primary porphyrias, only intermittent acute porphyria (IAP vide infra) is anything other than rare, and itself is uncommon. They may be divided clinically as follows:

(1) *Intermittent Acute Porphyria*

This is a dramatic disease. It appears usually in the third decade, and acute exacerbations are often precipitated by barbiturates. The sex incidence is equal, and inheritance seems governed by a dominant gene. Colic, vomiting, and constipation are reminiscent of lead poisoning. Peripheral neuritis is common, and irritability, termagantism, delirium, and hallucinations may occur. Fever, tachycardia, and moderate hypertension are common. Skin lesions, and haematologic abnormalities do not occur. Oliguria is the rule, and the urine is colourless, but as it contains large amounts of PBG and ALA it rapidly turns to the colour of port wine on standing. The diagnosis, however, depends upon chemical testing, not on any colour change.

Treatment is symptomatic. Pethidine may be used to control pain. Chloral hydrate or paraldehyde should be prescribed for sedation; barbiturates must be avoided, as they aggravate the condition and may precipitate paralysis.

(2) *Erythropoietic Photoporphyria*

It appears in childhood or adolescence, and its hallmark is dermal photo-sensitivity, presenting as solar urticaria or solar eczema. Skin reactions usually start within minutes of exposure to sunlight, and subside within 24 hours without permanent damage to the skin. The reaction has been shown to be due to a narrow band of light (400 mμ) near to the ultra-violet. This is identical with the maximum absorption band of the porphyrins.

The concentration of protoporphyrin is greatly increased in the erythrocytes and faeces. The stool may show red fluorescence with ultra-violet light.

(3) *Variegate Porphyria*

This is an hepatic type, and is common in South Africa. It is strongly familial, and its outstanding feature is skin sensitivity both to sunlight and mechanical trauma. Acute abdominal and neurological episodes may occur (vide supra, IAP) and the excretion of protoporphyrin and coproporphyrin in the faeces is continuously raised.

(4) *Congenital Erythropoietic Porphyria*

This is a rare inborn error of metabolism. It appears in childhood, and three-quarters of the cases are in males. It is inherited as a recessive, and a similar condition affects cattle, pigs, and possibly squirrels. Porphyrins are deposited in the bones, which are strained brown, and the teeth, which assume a lavender hue; there is a bright-red fluorescence with UVL. Porphyrins are also deposited in the skin, where they cause light sensitivity dermatitis. Histamine is released on exposure to sunlight, and a blistering eruption results. This heals with intense scarring, particularly over the nose and fingers, so that eventually scleroderma (p. 333) may be simulated. Hypertrichosis may also occur and there may be subacute haemolysis with splenomegaly. The urine is port-wine colour, and both urine and faeces contain large amounts of porphyrins, chiefly uroporphyrin I. Abdominal pains, and nervous manifestations are rare, and the patients are not sensitive to barbiturates.

Treatment is the avoidance of exposure to sunlight. Splenectomy has been performed in some cases with good effect.

CARCINOID TUMOUR

The argentaffin cells of the appendix (and elsewhere) may give rise to tumours which appear histologically to be malignant but which clinically seem relatively benign; hence the name, carcin-oid.

The tumours secrete a substance named *serotonin* (5-hydroxytryptamine, 5 H.T.) which stimulates smooth muscle. Normally it is detoxicated in the liver and probably the lungs, but if secondary hepatic carcinoid deposits have occurred, then high levels of 5 H.T. appear in the blood. This causes widespread disturbance of smooth muscle. In the bowel, watery diarrhoea is provoked. There is widespread cutaneous suffusion, most marked in the face, and punctuated by attacks of vivid flushing, lasting for a minute or two and often precipitated by alcohol. Stimulation of the smooth muscle in the bronchi may cause asthmatic spasm, with persistent wheezing. A thick white layer of fibrous tissue is deposited on the endocardium of the right side of the heart, causing pulmonary and tricuspid stenosis, and eventually leading to cardiac failure.

Some of the 5 H.T. in the body is converted into 5 hydroxy-indole acetic acid (5 H.I.A.A.), which is excreted in the urine and may be detected with Ehrlich's aldehyde reagent.

Treatment is unsatisfactory. Intestinal symptoms can sometimes be controlled by methysergide which blocks the action of S.H.T. The dose is 1–2 mg. three times daily. The course is variable, and patients may survive for ten years or more; the disease is always ultimately fatal.

AMYLOID DISEASE

Amyloid is an abnormal protein which may accumulate in the tissues around either reticulin or collagen fibres. It is commonly secondary to long-standing inflammation, for example, rheumatoid arthritis or tuberculosis, when it is perireticular in distribution. It may also complicate myelomatosis (p. 483) and is then pericollagenous. Rarely it is seen as a primary disease, which may be familial; in this case both types of deposition may be seen.

(1) In secondary amyloidosis infiltration occurs in the liver, spleen, kidneys, small intestines, arteries and skin. The heart is spared. More rarely endocrine glands, such as the adrenals or parathyroids are involved. The patient's already bad health grows worse, the skin takes on a waxy appearance, and diarrhoea and polyuria appear. Treatment is of the primary cause. There is some evidence that amyloidosis may be reversible in its early stages.

(2) When it complicates myelomatosis the kidney is specially involved, and a nephrotic syndrome may result.

(3) Primary amyloidosis is a rare disease affecting men and women equally, and occasionally familial. It occurs between 20 and 40, and may involve the heart, kidneys, muscles of swallowing and breathing, the peripheral nerves or the brain, the lymph nodes, liver and spleen, either singly or together. No treatment is very satisfactory but steroids (p. 572) are worthy of trial.

WILSON'S DISEASE (Hepatolenticular Degeneration)

Wilson's disease is a recessive metabolic disease which is characterized by degeneration of the basal ganglia, cirrhosis of the liver, and a brownish pigmented ring at the limbus of the cornea (Kayser-Fleischer rings). The disease is due to an increased absorption and/or a decreased excretion of dietary copper which leads to a progressive increase in the total body copper with consequent damage to the tissues of the brain, liver, and renal tubules.

Clinical Features. Wilson's disease is slightly more common in males than females and usually becomes clinically recognizable between the age of fifteen and thirty years. Except in young children in whom symptoms of cirrhosis of the liver are common, neurological symptoms predominate. Tremor and rigidity of the limbs are common presenting symptoms. Dysarthria is a frequent early symptom. Rarely, symptoms of cirrhosis of the liver may predominate and the patient die of liver failure in the absence of neurological signs. The disease is usually fatal within fifteen years of onset.

Laboratory Investigation. A decreased level of serum copper and ceruloplasmin associated with an increased urinary copper excretion is diagnostic. A normal level of ceruloplasmin does not exclude the diagnosis if Kayser-Fleischer rings are present. A low serum uric acid is common. Increased aminoaciduria is usual but not invariable.

Differential Diagnosis. The disease should be suspected in all disturbances of basal ganglion function and in all cases of juvenile cirrhosis of the liver. The presence of a Kayser-Fleischer ring is pathognomonic. Slit lamp examination is necessary in doubtful cases.

Treatment. This is directed towards removing the excess copper and decreasing dietary intake of copper. Penicillamine increases the urinary excretion of copper and is the treatment of choice (1·0–2·0 g. daily). Treatment may have to be continued indefinitely. Improvement in some patients may be striking.

FURTHER READING

Duncan, G. G. *Diseases of Metabolism*, Edited by Bondy, P. K. 6th edition. Saunders, Philadelphia, 1969.

Joslin, E. P., *et al. Treatment of Diabetes Mellitus*, 11th edition. Kimpton, London, 1971.

Thompson, R. H. S. and Wootton, I. D. P. *Biochemical Disorders in Human Disease*, 2nd edn. Churchill, London, 1970.

CHAPTER THIRTEEN

DISEASES OF THE ENDOCRINE GLANDS

HYPOTHALAMUS

It has long been known that diseases of this part of the brain were associated with disturbances of such profound functions as body weight, temperature regulation, sleep rhythm, water balance, and sexual function. The mechanisms by which such control are effected are only just emerging. It seems probable that within the hypothalamus there are discrete groups of cells capable of secreting hormones which have either inhibiting or stimulating effects on the pituitary and possibly other endocrine glands. The regulator of the activities of these centres seems to be the blood level of the hormone secreted by the glands themselves, acting cybernetically.

The messenger substances from the hypothalamus are secreted into its capillary bed and pass through portal veins to the pituitary. They have been extracted and partially analysed. They are substances of low molecular weight, probably polypeptides. They may be divided into those stimulating and those inhibiting pituitary function as follows.

Stimulating

Thyrotropine Releasing Factor (TRF)
Corticotropine Releasing Factor (CRF)
Somatotropic Releasing Factor (SRF)
Luteinising Hormone Releasing Factor (LRF)
Follicle Stimulating Hormone Releasing Factor (FRF)

Inhibiting

Prolactin-Inhibiting Factor (PIF)
Melanocyte Stimulating Hormone-Inhibiting Factor (MSH-IF)

A total deficiency of all these factors can be induced by section of the pituitary stalk, as is practised therapeutically in certain cases of malignant disease. Their production may be reduced in those diseases known to affect the hypothalamus, e.g. craniopharyngiomas, pinealomas, chromophobe adenomas and sarcoidosis. Overproduction is believed to occur in Cushing's syndrome, and to be responsible for some cases of precocious puberty.

The place of this new knowledge in clinical medicine at present is far from certain, but clearly the observations are of immense potential importance. It may offer an explanation for the observations of Nelson (1958) of the appearance of a chromophobe adenoma of the pituitary associated with skin pigmentation after bilateral adrenalectomy for Cushing's syndrome (p. 449). At operation both adrenal glands were found to be hyperplastic. After the appearance of the pigmentation, raised blood levels of ACTH and raised urinary levels of MSH were demonstrated.

THE PITUITARY GLAND

Introduction

There are three types of cell present which may be distinguished histologically—chromophobe, eosinophilic and basophilic. Each type may proliferate with typical consequences.

Chromophobe Adenoma

These tumours are uncommon but not rare and occur at any age and in either sex. They produce their effects by direct pressure on surrounding structures. The sella turcica is uniformly expanded, causing a bitemporal headache with a typical 'bursting' quality. There is pressure on the optic chiasma with early loss of visual acuity, proceeding to bitemporal hemianopia and optic atrophy. The olfactory nerves or their connections may be displaced, giving rise to anosmia. If the tumour becomes very large then it may behave as a space-occupying lesion (p. 287). Pressure on the *hypothalamus* causes some or all of a highly characteristic group of symptoms and signs.

(1) Weight gain.
(2) Somnolence.
(3) Polydypsia.
(4) Reduced B.M.R. and hypothermia.
(5) Low blood pressure.
(6) Scanty body hair.
(7) Loss of libido, reduced potentia sexualis.
(8) Disturbed menses, mammary hypoplasia.

To confirm the diagnosis it should be possible to demonstrate expansion of the sella turcica radiologically, and typical changes are seen in the visual fields. Treatment is by surgery and radiotherapy, and prognosis should be guarded.

Eosinophilic Adenoma

If the adenoma forms before the epiphyses have fused *gigantism* results; if they are already closed then *acromegaly* is produced. These syndromes frequently occur together. They have their counterparts in animal pathology. The Irish wolfhound has many of the features of gigantism, whereas the British bulldog is typical of acromegaly. Minor degrees of both abnormalities are common in any human population, but extreme examples are rare.

Gigantism

Giants are defined as people who are unusually tall as compared with other members of their population, this increased height being due to a pathological process. The elongation is due chiefly to disproportionately long arms and legs, and is usually associated with muscular weakness. The genitalia are small, and secondary sexual characteristics are poorly developed. Associated acromegalic features are common. Hyperphagia may occur. Diagnosis may be confirmed as in chromophobe adenomas. Treatment is by deep X-rays, and the prognosis is poor.

Acromegaly

This follows an insidious course over 20 to 30 years or longer. Early complaints are of easy tiredness, muscular aching, asthenia, excessive sweating, and tingling in the fingers from median nerve compression (p. 308). Later *progressive enlargement of the hands and feet* may be noticed, usually when buying gloves or shoes, or of the head when buying a hat. *Enlargement of the jaws* may cause dentures not to fit. All these symptoms occur so gradually that usually the diagnosis is not made for several years, and often only comes to light by chance. Later symptoms are of failure of secondary sexual characters, *amenorrhoea* in women and *loss of libido* and impotence in men.

Examination shows that the features are coarsened, with prominent supra-orbital ridges and jutting of the lower jaw. The bite may override, and the molar teeth become separated. The lips are thick, and the nose becomes large and bulbous. The skin is thickened and thrown into wrinkles and there is hypertrophy of the sebaceous glands and of hair follicles. Pigmentation may occur. The mucous membrane of the mouth is thickened, and the tongue is large, coarse, and thick. The hands are characteristic, and described as 'spade-like'; this appearance is caused by broadening and thickening of the fingers and palms. The volume of the larynx is increased, and the vocal cords thickened and elongated. This may cause a change in tone of the voice and some hoarseness. Kyphosis is progressive, and is due to enlargement of vertebrae. Osteoporosis rarely occurs. At post-mortem generalised splanchnomegaly is found.

Other endocrine disturbances may also be present. Menstrual irregularity in women is the rule, with loss of libido. In men there may be a transient phase of increased libido, but complete loss and gonadal atrophy eventually result. Persistent lactation in both sexes is occasionally (5 per cent) noticed. The thyroid gland is often enlarged, and the B.M.R. may be raised. Frank thyrotoxicosis is rare, however. Diabetes mellitus is frequent, and there may be evidence of hypothalamic disturbance.

The *diagnosis* is confirmed as for a chromophobe tumour, and treatment is by radiotherapy. Indications for treatment are visual failure, intractable headaches, and progressive development of distressing signs or symptoms. The results of treatment are not good and prognosis should be guarded. Death may result from intracranial extension of the tumour, diabetes mellitus or its complications (p. 405), heart failure, intercurrent infection, or hypopituitarism.

HYPOPITUITARISM (Simmonds' Disease)

Introduction. The commonest cause of pituitary failure is from necrosis following haemorrhage at the time of parturition. This accounts for over 80 per cent of all proved cases. Other causes are destruction by tumours, granulomatous lesions, trauma, and impairment of blood supply. It is much commoner in women than men. Effects are produced by a failure of secretion of hormones from the anterior lobe of the pituitary.

Clinical Features. The usual story is of a woman who some years before had a severe ante- or post-partum haemorrhage. Because of the failure of secretion of lactogenic hormone she was unable to breast-feed the child, and noticed painless subsidence of the breasts over the ensuing two or three weeks. This is followed by almost complete atrophy of the breast tissue, to some extent masked by subcutaneous fat. Gonadotrophic hormones also fail, both FSH and LH, causing regression of secondary sexual characteristics. The uterus withers to a tiny organ, and the cervix can be felt as a dimple only. The vagina also shrinks, and typically vaginal secretions fail; the special bacterial flora of the vagina disappear, and are replaced by those commonly found on the skin. Menstruation ceases, usually completely, but occasionally very minor bleeding occurs irregularly. There is loss of body hair, both pubic and axillary, except for a few sparse hairs on the labia majora. There is some loss of capital hair and of the eyebrows, but this may be caused by the concomitant hypothyroidism. At the same time the body's contour changes, so as to resemble the male outline. Loss of libido is complete.

Failure of secretion of other pituitary hormones leads to secondary failure of other organs.

(a) Growth hormone is not secreted, and at post-mortem generalised microsplanchnia is found.

(b) Melanocyte stimulating hormone (MSH) fails, causing widespread and highly characteristic depigmentation and pallor.

(c) Adrenocorticotropic hormone (ACTH) is not secreted, with consequent secondary adrenal failure. The appetite is poor, sweating is reduced, and there is striking loss of volition. Asthenia is marked. Hypoglycaemic attacks (p. 421) may occur, and the blood pressure is low.

(d) Failure of thyrotropic hormone (TSH) causes secondary myxoedema (p. 442). In some cases the myxoedematous facies, pallor, and asthenia lead to an erroneous diagnosis of a myopathy. Psychic changes are common, usually of a paranoid character, and normal female modesty is lost.

Special Investigations. The clinical picture when complete is so striking that confirmation is hardly needed. It should be noted that severe cachexia is not common, and its presence is not essential to the diagnosis. When less typical, however, the diagnosis may be confirmed by estimating the plasma cortisol (p. 448) which is very low. Normal values for men and women are 8–22 and 5–18 mg./24 hours respectively. In hypopituitarism and adrenal insufficiency they are greatly reduced. In hypopituitarism the values increase with ACTH. In the same way thyroid function (p. 442) is reduced, but will improve with TSH. The glucose tolerance test is abnormal, for slow absorption of sugar from the gut leads to hypoglycaemia and a flat curve (p. 408). Urinary FSH is very low or absent. Normochromic anaemia, leucopenia, and sometime eosinphilia are found.

Treatment. Much the best treatment is to achieve another pregnancy, when the remnants of the pituitary gland will increase in size and normal secretion may be restored. Unfortunately pregnancy is very difficult to accomplish in this condition. Failing this, the patients may be symptomatically improved by androgens (methyl testosterone 20–50 mg. sublingually daily), and cortisone (cortisone 25–50 mg. daily), or by ACTH. Some benefit from thyroxine (0·1–0·3 mg.), daily, but this should be given with caution.

Complications and Prognosis. Most of the patients with the disease live between 10 and 20 years from the onset and death in coma is the usual end. Expectation of life with proper treatment is normal Coma may be due to hypoglycaemia, hypoadrenalism or hypothermia. Blood sugar and electrolytes should be estimated at once, and the rectal temperature taken with a thermometer capable of recording as low as 85° F. The treatment of hypoglycaemia coma (p. 421) and Addisonian crisis (p. 451) are discussed elsewhere. Hypothermic coma is relieved by gradually warming the patient, either with relays of warm blankets or in a tepid bath. Heat cradles or other electric heating devices cause too rapid warming and are best avoided. Coma is often precipitated by intercurrent infection, which should always be treated seriously; during infections the patient should take supplementary cortisone (100–300 mg. daily).

THE THYROID GLAND

Introduction

Overaction of the gland produces the syndrome of hyperthyroidism; under-secretion causes myxoedema. Enlargement of the gland (goitre) may be associated with either of these conditions, or may occur in a euthyroid state.

Simple Goitre

If elemental iodine is not freely available for the iodination of tyrosine then excess of colloid is formed, and a *goitre* results. This may be because of geological insufficiency of iodine (Derbyshire neck, etc.), or because it is displaced by an excess of fluorine. It may also be rendered unavailable by substances occurring with it; this may explain the influence of water pollution on the distribution of goitre in the Himalayas. Or it may be prevented from following its physiological course by inborn errors of metabolism (*goitrous cretinism*) or the ingestion or absorption of toxic substances, for example cabbage stalk factor or resorcinol. Commonly the cause cannot be discovered.

Simple goitre occurs frequently in euthyroid adolescent girls and it is usually self limiting.

Treatment depends upon cause. Iodination of table salt has prevented goitres in most endemic areas.

THYROTOXICOSIS

Introduction. With the possible exception of the eye signs all the features of hyperthyroidism can be reproduced by the administration of thyroid hormone. None the less, two distinct clinical forms of the disease can be recognised, one associated with a soft, regular, diffuse enlargement, and the other with irregular enlargement of the gland from multiple adenomata. Distinguishing features are tabulated blow.

	Diffuse Goitre	*Nodular Goitre*
Age	Less than 35	Over 35
Neurological symptoms and signs	marked	not prominent
Eye signs	marked	uncommon
Cardiac symptoms and signs	not prominent	marked
Recurrence after surgery	not uncommon	rare

Clinical Features. (a) *Symptoms.* Common complaints are of increased irritability, emotional lability, tremor, sweating, intolerance for hot weather, and palpitations. There is usually loss of weight, and sometimes diarrhoea. Amenorrhoea is common in women; occasionally menorrhagia may occur. Hyperphagia is sometimes noticed, and occasionally muscular weakness and asthenia are prominent.

(b) *Signs.* Much can be learned by examining the eyes. They may be staring, with infrequent blinking, or frankly protruded, with dilated pupils. The upper lid may lag behind the globe as gaze is lowered, momentarily unmasking a rim of sclera above the cornea—so-called 'lid lag'. Other evidence of sympathetic overactivity may be found in the tremor, tachycardia, nervousness, and agitation, rarely progressing to true delirium. The eyelids may be pigmented and generalised pigmentation of Addisonism type may also occur. Weakness of ocular muscles may cause difficulty, particularly in upward gaze. This is associated with infiltration of the muscles with lymphocytes. Skeletal muscle is not spared; acute *thyrotoxic myopathy* is rare and causes rapidly developing muscular wasting and weakness which may end in death. Lesser degrees of chronic thyrotoxic myopathy are common, and cause wasting and weakness, especially of proximal muscle groups. Difficulty in climbing stairs is an early symptom. A myasthenia-like syndrome also occurs, responding to nothing but control of the thyrotoxicosis.

Tachycardia, with forceful overaction of the cardiac impulse and sometimes auricular fibrillation, usually paroxysmal (10 per cent) but occasionally constant (5 per cent), may occur. Heart failure may supervene.

There are other general signs of the disease. The patients are usually thin; uncommonly they are fat. The skin is warm and often damp from sweat, and both skin and hair are of a silky texture—in marked contrast to myxoedema. Dermatographia is common. There may be generalised lymphadenopathy, and rarely splenomegaly. Osteoporosis may occur, sometimes with collapse of vertebrae or rib fractures.

To be certain that a swelling is in the thyroid gland it must be shown to be situated deep to the sternomastoid muscles and to be attached to the larynx; that is to say, it should move with the larynx on swallowing. It may be associated with redness of the overlying skin, and systolic pulsation in the neck is usually obvious. A loud systolic bruit may be heard over the gland. Palpation is best made from behind, with the neck flexed. The gland may be diffusely enlarged, and soft, or irregularly nodular and harder. Retrosternal prolongation of the gland cannot readily be felt, but may displace the trachea. It is easily seen on lateral chest radiography.

Not all the signs described are usually present, and none is invariable. Many subtle clinical varieties of this common disease exist to tax diagnostic acumen.

Special Investigations. Laboratory studies show the B.M.R. to be raised, and the uptake of ^{132}I by the gland is increased (p. 444) as is the turnover of iodine as measured by the rate at which radioactive protein bound iodine (PB^{132}I) appears in the plasma. The serum protein bound iodine is increased, as is the saturation of thyroid-binding globulin by thyroxine, which may be measured by the tri-iodo-thyronine resin uptake (T_3) test. Food is absorbed rapidly from the intestine and the glucose tolerance test shows the 'lag' form (p. 408). Intermittent glycosuria is common, and excess creatinuria is usual. There may be an absolute lymphocytosis in the blood.

In doubtful cases the thyroid stimulating hormone (TSH) suppression test may be carried out. Its principle is that if normal subjects are given thyroid derivatives TSH is suppressed, and thyroid activity, as estimated by ^{132}I uptake, is greatly reduced. In hyperthyroidism this is not so, the gland behaving autonomously throughout.

All tests involving iodine may be vitiated if the patient has recently taken iodine preparations for diagnostic or therapeutic reasons: other drugs, in particular the contraceptive pill and pregnancy may cause similar effects.

Treatment. This is by means either of surgical removal of the gland, the use of drugs which interfere with the synthesis of thyroid hormone, or by using ^{131}I which is selectively concentrated in the gland and destroys it by local radiation. Each case must be considered on its merits, and the treatment of choice will occasionally be in doubt. Some indications and contra-indications for these various modes of therapy which are currently accepted may be stated.

(a) *Surgery.* Indications
       (1) Possibility of malignancy.
       (2) Marked pressure symptoms.
       (3) Retrosternal goitre.
       (4) Enormous goitres.
       (5) Refusal to accept medical treatment.
       (6) Sensitivity to antithyroid drugs.

(b) *Medical Treatment.*
  (1) Drugs.
      (i) Mild hyperthyroidism in young women, which is often self limiting.
      (ii) Patients too frail or too ill for surgical treatment.
      (iii) During pregnancy.
  (2) Radioactive (^{131}I) iodine.

When generally available this may be the treatment of choice for all patients in whom surgery is not indicated. Exceptions are pregnancy; failure to concentrate the iodine in the gland; and young patients, in view of the risk of malignant change in the gland many years later. Subsequent hypothyroidism is common, the incidence rising progressively during the years after treatment.

The *antithyroid drugs* currently used are propyl thiouracil, carbimazole and propranolol. Propyl thiouracil is given initially as 200–400 mg. daily. The effect is seen in about three weeks, after which the dose can be reduced to 50–100 mg. daily. Carbimazole is first given in a dosage of 10–40 mg. daily, later reducing to 15–5 mg. daily. It is slower acting than propyl thiouracil, and its maximal effects are not seen for about two months. Both drugs cause toxic reactions, carbimazole rather less readily than propyl thiouracil. They consist of skin rashes and blood dyscrasias, the most important of which is granulopenia. Recently propranolol (p. 118) has been used and seems particularly valuable where tachycardia is severe.

Thyrotoxicosis is not uncommon during pregnancy, and should be treated cautiously with propyl thiouracil and sedation.

Malignant Exophthalmos

Clinical Features. It is more common in males, and normally occurs in middle life. Evidence of hyperthyroidism is not usually marked, nor is the gland much enlarged. Proptosis is usually extreme, and frequently unequal. The changes which should arouse suspicion, however, are slight oedema of the eyelids, with inability to close them completely, chemosis of the cornea, oedema of the conjunctiva with hyperaemia and epiphora and photophobia. In the later stages frank ulceration of the cornea may occur. There may also be reduced mobility of the eye, usually impaired elevation, and inco-ordination of the recti and oblique muscles, causing diplopia. Pupillary reactions are normal, but there may be papilloedema and later optic atrophy.

Malignant exophthalmos is sometimes associated with clubbing of the fingers, and with *pretibial myxoedema*. This describes the occurrence of patches of myxoedematous tissue, usually over the shins, but sometimes in other parts of the body, and rarely confluent so as to give the appearance of elephantiasis to the leg. The patches are raised, purplish pink in colour, cold to touch and do not pit on pressure.

Treatment. Treatment of malignant exophthalmos is unsatisfactory. In an emergency the eye can usually be saved by temporary tarsorrhaphy; occasionally decompression of the orbit is necessary. No treatment is very good and most patients are left with unsightly exophthalmos and often diplopia, though thyroid hormone has been tried to attempt pituitary suppression. Recently some benefit has been obtained by the use of guanethidine eye drops (5%). Some rapidly progressive cases are improved by steroids in high dosage.

MYXOEDEMA

Introduction. The syndrome of myxoedema is much commoner in women than in men. It may result from primary failure of the thyroid gland, failure of secretion of thyrotropic hormone (TSH), or from excess loss of serum protein-bound iodine in the urine in nephrosis. The myxoedematous elements of advanced nephrosis are of interest, but are overshadowed by the renal disorder. Failure of TSH secretion is readily distinguished from primary myxoedema by the associated features resulting from failure of secretion of other pituitary hormones (p. 434) and by the effect of TSH injection on thyroid function.

Primary thyroid deficiency may occur for a number of reasons. The thyroid may fail to develop, causing cretinism; or there may be an inborn error of metabolism in the gland itself, causing goitrous cretinism. The gland may be destroyed by disease processes, such as acute thyroiditis, or by auto-antibodies (p. 327). It may be too fully removed surgically, or destroyed by radiotherapy. Its activities may be deranged by goitrogens, such as thiouracil, carbimazole, or resorcinol. Conditions of iodine deficiency may exist, so that an essential raw material for the manufacture of thyroid hormone is lacking. Most commonly, however, no cause for the gland's failure can be discovered; this type is commoner in the second half of life. The presence of thyroid auto-antibodies in some case suggests a relationship to Hashimoto's thyroibitis. Ten per cent of patients with spontaneous myxoedema also have pernicious anaemia.

Clinical Features. (a) *Symptoms.* Early symptoms are of *fatigue* and weakness, and of muscular cramps and aching. There is lethargy and drowsiness unrelieved by sleep. *Intolerance to cold* is common, and although appetite is poor the body weight increases. Memory is bad, and there is progressive *mental dulling* ending in dementia. The *voice is hoarse* and low pitched, and speech is thick and slow.

The hair falls out progressively, starting above the forehead, and the outer third of the eyebrows and body hair may become scanty. The carpal tunnel syndrome (p. 308) occurs frequently, and constipation may be profound. Menstrual disturbances are common. Menorrhagia or amenorrhoea may occur, with loss of libido and sterility.

(b) *Signs.* The face is pale, of a yellowish hue, and generally puffy, especially round the eyes. Eventually the whole body may be encased in myxoedematous tissue, which thickens and blunts the features but does not pit on pressure. The skin is dry, rough and cold, and the hair coarse and sparse. It falls progressively, and untreated patients become bald. The body temperature is lowered, and the pulse may be slow. Reduced blood pressure is the rule, but sometimes systolic hypertension occurs. The heart is enlarged, and the heart sounds muffled. Pericardial effusions may occur, sometimes with generalised oedema. Peripheral vasoconstriction is the rule, but despite this postural hypotension is common. Angina is an occasional complaint, and is sometimes relieved by treatment of the myxoedema. Anaemia is common. The absorption of food from the gut is delayed, and peristalsis is reduced, causing tympanites and constipation. Spontaneous hypoglycaemia may also occur, possibly from failure of mobilisation of glucose from liver glycogen, and there is marked sensitivity to morphine (as in liver cirrhosis) and sometimes deafness of a conduction type. Rarely there may be exophthalmos. The ankle jerks are sluggish and reduced.

Usually the gland cannot be felt. If it is large and soft, iodine deficiency should be suspected. If it is rubbery, the cause underlying may be Hashimoto's disease (p. 445); if it is iron hard, Riedel's thyroiditis.

Myxoedema Coma

Coma is unusual and occurs most frequently in elderly women with unrecognised myxoedema. It is of gradual onset. There is a general slowing down of all vital processes, so that the pulse is slow, breathing shallow, and the body cold and the temperature lowered. Convulsions may occur. Hypothermia (rectal temperature 80–90° F.), hypoxia, hypercapnia, hypoglycaemia and hyponatraemia may all play a part in its causation.

Treatment is by gradual heating of the body with relays of warm blankets and the maintenance of an adequate airway for the administration of oxygen. Tri-iodothyronine 0·02 mg. eight-hourly should be given because of its rapid tissue action, and also hydrocortisone mg. 100 I.V. eight-hourly. If hypotension is marked then a nor-adrenaline infusion should be given.

Prognosis is very bad; once coma has supervened, over two-thirds of all patients die.

Special Investigations. The diagnosis may be confirmed by measuring the basal metabolic rate (B.M.R.) which is reduced, or by estimating the amount of 131 iodine taken up by the gland. Uptake is uninfluenced by TSH in primary myxoedema, nor are auto-antibodies present. The serum protein-bound iodine is reduced as is the saturation of thyroid-binding globulin (p. 440). The E.C.G. shows typical changes (p. 146), and the serum cholesterol is markedly raised (250–500 mg./100 ml.). Achlorhydria occurs in about half of the patients, and there may be normochromic normocytic anaemia, more rarely macrocytic anaemia.

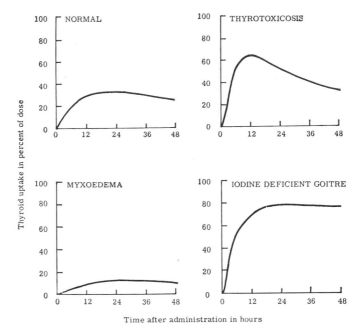

Time after administration in hours

THE UPTAKE OF RADIOIODINE TRACER DOSE IN THE THYROID GLAND
(After Veall and Vetter)

Treatment. All but a few patients respond excellently to 1-thyroxine (0·2–0·5 mg.). A word of caution must be given: the worse the condition appears and the more urgent treatment seems the smaller the initial dose should be. In very severe cases as little as 0·05 mg. should be given initially, the dose being doubled at weekly intervals until a maintenance level is reached. Most patients respond excellently, and require 0·1–0·3 mg. daily. If they do not then a trial with tri-iodothyronine (10–100 μg.) should be made; this is a rapidly acting drug, and therapeutic response may be used as a confirmation of the diagnosis.

The whole dose of thyroid, however large, may be given at one time. Failure to start treatment with low dosage may precipitate angina pectoris or left ventricular failure with pulmonary congestion.

Prognosis in cases diagnosed early is excellent. As long as thyroid hormone administration is continued they do well. Cases in which diagnosis has been delayed may develop coronary or cerebral atheroma, and very great delay in diagnosis may lead to irreversible mental changes.

SUBACUTE THYROIDITIS

Introduction. Occurs usually between the ages of twenty and fifty and is three times more common in women than in men. Frequently there is pre-existing goitre. Half of the patients have a brief infection of the upper respiratory tract immediately before the onset of specific symptoms, which may also follow many of the acute specific fevers.

Clinical Features. There are general signs of an infection, with dysphagia, hoarseness, non-productive cough, and pain in the region of the gland. This is swollen, hot, and tender, and may be adherent to overlying structures. Whole or part of the gland may be affected. The disease is self-limiting and most cases recover within a few months. Occasionally the general signs of disease improve, but the local evidence of involvement of the gland remains. Needle or drill biopsy is diagnostic.

Treatment. Initially bed rest, extra fluids, analgesics, and local cooling of the gland. If evidence of hyperthyroidism appears then propylthiouracil should be given. Steroids (prednisolone 5–10 mg. 3 times daily) are often of value.

HASHIMOTO'S DISEASE (Hashimoto's lymphadenoid goitre)

Introduction. It is uncommon, but not rare. Almost confined to women between the ages of twenty and fifty, it has occasionally been reported in identical twins. It usually presents as myxoedema (p. 442), but there is sometimes a short and mild hyperthyroid introduction to what is essentially a hypothyroid disease. The gland is symmetrically enlarged, firm, and rubbery, and microscopy shows dense infiltration with lymphocytic cells.

It was noticed that the E.S.R. was frequently raised, and this was shown to be due to excess of gamma globulins in the serum. These globulins also caused abnormal results if the empirical tests for liver function (p. 91) were made. More recently it has been shown that these gamma globulins are in fact auto-antibodies to the intracellular contents of the gland itself. Serological tests have now been developed to these antibodies, thus rendering the diagnosis more precise, and allowing identification of the disease in a number of patients with apparently uncomplicated non-goitrous myxoedema. Another recent observation is the association of Paget's disease of bone with Hashimoto's disease, and the frequent presence of auto-antibodies to the thyroid gland in systemic lupus erythematosus (p. 330).

Treatment. Large doses (0·5–1·0 mg. of l-thyroxine daily) are necessary; this causes reduction in size of the gland and restoration of the serum gamma globulin levels to normal. Prednisolone 5–10 mg. 3 times daily may be of value in resistant cases.

RIEDEL'S DISEASE (Riedel's woody or ligneous thyroiditis)

This is an excessively rare disease. In 42,000 thyroidectomies performed at the Mayo Clinic over 36 years only 20 cases were discovered. The hallmark of the disease is the extremely hard thyroid gland (*Eisenharte Tumoren*) and the invasion of the surrounding tissues by the disease process. Treatment is surgical, and the prognosis good.

THE ADRENAL GLAND

Introduction

There are two parts to the adrenal gland, the cortex and the medulla. The chief secretions from the medulla are adrenaline and nor-adrenaline, and from the cortex a number of steroid compounds. These steroids have three chief activities: virilisation, conversion of tissue proteins to glucose, and salt and water retention.

Pituitary and Adrenal Function Tests

This subject has been revolutionised by the fluorimetric assay of 11-hydroxycorticosteroids ('Cortisol') in the plasma. The levels vary throughout the 24 hours, and normal values are tabulated below. Patterns of secretion are of more importance than individual levels, and estimations are customarily made at 9.00 a.m., midday, and midnight.

Adrenal Suppression Test

Synthetic steroids given orally to normal subjects completely suppress the output of ACTH from the pituitary with consequent fall in adrenal function. In Cushing's syndrome it is usual to see no such effect; in some advanced cases a degree of suppression may be seen initially, but 'midday escape' is then usual.

Adrenal Stimulation Test

The adrenal can be stimulated directly by the intramuscular injection of Tetracosactrin.

Pituitary Stimulation Test

Intramuscular injection of Lysine-8-Vasopressin (L8V) causes direct stimulation of the pituitary.

Insulin Sensitivity Test of Pituitary Stress Response

Hypoglycaemia is induced with intravenous insulin. Plasma cortisol response is a measure of the integrity of the hypothalamus, pituitary, and adrenal glands and their connections.

VALUES OF PLASMA 11-HYDROXYCORTICOSTEROIDS (CORTISOL) MEASURED FLUORIMETRI-
CALLY IN NORMAL SUBJECTS AND THOSE WITH DISORDERS OF THE ADRENAL AND PITUITARY
GLANDS (MICROGRAMS/100 ML.)

	9.00 *a.m.*	*Mid-day*	*Midnight*
Healthy resting subjects	7–25	7–18	3–7
Normal adrenal suppression level (Dexamethasone 2 mg. orally produces suppression for up to 24 hours)	1·5–5	1·5–5	1·5–5
Cushing's Syndrome (p. 449) (Resting patient)	14–85+	14–85+	14–85+
Cushing's Syndrome (Dexamethasone Suppression)	Never below rest level for normal patients. If morning suppression occurs, midday or evening 'escape' is significant.		

Time in Minutes	0	30	60
Normal adrenal stimulation level (Synacthen 0·25 mg. i.m. after resting blood is drawn)	7–25 ·	30+	30+
Synacthen stimulation in abnormal adrenal function	No stimulation indicates adrenal malfunction (p. 428). Values above 40 indicate prolonged stress, or early Cushing's. Normal resting levels, but failure of response (or low response) is seen in adrenal hypofunction or adrenal hyperplasia (vide infra).		
Normal pituitary stimulation (10 units L-8-V i.m.)	7–25	30+	30+

If the pituitary gland is not functioning then plasma cortisol levels are greater with
Synacthen than with L-8-V. Similar results are seen in response to hypoglycaemia.

ADRENO-CORTICAL OVERACTION

Adreno-genital Syndrome

Excess secretion of androgens in women past puberty causes *virilisation.*
Hirsutism is marked, and the pubic hair is of masculine distribution. The
clitoris enlarges and the breasts shrink, and there is amenorrhoea. The
voice becomes deep, the muscles increase in size, and interests and behaviour become masculine. These changes are usually associated with
tumour formation or hyperplasia of the adrenal cortex. These may be distinguished by the administration of cortisone, which causes suppression of
hyperplastic adrenal glands, but has no effect upon adrenal tumours.
Rarer causes are a virilising ovarian tumour (*arrhenoblastoma*), and occasionally *hyperostosis frontalis interna*, a condition in which there is overgrowth of some of the bones of the skull, possibly causing pituitary stimulation.

Treatment of adrenal tumours is surgical. Hyperplasia may be suppressed
by the continued administration of cortisone, which leads to a dramatic
recession of the condition and subsequent restoration of normality·

PLASMA 11-HYDROXY CORTICOSTEROID (CORTISOL) LEVELS IN DISORDERS OF ADRENAL FUNCTION.

Cushing's Syndrome

Introduction. This is a rare but striking syndrome occurring most commonly in women between twenty and forty; no age is immune, however. Changes include a redistribution of body fat, so that the face is moon-shaped, the trunk fat, and a cervical pad of fat is present, whereas the arms and legs remain slender—the characteristic habitus being described as a 'lemon on toothpicks'. Polycythaemia rubra may occur, causing the face to be red or cyanosed. There is usually some degree of virilism, causing hirsutism, acne, and seborrhoea, and there is complete amenorrhoea. Protein is withdrawn from connective tissue, and converted into carbohydrate. This withdrawal of substance weakens the bones, and causes osteoporosis (p. 351) and pathological fractures (especially of the ribs); blood vessels are similarly affected, so that easy bruising and bleeding are the rule. The skin also suffers, and wide purple striae form over the abdomen and flanks. Carbohydrate metabolism is deranged, and glycosuria and hyperglycaemia are common. Frank diabetes mellitus (p. 405) sometimes results. Hypertension and oedema are frequent, and there is marked muscular weakness; these findings may be attributed to retention of sodium and loss of potassium. Polycythaemia causes a central cyanosis, and makes the abdominal striae even more livid. Psychological changes are sometimes marked and usually of a paranoid character.

The causes of the syndrome lie in oversecretion of adreno-cortical hormones. This may be because of a pituitary *basophil adenoma*, causing cortical hyperplasia, or from primary hyperplasia of the adrenals or tumour formation. Occasionally similar changes are seen with thymic or bronchial carcinomas.

Special Investigations. Increased quantities of 11-hydroxycorticoids and sometimes 17-ketosteroids are excreted in the urine (p. 453). Polycythaemia rubra occurs in about half the cases, and there is usually leucocytosis with lymphocytopenia and eosinopenia. In normal people the plasma *cortisol* level is high in the morning and low in the evening; in Cushing's syndrome this diurnal fluctuation disappears and the 10 p.m. level is above the upper limit of normal (7 μg./100 ml.).

Treatment. This is by excision of whole or part of the adrenals, with or without some replacement with cortisone. Prognosis is good in cases treated early in the disease, but about 10 per cent of those with no evidence of pituitary tumour before adrenalectomy develop signs of a pituitary adenoma after operation. Death results either from heart failure, cerebral haemorrhage, or from a separate carcinoma, which occurs more frequently than can be accounted for by chance alone.

Primary Aldosteronism (Conn's Disease)

This is a rare condition characterised by hypertension, sometimes malignant, leading to impaired renal function, and associated with periodic attacks of muscular weakness indistinguishable from familial periodic paralysis.

There may also be tetany, and severe paraesthesiae.

The level of potassium in the serum is reduced, and the urinary potassium excretion is increased. The total potassium content of the body is reduced, and there is a persistent alkalosis (p. 402). Serum and urinary aldosterone levels are increased. It is usually caused by an adrenal cortical adenoma. Treatment is surgical, and results have been good in the few cases so far reported.

OVER-ACTION OF THE ADRENAL MEDULLA (PHAEOCHROMOCYTOMA)

This too is a rare syndrome but a highly characteristic one. It occurs usually in the fourth and fifth decades, and is usually manifest by paroxysms of acute anxiety, with severe sweating, tachycardia, striking pallor and raised blood pressure. Tremor is marked, and Raynaud's phenomenon (p. 172) may occur. Headache is usual and there may be vomiting or even epileptic fits. During the attack there is hyperglycaemia, and there may be glycosuria.

The usual cause is an adrenal medullary tumour (*phaeochromocytoma*) which is secreting adrenaline and nor-adrenaline (in varying proportions). Similar attacks may occur in tabes dorsalis (p. 284), lead poisoning (p. 564). porphyria (p. 430) and rarely in peripheral neuritis from other causes. It is postulated that there is impaired innervation of the carotid body in all these conditions. Confirmation of the diagnosis of phaeochromocytoma may be made in various ways:

(1) There is undue sensitivity to histamine. If 0·05 mg. of histamine base is given intravenously the systolic blood pressure does not normally rise more than 12 mm. Hg. This figure is substantially exceeded in phaeochromocytomas.

(2) If 5 mg. of phentolamine (rogitine) are given intravenously the blood pressure should fall either to normal levels, or if it is initially very high, by 35 mm. Hg. systolic and 25 mm. diastolic within 20 minutes, in patients with phaeochromocytoma.

(3) By assay of catechol amines or vanilmandelic acid in a 24 hours urine specimen.

Phaeochromocytomas may be removed surgically, and are usually benign.

ADRENAL INSUFFICIENCY (Addison's disease)

Introduction. This insidious disease is uncommon. It is produced by gradual destruction of the adrenal glands by disease. It is commoner in men than women, can occur at any age but is most usual between the ages of twenty and forty. Tuberculosis used to be the commonest cause, but today takes second place to idiopathic atrophy. Very rare causes of destruction are secondary carcinomatous deposits, usually from the bronchus, or involvement by amyloid disease. Acute adrenal failure also causes a typical picture (p. 498).

Clinical Features. (a) *Symptoms.* Early symptoms are *languor, debility, nausea,* and *vomiting.* These are usually accompanied by some *weight loss* and a delicate melanin *pigmentation* of the skin and mucous membranes.

Spontaneous hypoglycaemic attacks may occur (p. 421) giving rise to periods of irrational behaviour or even coma. Colicky abdominal pains become frequent, and there may be constipation or diarrhoea. Asthenia becomes marked.

(b) *Signs.* On examination the patient presents a typical appearance. The body temperature may be reduced, and rectal temperatures should always be recorded. The pulse is rapid and of reduced force, and the *blood pressure low.* The heart sounds are soft, and pigmentation is apparent. This may be seen particularly in exposed areas, or those subjected to pressure. It also occurs in the mouth and vagina, the alveolae of the nipples, the axillae, the external genitalia, and in the skin creases and any scars that exist. It is accompanied by large numbers of dark melanin spots, the whole resembling the protective coloration of the shell of a coot's egg. It may be caused by oversecretion of MSH from the pituitary, and must be distinguished from similar, though usually less intense, pigmentation occurring genetically, or in association with pregnancy or thyrotoxicosis.

Special Investigation. Examination of the serum may show reduced levels of sodium and chloride ions with increase of potassium and urea. Despite this hyponatraemia sodium and chloride are freely present in the urine. The only other condition in which this occurs is salt-losing nephritis.

Complications. *Addisonian Crisis* may be precipitated by the stress of infection, infarction, fractures, or emotion. It leads to an intensification of the clinical and laboratory findings; the patient is usually admitted in stupor or coma. Urgent treatment is necessary to preserve life.

Treatment. Treatment may be considered under the headings of crisis, maintenance, and prophylaxis.

(a) *Crisis.* The foot of the bed should be raised, and an intravenous infusion of 500 ml. of normal saline (9 g./litre) containing 100 mg. of hydrocortisone should be given in less than half an hour, followed by 10 per cent glucose in normal saline. Further injections of hydrocortisone should be given as required. 1 million units of penicillin should be given at once. The duration of intravenous treatment must depend upon the patient's clinical state, but in general when vomiting ceases it is safe to revert to oral therapy. Progress should be measured clinically by the patient's consciousness, blood pressure, and pulse rate, and chemically by serum levels of sodium, potassium, and glucose. If hypoglycaemia is troublesome it may be treated by injecting 50 per cent glucose solution through the plastic tubing of the transfusion set. Care must be taken throughout to avoid pulmonary oedema, or water intoxication (p. 393).

RESULTS OF TREATMENT OF ADDISONIAN .CRISIS

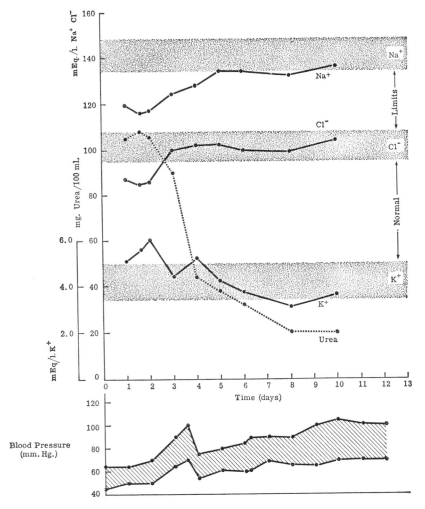

(b) *Maintenance*. Most patients do best with both cortisone and 9-alpha fluoro-hydrocortisone (Fludrocortisone). Usual doses are

(1) Cortisone 12·5–25 mg. twice daily.
(2) Fludrocortisone 0·2 mg. once or twice daily.

(c) *Prophylaxis*. All patients should carry a document stating clearly:

(1) The diagnosis.
(2) The exact doses of maintenance therapy.
(3) The steps to be taken if unusual stress occurs.

Many centres now provide patients with a pack containing an antibiotic and extra doses of steroids to be taken in an emergency.

Normal urinary excretion of adrenal hormones (units/24 hours)

	Male	Female	Units
17-Ketosteroids	8–22	5·5–18	mg.
17-Ketogenic steroids	5·8–22·5	5–16	mg.
	(12·0)	(9·3)	mg.
11-Hydroxycorticoids	4–14	4–10	mg.
	(7)	(6)	
Total Catechol Amines	up to 200		μg.
Vanilmandelic Acid	up to 8		mg.

THE TESTES

Testicular Insufficiency

Introduction. Testicular failure may occur with or without evidence of androgen deficiency. It may result from failure of secretion of follicle stimulating hormone (FSH) or because the testicles are unable to respond normally to it. The clinical picture is varied, depending on whether the testicular failure was pre-pubertal, pubertal, or post-pubertal. Testicular failure may only be detected by examination of a seminal specimen unless there is accompanying androgen deficiency. (Eunuchoidism.)

Clinical Features of Eunuchoidism. The patient is usually tall and thin, and the span exceeds the height. The distance from the pubic spine to the ground exceeds that from the pubic spine to the crown of the head. This results from the unchecked action of growth hormone on the long bones. The muscles are small, but not always weak, and the thyroid cartilage remains infantile, so that the voice is high pitched. There is no growth of beard, and no temporal recession of the hair line. Hair on the trunk is sparse, and there is little or no pubic or axillary hair. The penis and prostate are infantile.

Special Investigations. Primary and secondary testicular failure with eunuchoidism can be separated by estimating the amount of FSH in the urine. It is raised in about 40 per cent (hypergonadotropic) and lowered in 60 per cent (hypogonadotropic) of cases. In the second group further differentiation may be achieved by searching for other signs of pituitary failure (p. 437), or if the pituitary appears intact, by testicular biopsy, when a number of typical appearances may be seen on microscopy.

Treatment is by means of chorionic gonadotropin.

In the hypergonadotropic group (40 per cent) about 15 per cent fail before puberty, and 25 per cent at or about the time of puberty. *Prepubertal failure* may result from congenital abnormalities of the testis, or from infection or trauma during infant life. The scrotal contents are likely to be atrophied. *Treatment* is with androgens. *Pubertal testicular failure* (Klinefelter's syndrome, p. 3), is familial and despite its relatively late onset, probably represents an inborn error of metabolism. The testes are small, and biopsy shows the diagnostic appearance of hyalinisation of the seminiferous tubules. Depending on whether the onset is *early* or *late* in puberty the signs of eunuchoidism are more or less marked. If the onset is late in puberty they may be minimal, but gynaecomastia is severe. Treatment is by androgens and plastic surgery to the breasts.

Testicular Failure without Eunuchoidism. This presents as sterility. It is confirmed by counting the sperms and observing their forms in a seminal specimen. Azoospermia or oligospermia are strong indications for testicular biopsy, when certain classical appearances may be seen on microscopy. At present treatment is largely ineffective.

Male Climacteric

Usually occurs over the age of sixty-five and is thought to be associated with Leydig cell deficiency. Symptoms include anxiety, nervousness, palpitations, hot flushes, reduced libido, and impotence. The patients become easily tired, and there is muscular weakness and wasting. Levels of FSH in the urine are greatly raised. Treatment is with androgens, for example sublingual testosterone 25 mg. daily.

THE OVARIES

Introduction

Secretion by the ovaries may fail either by absence or reduction of progesterone from the corpus luteum, by anovulation, or by failure of oestrogens. This last may occur before or after puberty.

Progesterone Deficiency

This causes poly- or hypermenorrhoea, with sterility or frequent abortion. Temperature records show less than 11 days between the 'dip and rise' which occur at the time of ovulation and the onset of bleeding; the normal interval is 11 to 14 days. Vaginal smears and endometrial biopsy show an inadequate luteal phase of menstruation, and urinary pregnandiol (the excretory end product of progesterone metabolism) is reduced below 3 mg./24 hours. Treatment is unsatisfactory, but consists in giving progesterone and oestrogens in the post-ovulatory phase of the menstrual cycle.

Anovulation

This causes sterility, and may be identified by the absence of the 'dip and rise' in temperature in the middle of the menstrual cycle. Endometrial biopsy shows only oestrogenic changes. If ovulation has failed due to lack of pituitary gonadotrophin it may be induced by clomiphene citrate, which stimulates the pituitary to increase gonadotrophin production.

Oestrogen Failure

Clinical Features. The subject reaches chronological maturity without the appearance of female secondary sexual characteristics. Examination shows an infantile (length of cervix greater than that of body) uterus, with small and underdeveloped vagina and breasts. Pubic and axillary hair is sparse, and there is a tendency to fatness. Skeletal growth is deranged; unless there is a coincident somatic growth defect (Turner's syndrome, vide infra) there is delayed fusion of epiphyses and overgrowth of the long bones. Radiographs show retarded bone age, and the gynaecoid formation of the pelvis does not occur.

Special Investigations. These changes may be due either to partial or complete pituitary failure (p. 437), or to inability of the ovary to respond to follicle stimulating hormone (FSH). They may be separated by studying FSH levels in the urine; these are decreased if the pituitary is at fault, increased if it is the ovary.

Trauma, irradiation, and inflammatory or neoplastic disease may all damage the ovaries, or there may be ovarian agenesis.

Turner's Syndrome (Gonadal dysgenesis, p. 3).

These patients appear as small women, and are psychically orientated as such; they are in fact genetic males in whom there has been complete testicular agenesis. In this connection it is interesting to note that if male embryos of rabbits or mice are castrated before the genital tract has differentiated they apparently develop into females. As no ovaries are present, however, no secondary female sexual characters can appear.

Clinical Features

    (1) Hypogonadism (p. 453).
    (2) Short stature; they are all under 5 feet.
    (3) Congenital abnormalities include short neck, webbed neck, Klippel-Feil deformity, cubitus valgus, and congenital heart disease, especially coarctation of the aorta; abnormalities of the urinary tract, deafness, mental deficiency, and Mongolism.

It may be confirmed by demonstrating high levels of gonadotropins (FSH) in the urine. No treatment is satisfactory, but secondary sexual characteristics can be induced with oestrogens, and menstruation produced with oestrogens and progesterone.

Female Climacteric

Is caused by involution of the ovaries, and is associated with regression of the vagina, uterus, and breasts, and with osteoporosis, sometimes marked (p. 351). There are usually vasomotor symptoms, such as hot flushes, sweating, and sudden feelings of intense heat ('hot flashes'). Frequently psychogenic complaints are prominent. Disturbed menstruation frequently proceeds amenorrhoea. Many women pass the climacteric without undue disturbance. Symptoms can usually be allayed by reassurance, sedation, and supportive interviews. Oestrogen replacement (stilboestrol 0·2 mg. daily or ethinyloestradiol 0·01 mg. daily) is sometimes necessary if these measures prove inadequate.

More serious complications, such as the mental disturbance, arthritis and osteoporosis which may occur are dealt with elsewhere.

Stein-Leventhal Syndrome

This is an interesting syndrome, presenting usually as obesity and sterility. Menstruation is anovular, and various menstrual irregularities, including amenorrhoea, oligomenorrhoea, and menorrhagia have been reported. There is usually evidence of moderate virilisation (vide infra). Both ovaries are enlarged to 4 to 5 times the normal size and shows polycystic changes. Treatment is by wedge-resection of the affected ovaries, or by administration of clomiphene.

Feminising Syndromes

They can usually only be diagnosed in the prepubertal or post menopausal female when they cause the appearance of female secondary sexual characteristics. In males there is a disappearance of male characteristics and the appearance of female ones in their place, notably gynaecomastia and female distribution of pubic hair. They are caused by excess of circulating oestrogens, either from their ingestion for therapeutic reasons, from over-secretion by ovarian tumours (granulosa cell or theca cell), or from the adrenal glands. Some cases of Cushing's syndrome (p. 449) in males may show female characters. In cases of advanced liver disease the oestrogens are not properly conjugated, and striking feminisation may result. Gynaecomastia may be marked in Klinefelter's syndrome (p. 454) occurring late in puberty.

Virilising Syndromes

In male prepubertal children they induce the precocious appearance of masculine secondary sexual characteristics. There is no typical syndrome recognised in adult males. In females virilisation results (p. 447). The syndrome is caused by an excess of circulating androgens, either from hormone secreting tumours of the adrenal or testis, or by adrenal hyperplasia. Rarely they are produced by arrhenoblastomas of the ovary. Seventeen keto-steroid excretion is increased in the urine.

Oral Contraceptives

There is no doubt that these preparations are the most efficient method of contraception. They are widely used in the U.K. today, and pregnancy rates of 0·1 to 1·0 per 100 'woman years' are quoted. Complications (vide infra) do occur, but their exact frequency is hard to determine. It is probably very low indeed.

Details of available preparations may be found in the Prescribers Journal, vol. 10, no. 1, p. 1 (1970). Most are mixtures of oestrogens and progesterone, some contain progesterone alone. They act by inhibiting the pituitary gonado-trophins. There is some evidence that venous thrombosis and subsequent embolism is related to the oestrogen rather than the progesterone component.

They are completely contra-indicated in patients with liver disease or with carcinoma of the breast or the cervix. The presence of severe varicose veins, obesity, diabetes, hypertension or a previous history of venous thrombosis or embolism are relative contra-indications; and because of their water retaining action these preparations should be prescribed with caution in the presence of heart or renal disease, and epilepsy.

FURTHER READING

Hall, R., Anderson, J., and Smart, G. A., *Fundamentals of Clinical Endrocrinology*, Pitman Medical Publishing Co., London, (1968).

Williams, R. H., *Textbook of Endrocrinology*, Saunders Publishing Co., London, (1968).

CHAPTER FOURTEEN

DISORDERS RESULTING FROM VITAMIN DEFICIENCIES

Introduction

Serious illnesses from vitamin deficiencies are rare in the Western world today. They are still sadly common in the underdeveloped countries. In this country their appearance is usually conditioned by some extra factor, neglect of an infant or elderly person, insanity, gastrointestinal disease causing impaired absorption, alcoholism, or drug addiction. Deficiency of the accessory food factors known to be synthesised by bacteria in the gut (folic acid, nicotinic acid, riboflavin, and vitamin K) may be induced by antibiotic therapy. Certain groups of the population, for instance pregnant or lactating women, growing children, or children suffering from protracted febrile illnesses are specially at risk. Closed communities are at the mercy of cooks.

Although described separately they commonly occur together. Treatment must always include the resumption of a normal diet, and where doses of vitamins for treatment are quoted they are intended as supplements to such a diet.

VITAMIN A DEFICIENCY

Deficiency occurs endemically in the Middle East, rarely in this country, Symptoms are (1) *Night blindness* (Hemeralopia) from affection of visual purple; (2) *Xerophthalmia*, drying and thickening of the conjunctiva, progressing to (3) *Keratomalacia*, softening and inflammation of the cornea, leading to opacity and blindness; (4) *Follicular keratosis* (phrynoderma). the blocking of skin follicles with horny plugs leading to dryness and roughness of the skin surface. Similar changes are seen in myxoedema.

For details of treatment, etc., see table.

VITAMIN D DEFICIENCY

Introduction

In infants deficiency causes rickets, in adults osteomalacia. Rickets results from the combination of low calcium diet, lack of sunshine and vitamin D deficiency. In adults, prolonged dietary inadequacy, pregnancy, and lactation are important contributory causes. Osteomalacia is endemic in underdeveloped countries, but extremely rare now in the Western world.

Clinical Features. Osteoid is prepared at the growing ends of bones, where it heaps up and causes tender swellings which do not become calcified. This is particularly apparent in the skull (*fronto-parietal bosses*), the ribs (*rickety rosary*), and the distal ends of the long bones, particularly at the wrist. Failure of calcification also causes softening of the bones so that they bend under stress; this shows clearly as a sulcus at the line of attachment of the diaphragm (Harrison's sulcus), and in the legs (*genu valgum,* or *varum*). *Dentition* is similarly delayed and defective. The muscles are generally hypotonic; there is delay in walking and standing, with weakness, lordosis, and abdominal protuberance. If the serum calcium is low, *tetany* (p. 344) may result.

For details of treatment, etc., see table.

Overdosage

Symptoms are anorexia, nausea, thirst, vomiting, polyuria and drowsiness. Calcium and phosphorus levels in the serum and urine may be elevated, and tissue calcification may occur. Calcification of the kidneys may lead to hypertension and uraemia.

VITAMIN K

Deficiency causes hypoprothrombinaemia (p. 474).

VITAMIN B DEFICIENCY

(a) **Thiamine deficiency** is much more likely to occur in the presence of achlorhydria and when a high proportion of the dietary calories are provided by carbohydrate.

Clinical Manifestations

(1) *Polyneuritis* (Dry beri-beri) (p. 312), less commonly myelitis. The neuritis is always associated with extreme tenderness of muscle.

(2) *Cardiac failure* with oedema, cardiac enlargement, usually regular rhythm, and circulatory hyperkinesis (high output failure). (Wet beri-beri.)

(3) *Wernicke's Encephalopathy* (p. 311), in which confusion, ataxia, nystagmus, squint, and diplopia are common.
(Treatment, etc., see table.)

(b) **Riboflavine deficiency** causes widespread affection of the mucous membranes and skin, presenting as:

(1) *The tongue is sore and magenta coloured.*

(2) *Angular stomatitis,* painful red fissures at the angles of the mouth.

(3) *Cheilosis,* a stripping of the superficial epithelium at the line of closure of the lips.

(4) *Vascularisation of the cornea,* spreading in from the periphery and visible initially only on slit-lamp microscopy, later to the naked eye.

(5) Eventually *keratomalacia* with corneal opacity may develop.

(6) *Seborrhoeic dermatitis* of the naso-labial folds, ears and chest.

Vitamin	Solubility	Clinical Deficiency Disorder	Test for Deficiency	Prophylaxis (Daily)	Therapy (Daily)	Natural Sources
A	Fat	Xerophthalmia Keratomalacia Night blindness Follicular keratosis	Serum carotene levels	2,500–5,000 i.u.	10–25 000 i.u.	Eggs, milk, butter, vitaminised margarine, fish liver oils, coloured vegetables
D	Fat	Bone changes Hypotonia Tetany	Radiography of bones, serum alkaline phosphatase serum calcium serum phosphate	Calcium-containing foods. 400 i.u. daily, calciferol 3,000 i. units	3–5,000 i.u.	Eggs, milk, butter, vitaminised margarine, fish liver oils
K	Fat	Hypoprothrombinaemia (p. 474)	Serum prothrombin time	1–2 mg.	5–10 mg.	Spinach, cabbage, kale, cauliflower, synthesised in gut
B Thiamine (B₁)	Water	Beri-beri, dry or wet, Wernicke's encephalopathy (p. 311)	Pyruvate tolerance test	1–1·6 mg.	50–100 mg.	Whole grain cereals, yeast, liver
Riboflavine (B₂)	Water	Rubiolation of cornea, Keratomalacia, Cheilosis Angular stomatitis Magenta tongue, Seborrhoeic dermatitis	Slit-lamp microscopy of Cornea	1·4–2·5 mg.	5–15 mg.	Milk, eggs, butter, liver, yeast
Nicotinic acid (Niacin)	Water	Pellagra		10–16 mg.	100–500 mg.	Whole grain cereals, excluding maize
Pyridoxine (B₆)	Water	Peripheral neuritis Anaemia in infants		1–2 mg.	10–50 mg.	Whole grain cereals, yeast
Cyanocobalamin (B₁₂)	Water	Pernicious anaemia (p. 469)	Serum B₁₂	2–4 µg.	(See p. 461)	Whole grain cereals
C	Water	Scurvy	Vit. C content of white blood cells	70–150 mg.	500–1,000 mg.	Green vegetables, fresh fruit, oranges, tomatoes, blackcurrants

(c) **Nicotinic Acid deficiency** causes the clinical syndrome of *pellagra*.

Clinical Features

(1) *Dementia* (p. 43).

(2) *Diarrhoea*, which is intractable and may lead to potassium deficiency (p. 395).

(3) *Dermatitis.* This consists of a scaly pigmentation of the exposed skin surfaces. The tongue is affected, and has been likened to 'raw beef'. Pellagra is a disease of maize eaters. Secondary deficiency may occur in gastrointestinal disorders and with carcinoid tumours.
(Treatment, etc., see table.)

(d) **Pyridoxin deficiency** is a rarity. Artificially fed infants given a pyridoxine deficient diet develop an anaemia with all the characteristics of iron deficiency except that it responds only to pyridoxine. They may also have convulsions. In adults, where deficiency may occur as a side effect of isoniazid administration, cheilosis, glossitis, weakness, peripheral neuritis and increased susceptibility to infection may occur.

(e) **Cyanocobalamin deficiency** causes pernicious anaemia (p. 469). Peripheral neuritis, subacute combined degeneration of the cord, optic atrophy, and dementia may also occur, either in association with the anaemia or separately.

VITAMIN C DEFICIENCY

Introduction

Scurvy is seen mainly nowadays in elderly people living alone on a diet which contains no fruit or vegetables. The diet must be grossly deficient in ascorbic acid for some six months before symptoms appear.

Clinical Features. Patients feel generally ill. Signs are produced by *spontaneous haemorrhages*. These occur most frequently in the gums, which bleed at a touch, especially the interdentate papillae (*scurvy buds*). *Teeth* become loose and infected, and *foetor oris* is marked. Perifollicular haemorrhage may cause *skin purpura*, and derangement of the hairs (corkscrew hairs). Later there may be large spontaneous haemorrhages, into muscles or joints, or subcutaneous (*ecchymoses*). There is deficient haemoglobin synthesis, causing anaemia, and impaired collagen formation which gives rise to delayed wound healing.
(Treatment, etc., see table.)

FURTHER READING

Wohl, M. G., and Goodhart, R. S. *Modern Nutrition in Health and Disease,* 4th edition., Henry Kimpton, London, 1968.

CHAPTER FIFTEEN

DISORDERS OF THE BLOOD

ANATOMY AND PHYSIOLOGY

Blood contains three types of cell, red blood corpuscles (erythrocytes), white blood corpuscles (leucocytes), and platelets (thrombocytes). These cells are formed mainly in the bone marrow and normally the speed of production is regulated to ensure that just sufficient numbers of each type of cell are delivered into the peripheral blood each day to replace those which have worn out and have been removed.

Red Blood Corpuscles

The parent cell in the bone marrow is the erythroblast, a large cell which has deeply basophilic cytoplasm, contains no haemoglobin and has one or more nucleoli in its nucleus. In the presence of adequate supplies of vitamin B_{12} and folic acid the erythroblast produces by division a smaller cell with a denser nucleus; this is the early normoblast, which still has basophilic cytoplasm. Haemoglobinisation of the cell occurs at this stage and the cytoplasm changes from the blue colour of the primitive cell through a polychromatic phase to the pink of the mature normoblast, which now has a very dense pyknotic nucleus. Disintegration of the nucleus transforms the normoblast into the young erythrocyte or reticulocyte, so-called because supra-vital staining with cresyl blue reveals a fine reticulum of polychromatic material in the cytoplasm. The fully mature erythrocyte contains no such reticulum and therefore a reticulocyte count gives a valuable indication of the rate of new red cell production. In health no nucleated red cells appear in the peripheral blood.

In the absence of adequate supplies of vitamin B_{12} or folic acid there is failure of maturation beyond the erythroblast-early normoblast phase and these large primitive cells become prematurely haemoglobinised. Anaemia characterised by large cells and a high haemoglobin content (macrocytic and hyperchromic) is the result. Iron is an essential element in the haemoglobin molecule so that iron deficiency leads to shortage of haemoglobin, but it does not interfere with the normal maturation of the red cells. Although less haemoglobin is put into each cell, the cells are smaller and thinner than normal, and the cell haemoglobin *concentration* is unaltered. The cells appear small and pale (microcytosis and hypochromia).

Small amounts of thyroid hormone, ascorbic acid, and copper are also required for efficient red cell production.

The life of each red cell in the circulation is about 120 days. At the end of that time it is broken down by cells of the reticulo-endothelial system, mainly in the bone marrow, spleen, and liver, the haemoglobin being split into two fractions. One of these contains the iron atoms and is returned to the bone marrow for re-synthesis into new red cells, forming by far the biggest source of the iron used for this purpose; the non-iron-containing fraction constitutes the bile pigment bilirubin and is transported in the blood to the liver for excretion.

White Blood Corpuscles

(1) *The Granular Series*

The parent cell in the bone marrow is the myeloblast, a large cell with basophilic non-granular cytoplasm and a nucleus containing several nucleoli. From this is formed a smaller cell without nucleoli called the myelocyte, which acquires granules in its cytoplasm as it matures. The nucleus gradually condenses, becoming first kidney-shaped (at which stage the cell is known as a metamyelocyte) and then lobulated. The cell is now a mature granulocyte, and is classified as neutrophil, eosinophil, or basophil according to the staining reaction of the granules in its cytoplasm. As the cell becomes older it acquires more lobes in its nucleus.

Normal blood contains 2,000–7,500 neutrophil granulocytes, 0–400 eosinophils and 0–200 basophils per cu. mm.

(2) *The Lymphocyte Series*

The parent cell is the lymphoblast, found in lymphoid tissue throughout the body as well as in the bone marrow. It looks very like a myeloblast, but can usually be distinguished by the company it keeps: i.e., it breeds lymphocytes and not granulocytes. From the lymphoblast are derived the large and small lymphocytes, cells with clear blue cytoplasm and dense nuclei; the small ones are probably the more mature cells.

The normal lymphocyte count is 1,000 to 3,500 per cu. mm.

(3) *The Monocyte Series*

The monoblast, which also closely resembles the myeloblast, is derived from reticulum cells and gives rise to the monocyte, a cell with cloudy blue cytoplasm containing a few small red granules, and a kidney-shaped nucleus.

The normal monocyte count is 0–800 per cu. mm.

The Platelets

The parent cell is the megakaryocyte found in the bone marrow, a very large cell with multilobulated nucleus and granular cytoplasm. The platelets formed from it are small (2–4 μm.) bodies containing blue or purple granules but no nucleus.

The normal platelet count is 150,000–350,000 per cu. mm.

ANAEMIA

Definition

Anaemia is a condition of diminished oxygen-carrying capacity of the blood due to a reduction in the numbers of red cells or in their content of haemoglobin, or both.

Symptoms and Signs of Anaemia

The symptoms and signs due to the diminished oxygen-carrying capacity of the blood are common to all types of anaemia. They include general tiredness, shortness of breath on exertion, giddiness, headache, pallor (especially pallor of the mucous membranes and of the palms of the hands), palpitations, oedema of the ankles, and occasionally in older people angina pectoris (see p. 155).

Causes of Anaemia

The anaemias can be classified primarily into two groups:

(1) those due to some failure in the quality or quantity of new red cells being produced in the marrow, and

(2) those due to excessive loss of red cells from the circulation, either from acute or chronic haemorrhage or from abnormal haemolysis.

There is frequent overlap between these two groups since haemorrhage leads to iron deficiency, which is by far the commonest cause of the anaemias in group (1). The classification is useful for descriptive purposes, however, and can be amplified as follows:

(1) Deficient Red Cell Production

(a) Iron deficiency anaemia.

(b) Vitamin B_{12} or folic acid deficiency.

   (i) Pernicious anaemia (Addison's anaemia)

   (ii) Failure of absorption of vitamin B_{12} or folic acid due to disorders of the gastrointestinal tract such as sprue, idiopathic steatorrhoea, and after gastrointestinal operations.

   (iii) Tropical nutritional macrocytic anaemia.

   (iv) Macrocytic anaemia of pregnancy.

(c) The anaemia of myxoedema from lack of thyroxin.

(d) The anaemia of scurvy from lack of vitamin C.

(e) Impairment of erythroblastic activity in bone marrow:

   (i) Aplastic anaemia.

   (ii) Invasion of bone marrow in leukaemia, metastatic malignant disease, Hodgkin's disease, myelomatosis, and myelosclerosis.

   (iii) Probable toxic effect on erythroblasts in uraemia, chronic infections, malignant disease, and certain collagen diseases.

(2) Excessive loss of red cells

(a) Haemorrhage.

(b) Abnormal haemolysis:

(i) Due to congenital defects in the red cells, in familial acholuric jaundice, and sickle-cell anaemia.

(ii) Due to acquired haemolysins in the blood, either of unknown cause or in incompatible blood transfusions, septicaemias, malignant disease, and erythroblastosis foetalis.

INVESTIGATION OF ANAEMIA

Haemoglobin

The average haemoglobin content of normal blood is 14·8 g. per 100 ml., which is consequently taken as the arbitrary 100 per cent level in most laboratories. There is still no general agreement on this point, however, and to prevent confusion the haemoglobin should always be expressed in grams per 100 ml., the percentage figure being given in addition if desired.

Red Blood Count

The red count has a wide physiological range between about 4–6 million per c.mm. Calculation of the haematological indices outlined below is based on the assumption that the normal red count is 5 million and that 100 per cent haemoglobin is 14·8 g. per 100 ml.

Haematocrit Value (or packed-cell volume)

This is the volume occupied by the red cells in 100 ml. of centrifuged blood and is normally about 45 ml. per cent.

Mean Corpuscular Haemoglobin Concentration (M.C.H.C.)

This value has been used for many years as a measure of concentration of haemoglobin within the red cells and a low value was taken as an indication of iron deficiency anaemia.

It is obtained from the formula

$$\frac{\text{Hb in grams/100 ml.}}{\text{Packed cell volume/100 ml.}} \times 100$$

The low values found in iron deficiency have however been shown to be due to the loose packing of the irregularly shaped erythrocytes when the packed cell volume is estimated by centrifugation. It is not really an estimate of cell haemoglobin concentration. If the packed cell volume is obtained from the red cell count and the mean corpuscular volume (as occurs with the Coulter 'S' Counter), a normal M.C.H.C. will be found in iron deficiency.

The haematological diagnosis of iron deficiency anaemia depends on the finding of a low M.C.V. and M.C.H. which is associated with small and irregular hypochromic erythrocytes on the stained smear (due to cells being small and thin, rather than having a low haemoglobin concentration). In addition the serum iron will be low and the bone marrow will show absence of stainable iron.

Mean Corpuscular Volume (M.C.V.)

This is the average volume of a single red cell in cubic microns and is obtained by dividing the packed-cell volume in ml. per 1,000 ml. blood by the red cells in millions per c.mm. The normal range is 78–94 cu. μm. With the Coulter 'S' counter the M.C.V. is measured directly and is not derived from the packed cell volume obtained by centrifugation. The M.C.V. gives an indication of the size of the red cell in three dimensions.

The **Mean Corpuscular Diameter** (M.C.D.), on the other hand, being obtained by measurement of the diameter of the red cells in a stained film, gives an indication of the size of the cells in two dimensions only and takes no account of their thickness. The average normal M.C.D. is 7·2 μm, with a range of 6·7 to 7·7 μm.

Colour Index

This is obtained by dividing the haemoglobin percentage by the red cell count (expressed as a percentage of the normal figure of 5 million) and therefore indicates the mean haemoglobin content of a single red cell. The normal figure is 1, with a range of about 0·9 to 1·1. Since a normal red cell contains as much haemoglobin as it can hold a high colour index, indicating that each cell contains more haemoglobin than normal, also implies that the cells are bigger than normal.

IRON DEFICIENCY ANAEMIA

Iron Metabolism

In normal men the amount of iron excreted daily does not exceed 1–1·5 mg. Iron absorption from the upper small intestine is limited by a mucosal block mechanism, just enough being absorbed to replace the amount lost, the total body iron thus being kept fairly constant at about 4–5 g. Iron is transported in the plasma in combination with a specific fraction of the β globulin, which when fully saturated can unite with some 300–350 μg. iron per 100 ml. The normal plasma iron level, however, is only about 100 μg. iron per 100 ml., which represents approximately one-third saturation of the iron-binding capacity of the plasma. The body's reserve stores of iron, contained mainly in the liver, are about 1·5 g.; this provides enough iron for the replacement of about 3 to 4 pints of blood. Normally the iron used in haemoglobin synthesis for new red cells is nearly all provided by the catabolism of haemoglobin from old red cells and very little has to be drawn from the reserve stores.

The average daily loss of iron is at least doubled in women during the reproductive period of life by menstruation, pregnancy, and lactation. To remain in iron balance they must therefore absorb daily some 2–3 mg.

instead of 1–1·5 mg. and to ensure this absorption a diet containing at least 15 mg. iron is essential. A similar iron intake is advisable for growing children, but for everyone else 5–10 mg. daily is probably adequate.

Aetiology

(a) The most important cause of iron deficiency is *haemorrhage*. If a pint of blood is withdrawn weekly from a healthy young man the blood count remains normal for about a month. By that time, however, the reserve stores of iron are exhausted and if bleeding continues at the same rate there is a shortage of iron and therefore of haemoglobin for the new red cells being poured out by the marrow. Signs of iron deficiency, therefore, rapidly appear in the blood. Clinical iron deficiency may be the result of acute haemorrhage of the same order, frequently from haematemesis or melaena, but much more often it is a consequence of chronic blood loss. Menorrhagia is by far the most important factor and its ill-effects are commonly enhanced by previous depletion of the reserve stores of iron by pregnancy and lactation. This is why iron-deficiency anaemia is seen mainly in women.

(b) *Dietary deficiency of iron* occurs in those who, usually from either poverty, ignorance, or food-fad, do not eat enough of the main iron-containing foods, meat, eggs, and green vegetables. The deficiency is serious particularly in women who, as explained above, have high iron requirements.

(c) Impaired absorption of iron may be the result of achlorhydria, gastrectomy, and short-circuit operations involving the small intestine, or the malabsorption syndrome (coeliac disease, sprue, and idiopathic steatorrhoea).

Clinical Features

In addition to the usual symptoms and signs of anaemia, patients with iron deficiency often have brittle, spoon-shaped nails (*koilonychia*) and a very smooth tongue. The latter change is due to atrophy of the filiform papillae. Similar atrophic changes in the mucous membrane in the upper part of the oesophagus, and the development of a curious 'web' of delicate tissue which partially obstructs the lumen and causes dysphagia, occasionally develop and complete the picture of the *Plummer-Vinson syndrome*. The spleen is sometimes palpable.

Blood Count. Since lack of iron leads to shortage of haemoglobin but does not retard the production of red cell envelopes, less haemoglobin is put into each red cell. The red blood count is only slightly lowered, therefore, but the haemoglobin level is reduced; the colour index is consequently low and the red cells are small in size as well as hypochromic. In a patient with untreated iron-deficiency anaemia a reticulocyte count above 1 per cent, indicating increased turnover of red cells, suggests that haemorrhage has been an important aetiological factor. The untreated patient is also likely to have a fasting serum iron level below 50 μg. per 100 ml. and the unsaturated iron-binding capacity of the serum will be in the range of 300–400 μg. per 100 ml.

Treatment. It is important wherever possible to deal with the various factors which have led to the iron deficiency at the same time as the latter is corrected. In practice this usually means arranging appropriate treatment for menorrhagia or gastrointestinal bleeding and giving advice about diet. For correcting the iron deficiency it is nearly always satisfactory to give *iron by mouth* and since ferrous sulphate is the cheapest effective preparation it is the one which should be chosen for routine use. There is some evidence that absorption of iron is better if it is not given on a full stomach, so that a good prescription is tab. ferrous sulphate 200 mg. four times daily between meals. Ascorbic acid 50 mg. twice daily, is sometimes given in the belief that it aids iron absorption; the giving of dilute hydrochloric acid for this purpose is no longer thought to be of any value. If ferrous sulphate causes gastrointestinal upset (nausea, diarrhoea, or constipation) tab. ferrous gluconate 600 mg. four times daily may be given instead.

Parenteral iron therapy is indicated:

(1) when there is a serious impairment of absorption,

(2) when severe iron deficiency has to be corrected quickly during pregnancy, and

(3) rarely when real or imagined intolerance of oral preparations makes effective treatment by mouth impracticable.

Either iron sorbitol citric acid complex ('Jectofer') or iron dextran ('Imferon') may be given intramuscularly and are usually effective and well tolerated. Each contains 50 mg. iron in 1 ml. The injections cause local pain and may result in staining of the skin which is transient with 'Jectofer' but permanent with 'Imferon'. After a test dose of 25 mg. injections of 100 mg. may be given daily or at longer intervals to a total of 1–2 g. Total dosage is calculated from the fact that about 50 mg. is required to raise the haemoglobin by 1 per cent. Toxic effects are rare if single doses do not exceed 100 mg., but 'Jectofer' may cause fever, vomiting, disorientation, temporary loss of taste, a metallic taste in the mouth and local urticaria, and 'Imferon' fever, allergic reactions, lymph-node enlargement and arthralgia.

SIDEROBLASTIC ANAEMIAS

These are rare disorders in which varying numbers of hypochromic microcytic red cells are found in the blood and normoblasts containing an excess of iron-containing granules appear in the marrow. There are also increased iron stores in the reticulo-endothelial system and in parenchymatous organs such as the liver, pancreas and heart; the serum iron level is raised and there is complete or almost complete saturation of the iron-binding protein. Kinetic studies may show increased iron turnover but impaired iron utilisation.

Congenital Sideroblastic Anaemia

This is usually inherited as an X-linked trait and is therefore seen mainly in male patients; it sometimes responds to large doses of pyridoxine, though there is no evidence of pyridoxine deficiency.

Acquired Sideroblastic Anaemia

This may be related to underlying disease such as carcinomas, Hodgkin's disease, leukaemia or rheumatoid arthritis, or may be a side-effect of drugs such as isoniazid and cycloserine which interfere with pyridoxine metabolism.

Treatment. Pyridoxine 50–200 mg. daily should always be given for 2 months and then if there is no response steroid therapy may be tried. Since the iron overload may have serious consequences (see Haemochromotosis, p. 88) iron therapy should be avoided and blood transfusions should be given sparingly.

ANAEMIAS DUE TO VITAMIN B$_{12}$ OR FOLIC ACID DEFICIENCY

Pernicious Anaemia (Addison's anaemia)

Aetiology. This is primarily a disease of the gastric mucosa, which in middle age or beyond fails to produce hydrochloric acid, pepsin and Castle's intrinsic factor. The cause of this failure is not known, but present evidence suggests that it is probably due to an inherited constitutional weakness; thus there is a significant familial incidence and the disease has been shown to be commoner in people of blood group A than blood group O. Gastric cytoplasmic antibodies can be demonstrated in over 80 per cent of patients, indicating a defect in the body's 'self-recognition system'. B$_{12}$ in the diet is not absorbed in the absence of gastric intrinsic factor. The disease is very rare below the age of thirty. These patients often have prematurely grey hair.

Clinical Features. The onset is very insidious and frequently the patient does not consult his doctor until the red cell count has fallen to 1–2 million per c.mm. or even lower. This observation alone may suggest the diagnosis, since counts as low as this in the absence of severe symptoms are very rarely found in other anaemias. In addition to the symptoms common to all anaemias (p. 464), the patient may complain of recurrent soreness of the tongue and very rarely the symptoms of subacute combined degeneration of the cord (p. 313) may be the first indication of the disease. Fever is often present, but significant loss of weight is unusual. Abdominal pain and diarrhoea are common.

Examination shows pallor and in advanced cases the faint lemon-yellow colour of haemolytic jaundice due to rapid breakdown of the abnormal red cells in the circulation. About half the patients have a red raw-looking and smooth tongue. A haemic cardiac murmur, nearly always systolic in timing, can often be heard and retinal haemorrhages are sometimes present. The spleen is palpable in about 60 per cent of patients.

Investigations. *Gastric analysis* invariably reveals pentagastrin-fast achlorhydria, so that if any HC1 is found in samples aspirated from the stomach after the subcutaneous injection of pentagastrin 6 μg./kg. or histamine 40 μg./kg. the diagnosis must be discarded.

Blood Picture. There is severe reduction in the red count but only moderate reduction in haemoglobin percentage, so that the colour index is high, and raised M.C.D. and M.C.V. values (p. 466) show that the cells are macrocytic. Examination of the stained film shows abnormal variations in size, shape, and staining reaction and immature nucleated cells, usually normoblasts but sometimes haemoglobinised megaloblasts, may be seen. There is usually a low total white count of about 3,000–4,000 per cu.mm., the reduction affecting mainly the granulocyte cells, which also show a shift to the right (a predominance of older cells). In severe cases the platelets may also be decreased.

Bone marrow examination shows the presence of large numbers of haemoglobinised megaloblasts.

The Schilling Test. Vitamin B_{12} labelled with radioactive cobalt is given by mouth and within an hour 1,000 μg. of ordinary B_{12} is injected intramuscularly to flood the body's stores and ensure excretion by the kidneys of any of the B_{12} absorbed. The urine is collected for 48 hrs. and its content of radioactive B_{12} estimated. Normal people eliminate 15–50 per cent of the given dose in the urine, but patients with pernicious anaemia less than 10 per cent.

The Serum level of Vitamin B_{12} is reduced (normal 150–850 pg./ml.).

Treatment must continue for life since the gastric atrophy is permanent. This fact should be impressed on the patient as soon as the diagnosis is made, for if the blood count is allowed to fall below normal at any time there is grave danger that irreversible changes of subacute combined degeneration of the cord will develop. Vitamin B_{12} is administered intramuscularly as cyano-cobalamin or hydroxy-cobalamin. There is a good deal of individual variation in the dosage required, but average doses are 100–1,000 μg. of vitamin B_{12} (cyano-cobalamin) every day until the blood count is normal, followed by a similar amount once every 2 to 4 weeks for maintenance. The patient's progress must of course be followed by regular blood counts. At the start of treatment there is an outpouring of new young erythrocytes into the circulation, so that the reticulocyte count rises sharply to reach a peak by about the seventh day. The degree of rise in the reticulocyte count varies with the severity of the anaemia before treatment; when the initial red count has been very low it may reach 40 or 50 per cent. If no reticulocyte crisis occurs in response to treatment the diagnosis should be reconsidered.

Complications. *Subacute combined degeneration of the spinal cord* is by far the most important complication and is discussed on p. 313.

Carcinoma of the stomach occurs more often in patients with pernicious anaemia than in the general population and some authorities advocate annual barium meal examination or even annual gastroscopy for its early detection in such patients. It is probably an adequate precaution, however, to perform such investigations only when there is some special indication such as an unexplained rise in the sedimentation rate.

Other Macrocytic Anaemias

Macrocytic anaemia, haematologically similar to pernicious anaemia, and resulting also from lack of adequate supplies of B_{12} or folic acid in the bone marrow, may be seen under the following circumstances:

(a) Dietary deficiency, mainly of folic acid but affecting B_{12} too, occurs only in association with gross general malnutrition and has been reported mainly from India as tropical (or nutritional) macrocytic anaemia.

(b) Lesions of the gastrointestinal tract may impair the absorption of B_{12} and folic acid. Thus macrocytic anaemia is sometimes found in patients with carcinoma of the stomach, after total gastrectomy, after operations on the small gut, particularly when multiple anastomoses or blind loops have been formed, and in patients with the malabsorption syndrome (coeliac disease, sprue, and idiopathic streatorrhoea).

(c) Diffuse disease of the liver is occasionally accompanied by macrocytic anaemia, presumably as a result of impaired storage of vitamin B_{12}.

(d) Macrocytic anaemia, which usually responds to treatment with tablets of folic acid 10 mg. daily, sometimes occurs for reasons unknown during the later months of pregnancy.

HAEMOLYTIC ANAEMIAS

Abnormally rapid breakdown of the red cells in the circulation leads to an increase in the level of bilirubin in the serum, causing latent or overt jaundice, and to an increased excretion of urobilinogen in the urine and faeces. The compensatory increase in the rate of erythropoeisis in the bone marrow causes an outpouring of new red cells into the circulation, so that a high reticulocyte count is another characteristic feature of haemolytic anaemia.

Causes. Excessive haemolysis may be due to:

    (1) hereditary abnormalities in the erythrocytes, as in acholuric jaundice,

    (2) haemolysins in the blood, or

    (3) toxic or infective factors.

HEREDITARY ABNORMALITIES IN THE RED CELLS

(1) Acholuric Jaundice

This rare disease is usually inherited as a Mendelian dominant, being passed directly from parent to child. The sexes are affected equally. Red cells from a patient with acholuric jaundice are destroyed at a greatly increased rate when transfused into normal people, whereas normal red cells survive for the expected time when transfused into patients with acholuric jaundice. Furthermore haemolysins cannot be demonstrated in the blood. The defect therefore lies in the red cells themselves, which are smaller in diameter (about $5 \cdot 6$–$6 \cdot 2$ μm.) and more spherical in shape than normal erythrocytes (*microspherocytes*) and remain in the circulation on an average for only fifteen days instead of the normal 120 days. The mean corpuscular volume and mean corpuscular haemoglobin concentration are usually normal. There is always a high reticulocyte count of 10–20 per cent, rising to 50 per cent or more during haemolytic crises. The red cells show an increased fragility in salt solutions, haemolysis starting at a salt concentration of $0 \cdot 75$ per cent and being complete at $0 \cdot 4$ per cent (normal range $0 \cdot 45$ to $0 \cdot 3$ per cent).

Clinical Features. Yellowness of the skin is usually noted during the first few years of life, but apart from this symptoms are few and slight except during the so-called haemolytic crises when the patient becomes pale, weak, and febrile. Slow spontaneous recovery usually occurs in about a month. It is now thought that some of these attacks are not episodes of increased haemolysis but of temporary marrow aplasia, since the reticulocyte count may fall and the jaundice become lighter.

The spleen is nearly always palpable and may extend to the umbilicus. About 60 per cent of patients have gallstones of 'metabolic' type, which are precipitated from the excess of bilirubin excreted in the bile; they contain pigment and calcium but no cholesterol. Cholecystectomy is, however, rarely necessary. A curious but important symptom is intractable ulceration of the legs which heals only after splenectomy.

Treatment. Splenectomy is a very satisfactory treatment which nearly always leads to permanent symptomatic cure.

(2) Sickle-cell Anaemia

This disease, which is practically confined to negroes, is inherited as a Mendelian dominant. The essential fault is an abnormal haemoglobin in the red cells which causes the latter to assume a sickle shape at the lower end of the physiological range of oxygen tension. The abnormal shape of the red cells leads to increased blood viscosity and tends to promote capillary thrombosis.

The illness presents as a chronic haemolytic anaemia, sometimes with acute crises and sometimes with thrombotic episodes, and the diagnosis is confirmed by demonstrating sickling of the red cells in a sealed preparation of blood in which the oxygen tension has been reduced. There is no effective treatment apart from transfusion for severe anaemia.

(3) **Cooley's anaemia** (thalassaemia major), due to Mendelian dominant homozygous inheritance of a metabolic fault leading to continued production of foetal haemoglobin, is found in Mediterranean peoples and usually leads to death in childhood from haemolytic anaemia. Splenectomy some-

times reduces the need for transfusion, but there is no generally effective treatment.

Thalassaemia minor, due to heterozygous inheritance of the same gene, is usually symptomless and is detected only by routine blood examination. (4) **Non-Spherocytic Anaemia.** In two members of this group specific enzyme defects have been demonstrated: (a) deficiency of red cell pyruvate kinase, inherited as a recessive character, and (b) deficiency of glucose-6-phosphate dehydrogenase, with sex-linked recessive inheritance.

HAEMOLYTIC ANAEMIA DUE TO CIRCULATING HAEMOLYSINS

Acquired Haemolytic Anaemia

This disease is due not to abnormalities in the red cells but to the presence of haemolysins in the blood, because:

(1) when compatible cells from patients with acquired haemolytic anaemia are transfused into normal people they survive for a normal time, whereas normal cells are quickly destroyed when transfused into patients with acquired haemolytic anaemia, and

(2) the *Coombs' test* is nearly always positive, either the direct Coombs' test demonstrating the presence of antibody adsorbed to the red cells or the indirect Coombs' test indicating a free antibody in the blood.

Acquired haemolytic anaemia, which may present in acute, subacute, or chronic clinical forms, may be seen in patients with chronic infections such as tuberculosis, syphilis, or malaria, with malignant disease, or with leukaemia or the reticuloses. Frequently, however, the underlying cause is never discovered.

Treatment. The abnormal haemolysis can usually be controlled by giving corticosteroids, which are therefore life-saving in this disease. The drug may have to be continued indefinitely, however. (See p. 572 for dangers of long-term therapy.) Dosage is very variable; the smallest daily dose which will prevent haemolysis and therefore drop in haemoglobin should be given. Splenectomy is of benefit in some patients. The abnormal haemolysis sometimes stops if the underlying cause can be treated.

TOXIC AND INFECTIVE HAEMOLYTIC ANAEMIA

Very rarely haemolytic anaemia may occur in association with severe infections, such as streptococcal or staphylococcal septicaemia or as a result of poisoning with lead or dinitro-benzene or from idiosyncrasy to drugs such as sulphonamides, amphetamine, or potassium chlorate. The presence of large numbers of Heinz bodies in red cells strongly suggests haemolytic anaemia due to chemical poisoning.

THE HAEMORRHAGIC DISEASES

A tendency to abnormal bleeding may result from:

(1) **A coagulation defect,** or lack of one of the various substances in the blood which are necessary for the formation of a firm blood-clot when blood is shed (e.g. haemophilia).

(2) **Thrombocytopenia,** which may be either idiopathic or symptomatic of some disease of the bone marrow such as leukaemia or aplastic anaemia, or

(3) Some abnormality in the **capillaries.**

Diseases in group (1) lead to persistent bleeding after injury or trauma; groups (2) and (3) constitute the *purpuras*, which are characterised by spontaneous bleeding from mucous surfaces and into the skin, causing a purpuric eruption (petechiae or ecchymoses). Purpuric spots are easily recognised since, the blood being extravascular, they do not fade on pressure.

COAGULATION DEFECTS

Physiology of Blood Coagulation

The immediate arrest of haemorrhage after injury to small blood vessels is due to vaso-constriction and plugging of the leaks by aggregations of platelets which control the bleeding until a firm blood-clot forms. Coagulation is a complex process initiated by contact of the blood with a water-wettable surface and involves the interaction of many coagulation factors; the nomenclature of these factors has now been standardised internationally, using Roman numerals:—

Factor	Synonym
Factor I	Fibrinogen
Factor II	Prothrombin

(Factor III was originally tissue thromboplastin; Factor IV calcium; and Factor VI the activated form of Factor V; these terms are now seldom used.)

Factor V	Labile factor
Factor VII	Stable factor
Factor VIII	Anti-haemophilic globulin
Factor IX	Christmas factor
Factor X	Stuart-Prower factor
Factor XI	
Factor XII	Hageman factor
Factor XIII	Fibrin stabilising factor

Contact with a water-wettable surface leads to a molecular rearrangement of factor XII which thus acquires enzymatic properties and by interaction with factors XI, IX and VIII converts factor X to its active form.

Activated factor X with factor V and the platelet factor form prothrombinase, which converts prothrombin to thrombin; interaction of thrombin with fibrinogen in the presence of factor XIII leads to the formation of fibrin, which provides the framework of the blood clot. Retraction of the blood clot, which helps to draw the edges of the wound together, is due to shortening of the fibrin strands by the action of a protein liberated from the platelets.

In haemophilia and allied states the initial arrest of haemorrhage takes place normally but failure of a firm blood clot to form results in bleeding an hour or so after the injury when the vasoconstriction passes off. This also explains why in these conditions the coagulation time is prolonged, but the bleeding time is typically normal.

INVESTIGATION OF PATIENTS WITH A HAEMORRHAGIC DISEASE

Hess's Test. The sphygmomanometer cuff is placed round the upper arm and the pressure maintained halfway between the systolic and diastolic pressures for five minutes. A positive test, shown by the appearance of numerous purpuric spots on the arm below the level of the cuff, is found in patients with capillary defects and with severe thrombocytopenia.

Platelet Count. Purpura is usually present when the platelet count is below about 40,000 per cu.mm. Such patients also have a prolonged bleeding time and poor clot retraction.

Clot Retraction. Poor clot retraction is seen in patients with low platelet counts or more rarely when there is deficient blood fibrinogen.

Bleeding time is increased when the platelets are deficient. The lobe of the ear is pricked with a needle and the blood absorbed every 30 seconds on a piece of blotting paper which is not allowed to touch the skin. By this method the normal bleeding time is two to five minutes.

Coagulation time is increased in haemophilia and the allied coagulation-defect states. By *Lee and White's* method, using venous blood, the normal coagulation time is four to ten minutes, but a control with normal blood should always be performed as there is a wide variation in results according to the precise conditions of the test.

Haemophilia

Deficiency of anti-haemophilic globulin in the plasma is inherited as a sex-linked recessive character, appearing only in males and transmitted to them by clinically normal female carriers. All the sons of haemophiliacs are free from the haemophiliac gene and all the daughters are carriers. When a female carrier marries a normal man half the sons are haemophiliacs and half the daughters are carriers. In practice, only two out of three haemophiliacs know of other bleeders in their families so that a typical pedigree must not be regarded as an essential diagnostic criterion.

The common *symptoms* are persistent bleeding after cuts and abrasions, and after extraction of teeth (of first or second dentition), and bleeding into joints, particularly the knee joint. The severity of the haemophilic state is very variable, depending on the degree of deficiency of anti-haemophilic globulin. In severe cases major operations are very hazardous, probably carrying a mortality of about 50 per cent.

Treatment. Until the bleeding stops enough anti-haemophilic globulin (AHG) must be given I.V. daily to maintain at least 20–30 per cent of the level found in the plasma of normal people. In the past fresh plasma transfusions had to be given, since AHG rapidly disappears from stored blood or plasma; but now a cryoprecipitate of human plasma is available which can be stored frozen and enables the AHG from a pint of plasma to be given in a 20 ml. injection. This can be given to outpatients and haemophiliacs should be encouraged to attend for treatment as soon as any bleeding starts. However, they should be admitted to hospital for dental extractions and must be given AHG before operation as well as afterwards. Tooth sockets should be packed lightly with a preparation of thrombin or Russell viper venom (Stypven); this can be done most effectively with the aid of a dental splint made before the extraction.

Christmas disease has the same inheritance and clinical features as haemophilia, but the Christmas factor (which is present in normal serum) is much more stable than anti-haemophilic globulin and stored blood can be used in treatment.

Von Willebrand's disease is a rare disorder inherited as an autosomal dominant trait (and occurring therefore in both sexes) in which there is deficiency of factor VIII, but in contrast to true haemophiliacs the patients also have purpura of the skin and mucosae and a prolonged bleeding time, presumably due to an associated abnormality of the capillaries or platelets. Treatment is as for haemophilia.

Factor V deficiency is inherited in some families as a dominant trait but is extremely rare.

Factor VII deficiency is seen in patients under anticoagulant therapy and occasionally in advanced liver disease.

Prothrombin is produced in the liver from vitamin K. Vitamin K is synthesised by certain bacteria in the intestines and is also present in a number of vegetable foods; it is not absorbed properly in the absence of bile salts. Clinical prothrombin deficiency is seen in two groups of patients: newborn babies in whose intestines the vitamin-K-forming organisms have not yet become established (*haemorrhagic disease of the newborn*); and patients with *obstructive jaundice* whose intestine contains no bile salts. The former variety can be largely prevented by giving vitamin K 5 mg. intramuscularly daily to the expectant mother for a few days before delivery. Patients with obstructive jaundice should receive similar treatment, particularly if any surgical operation is contemplated, as otherwise serious haemorrhage may occur.

THE PURPURAS

Essential Thrombocytopenia (Idiopathic thrombocytopenic purpura)

This rare disease occurs mainly in adolescents and young adults, particularly girls, and is characterised by episodes of skin purpura and bleeding from such sites as the nose, uterus, and alimentary tract. Absence of joint pains is a useful point of distinction from anaphylactoid purpura. The platelet count is low (usually below 40,000 per cu.mm.), the bleeding time is prolonged, clot retraction is poor, but the coagulation time is normal. Hess's test is strongly positive. Gross enlargement of the spleen is uncommon, but in about one-third of the patients it becomes just palpable. As a result of haemorrhage haematological signs of iron deficiency often develop. Cerebral haemorrhage may occur.

Aetiology is obscure. There appears to be a defect in capillary endothelium. In some patients the platelet deficiency seems to be due to a splenic action, which either destroys the platelets or inhibits their release from the bone marrow; in other patients they appear to be destroyed by circulating antibodies (cf. acquired haemolytic anaemia).

Treatment. The effect of steroid therapy should first be tried, but if a complete remission does not occur or if relapse follows withdrawal of the drug splenectomy should be performed without delay. Results of operation are less satisfactory when the disease has been present for more than 12 months.

Purpura due to Capillary Damage

Purpura may be seen in any of the *acute specific fevers*, particularly meningococcal infections. It may also result from *drug sensitivity*; sedormid is the most notorious offender, but other well-known drugs which may cause it are quinine, quinidine, belladonna, phenobarbitone, thiouracil, chlorpromazine, isoniazid, sodium salicylate, carbromal, and the heavy metals. In certain drug purpuras a circulating antibody causing lysis of platelets has been demonstrated; such patients have a thrombocytopenia. Withdrawal of the drug is usually sufficient treatment, but if not steroid therapy may be helpful. *Senile purpura* is common in elderly people, possibly as a result of degenerative changes in the capillary endothelium. The purpura of *scurvy* is due to nutritional changes in the capillary endothelium.

Anaphylactoid purpura (the Schönlein-Henoch syndrome) is characterised by purpura and allergic manifestations, namely urticaria, joint pains and swelling, and angio-neurotic oedema which affects not only the subcutaneous and submucous tissues but also the gut, causing intestinal colic and sometimes rectal bleeding. Classically Henoch's purpura was associated with abdominal colic and Schönlein's purpura with joint pains, but it is now recognised that the two groups often overlap.

Treatment. Subcutaneous adrenaline, 0·5 ml. of a 1/1,000 solution, and oral antihistamines should be given. If the symptoms persist corticosteroid therapy is usually effective.

APLASTIC ANAEMIA

This rare disease, which usually occurs in young adults, is the result of destruction of those cells in the bone marrow which produce the red cells, the white cells, and the platelets. A similar process affecting only the granular leucocytes is termed *agranulocytosis*. Death or destruction of the parent bone-marrow cells is sometimes a toxic reaction to certain drugs, notably amidopyrin, sulphonamides, heavy metals such as gold or arsenic, thiouracil, chloramphenicol, or tridione; or to certain industrial poisons such as benzole and its derivatives. It may also result from excessive exposure to X-rays or radio-active materials. Frequently, however, the cause is unknown (idiopathic aplastic anaemia, or idiopathic agranulocytosis).

Clinical Features. Failure in production of red cells causes the gradual development of the symptoms and signs of anaemia; diminished or absent output of granulocytes impairs the body's defences against infection, leading to painful ulceration of the throat and fever; and scarcity of platelets in the blood causes purpura and bleeding from different parts of the body.

Treatment consists in removal of the cause, if possible; fresh blood transfusion repeated as often as necessary for the correction of the anaemia; and the administration of penicillin or other suitable antibiotic to combat infection. Transfusion may have to be repeated at regular intervals for months or even years, but occasionally the affected bone-marrow cells eventually recover and the patient is restored to normal health.

Hypersplenism is a condition in which there is progressive decline in the numbers of red cells, white cells, and platelets in the peripheral blood (or any combination of the three) associated with splenomegaly of varied aetiology. The bone-marrow shows not aplasia but hyperplasia. The spleen appears to be exerting some inhibitory effect on the maturation or release of cells from the bone marrow and splenectomy is frequently followed by clinical cure.

LEUKAEMIA

Leukaemia is a disease characterised by abnormal proliferation of leukopoietic tissue throughout the body. The cause is not known, but it is now generally regarded as a neoplastic process. The risk of developing it is increased by exposure to excessive radiation: there was a twentyfold increase in its incidence among survivors of the Hiroshima and Nagasaki atomic explosions; the incidence is some six times higher in patients with ankylosing spondylitis who have been treated with radio-therapy than in the general population; and radiologists have an incidence several times higher than other doctors. The risk to doctors generally, however, appears to be about twice that to the general population and in the latter the number of cases per million has doubled in the past twenty years.

Leukaemia is classified according to the type of leukocyte affected into lymphatic, myeloid, and monocytic varieties. It is also subdivided into acute and chronic types according to the speed of the clinical course.

Acute Leukaemia

Acute lymphatic, acute myeloid, and acute monocytic leukaemia present similar clinical pictures so that one description suffices for all. It may occur at any age but is most common in childhood and boys are affected more often than girls. At the start about one-third of the cases are aleukaemic (that is, have no excess of leukocytes in the peripheral blood); there may indeed be leucopenia and this with the low red cell and platelet counts may lead to a mistaken diagnosis of aplastic anaemia. Recurrent infective lesions and purpuric manifestations may occur in this phase, which may last for a few months, but when the leukaemia becomes manifest the course is usually short. More often the onset is sudden, with fever, sore throat, and bleeding from the mouth, nose, or elsewhere and it quickly becomes clear that the patient is gravely ill. Typically there is a total white count of some 20,000 to 50,000 per cu.mm. of which about 90 per cent are blast cells (lymphoblasts, myeloblasts, or monoblasts). There is always severe reduction in the red cell and platelet counts. The diagnosis can be confirmed by examination of the bone marrow. With modern treatment a remission can be induced in 50 per cent of children with acute leukaemia and the median survival in this group is now about 12 months. The incidence of remission in adults is only about 15 per cent, probably because in them the lymphoblastic type of acute leukaemia is less common.

Chronic Myeloid Leukaemia

Chronic myeloid leukaemia occurs mainly between early adult life and middle age and is rather more common in men than in women. Slowly progressive tiredness due to anaemia is usually the presenting symptom, or the patient may complain of a dragging sensation in the abdomen due to the enlarged spleen. The spleen attains a larger size in this disease than in any other seen in temperate climates and may extend into the right iliac fossa. The B.M.R. is increased and this may partly explain the nervousness, night sweats, and loss of weight which are sometimes prominent symptoms. Leukaemic infiltration of the skin sometimes occurs, and pruritus may be a troublesome symptom even when no lesions can be seen or felt. In men painful priapism, due to thrombosis in the corpora cavernosa, may be an early symptom. *Blood count* typically shows a total white count between 100,000 and 500,000, of which some 50 to 70 per cent are polymorphonuclears and 10 to 20 per cent myelocytes, and there is always moderate to severe anaemia. The *diagnosis* is usually easy in view of the enormously enlarged spleen and typical white count, but confirmation may be obtained by marrow examination.

Chronic Lymphatic Leukaemia

Chronic lymphatic leukaemia is nearly always seen in men of late middle age. The patient complains of slowly developing tiredness, due to associated anaemia, and the spleen, liver, and lymph nodes in the neck, axillae, and elsewhere are found to be enlarged. The spleen, however, does not attain the enormous size seen in chronic myeloid leukaemia. As in the latter disease the B.M.R. is raised. Priapism does not occur, but impotence is a common symptom. Infiltration of the skin may result in eruptions of various types. The blood count usually shows a total white count of up to 100,000 of which 80–90 per cent are small lymphocytes and there is always an associated anaemia.

Treatment of Leukaemia

The object of treatment is the destruction of abnormal leucocytes and the suppression of abnormal leucocyte proliferation. The drugs used fall into three groups:

(a) *Antimetabolites*, which compete directly with substances which are taken up by the cell for its metabolism. Thus, 6-mercaptopurine inhibits the uptake of purines and methotrexate the uptake of folic acid.

(b) *Alkylating agents*, which combine chemically in vivo with the chromosomes and so kill the cells or prevent their division. This group includes chlorambucil, cyclophosphamide and busulphan.

(c) *Corticosteroids*. The way in which steroid therapy exerts its beneficial effect in leukaemia is not understood

(d) The *Plant Alkaloids* vinblastine and vincristine interfere with mitotic spindle function.

Apart from the corticosteroids all these drugs cause severe bone marrow depression and throughout the treatment frequent blood counts must be done. It has been shown that better results are obtained when combinations of drugs are given than when they are given singly or successively, presumably because the malignant cells develop drug resistance less easily (c.f. anti-tuberculous chemotherapy, p. 227); and leaving intervals between courses allows the normal cells in the marrow and gastro-intestinal tract to recover and permits more of the effective agents to be given without increasing the toxic effects.

Ideally treatment should be controlled by a physician with special experience in this complex and rapidly changing subject.

Acute Lymphoblastic Leukaemia

At present the best combination for inducing remission is vincristine with prednisone; only 10% of patients fail to respond and they may be tried on various combinations of 6-mercaptopurine, methotrexate, cyclophosphamide or chlorambucil.

Acute Myeloblastic Leukaemia

Treatment is much less satisfactory than for the lymphoblastic type, but has been improved by the introduction of cytosine arabinoside and daunorubicin which are given in combination with either 6-mercaptopurine or prednisone for inducing remission. Methotrexate is used for maintenance therapy.

Symptomatic Treatment. Transfusion is often required for severe anaemia in acute leukaemia and occasionally in the chronic types. Penicillin or other appropriate antibiotic should be given in large doses for infective lesions in the mouth or elsewhere. In the chronic leukaemias local lesions such as painful splenomegaly may be relieved by radiotherapy.

THE RETICULOSES

Hodgkin's Disease (Lymphadenoma)

The cause of Hodgkin's disease is unknown, but it is probably a malignant process. Most of the patients are young adults, though it can occur at any age, and men are affected about twice as often as women.

Clinical Features. The first symptom is usually the painless enlargement of a group of lymph-nodes, particularly in the neck but sometimes in the axillary or inguinal regions. At first the nodes feel firm, rubbery, and discrete, but later they often become matted together. In other patients mediastinal or abdominal lymph nodes enlarge before those in accessible peripheral situations and the patient may present with cough, dyspnoea, or pain in the chest or abdomen; such patients may have fever of the Pel-Ebstein type, which occurs in waves lasting a week or two separated by afebrile intervals of varying length. As the disease progresses general malaise and weakness become severe, anaemia develops, evening fever is usual and night sweats common. An interesting symptom of unknown cause is severe pain after taking even small quantities of alcohol; though usually associated with Hodgkin's disease, this phenomenon does occur in other conditions, for example pancreatic carcinoma. In the majority of patients the spleen and liver eventually become enlarged. Almost any organ may be infiltrated with Hodgkin tissue: relatively common examples are bone, leading to severe pain in the spine, pelvis, or ribs; the nervous system, causing peripheral nerve palsies or cord compression; and the skin, frequently causing severe pruritus and rarely a nodular eruption.

Diagnosis can be established with certainty only by lymph-node biopsy.

Treatment. *Deep X-ray therapy* is the treatment of choice, particularly when the disease is limited to one or two areas; of patients given radiotherapy for disease localised to one group of nodes about three quarters survive for five years and a third for 15 years. Occasionally, permanent cure appears to be achieved. It is important that not only the affected nodes should be irradiated but all contiguous groups of lymph nodes as well.

Eventually, however, the disease usually recurs and becomes widely disseminated and then some form of chemotherapy is indicated. It is usual to start with some form of nitrogen mustard and most physicians now prefer *cyclophosphamide* to the original mustine hydrochloride. It may be given I.V. to a total of 2·0 g. over 10 days followed by 150 mg. daily by mouth until severe leucopenia or other side-effect appears. The most common of these is alopecia; the hair re-grows when the drug is stopped. When the disease no longer responds to cyclophosphamide *vinblastine sulphate* (Velbe) may be given and appears more likely to induce a remission in patients who have already responded to one of the nitrogen mustards. It is given in weekly I.V. injections of about 10 mg. (0·1–0·2 mg./Kg.). It causes leucopenia and, if the dose is too high, paralytic ileus. Peripheral neuropathy also occurs. When vinblastine has to be stopped on account of toxicity or loss of effect procarbazine (Natulan) may be given by mouth, the dose being slowly increased from 50 mg. to 250 mg. per day. This drug causes nausea and vomiting; it should be given after meals and an antiemetic such as prochlorperazine 5 mg. t.d.s. or chlorpromazine 25·0 mg. t.d.s. is indicated.

As an alternative to giving cytotoxic drugs in sequence, a number of drugs may be given together and the course of treatment repeated at intervals, even if the patient appears to be in a remission. This method seems to be giving superior results and may well be the treatment of choice. A typical course for an adult is:—

Mustine 6 mg./m^2 I.V.	Day 1 and 7.
Vinblastine 10 mg. I.V.	Day 1, 7 and 14.
Procarbazine 100 mg. orally.	Day1–14 inclusive.
Prednisolone 40 mg. orally	Day 1–14 inclusive.

The courses are repeated at four week intervals to a total of six courses. Smaller doses are required if the white count is low.

In the later stages of the disease blood transfusion is often needed for anaemia. A corticosteroid such as prednisolone in doses up to 40 mg. daily as well as its antitumour action may improve the general sense of well-being and is particularly indicated if evidence of an acquired haemolytic anaemia is found.

Lymphosarcoma and Reticulum Cell Sarcoma

These two malignant lymphoid tumours have a close clinical similarity to Hodgkin's disease and the differential diagnosis can be made only by lymph-node biopsy. Occasionally in the later stages of lymphosarcoma the blood picture of acute lymphatic leukaemia eventually emerges; and in any of the reticuloses associated with splenomegaly an acquired haemolytic anaemia sometimes develops.

Prognosis. Both lymphosarcoma and reticulum cell sarcoma tend to run a more rapid course than Hodgkin's disease and the average survival time is little more than two years.

Treatment. This is as for Hodgkin's disease (p. 481), but chlorambucil by mouth is perhaps more effective in this group. It is given in doses of 0·2 mg. per kg. body weight daily for three or four weeks, after which unless there is severe bone-marrow depression treatment may be continued at half the dosage for a further month or so.

POLYCYTHAEMIA RUBRA VERA (Erythraemia)

This is a disease of middle age and is commoner in men. It is characterised by hyperplasia of the erythroblastic, leucoblastic, and megakaryocytic tissue of the bone marrow; and although the clinical picture is dominated by the greatly increased number of red cells in the peripheral circulation, there may eventually be exhaustion of the marrow cells, leading to aplastic anaemia, or the leucoblastic tissue may continue to proliferate as the erythroblasts die out, so that the final picture may be that of frank leukaemia.

It is now recognised that in a small proportion of patients with polycythaemia (about 9 per cent) there is an underlying renal lesion, neoplasm, cyst or hydronephrosis. In such patients there is presumably increased production of erythropoeitin by the kidney. Nephrectomy may cure the polycythaemia.

Clinical Features. The patient usually complains of headache, dizziness, and tiredness and has a very plethoric cyanosed appearance. The spleen is nearly always palpable. Congestion of the capillary bed leads to haemorrhage from various sites (for example, after dental extraction), while arterial thromboses in the brain, limbs, and elsewhere are also common, no doubt as a result of the increased blood viscosity. There is also an increased incidence of peptic ulcer and of gout.

The *red count* may be up to 10,000,000 per cu.mm. or even higher with an equivalent increase in the haemoglobin level. The white count is usually raised to about 20,000 per cu.mm. and the platelet count to 500,000 per cu.mm. or more.

Treatment. The treatment of choice is an intravenous injection of radioactive phosphorus (^{32}P) in a dosage of 5–7 millicuries. This is usually followed by very satisfactory clinical remission, but the patient must be carefully followed up as further treatment is often necessary after about three years. Alternatively, the patient may be kept symptom-free by regular venesection of a pint or so of blood every three or four weeks.

MYELOMATOSIS

This is a neoplastic proliferation of plasma cells in the bone marrow and rarely in other organs such as the liver, spleen and lymph-nodes, occurring mainly in late middle-age. It is more common in men than in women.

Clinical Features. The commonest initial symptom is bone pain, often in a rib or vertebra, but sometimes the first indication is an unexplained anaemia or fever or rarely a bleeding tendency due to thrombocytopenia.

There are seldom any abnormal physical signs; splenomegaly and enlarged lymph-nodes are very rare. Radiographs of the skeleton may show generalised demineralisation or characteristic punched-out osteolytic lesions particularly affecting the skull, ribs and vertebral column. Pathological fractures and collapse of vertebrae may occur. Anaemia from impaired erythropoeisis is usual and haemolytic anaemia may develop; ultimately thrombocytopenia is the rule. Plasma cells rarely appear in the peripheral blood.

The plasma cells produce an abnormal protein which on electrophoresis is found to move with the beta or gamma globulins. This protein is responsible for the very high sedimentation rate which is frequently found and in about one-third of the patients is associated with Bence-Jones protein in the urine; this precipitates when the urine is heated to about 70° C., but re-dissolves before boiling point is reached. Myeloma proteins are mono-clonal: i.e., in any individual patient they belong to a single immunoglobulin class (see Table, p. 321). The IgM proteins are referred to as macroglobulins. Bence-Jones proteins are made up of the light polypeptide chains of immunoglobulins. Proteinuria often occurs in myelomatosis even in the absence of Bence-Jones protein. Progressive renal failure may ensue, apparently due to plugging of the renal tubules by casts; such obstruction may be precipitated by intravenous pyelography, which should therefore be avoided. A few patients also have renal amyloidosis, while in others hypercalcaemia may lead to further damage to the kidneys.

The diagnosis can usually be established by marrow examination. The prognosis is very variable, but most patients die within two years.

Treatment is unsatisfactory. The best drug is probably *melphalan*. The dose is 10 mg. daily for seven days, followed if there is no bone marrow depression by maintenance treatment with 2·0 mg. daily. A close watch must be kept for leucopenia or thrombocytopenia. As an alternative cyclophosphamide combined with steroids may be useful; prednisolone is indicated in particular if there is haemolytic anaemia. The pain from local involvement of bone can be relieved by radiotherapy, and transfusion may be required to correct anaemia.

FURTHER READING

Whitby, L. E. H., and Britton, C. J. C. *Disorders of the Blood*, 10th edition. Churchill, London, 1969.

Wintrobe, M. M. *Clinical Haematology*, 6th edition. Kimpton, London, 1968.

CHAPTER SIXTEEN

INFECTIOUS DISEASES

DEFINITION. Although the term 'infectious disease' might logically be applied to any illness which results from invasion of the body by a micro-organism, its use is customarily restricted to those diseases which spread by direct contact from patient to patient. This chapter therefore deals mainly with those diseases for which isolation or 'barrier nursing' is required to prevent spread of infection.

INFECTION AND IMMUNITY

The result of any infection depends partly on the virulence and numbers of the invading organisms and partly on the state of the patient's defences against them. The state of his defences depends partly on his *natural immunity*, which may be good or bad according to his race and heredity and may have been reduced by such factors as malnutrition, worry, and over-work, and partly on *acquired immunity* resulting from previous infection or prophylactic inoculation with this particular organism. Such inoculations given to stimulate the formation of antibodies constitute *active immunisation*, and are widely used in the prevention of such diseases as smallpox, diphtheria, tetanus, enteric fever, and poliomyelitis. *Passive immunisation* means conferring temporary protection against a disease by injecting serum containing the specific antibodies; such serum is obtained from humans who have recovered from the disease or from horses actively immunised for this purpose.

Carriers. Some people after recovering from an infectious disease continue to harbour the specific organisms and may transmit them from time to time to susceptible persons, either by direct contact or by infecting food or water. This carrier state is particularly important in the spread of enteric fever.

Routes of Infection. The invading organism usually gains access to the patient either in inspired air ('droplet infection') or in contaminated food or drink.

Incubation Period. This is the time which elapses between the access of organisms to the tissues of a susceptible individual and the onset of the first clinical symptoms. Its duration varies widely in the different infectious diseases, but remains fairly constant in each of them. The approximate length of the incubation period of the common specific fevers is:

Less than 7 days	Cerebrospinal meningitis
	Diphtheria
	Scarlet fever

10 to 14 days	Measles
	Whooping cough
	Smallpox
	Enteric fever
14 to 21 days	
(usually nearer *21*)	Chicken-pox
	German measles
	Mumps

The incubation period is occasionally helpful in diagnosis if the date of exposure to a particular infection is known. The period of *quarantine* or isolation of contacts, used in serious diseases such as smallpox and where there is some special risk, is obtained by adding a few days (to be on the safe side) to the known incubation period.

Stage of Invasion. At the end of the incubation period the infecting organism or its toxic products become distributed throughout the body and give rise to the symptoms and signs of the disease. Common to all infectious diseases are fever, headache, general malaise, loss of appetite, dry furred tongue, hot dry skin, and scanty highly coloured urine; but in addition each has special features, which in many include a typical rash, which enable diagnosis to be made.

Barrier Nursing

To prevent direct transmission of organisms from patients with proven or suspected disease to other patients the technique known as 'barrier nursing' is employed. Preferably the patient is isolated in a separate room; if he must remain in a general ward the space between the adjoining beds is increased and a screen placed at the foot of the bed serves as a reminder that barrier precautions are being observed. Gowns are provided for all medical and nursing staff attending the patient; these may be hung within the 'barrier' with the 'dirty' side outermost or outside the barrier with the 'dirty' side turned inwards. The hands must be washed before removing the gown and again after leaving the barrier. For diseases spread by droplet infection masks should also be worn. To prevent indirect transmission of infection the patient's cutlery, crockery, and linen are kept separate, everything that has been near him being considered a possible source of infection.

Scheme of Prophylactic Inoculations for Children

Age	*Vaccine*	*Interval*	*Notes*
During first year of life	Diph/Tet/Pert & first dose of oral Polio vaccine		The first dose should not be given before 3 months; a better immunological

Age	Vaccine	Interval	Notes
	Diph/Tet/Pert & 2nd dose of oral Polio vaccine	Preferably after an interval of 6–8 weeks.	response is obtained if it is not given until 6 months of age.
	Diph/Tet/Pert & 3rd dose of oral Polio vaccine.	Preferably after an interval of 6 months	
During second year of life	Measles vaccine	After an interval of not less than 3–4 weeks.	
At 5 years old or school entry	Diph/Tet and oral Polio vaccine		These may be given at 3 years to children at nursery school, day nurseries or homes.
Between 10–13 years of age	B.C.G. vaccine		For tuberculin negative children.
At 15–19 years or on leaving schoool	Polio vaccine Tetanus toxoid Smallpox re-vaccination.		

Antigens for primary immunisation are now given later, at an age when antibody responses are no longer depressed by the presence of maternal antibody and the child is able to make antibody more efficiently.

Precautions. Routine vaccination of chidlren against Smallpox is no longer recommended in the U.K. since the risk of contracting the disease is now less than the risk of developing a serious complication of vaccination. *Encephalopathy* is a rare complication of whooping-cough vaccination and it is more likely to occur in infants with a history of convulsions, such children should be given combined diphtheria and tetanus vaccine instead of triple vaccine. Children with a history of asthma, hay fever, or eczema have a high incidence of *allergic reactions* after injections; they must be kept under observation for an hour after inoculation, therefore, and adrenaline must be immediately available for injection if needed. When a severe local reaction occurs after the first injection of triple vaccine it is probably the whooping-cough component which is responsible and for the subsequent injections it may be advisable to use only the combined diphtheria and tetanus vaccine.

When does the Rash come Out?

It is important to remember the day of the disease on which the specific eruption usually appears in the exanthemata. The following is a useful mnemonic:

	Disease	*Rash appears on*
Really	**Rubella**	1st day
Sick	**Scarlet Fever**	2nd day
People	**Small Pox**	3rd day
Must	**Measles**	4th day
Take	**Typhus**	5th day
No	**Nil**	—
Exercise	**Enteric**	7th day

BACTERIAL INFECTIONS

DIPHTHERIA

Diphtheria is an infection of the throat, nose or larynx (or occasionally the skin) and although the organism, C. diphtheriae, remains localised to this site, it produces a powerful exotoxin which becomes widely distributed and may cause serious or fatal effects on other parts of the body. The amount of exotoxin produced by different strains of the organism varies a good deal and that is one reason why some patients are much more severely ill than others. Another reason for the variation in clinical severity is the state of the patient's immunity at the time of infection.

Immunity. Immunity to diphtheria may be acquired in three ways:

(1) After recovery from an attack of the disease.

(2) After repeated subclinical infection, that is, as a result of coming into contact from time to time with organisms insufficient in either numbers or virulence to cause a full-scale attack of diphtheria.

(3) As a result of active immunisation by inoculation. It is because of the widespread inoculation of children that this killing disease is much less common than it used to be; if immunisation were universally practised, as it should be, there would be no cases.

The Schick Test is used to detect whether an individual has immunity against diphtheria. Diphtheria toxin 0·2 ml. is injected into the skin of the left forearm and 0·2 ml. of the same toxin which has been heated to 70° C. to destroy its potency is injected into the skin of the right forearm as a control. The result is read in 5 to 7 days, as follows:

Positive. An area of redness and swelling at the site of injection on the left arm, with no reaction on the right (control) arm. This indicates that the person tested has no antitoxin with which to neutralise the toxin injected; in other words, he is *susceptible* to diphtheria.

Negative. No reaction in either arm. The injected toxin has been neutralised by anti-toxin and the subject is therefore *immune* to diphtheria.

Positive plus 'Pseudo Reaction'. There is redness and swelling on both arms, but more on the left (test) arm than on the right (control) arm. The reaction on the right arm and part of the reaction on the left are due to some factor in the injection other than the actual toxin; the extra reaction on the left must be due to unneutralised toxin and the subject is therefore *susceptible* to diphtheria.

Negative plus 'Pseudo Reaction'. There is equal redness and swelling on both arms; the subject is *immune* to diphtheria.

Active Immunisation

All children should be immunised against diphtheria. The Schick test is used on adults who are exposed to special risk of infection, for example nurses and medical students, and those shown to be susceptible are immunised.

Immunisation of children may be effected by three injections of alum-precipitated toxoid (A.P.T.), but it is better to give a combined triple vaccine against diphtheria, whooping cough, and tetanus. The first dose of 0·3–0·5 ml. of A.P.T. is given between three and nine months, the second of 0·5 ml. is given four weeks later and the final boosting dose of 0·2 ml. at the age of four. Adults are immunised in the same way, but if the preliminary Schick tests show a 'positive plus pseudo' result unpleasant reactions may follow the use of A.P.T. and it is better to use toxoid-antitoxin floccules (T.A.F.). This is given in three doses of 1 ml. each at intervals of two weeks and rarely causes any side effects.

Clinical Features of Diphtheria

Diphtheria is classified clinically according to the exact site of infection. The commonest variety is *faucial* diphtheria, in which the characteristic membrane of the disease forms in the throat. There is a short incubation period of only three or four days from exposure to infection. Points which help to distinguish diphtheria from streptococcal tonsillitis are:

(1) The throat is not so sore and the temperature usually not so high, but the general exhaustion and toxaemia are much greater.

(2) The lymph-nodes in the neck are usually enlarged to a greater extent, in severe cases causing a collar of swelling sometimes referred to as the 'bull-neck'.

(3) The exudate in the throat is not confined to yellowish spots on the tonsils, but forms a continuous greyish sheet of membrane which often extends forwards over the soft palate and

backwards on to the pharyngeal wall and is so firmly adherent that any attempt to wipe it off leaves a bleeding surface.

Less common and more difficult to diagnose are *nasal diphtheria*, in which the membrane is confined to the nose, where it may lead to a blood-stained nasal discharge; and *laryngeal diphtheria*, a very dangerous form in which the membrane on the larynx may obstruct breathing and necessitate emergency tracheotomy. *Cutaneous diphtheria* is very rare in this country, but in troops serving in the East during the war it was a common cause of so-called 'jungle-sores' or 'desert-sores', the true nature of which was often not appreciated until the development of post-diphtheritic paralysis.

Complications

The complications of diphtheria are due to the effects on the heart and nervous system of the exotoxin absorbed from the lesions in the upper respiratory tract or skin.

Carditis may occur during the second week and is characterised by vomiting, a greyish pallor, a weak rapid pulse, low blood pressure, diminished urinary output, usually with some albuminuria, and sometimes pain over the heart. Conduction defects such as heart block may be found. Sudden death is not uncommon in these cases, but no permanent cardiac lesion results in patients who recover.

Paralysis. Paralysis of the palate is the commonest type and causes a nasal voice and regurgitation of food through the nose. It usually appears in the second or third weeks and may extend to the pharyngeal muscles, causing difficulty in swallowing, or rarely to the intercostal muscles or diaphragm, causing weakness in breathing and necessitating treatment with a mechanical respirator. There is sometimes paralysis of the ciliary muscle, causing difficulty in reading, and lateral rectus (sixth nerve) palsy is not uncommon. Towards the fifth or sixth weeks peripheral neuritis may occur, causing weakness in the limbs of varying degree. Complete recovery from all types of diphtheritic weakness occurs, but may take as long as six months.

Treatment

Antitoxin and Antibiotics

Although a throat or nasal swab should always be taken whenever diphtheria is suspected, the disease is so dangerous that treatment must invariably be started at once without waiting for the result of the culture. The most important measure is the immediate administration of antitoxin. The dose varies from about 8,000–100,000 units, according to the severity of the infection and it is usual to give half the total dose intramuscularly and then if there has been no serum reaction within 15 to 30 minutes to give the remainder, warmed to body temperature, by slow intravenous injection. The latter route should be avoided, however, in patients giving a history of allergic phenomena, owing to the serious risk of fatal anaphylaxis; and any patient who develops vomiting, wheezing, urticaria, or collapse must be given 0·5 ml. of 1:1000, adrenaline subcutaneously without delay and an antihistamine, for example promethazine 25 mg., by slow intramuscular injection. It is usual also to give intramuscular benzyl penicillin, 100,000 to 500,000 units every four hours with erythromycin 250 mg. four-hourly, but it should be stressed that these are less important than the antitoxin.

Nursing

The patient is nursed flat in bed with only one pillow and as complete rest is essential everything, including feeding, must be done for him. In patients with acute carditis these conditions may have to be maintained for some two or three months. Local treatment of the throat probably does more harm than good, but ordinary cleanliness of the mouth is important. If palatal and pharyngeal paresis occur tube-feeding may become necessary.

Control of Outbreaks

When a case of diphtheria occurs in a closed community such as a school or a hospital ward the parents and medical officer of health are notified and the patient is transferred to an infectious diseases hospital. The parents of contacts are also notified and combined active and passive immunisation of the latter is carried out. Antitoxin 1,000 units is given into the deltoid of one arm and the first 0·5 ml. of A.P.T. into the other. Four weeks later the second injection of 0·5 ml. of A.P.T. completes the procedure.

Sometimes an outbreak of diphtheria can be traced to a healthy *carrier* and it is important that his infection be eradicated to prevent further spread of the disease. This can sometimes be achieved by giving large doses of penicillin, 2–4 million units daily, combined with sulphadimidine 4–6 g. daily for up to a week. If the infection persists tonsillectomy may be indicated.

WHOOPING COUGH (pertussis)

Whooping cough is an infection of the respiratory tract by either Bordetella pertussis or a virus. In this country at present it is the most serious of the acute specific fevers of childhood, not only causing many deaths in young children, particularly under the age of twelve months, but also occasionally leading to serious damage to the bronchi and lungs (see bronchiectasis, p. 199). Asthma in childhood also sometimes dates from an attack of whooping cough. Infants receive no passive immunity from the mother and are therefore susceptible to the infection from birth.

Clinical Features. After an incubation period of about 7 to 14 days the child develops what is thought at first to be an ordinary cold on the chest, but within a week of onset the paroxysms of coughing have usually become so severe and typical that the diagnosis is obvious. A characteristic paroxysm consists of a deep inspiration followed by a rapid series of explosive coughs during expiration. The tongue protrudes, the face and lips become deeply cyanosed and the attack may end with the inspiration of air through a partially closed glottis, producing the classical whoop. Paroxysm may follow paroxysm until a little sticky mucus is expectorated or until the child vomits and sinks back exhausted. During the spasms of coughing the tongue may be abraded against the lower incisors, causing a traumatic ulcer on the fraenum; rectal prolapse, hernia, and haemorrhage, particularly under the conjunctiva, may also be induced.

In young infants, however, cough is often not such a prominent symptom. Instead, procedures such as feeding or changing may induce cyanotic attacks, in which the child becomes flaccid, blue, and alarmingly lifeless. There may also be frequent vomiting. Furthermore, immunised subjects may have a mild form of the disease without the typical paroxysmal cough or whoop. The diagnosis may remain very obscure until the appearance of a few feeble whoops at the end of attacks. The preliminary catarrhal stage is short in duration but highly infectious; the paroxysmal stage and whooping may continue for many weeks but the infectivity is now very slight.

Diagnosis. The paroxysmal coughing is virtually diagnostic, but bacteriological confirmation may be obtained by isolation of B. pertussis on 'cough plates' (a Petri dish held in front of the patient's mouth) or better, by taking a post-nasal swab. B. pertussis does not grow readily, however, and special culture media are essential. It is now thought that patients with negative cultures have virus infection. The blood count shows a lymphocytosis, but young children have a high lymphocyte count in health so that no significance should be attached to a count of less than 70 per cent of 20,000.

Complications. Acute bronchitis and *broncho-pneumonia* are the most serious complications and account for most of the deaths which occur in infancy and in old age. *Collapse* of broncho-pulmonary segments, or less often of lobes of the lung, from plugging of bronchioles or bronchi by sticky mucus may lead to bronchiectasis if allowed to persist. A radiograph should be taken, therefore, and appropriate physiotherapy instituted if necessary. *Otitis media* is the other common infective complication. *Convulsions* occur more often in whooping cough than in any of the other specific fevers. *Spontaneous pneumothorax* may occur.

Treatment. Chloramphenicol given in full dosage (25 mg./lb. body weight/day) to infants under six months within seven days of the onset may prevent further development of the disease, and the same drug may be given later if broncho-pneumonia develops. Feeding is often a problem; the diet is most likely to be retained if given after an episode of vomiting. Cyanotic attacks in infants should be treated by freeing the airway and re-establishing breathing by gentle pressure on the chest. It may also be advisable to nurse such a child in an oxygen tent. Phenobarbitone 8–32 mg. has a calming effect and may reduce the number of paroxysms and ephedrine 16–32 mg. relieves or prevents bronchial spasm; the latter may be prescribed conveniently in mist. bellad. et ephedrine pro inf. N.H.F. 4–8 ml. Eumydrin given as a 0·6 per cent alcoholic solution in drops may also help to relieve the cough spasms.

Prophylactic Inoculation. Suspended whooping cough vaccine may be given subcutaneously or intramuscularly. It is best given as a combined triple vaccine against diphtheria, whooping cough, and tetanus (p. 486).

SCARLET FEVER

When seen in historical perspective many infective diseases go through periods of increased or decreased severity, and scarlet fever at the present time is a much less serious illness than it was in the first two decades of this century. It is a haemolytic streptococcal infection which is distinguished from other diseases due to the same organism by its typical rash; this rash indicates that the streptococcus concerned is of a strain which produces a special erythrogenic toxin and that the patient is susceptible to its action.

The **Dick test** is performed by injecting 0·2 ml. of erythrogenic toxin into the skin of the forearm, no control injection in the other arm being necessary. A red swollen area at the site of injection in twenty-four hours shows that the person tested is *susceptible* to the toxin (Dick positive); no reaction shows that he is *immune* (Dick negative). The test is little used at the present time.

Clinical Features. After a short incubation period of less than a week the illness starts abruptly with sore throat, fever, shivering, and often vomiting. Small children may not complain of sore throat, but examination shows that the tonsils and fauces are very red and swollen and the tonsils may be covered with patches of soft, yellowish exudate. At first the tongue is covered with a white fur, which peels off from the edges during the next two or three days, leaving a clean surface with enlarged red papillae—the 'strawberry' or 'raspberry' tongue.

The *rash* appears on the second day and is described as a punctate erythema; the skin is a bright scarlet colour and on close inspection is seen to be covered with minute red spots. It appears first behind the ears and on the side of the neck and spreads rapidly over the whole body, but avoiding the area round the mouth (giving the so-called 'circum-oral pallor') and tending to be particularly heavy in flexures such as the axillae, cubital fossae, and groins. After about a week 'pin-hole desquamation' of the skin starts: little round pieces of dead skin flake off, temporarily leaving small holes in the superficial layers of the epidermis.

Septic Scarlet Fever, in which there is suppuration of cervical lymph-nodes as well as extensive septic infection in the throat, and **Toxic Scarlet Fever,** in which there is overwhelming toxaemia characterised by circulatory failure, delirium and stupor with minimal faucial reaction and rash, are severe and often fatal forms of the disease fortunately rare at the present time.

Complications. Local spread of infection may cause peritonsillar abscess (quinsy), retropharyngeal abscess, sinusitis, and cervical adenitis while aspiration may cause bronchitis and pneumonia, but none of these is common nowadays.

Late complications, occurring some three weeks after the original illness, are those which may follow any streptococcal tonsillitis, namely acute nephritis, rheumatic fever and anaphylactoid purpura.

Treatment. For the mildest form of the disease oral penicillin (phenoxymethyl penicillin) 250 mg. four times daily or phenethicillin 125 mg. four times daily is satisfactory. For more severe infections benzyl penicillin 250,000 to 1,000,000 units once or twice daily should be given intramuscularly and gravely ill patients should receive in addition refined scarlet fever antitoxin intramuscularly, the dose varying from 10,000 to 30,000 units according to the severity of the infection. To ensure eradication of haemolytic streptococci and minimise the risk of acute nephritis and rheumatic fever it is wise to continue penicillin therapy for ten days.

ENTERIC FEVER

Enteric is the name applied to a group of diseases which consists of typhoid fever and paratyphoid A, B, and C. They are due to closely related salmonella organisms, short thick motile gram-negative bacilli which can be distinguished from most of the non-pathogenic organisms of the coli-typhoid group by their inability to ferment lactose. Typhoid and paratyphoid B occur all over the world, the latter being the most common of the enteric fevers in this country; paratyphoid A is found mainly in the East; paratyphoid C is rare.

Method of Spread. Enteric fever is spread by contamination of food or water by excreta from carriers or from patients with the disease. It is therefore prevalent in countries whose standards of sanitation are low and armies on active service in the tropics are at special risk. The sharp reduction in the incidence of the disease which occurred in this country at the end of the nineteenth century was due to the introduction of methods of sewage disposal which prevent access to the water supplies. In countries with good sanitation outbreaks can usually be traced to unsuspecting carriers of the disease who are engaged in the handling of foodstuffs.

Clinical Features. After an incubation period of about a fortnight there is usually a gradual onset of *headache, aching* in the limbs, *tiredness, cough,* and *fever,* which typically rises in 'step-ladder' fashion by about one degree (F.) each day to reach a height of perhaps 103–104° F. towards the end of the first week. For the next week, or sometimes much longer, the temperature continues at this high level, showing very little variation throughout the twenty-four hours. The pulse usually does not show the increase in rate which accompanies most febrile illnesses, a *relative bradycardia* of less than 100 per minute being frequently maintained through the whole course of the illness. *Cough* and signs of bronchitis or even broncho-pneumonia are common in the first few days and may dominate the clinical picture at this stage.

In suspected cases watch must be kept about the end of the first week for the appearance of the characteristic *rash*. In typhoid this consists of a few 'rose-spots', which can easily be overlooked but which nevertheless are very typical of the disease. They occur particularly on the abdomen or chest and appear for a few days in a succession of crops of tiny pink spots, each not more than 1–2 mm. in diameter and each one lasting for only 24 hours or so. It is useful, therefore, to make a ring with a skin pencil round each spot seen so that the next day if any new ones have appeared it is clear at a glance that they are a new crop. In paratyphoid the rash is often much more profuse and may be composed of much larger less clearly defined elements which tend to coalesce with each other, producing an eruption rather like that of measles. The spleen often becomes palpable at about the same time as the rash appears.

Most patients are constipated during the first few days, but towards the end of the second week the abdomen becomes distended and *diarrhoea* sets in. By this time if the attack is a severe one the patient is very gravely ill and may pass into the 'typhoid state', in which he remains throughout the 24 hours in what has been called a 'coma-vigil', drowsy and confused but continually muttering to himself, plucking at the bedclothes. and groping for non-existent objects. The faeces are now fluid and light yellow in colour ('pea-soup stools') and up to twenty may be passed in 24 hours.

Gradual improvement usually occurs during the third and fourth weeks; the temperature settles by lysis, the diarrhoea stops, the mind becomes clearer and the other symptoms also slowly disappear. Very occasionally relapse occurs in convalescence: the writer has seen one patient before the antibiotic era who went through the whole course of typhoid fever three times within six months before making a complete recovery.

Diagnosis

Blood culture is by far the best way of establishing the diagnosis, and as the organisms circulate in the blood only during the first week it is extremely important that blood should be taken for culture as early as possible, preferably during the first three days.

Blood count typically shows a leucopenia, but this is not a constant finding, particularly in paratyphoid, and in the presence of bronchitis or other complication there may even be a slight leucocytosis.

Agglutinations (Widal test). As a rise in the agglutinin titre during the illness is the most important evidence of active infection, blood should be taken for this estimation at the same time as the initial blood culture during the first few days, and again during the second week. Quite high titres of 'H' (flagellar) agglutinin may be found in the blood of healthy people who have been inoculated with T.A.B., but a rising titre of 'O' (somatic) agglutinins is usually indicative of enteric infection. A high titre of 'Vi' (virulence) agglutinin is also usually significant.

Complications. The two most serious complications of typhoid are liable to occur during the third week of illness, when sloughs separate from the

Peyer's patches in the ileum leaving deep ulcers which may *perforate* or cause serious *haemorrhage*. Such *perforations* are easily overlooked clinically. By the time they occur the patient is in such a weak state that very little peritoneal reaction takes place and nothing approaching the dramatic pain and tenderness of the patient with a perforated peptic ulcer is to be expected; the only clue may be a sudden worsening of the general clinical condition, with a fall in the temperature and a rise in the pulse and respiration rates and the appearance of minimal abdominal tenderness. Before the days of antibiotics surgical closure of the perforation gave the only hope of recovery, but patients receiving chloramphenicol can usually be treated conservatively. *Haemorrhage* is more common than perforation; it is suggested by sudden faintness, pallor, and sweating, and diagnosed by the appearance of bright-red blood in the next stool passed. Transfusion is occasionally necessary but surgery never.

Venous thrombosis, particularly in the femoral vein, is common.

Parotitis is a dangerous complication which should be prevented by careful attention to the hygiene of the mouth.

Cholecystitis, with the subsequent formation of gall-stones containing salmonella typhi, and *acute arthritis*, are rare complications.

Typhoid abscesses in bone and periostitis causing the stiff and painful *typhoid spine* are very rare sequelae which may appear years after the original infection.

Treatment. The prognosis of typhoid has been greatly improved since the introduction of chloramphenicol, which is usually very effective. A satisfactory scheme of dosage for an adult is 1·5 g. twice daily for the first five days, then 0·75 g. twice daily for a week, and finally 1 g. daily for a few more days. Agglutination titres are lower and relapses more common than in untreated patients but the relapses usually respond satisfactorily to further courses of chloramphenicol. Subsequent development of the carrier state is no commoner in treated than in untreated patients, but chloramphenicol usually fails to eradicate the organisms from carriers and for this purpose cholecystectomy remains the most useful measure.

Ampicillin, in doses of 8 g. daily, is also effective but rather slower in producing a response than chloramphenicol.

Patients with typhoid must of course be nursed with strict barrier precautions. They should be given a high-calorie low-roughage diet.

Prophylactic immunisation against the enteric fevers is achieved by giving T.A.B.C. vaccine intramuscularly, 0·5 ml., followed a week later by a second inoculation of 1 ml. Those living in endemic areas should receive 'booster' doses of 0·5 ml. annually.

STAPHYLOCOCCAL FEVER

Staphylococci may invade the bloodstream from abscesses in any part of the body, the most common primary lesions being skin boils and carbuncles, lung abscess, osteomyelitis, and renal carbuncle. Factors tending to promote bloodstream invasion are the early incision of abscesses and attempts to evacuate pus by squeezing, and general debility due to chronic fatigue, malnutrition, or serious underlying disease such as diabetes or leukaemia.

Outbreaks of antibiotic-resistant staphylococcal infection have become a serious menace in hospital wards in recent years, the organism being disseminated by contact with such articles as blankets and bed-curtains, and by healthy carriers.

Clinical Features. The initial staphylococcal lesion may be an apparently trivial one, unsuspected by the patient as the source of his subsequent severe illness. The onset of septicaemia is heralded by *rigors* and *fever* which is usually high and remittent or intermittent in type. Profuse *sweats* are common and sometimes there is a relative bradycardia. Metastatic *abscesses* develop in various sites, notably the lungs, joints, muscles, and skin, and purpura is also common. Bacterial endocarditis should be suspected when there are changing cardiac murmurs and when septicaemia persists in the absence of obvious staphylococcal lesions elsewhere. Some anaemia and leucocytosis are usual and the diagnosis is clinched by a positive *blood culture.*

Treatment. In spite of modern antibiotic therapy the mortality rate is still high. When staphylococcal septicaemia is suspected clinically, blood should be taken for culture and treatment started with benzylpenicillin 10 mega units daily together with cloxacillin 4·0 g. daily. Treatment should be continued for at least two weeks, (six weeks if endocarditis is suspected). If a satisfactory response is not obtained, sodium fusidate 500 mg. thrice daily should be added to the treatment. If blood culture reveals other organisms antibiotic treatment should be adjusted accordingly.

CEREBROSPINAL FEVER (Meningococcal meningitis)

This disease is endemic throughout the world and in this country it is seen mainly during the winter months. From time to time epidemics occur, usually localised ones in residential institutions such as military barracks. Sporadic cases are commonest in infancy, while outbreaks affect adolescents and young adults.

Transmission is by droplet infection from patients and carriers and in susceptible contacts the meningococcus enters the bloodstream from the nasopharynx, causing a septicaemia. Usually, but not always, the infection then becomes localised to the meninges.

Clinical Features

(1) **Usual Meningitic Form.** After an incubation period of two or three days the illness starts rather suddenly, often with a shivering attack or rigor, followed by fever, severe headache, and vomiting. Convulsions are common in children. Within a few days signs of acute meningeal irritation develop: these are *neck rigidity* and a positive *Kernig's sign.* About 30 per

cent of patients have a macular rash which rapidly becomes purpuric and is of great help in clinical diagnosis. Although the eruption may be profuse, there are frequently only a few lesions which are easily overlooked unless a careful search is made for them.

Diagnosis is established by lumbar puncture, which reveals turbid fluid under increased pressure. The fluid contains large numbers of polymorphs, and meningococci can be demonstrated either by microscopy of a stained film or on culture.

(2) **Fulminating Meningococcal Meningitis.** This rapidly fatal but fortunately rare form starts very abruptly with high fever and within a few hours the patient is in coma with signs of acute meningitis and a profuse petechial rash. In spite of treatment death usually occurs within 24 to 48 hours.

(3) **Waterhouse-Friderichsen Syndrome.** Also fortunately rare, this syndrome is the result of bilateral adrenal haemorrhages accompanying the purpura of acute meningococcal (and other) septicaemias and is usually seen in children. Acute adrenal insufficiency leads to vomiting, collapse, and low blood pressure. Cortisone 200–300 mg. daily must be given in addition to antibiotic therapy but rarely averts the fatal outcome.

(4) **Chronic Meningococcal Septicaemia.** This curious, recurrent, and often puzzling disease, which has become much rarer since the introduction of the sulphonamides and antibiotics, causes little constitutional upset but presents with bouts of low fever, accompanied by headache, joint pains, and a maculo-papular rash on the trunk and limbs. On the legs the eruption may mimic erythema nodosum and sometimes, though not always, it contains purpuric elements. Such attacks may recur at varying intervals over a period of many months. The diagnosis is confirmed by isolation of the meningococcus on blood culture.

Treatment. The meningococcus is sensitive to both the sulphonamides and penicillin. Suitable dosage of sulphadiazine for an adult is 1·5 g. four-hourly for two days, then 1 g. four-hourly for two days, and finally 1 g. six-hourly for three or four days. During this time it is particularly important to maintain an adequate fluid intake. Patients who are gravely ill or vomiting should be given 1 g. by slow intravenous injection every four hours and in addition should receive benzyl penicillin 1 million units intramuscularly every four hours. Penicillin alone is not satisfactory for the treatment of meningitis, however, in view of its poor penetration of the blood-brain barrier.

VIRUS INFECTIONS

SMALLPOX (Variola)

There are three varieties of the smallpox virus. The first causes true Asiatic smallpox (*variola major*), which has a high mortality rate; the second causes a much milder disease (alastrim or *variola minor*); and the third is the one used for vaccination, which, though it retains the power to stimulate immunity against smallpox, can no longer itself cause a serious disease.

Routine vaccination of children is no longer recommended in the U.K. since the risk of contracting small pox is now less than the risk of a serious complication of vaccination, which is given therefore only to people at special risk, such as doctors and nurses, and those travelling to endemic areas.

Clinical Features. After an incubation period of about a fortnight (exactly 12 days in most patients) there is sudden onset of headache, fever, shivering, severe pain in the back, and generalised aching in the limbs. In the most severe cases a prodromal purpuric rash may be seen almost from the start, but the true eruption of smallpox does not appear until the third day. Mucosal lesions are often the first to appear and may be very extensive in the mouth and throat. When the disease is very severe the skin of the whole body may be covered by the rash (confluent smallpox), but usually it can be seen that the peripheral parts of the limbs are more thickly covered with spots than the proximal limb segments and the trunk. Each spot starts as a red discoloration (a *macule*), but within about 24 hours it becomes thick and raised so that it can be felt with the finger (a *papule*). About three days later the centre of the papule becomes soft and filled with clear serous fluid, so that it is now a *vesicle*; and secondary infection of the fluid with pyogenic bacteria changes it in a few days into pus, so that the lesion now becomes a *pustule*. All the spots go through this series of changes at approximately the same time. A day or two after the appearance of the rash the patient's temperature may come down and his general condition improve, but a few days later, when the lesions have become pustular, the fever returns and he again becomes gravely ill. Most of the deaths (up to 25 per cent of the patients in some epidemics of variola major; 16 out of 64 patients in one outbreak dealt with by the writer) occur during the pustular stage, though in the most severe but fortunately rare form of the disease (*haemorrhagic smallpox*) death occurs within 48 hours of the onset with signs of bleeding into internal organs and from various mucosal surfaces. In patients who recover, the temperature slowly settles over a period of a week or so as the pustules gradually dry off into crusts and scabs. Since the crusts contain living virus, the patient has to be kept in isolation until they have all come away: this may take several weeks, the last to separate being the deep-seated scabs in the palms of the hands and soles of the feet.

Modified Variola Major and Variola Minor. Variola major modified by partial immunity from past vaccination and variola minor are relatively trivial illnesses with only slight constitutional upset and a rash which may be very difficult to distinguish from that of chicken-pox.

Diagnosis. In distinguishing mild smallpox from chicken-pox the following points are helpful:

> (1) The lesions of chicken-pox are set more superficially in the skin and tend to be smaller.

(2) In chicken-pox the lesions are more profuse on the trunk than on the extremities; the reverse is true of smallpox.

(3) In chicken-pox the eruption appears in a series of crops, so that at any one time lesions at different stages of maturity can be found; in smallpox the lesions are all at the same stage.

(4) Recent successful vaccination excludes smallpox.

(5) The diagnosis of smallpox can be confirmed by demonstrating virus elementary bodies in fluid obtained from vesicles and in the blood in the pre-emptive stage.

(6) Complement-fixation and set-diffusion tests can be used to demonstrate antigen in material from lesions and, later in the illness, antibodies in the blood.

Complications include broncho-pneumonia, otitis media, conjunctivitis, corneal ulceration and resultant opacity, cardiac failure, and encephalitis.

Treatment. There is no specific therapy against the virus of smallpox, but the stage of secondary pyogenic infection can be cut short by the administration of a suitable antibiotic. Penicillin by injection or one of the tetracyclines by mouth may be given for this purpose and if necessary changed later when the *in vitro* sensitivities of the organism isolated from the lesions have been established. Skilled nursing is of great importance, particular attention being paid to the care of the mouth, eyes, and skin.

Action to be taken when Smallpox is suspected

(1) The medical officer of health must be notified immediately.

(2) If the diagnosis is confirmed the patient is transferred at once to a special smallpox hospital.

(3) All members of the hospital staff and all who have been in contact with the patient must be vaccinated or revaccinated. N-methylisatin-thiosemicarbazone ('Marboran') given by mouth to contacts within the incubation period has been reported as giving remarkable protection and may replace vaccination for this purpose. The dose is 1·5–3 g. twice daily for four days.

In addition the medical officer of health will take further action to trace the source of infection and to prevent further spread; this will include disinfection of the patient's house and keeping his family and other contacts under supervision for at least 16 days.

Prevention by Vaccination

Edward Jenner introduced vaccination at the end of the eighteenth century after noting that milkers who had had cowpox (vaccinia) appeared to be immune to smallpox. This is because the virus of smallpox is attenuated by passage through the cow, though it retains its antigenic properties.

Technique of Vaccination. Fresh glycerinated calf lymph is obtained from the public health laboratory service and stored in a refrigerator.

Secondary infection is least common when the vaccination is performed over the deltoid area. The skin at the chosen site is cleaned with soap and water and dried with a sterile towel; alternatively ether or acetone may be used, but spirit and iodine should be avoided as they may kill the virus and so prevent the vaccination taking. Using a rubber bulb a drop of lymph is ejected from the capillary tube on to the prepared area of skin and a sterile Hagedorn needle, held parallel to the skin, is moved rapidly up and down through the lymph, just sufficient pressure being applied to penetrate the epidermis at the point of the needle. This is the *multiple pressure technique*, which is superior to the old scratch method as it limits the depth of penetration of the virus into the skin and reduces the incidence of complications. About 10 pressures are recommended for primary vaccination and 30 pressures for revaccination. After a few minutes (during which time the area should not be exposed to direct sunlight) excess lymph is dabbed off and a dry sterile dressing is applied.

Results of Vaccination. Successful vaccination may be indicated by three types of reaction:

(1) The *primary reaction* (obtained in people who have not been vaccinated before) is the appearance by the third or fourth day of a papule which develops through a vesicular stage to become a pustule by the seventh day (when the result is read). During this week there may be fever, malaise, and axillary adenitis. A scab forms in the second week and separates in the third week, leaving a permanent pitted scar.

(2) The *accelerated reaction* is seen in people with partial immunity. The lesion goes through its stages more quickly and may never become pustular.

(3) The *immune reaction*, seen in people with a higher degree of immunity, consists simply of a small itchy papule on the second or third day which disappears without becoming vesicular.

Complications of Vaccination are very rare and particularly so in infancy.

Encephalitis (see p. 508) is much the most serious and has a mortality of about 50 per cent. Its incidence is about 1 in 100,000 vaccinations.

Generalised vaccinia, in which lesions occur on the skin all over the body from widespread dissemination of the virus, is also very rare except in people with eczema, who should not be vaccinated unless exposed to special risk.

Secondary infection of the vaccination site and *accidental inoculation* of other areas of skin by scratching are commoner and less serious complications.

Foetal mortality is high in women vaccinated during the first three months of pregnancy and this time should consequently be avoided for vaccination whenever possible.

CHICKEN-POX (Varicella)

The virus of chicken-pox is identical or closely allied to the virus of herpes zoster (shingles); susceptible children who come into contact with shingles frequently develop chicken-pox, while less often adult contacts of the latter disease may develop shingles.

Clinical Features. After an incubation period of up to three weeks the illness may start with a day of vague malaise, headache, fever, and a transient prodromal rash, before the specific eruption appears, but more often the rash is the first sign of the disease. Vesicles appear first in the mouth and throat and soon rupture, leaving ulcers which may cause a good deal of pain and difficulty in swallowing. The skin rash, unlike that of smallpox, is most profuse on the trunk and sparsest at the periphery of the limbs; and instead of all the lesions going through their various stages together, the spots appear in a succession of crops over several days, so that at any one time papules, vesicles, pustules and crusts can be seen together. The papules develop within a few hours into small round vesicles containing clear fluid set in the superficial layers of the skin. Within two or three days they become pustules and then dry up into crusts.

Constitutional upset is usually slight, though the enanthem (mucosal lesions) may cause much discomfort and the exanthem (skin rash) much itching. The disease is more severe in adults, who may develop patchy consolidation in the lungs and may subsequently be found to have scattered calcified opacities on chest X-ray.

Complications are unusual. Secondary infection may lead to boils, impetigo, cellulitis, or conjunctivitis. More serious but very rare are polyneuritis, transverse myelitis, and encephalitis.

Diagnosis from smallpox; see p. 499.

Treatment is purely symptomatic. Irritation of the skin can be relieved by the application of calamine lotion containing 1–2 per cent phenol, or by warm boracic baths, and anti-histamine tablets may be helpful.

MEASLES (Morbilli)

Next to whooping cough this is the most serious of the infectious fevers of childhood at the present time. Passive immunity from the mother prevents infection in the first three months of life, but thereafter the child becomes highly susceptible.

Clinical Features. About ten to fourteen days after exposure to infection there develops what appears to be a common cold, with fever, running nose and eyes, sneezing, and cough. Examination of the mouth, however, reveals an eruption of tiny white spots like grains of salt set on a slightly reddened base, usually best seen on the mucous membrane inside the cheeks opposite the molar teeth. These are *Koplik's spots* and they are diagnostic of measles. If they are overlooked the erroneous impression that the child simply has a cold may appear to be confirmed on the third day, when the temperature may come down to normal, but this opinion is finally refuted on the fourth day, when the rash appears on the skin.

Transient prodromal rashes are sometimes seen during the first three days, but the true *morbilliform eruption* appears on the fourth day as pink macules, about 3–5 mm. in diameter, which first appear behind the ears and quickly spread over the face, trunk, and limbs. Within a day or two the lesions enlarge and become papular, many of them coalesce into large, irregular, blotchy areas, and their colour gradually changes to a darker red. The temperature rises again with the appearance of the rash and continues for several days before finally subsiding as the lesions fade.

Complications are mainly due to secondary bacterial infection of the respiratory tract. *Broncho-pneumonia* is the most serious of them, particularly in very young children, and should always be suspected in a severely ill child with a persistent cough. *Otitis media* is fairly common. *Corneal ulceration* and potential blindness should be prevented by careful treatment of any conjunctival inflammation which occurs.

Treatment. The virus of measles is not susceptible to any form of specific treatment, but antibiotics are of value for the prevention and cure of secondary bacterial complications. Save in the mildest cases it is probably wise to give a course of penicillin, starting with the appearance of the rash and continuing for up to a week. Procaine penicillin 300,000 units twice daily may be given intramuscularly, but phenoxymethyl penicillin 250 mg. six-hourly, is almost as satisfactory and avoids the necessity of injections.

Prevention. Effective Measles vaccines are now available and the best course for inducing *active immunity* is probably to give 0·5 ml. killed vaccine intramuscularly followed by 0·5 ml. of live vaccine one month later. A rise in temperature may occur after live vaccine and it should not be given to children under 9 months, to pregnant women or to patients with infective or neoplastic disease. Rapid *passive immunisation* lasting two or three weeks can be achieved by the intramuscular injection of gamma globulin, from 150 to 900 mg. during the first five days after exposure to infection. Large doses prevent the attack of measles; smaller doses have the advantage that, although an attack of measles may occur, it will be mild one and recovery from it will leave lifelong immunity.

GERMAN MEASLES (Rubella)

This is a less infectious disease than true measles and even in towns many people reach adult life without acquiring it. It causes little constitutional upset and is never fatal, but when acquired by women in the first four months of pregnancy it may lead to developmental defects in the foetus. Cataract, glaucoma, disorders of retinal pigmentation, deaf mutism, and congenital heart disease are the lesions commonly caused. There is also an increased incidence of abortion, miscarriage, and stillbirth, but foetal injury is not inevitable and a proportion of women who have had rubella early in pregnancy do produce healthy live babies. It is now recommended that girls who have not had Rubella should be given a single dose of live attenuated rubella virus, Cendehill strain, between the ages 11–14. No other vaccine should be given within 3–4 weeks. This vaccine must not be given to pregnant women because of the risk of foetal damage, or to patients with Hodgkin's disease or leukaemia or to those on immuno-suppressive therapy.

Clinical Features. After an incubation period of two to three weeks the rash is usually the first indication of the disease, and takes the form of small pink macules and papules which remain distinct units and do not run together as in true measles. There are no Koplik's spots in the mouth. The only other notable feature is generalised lymph-node enlargement, affecting particularly the nodes at the back of the neck. There are rarely any general symptoms of illness and the rash usually fades in two or three days. In adults a transient mild arthritis is common.

No **treatment** is needed. The disease may be prevented in women in early pregnancy who have been exposed to infection by giving high-titre immunoglobulin if available.; protection lasts for three weeks. Ordinary gamma globulin is of little value.

MUMPS (Epidemic parotitis).

Mumps is a relatively trivial illness in young children, but if contracted after puberty it may have serious complications. There are undoubted advantages, therefore, in 'getting it over' early in life, and only if a child is in a weak state of health from some other illness should any steps be taken to isolate him from this infection.

Clinical Features. After an incubation period of three weeks or a little longer the patient develops fever, malaise, and stiffness in the jaw, and examination reveals swelling of one or more of the salivary glands. Usually the parotid glands are affected and fill out the hollow between the angle of the jaw and the mastoid process. Sometimes the submandibular glands are affected too, or occasionally they are involved alone. There is no rash and usually the fever and glandular swellings subside within a few days.

Complications are almost confined to adolescent and adult patients and usually arise a few days after the swelling of the salivary glands.

Orchitis is the commonest complication, being seen in about 25 per cent of patients. It is usually unilateral and causes severe pain and swelling of the testicle. Very rarely it may be bilateral and result in sterility.

Oophoritis is less common and causes severe lower abdominal pain and vomiting.

Prostatitis should be suspected in patients with unexplained fever and perhaps some frequency of micturition.

Mastitis, causing pain and swelling of the breast, may be seen in either sex.

Pancreatitis is characterised by severe upper abdominal pain, fever and vomiting.

Meningitis. Routine lumbar puncture in patients with mumps usually reveals a pleocytosis in the C.S.F., so that invasion of the nervous system by the virus is common, but in only about 10 per cent of cases is there clinical evidence of meningitis (headache, fever, vomiting, and neck rigidity). These symptoms usually subside within two or three days and the prognosis is excellent.

Encephalitis, characterised by severe headache, fever, vomiting, perhaps cranial nerve palsies, drowsiness, and coma, is much more serious and carries a mortality of about 50 per cent.

Treatment. There is no specific treatment and no method of inducing either active or passive immunity has yet been shown to be effective. However, patients with orchitis gain relief from systemic steroids.

ORNITHOSIS (Psittacosis)

This virus is acquired by contact with infected birds, who do not themselves necessarily appear ill. Originally described in parrots, it can, however, be transmitted by other birds, including canaries and budgerigars.

Clinical Features. After an incubation period of one to two weeks there is gradual onset with cough, fever, headache, backache, and general malaise. The pulse usually remains low in relation to the temperature, but in fulminating cases with high fever and delirium rising pulse and respiratory rates indicate a poor prognosis. Though clinical signs of pulmonary consolidation are often absent, radiographs usually show evidence of pneumonia spreading out from the hilum of the lung. The white blood count is low or normal.

The disease acquired from parrots is often more severe than that spread by other birds. Convalescence is usually slow and prolonged.

Diagnosis may be confirmed by a complement fixation test using psittacosis antigen.

Treatment. Tetracycline is the drug of choice and should be given in doses of 0·5 g. four-hourly for a week. In view of the possibility of case to case transmission by droplet infection the patient should be nursed on barrier precautions.

GLANDULAR FEVER (Infectious mononucleosis)

The infective agent causing glandular fever has not yet been isolated, but it is thought to be a virus. It is a common disease, seen mainly in young adults, but its infectivity is low, though small outbreaks occur quite often in hostels and similar institutions. Patients in general wards should be nursed on barrier precautions.

Clinical Features. The main symptoms are fever, which is usually low and long-continued, lassitude, general malaise, and sometimes sore throat, but the severity and course of the disease are very variable. Some patients simply feel a little tired for a week or two, while others are gravely ill with high fever, headache, and severe sore throat; and although this acute stage does not usually last for more than a week or so, general debility and depression may persist for up to six months. The prognosis, however, is excellent; the disease is never fatal and all patients make a complete recovery. Examination usually reveals enlarged lymph nodes in the neck and elsewhere and the spleen can often be felt. Many patients have a transient macular rash and palatal petechiae are common.

Subclinical hepatitis is very common but actual jaundice infrequent. E.C.G. evidence of myocarditis has been reported in 16 per cent of patients. Acute abdominal pain simulating appendicitis, benign lymphocytic meningitis, transient thrombocytopenic purpura and rupture of the spleen are rare manifestations.

Diagnosis depends on:

(1) The *white blood count* which after an initial leucopenia is usually raised with an excess of monocytes and lymphocytes, many of which are seen in the stained film to have a characteristic abnormal appearance ('glandular fever cells').

(2) The *Paul-Bunnell* test is positive in about 90 per cent of cases. It depends on the fact that in glandular fever the serum contains an unknown factor which agglutinates sheep's red cells. Occasional false positive results occur, but a titre of 1:64 or higher, and particularly a rising titre during the illness, may be taken as significant.

Treatment. The duration of fever and debility may be reduced by a week's course of prednisolone, starting with 40 mg. daily, but this should be reserved for severely ill patients. There is no specific treatment, and prolonged convalescence is often necessary.

INFLUENZA

Of the three strains of influenza virus, A is more common than B and C is rare. There is no correlation between the clinical severity of the illness and the strain of virus and no cross-immunity between the strains. Variation in the antigenic structure of the virus occurs from time to time and limits the effectiveness of vaccines. Epidemics of influenza A tend to occur every two to three years and influenza B every four to five years. Factors leading to occasional pandemics, as in 1918 and 1957 (the 'Asian flu') are unknown. Between epidemics the virus is probably kept going in a chain of sporadic infections in man; some of these may be subclinical. Transmission is by droplet infection.

Clinical Features. After an incubation period of one to two days there is sudden onset with fever, shivering, headache, profound malaise, and severe aching in the back and limbs. Cough, sneezing, and upper respiratory catarrh are usually relatively slight. Remittent fever and general prostration continue for up to a week and the temperature settles by lysis. In some patients convalescence is very slow and post-influenzal debility and depression may persist for months.

Influenzal pneumonia. Particularly in the 1918 pandemic pneumonia was a common complication and a common cause of death, but in recent years it has been comparatively rare. It is due to secondary bacterial infection with H. influenzae, staphylococci, streptococci, or pneumococci.

Treatment. There is no specific treatment, though the appropriate chemotherapy should of course be given for any bacterial complication. Aspirin 0·6 g. four-hourly helps to relieve symptoms during the febrile stage.

Prophylaxis. Vaccines containing inactivated strains of A and B virus give partial immunity for about six months and are of limited value if given just before an epidemic.

EPIDEMIC VOMITING

This very common virus infection typically causes small outbreaks of several cases in a family.

Clinical Features. Onset is abrupt with nausea and vomiting and sometimes there is mild fever and diarrhoea as well. Constitutional upset is very mild and complete recovery usually occurs within two days.

Diagnosis is usually obvious from the occurrence of multiple cases and the short duration of symptoms and no *treatment* is necessary.

OTHER VIRUS CONDITIONS

In addition to the well-recognised virus diseases, it is now realised that there are several groups of viruses which may cause a variety of clinical syndromes. Among the most common are:

COXSACKIE AND ECHO VIRUS GROUP

These viruses may cause:

(a) **Meningitis** (Benign lymphocytic)

This presents with fever, headache, nausea and a stiff neck. The cerebrospinal fluid contains a hundred or so cells per c.mm. which are predominantly lymphocytes.

(b) **Epidemic Myalgia** (Bornholm disease) (p. 316).

ADENOVIRUS GROUP

An acute upper respiratory tract infection which is sometimes no more than a common cold, but it may be a more severe influenzal-like illness with fever, sore throat, cough, and sometimes painful enlargement of the lymphatic glands. Areas of pneumonic consolidation and concomitant conjunctivitis have been reported.

HAND, FOOT AND MOUTH DISEASE

Th:s infection with Coxsackie A viruses is distinct from foot and mouth disease of animals, which is caused by another picornavirus. It is seen mainly in young children, but adults in the family are often affected too. It occurs mainly in summer and autumn.

Clinical Features. After an incubation period of 3–6 days there is a mild febrile illness lasting only a few days. On the second or third days a maculopapular rash, later becoming vesicular, appears on the fingers, toes and lateral borders of the feet and painful ulcers develop in the mouth. These lesions heal within about a week.

Diagnosis. The clinical picture is quite characteristic but if necessary the diagnosis can be confirmed by virus studies. The virus may be present in the faeces for several weeks after infection.

POST-INFECTIOUS ENCEPHALITIS AND ENCEPHALOMYELITIS

This condition is a very rare sequel to acute specific fevers such as whooping cough, measles, and mumps and less often to others such as chicken-pox, German measles, scarlet fever, and glandular fever; it is no commoner after severe than mild attacks. It also sometimes follows vaccination and other immunising procedures. It has been suggested that the underlying cause may be an antigen-antibody reaction and sometimes improvement does seem to follow treatment with ACTH or cortisone.

Clinical Features. Symptoms appear within a week or two of the onset of the original infection or vaccination. Headache, malaise, vomiting, irritability, drowsiness, or coma are common; other patients present with fits or sudden paresis mimicking a cerebral vascular accident; while in others the clinical picture is dominated by signs of meningitis, cranial nerve palsies, and transient lower motor neurone weakness in the limbs. Mortality is highest, about 50 per cent, in encephalitis following smallpox or vaccination, but even in the other groups it does not fall below 10 per cent and is often higher. Moreover, many of those who recover are left with a disability such as hemiplegia, cranial nerve palsies, mental defect, or a Parkinsonian syndrome.

INFECTIVE DISEASES for which barrier nursing is unnecessary.

WEIL'S DISEASE (Epidemic spirochaetal jaundice)

The causal organism, Leptospira icterohaemorrhagiae, is excreted in the urine of infected rats. Man acquires the infection either by ingesting food or drink contaminated by rat urine or by immersion in contaminated water, since the spirochaete is able to gain entry through the nasal mucosa or through minor skin abrasions. In this country leptospirosis is therefore mainly seen as an occupational disease of people working in damp rat-infested places, notably sewer workers, miners, canal and dock-workers, farm-hands and fish-cleaners.

Clinical Features. After an incubation period of between one and two weeks there is rapid onset of fever, headache, pains in the back and limbs. Injection of the conjunctivae is often a very striking feature. The name 'ictero-haemorrhagiae' implies jaundice and purpura, but clinical jaundice is seen in only about 75 per cent of patients; it appears during the first week. Features which help in distinguishing the disease from infective hepatitis are the profound prostration, heavy albuminuria, purpuric rash, and some-times haemoptysis, haematemesis, melaena, or bleeding from the gums. There is usually a leucocytosis. Some patients develop signs of meningeal irritation and some proceed from oliguria to anuria and uraemia; the mor-tality rate is about 15 per cent.

Diagnosis is established by identifying the spirochaete by dark-ground illumination of specimens of blood taken during the first few days or urine during the third week. The organism can also be isolated by intraperitoneal inoculation of guinea-pigs with blood or urine. A rising titre of serum agglutinins also occurs but does not give diagnostic information until the clinical illness is more or less over.

Treatment. To be effective penicillin must be given early in the illness, in large doses such as 3 million units six-hourly. If there is no improvement after three days oxytetracycline $1 \cdot 5$ g. six-hourly may be given a trial. Antileptospiral serum is also effective if given during the first few days; it is injected either intravenously or intramuscularly in doses of 20–40 ml.

BRUCELLOSIS (Undulant fever; Malta fever)

The causative organism is a gram-negative cocco-bacillus which is transmitted to man in infected milk. In this country the usual infecting organism is Brucella abortus, which is prevalent throughout the world and is transmitted in cow's milk. Brucella melitensis is transmitted in goat's milk and is found particularly in the Mediterranean area, where it causes Malta fever. Brucella suis infects pigs and is rarely transmitted to man.

The disease is an occupational hazard of farm workers and slaughtermen since infection can be acquired through the skin and mucosae, but others may be infected by drinking unpasteurised milk. There is reason to think it may be more common in this country than is generally realised.

Clinical Features. Typical undulant fever has an incubation period of between one and three weeks, followed by headache, malaise, anorexia, constipation, and a bout of fever which usually settles by lysis after about ten days. Cough and profuse sweating are common and the spleen is usually palpable. After the temperature has been normal for a few days another bout of fever begins and these febrile episodes may continue recurring at short intervals for many months. During the course of the illness arthritis is common. One joint is usually affected at a time, the pain and swelling subsiding after a few days and then appearing elsewhere. The joints most often affected are the hip, knee, shoulder, ankle, and wrist, but occasionally the small joints of the fingers and toes or of the spine may be involved. Peripheral neuritis, orchitis, and albuminuria are less common complications.

Abortus fever as seen in this country is on the whole clinically milder and sometimes takes such a prolonged and insidious course that the more appropriate label *chronic brucellosis* is often used. Recurrent bouts of drenching night sweats without serious general ill-health should always suggest this diagnosis and the other clinical features mentioned above may also be seen.

Diagnosis. *Blood culture* is the most satisfactory way of establishing the diagnosis, but the organism is difficult to isolate (even under increased CO_2 tension) so that sterile cultures do not rule out this disease. *Urine culture* is occasionally positive. A rising *agglutinin titre* during the illness is helpful; dilutions up to 1:5,000 should be tested, since agglutination may be found in the higher dilutions but absent in the lower ones. The brucellin skin test is of doubtful value. The *blood count* usually shows a leucopenia and perhaps mild anaemia.

Treatment. Tetracycline 0·75 g. six-hourly and intramuscular streptomycin 0·75 g. twice daily, with a vitamin B preparation such as becosym forte two tablets three times daily, should be given for two weeks. A second course of treatment may be necessary for patients with chronic brucellosis.

Prevention of infection may be achieved by attention to personal hygiene by those handling cattle, pigs, and goats; pasteurisation of milk; a clean water supply; and disinfection of excreta, particularly urine, from patients with the disease.

TETANUS

It is estimated that in Britain each year this preventible disease is contracted by 200–300 people and kills half of them. Clostridium tetani is a normal inhabitant of the alimentary tract of horses and sheep, so that its spores are particularly prevalent on cultivated land, and as it is a strict anaerobe it thrives especially in deep penetrating wounds contaminated with soil or road dust. The wound, however, may be a trivial one which heals before the tetanic symptoms appear. These are due to a powerful exotoxin which is absorbed by muscle end-plates at the site of infection and travels along motor nerves to the central nervous system.

Clinical Features. The incubation period is very variable and is important in prognosis: tetanus appearing within a few days of a wound is usually fatal, while if symptoms are delayed for two or more weeks the disease is likely to be mild. Local muscular weakness near the site of infection, attributable to the action of the toxin on the motor end-plates, may precede the generalised spasms. These are usually heralded by trismus (hence the term lockjaw), which may be accompanied by spasm of the facial musculature causing the classical 'risus sardonicus'. Tonic spasm spreads to the trunk, causing opisthotonus and board-like rigidity of the abdomen. Fever is commonly present.

The *paroxysmal stage* starts in severe cases within two days of the appearance of trismus; the longer it is delayed the better the prognosis. Paroxysms are precipitated by stimuli such as feeding and other nursing attentions, clinical examination or even simply external noises. The whole body is thrown into painful spasm, with arching of the back, extension of the limbs and clenching of the teeth; this may subside after a few seconds or persist for several minutes. In severe cases the paroxysms recur with increasing frequency until death occurs from exhaustion.

Treatment. (a) The patient should be nursed in a quiet room with shaded light. Intravenous *antitoxin* 200,000 units should be given providing there has been no reaction to a subcutaneous test dose of 1,500 units. Allergic subjects should be given a preliminary dose of 150 units (0·1 ml.), followed by 1,500 units half an hour later. If a reaction occurs intravenous administration must be avoided, but gradually increasing doses may be given intramuscularly, each accompanied by 1:1,000 adrenaline 0·5 ml. A syringe containing adrenaline must always be at hand when intravenous antitoxin is given. All patients should be given intramuscular antitoxin 25,000 units daily throughout the rest of the illness to deal with new toxin produced at the site of infection; antitoxin unfortunately has no action on toxin which has become fixed in nerve tissue.

(b) *Wound Toilet.* An hour after the antitoxin has been given surgical debridement of the wound should be carried out under light general anaesthesia.

(c) *Antibiotic Therapy.* As a prophylaxis against broncho-pneumonia procaine penicillin 450,000 units and benzyl penicillin 500,000 units should be given twice daily.

(d) *Control of Muscular Spasms.* For successful management of severe cases continuous skilled medical supervision throughout the 24 hours is necessary. Intravenous succinylcholine 0·2 per cent at a rate of 1–1·5 ml. (2–3 mg.) per minute controls most of the spasms, but occasionally much faster administration is needed for a few seconds and at these times respiration ceases and the lungs must be inflated with oxygen delivered through an anaesthetic machine. For the latter purpose tracheal intubation should be carried out as soon as satisfactory relaxation has been obtained and later a tracheotomy may be done. The foot of the bed should be blocked to prevent accumulation of secretions in the air passages, which are cleared every hour by a sucker attached to a catheter which is passed through the tracheotomy tube. From time to time the patient is allowed to come round so that an attempt may be made to feed him, but in the early stages this must be done through an intragastric tube. Intravenous therapy to maintain fluid and electrolyte balance is also essential.

Prophylaxis. *Active immunisation* if generally adopted could wipe out this disease. Tetanus toxoid should be given to all children in the combined triple vaccine with diphtheria and pertussis (see p. 486). Alternatively tetanus toxoid alone may be given in three doses of 1 ml., the second six to twelve weeks after the first and the third six to twelve months after the second. If an individual actively immunised in this way receives a wound he should be given a further dose of toxoid instead of antitetanic serum.

Passive immunisation. Antitetanic serum confers passive immunity for some four weeks, but occasionally causes anaphylatic reactions which may be fatal. In view of this danger, A.T.S. should not be given to allergic subjects, or to those who react to a test dose of 150 units (0·1 ml.) subcutaneously and may be omitted in patients with perfectly clean superficial wounds. On the other hand, pitchfork wounds and gunshot wounds involving the colon incur such a risk of tetanus that A.T.S. must be given even if there is a history of allergy; for details of administration see p. 511.

CAT-SCRATCH FEVER

This disease, whose causative organism has not yet been isolated, is transmitted by the scratch of apparently healthy cats.

Clinical Features. A few days after the scratch a small indolent ulcer or sore may appear at the site of inoculation and a week or two later the regional lymph nodes become very enlarged. There may be some fever at this stage but constitutional upset is slight. The affected lymph nodes sometimes suppurate, but recovery without serious complications or sequelae is the rule though adenitis may persist for some months. The white blood count is normal and aspirated pus is sterile.

Treatment. A course of tetracycline, 250 mg. six-hourly for five days, may prevent suppuration.

ACTINOMYCOSIS

The organism Actinomyces bovis occurs in pus as 'sulphur granules' of up to 1 mm. in diameter and is anaerobic. The disease is much more common in men than in women.

Clinical Features. There are three clinical varieties:

(1) *Actinomycosis of the jaw* is the commonest type. Infection through the mucous membrane of the gum leads gradually to woody induration of all the tissues of the jaw and overlying skin, through which multiple sinuses eventually discharge. There is little pain or constitutional upset and the regional lymph nodes are not usually involved.

(2) *Ileocaecal actinomycosis* causes a hard irregular mass in the right iliac fossa and in time fixation to the overlying skin and sinus formation

occur. The disease may spread to the liver, spleen, and other organs and is frequently fatal.

(3) *Actinomycosis of the lung* is the least common type. Cough, dyspnoea, fever, and pain in the chest occur and in the later stages induration and sinuses appear in the chest wall.

Diagnosis depends on identification of the 'sulphur granules' in the pus.
Treatment consists of the administration of penicillin in high dosage for a prolonged period and surgical eradication of the disease wherever possible.

FURTHER READING

Burnett, Sir Macfarlane. *Natural History of Infectious Diseases*, 3rd edition. Cambridge University Press, London, 1962.

CHAPTER SEVENTEEN

TROPICAL DISEASES

MALARIA

Malaria is by far the commonest and most important of the tropical diseases and is responsible for some millions of deaths each year. It is prevalent in areas where there are both anophelene mosquitoes and enough warmth and humidity to allow the parasite to develop in them. There are four varieties of human malaria, due to infection respectively with Plasmodium vivax (benign tertian malaria), Plasmodium falciparum (malignant tertian malaria), Plasmodium malariae (quartan malaria), and Plasmodium ovale (benign tertian malaria). P. vivax is responsible for most of the malaria seen in India and South-east Asia; P. falciparum is the common malarial parasite in Africa; P. malariae and P. ovale are both comparatively rare.

Life-cycle of the Malarial Parasite. Sexual forms of the plasmodium (*gametocytes*) circulate in the blood at a certain stage of malaria and when they are ingested into the stomach of an anophelene mosquito the male and female gametocytes unite, penetrate the stomach wall and form an oocyst. After some one to three weeks (the time varying with the temperature) *sporozoites* are liberated from the oocyst, find their way to the salivary glands and so back to the bloodstream of man. They quickly disappear from the blood to enter liver cells, where the pre-erythrocytic stage of development takes place. After $8\frac{1}{2}$ days (P. vivax) or $6\frac{1}{2}$ days (P. falciparum) numerous *merozoites* are liberated and enter circulating red blood corpuscles, or, in the case of P. vivax, P. malariae, and P. ovale infections—but not P. falciparum—they may enter new liver cells. In the latter site they may lie dormant for many months and are probably responsible for the relapses which are common in these three infections but do not occur in P. falciparum (malignant tertian) malaria. In the red cell the merozoite develops first into a ring form, then by asexual reproduction into a *schizont* from which a new batch of merozoites (the number varying with the species) are liberated into the blood on rupture of the red cell. This asexual reproduction takes some 48 hours in the tertian malarias and 72 hours in quartan malaria, the characteristically spaced rigors and fever occurring when the new shower of merozoites enters the blood. Each merozoite enters a new red cell and several cycles of schizogony usually occur before some merozoites invading red cells develop not into schizonts but into male or female gametocytes. The cycle is then complete.

Clinical Features. For the first few days there is usually either continuous or remittent fever with general malaise, headache, and vomiting, but by the end of a week the typical periodicity, with rigors on every alternate or every third day, is often becoming apparent. In relapses it may be a striking feature from the beginning. In some patients, however, no regular pattern ever emerges, probably because they harbour two or more 'families' of parasites at different stages of development. The typical attack of malaria starts with a cold stage with shivering or *rigors*, lasting from a few minutes to a couple of hours, followed by a *hot stage* in which the patient has a severe headache, vomiting, a hot dry skin, and high fever, and finally profuse *sweating* for an hour or two brings down the temperature and the patient feels better. He may then remain well, with a normal temperature, until the next attack two or occasionally three days later. By the time the patient has had two or three rigors his spleen has often become palpable. Some patients develop a crop of herpes febrilis on the lip or face with each relapse of malaria.

Diagnosis depends on finding the malarial parasite in a thick blood smear and then identifying the species in a thin blood film. Recognition of the plasmodium can be learnt only by practical study, however, and no description of its various forms will be given here.

Complications of Malignant Tertian (Subtertian) Malaria

These occur only in people with little or no acquired immunity to malaria; they are therefore seen particularly in visitors to malarious areas who have not taken a prophylactic antimalarial drug and in people living in areas where there is good malaria control who nevertheless acquire the infection.

(1) *Cerebral malaria.* Red cells containing P. falciparum sometimes adhere to capillary walls in sufficient numbers to impair blood flow and cause disturbances in cerebral function from anoxia. *Clinically* cerebral malaria usually presents with high fever and drowsiness, often rapidly proceeding to coma, or there may be epileptiform fits and hemiplegia or other evidence of focal cerebral lesions. There is a high mortality and treatment must be started at the earliest possible moment, even while awaiting confirmation of the diagnosis from the blood film examination.

(2) *Blackwater fever* is a variety of acute haemolytic anaemia with haemoglobinuria seen in patients with malignant tertian (falciparum) malaria who have been treated, often rather irregularly and inadequately, with quinine. It has therefore become extremely rare now that quinine has been largely superseded by the newer antimalarial drugs. The patient complains of headache, fever, rigors, and vomiting; he may become jaundiced within 24 hours or so; and he passes dark urine containing oxyhaemoglobin or methaemoglobin. In severe cases oliguria or anuria may occur and haemodialysis may be life-saving.

Relapses

Relapses of P. vivax and P. ovale infection commonly recur for two years after the patient leaves a malarious area, but are rare thereafter;

P. malariae (quartan) infection may recur for five years or longer. Falciparum malaria does not relapse.

Treatment

(1) *Acute attacks of malaria.* The drug of choice is chloroquine, which is put up in 250 mg. tablets containing 150 mg. base. The initial dose is four tablets, followed by two tablets in six hours and two tablets on each of the next two days. Patients who are gravely ill or vomiting should be given intravenous chloroquine sulphate 200 mg. (base) in 5 ml. distilled water and this dose may be repeated in eight hours if necessary.

Other drugs which may be used are amodiaquine dihydrochloride dihydrate 600 mg. (base) by mouth, followed by 400 mg. (base) daily for two days; mepacrine hydrochloride 300 mg. by mouth three times daily the first day, 200 mg. three times daily on the second day, and 100 mg. three times daily for the next five days; or quinine sulphate or dihydrochloride 650 mg. three times daily for a week. Quinine should be avoided, however, in falciparum infections in view of the danger of precipitating blackwater fever.

(2) *Prevention of relapses.* The most effective drug for eradicating pre-erythrocytic forms of P. vivax and P. malariae from the liver is primaquine diphosphate 7·5 mg. of base (1 tablet) two or three times daily for two weeks. This course may be started at the same time as the chloroquine course described above.

(3) *Suppressive therapy.* The following are recommended for suppressing malaria during residence in an endemic area. Administration should start as soon as the area is entered and continue for four weeks after it has been left. Clinical malaria may. of course. appear thereafter.

    (a) Proguanil monohydrochloride 100 mg. daily, or

    (b) Pyrimethamine 1 tablet (25 mg.) weekly.

    (c) Chloroquine phosphate 500 mg. weekly may be advised in areas where parasites are known to be resistant to drugs (a) and (b), but should be avoided for routine use to prevent the development of chloroquine-resistant strains.

Malaria Prevention may be achieved by:

(1) Measures to prevent the breeding of anophelene mosquitoes.

(2) Protecting humans from mosquito bites by:

    (a) Mosquito-proofing of houses and other buildings by fitting wire-meshing to windows and doors and regular spraying with D.D.T.

    (b) Sleeping under mosquito nets.

    (c) Wearing protective clothing and applying a repellent lotion to exposed parts, particularly when going out at night.

AMOEBIASIS

Although infection with the protozoon Entamoeba histolytica is not confined to hot climates, clinical amoebiasis is very much more common in tropical countries where relatively low standards of hygiene permit faecal contamination of food.

Entamoeba histolytica is found in man in a vegetative form, which exhibits active amoeboid movements, and a non-motile cystic form. The vegetative forms invade the wall of the colon producing ulcers with undermined edges separated from each other by areas of healthy mucosa. From the colon amoebae may be carried in the portal bloodstream to the liver to cause amoebic hepatitis or so-called amoebic abscesses. In the lumen of the gut the amoebae encyst and develop a tough outer envelope; it is these cysts passing out in the faeces which are infective to other humans. If amoebae are swallowed they are destroyed by the digestive juices of the upper alimentary tract, but the cysts are able to survive until they reach the large bowel, where they develop into the mature vegetative form.

Clinical Features

Clinically amoebiasis may present in several different ways:

(1) **Acute Amoebic Dysentery.** This is usually more insidious in its onset than bacillary dysentery and there is less fever and constitutional upset. The patient complains of lower abdominal colic and has frequent loose motions containing blood and mucus. Diagnosis is readily established by microscopic examination of a specimen of mucus from a freshly passed stool, which reveals active vegetative forms of Entamoeba histolytica (see below).

(2) **Chronic Amoebic Colitis.** Many patients never develop acute dysenteric symptoms, but pass rather gradually into a state of vague ill-health; they lose weight, complain of general tiredness and irritability and suffer recurrent exacerbations at varying intervals in which they pass a number of loose motions, usually in the morning, with a good deal of colic and flatulence. The stools usually contain mucus but no blood. Examination often reveals thickening and tenderness of the caecum, and during exacerbations appendicitis may be closely mimicked.

Diagnosis remains in doubt until the organisms have been identified and they may be much more elusive than in the acute dysenteric form of the disease. As the cysts are much more difficult to identify than the active amoebae, and as the latter rapidly lose their motility when the stool becomes cool, arrangements should be made for the patient to pass the specimen near the laboratory where it is to be examined. A small portion of mucus is selected, mixed with a little saline on a slide, covered with a cover slip, and quickly searched with the 2/3 microscope objective. A higher power is used for final identification of the Entamoeba histolytica which, in contrast to the non-pathogenic entamoeba coli, shows very active amoeboid movements and contains ingested red blood cells in its cytoplasm. Cysts of Entamoeba histolytica are pearly white in appearance and contain four nuclei and a greenish refractile chromatoid bar; they can be identified with certainty only by pathologists with wide experience of this type of work.

Sigmoidoscopy may reveal deceptively small-looking ulcers (they are flask-shaped in section and may extend quite widely into the submucosa) separated by areas of normal mucous membrane. This is in contrast to bacillary dysentery and ulcerative colitis, both of which show a generally inflamed mucosa. In the more chronic cases, however, the lesions are often confined to the caecum and ascending colon, so that the rectum and pelvic colon appear normal, but even in these patients sigmoidoscopy may be very helpful in diagnosis by providing a fresh specimen of mucus for microscopy.

(3) **Hepatic Amoebiasis.** Though usually a complication of acute amoebic dysentery, amoebic hepatitis is sometimes seen in endemic areas in people who give a history of only slight recurrent looseness of the stools. The patient presents with fever and pain in the right upper quadrant of the abdomen. Examination reveals an enlarged and tender liver, and there is often impaired resonance at the right base and a high immobile diaphragm on radiological screening. There is usually a leucocytosis but jaundice is very rare. Chloroquine provides a therapeutic test of the diagnosis; the inflammation rapidly resolves when it is given and the temperature should be normal after two or three days. If not, either the diagnosis is wrong or there is an associated amoebic abscess in the liver.

(4) **Amoebic Abscess in the Liver.** Pathologically the difference between amoebic hepatitis and amoebic abscess in the liver is probably simply a matter of degree; the 'abscess' contains the debris of necrotic liver tissue, but no pus cells. Such an abscess may develop many months or even years after the original infection. It may also be clinically silent until a late stage, as in a patient of the writer's, an army sergeant in a combatant unit who remained symptom-free and on active service until admitted to hospital following the rupture of a large liver abscess into the peritoneal cavity. This latter event is very unusual; more commonly the abscess points upwards and may rupture into the pleura, or into the lung and bronchus with subsequent expectoration of sputum aptly likened to anchovy sauce.

Treatment. Metronidazole is a safe and effective amoebicide which has replaced emetine as the drug of first choice in this disease. It is given by mouth in doses of 400–800 mg. t.d.s. for 10 days. Older regimes of treatment such as the following are still occasionally used:

Days 1–3 : Emetine hydrochloride 60 mg. intramuscularly daily.
Days 1–5 : Oxytetracycline 250 mg. six-hourly.
Days 6–16: Emetine bismuth iodide 0·2 g. daily by mouth.
Days 14–35: Diodoquin tablets 0·6 g. three times daily.

Emetine by injection may have toxic effects on the myocardium, so that patients must be kept in bed while it is being given and the treatment should be stopped if tachycardia, fall in blood pressure or flat T waves in the electrocardiogram appear. T minimise the vomiting caused by E.B.I the drug should be given in gelatin capsules (which prevent gastric irritation) and preferably last thing at night combined with an anti-histamine such as promethazine 25 mg. and a sedative such as amylobarbitone 200 mg. in the hope that the patient may 'sleep through his nausea' and so retain the drug.

Treatment of Hepatic Amoebiasis. Amoebic hepatitis usually responds quickly to emetine by injection, but chloroquine is the drug of choice for this condition since it is less toxic and even more effective. Chloroquine is a relatively feeble amoebacide, of no value in intestinal amoebiasis; it is effective in hepatitis because it is concentrated some thirty times in the liver. An adult should be given 600 mg. of base (4 tablets), followed by 2 tablets six hours later and then 2 tablets daily for two to three weeks. Failure of the temperature to settle a few days on this treatment suggests that there is a large abscess in the liver which requires aspiration.

VISCERAL LEISHMANIASIS (Kala-azar)

This disease is endemic in the Far East, India, East Pakistan, the Middle East, the Sudan, Kenya, the Mediterranean seaboard and parts of South America. The causative organism is the protozoon Leishmania donovani, which is transmitted from man to man by sandflies of the genus phlebotomus and parasites reticulo-endothelial cells in the liver, spleen, bone marrow and occasionally lymph nodes.

Clinical Features. After an incubation period which is usually several months but may be as long as three years, the illness usually starts insidiously and runs a long chronic or relapsing course. There are bouts of fever lasting from a few days to a few weeks; these are accompanied by night sweats and separated by apyrexial phases of variable length. Meanwhile the spleen slowly and progressively enlarges until eventually it may extend into the right iliac fossa. Hepatomegaly of lesser degree is common and occasionally there may be enlarged lymph nodes too. The blood count reveals anaemia and leucopenia. In the later stages the patient may become grossly wasted.

Diagnosis is established by identifying the parasites. These are rarely found in peripheral blood films, but more often in smears of bone marrow or splenic pulp obtained by percutaneous aspiration. The formol-gel and Chopra tests are useful ancillary investigations, but are not specific since they are positive in all conditions characterised by a raised serum globulin level.

(1) *Formol-gel test.* Add one drop of commercial formalin to 1 ml. of serum. The test is positive if the serum becomes opaque in 10–30 minutes.

(2) *Chopra test.* Add a few drops of 4-per-cent solution of a pentavalent antimony preparation to a 10-per-cent solution of serum in distilled water. The test is positive if the mixture becomes opaque within a few minutes.

Treatment

Pentavalent antimony compounds have replaced trivalent preparations since they are much less toxic. *Sodium antimony gluconate* is given intravenously, 0·3–0·6 g. daily dissolved in 6–10 ml. of sterile distilled water, for three to ten days. Alternatively the aromatic diamidine *pentamidine isethionate* is another effective drug which may be given if the patient fails to respond to the antimony preparation, or relapses. The dose is 2–4 mg. per kg. body weight dissolved in 5–10 ml. sterile distilled water and given by daily intravenous injection for ten to fourteen days.

Cutaneous Leishmaniasis

Within two years of receiving treatment for kala-azar some patients develop depigmented patches, usually on the face, shoulders and upper part of the chest, and later papular lesions may appear on these areas. The condition usually responds to a further course of treatment.

Trypanosomiasis (Sleeping-sickness)

This disease, which is endemic in tropical Africa, is due to infection with the flagellated protozoa Trypanosoma gambiense or T. rhodesiense. The organisms are spread from man to man by the tsetse fly, in which part of their life cycle occurs, and wild game also probably provide a reservoir of infection.

Clinical Features. The early symptoms are fever, anaemia, enlarged and tender lymph nodes in the neck and elsewhere, splenomegaly, and pleomorphic skin rashes, but eventually the central nervous system is invaded and lassitude and somnolence, often with dysarthria, tremors, and fits, now dominate the clinical picture. Patients who develop these neurological symptoms run a slowly downhill course over a period of months or years and invariably die if untreated.

Diagnosis is established by identifying the trypanosome in smears of blood, bone marrow, or material obtained by lymph-node puncture.

Treatment. (1) Cases without C.N.S. Involvement. If the C.S.F. shows no increase in globulin or lymphocytes the relatively toxic drug tryparsamide need not be used. Instead a course of eleven weekly intravenous injections of *suramin* is given, starting with a test dose of 200 mg. and if there is no reaction giving 1 g. at each subsequent injection. This drug may cause renal damage, so that the urine should be tested for albumen before each injection. Vomiting and skin rashes are other side-effects. If suramin has to be abandoned on account of toxicity or failure to cure a course of *pentamidine isethionate* should be given as for kala-azar.

(2) **Cases with C.N.S. involvement,** as shown by neurological signs or C.S.F. changes. Melarsoprol (Mel.B), a trivalent arsenical which crosses the blood-brain barrier, has largely replaced tryparsamide because of the latter's toxicity and the increasing emergence of trypanosomes resistant to it. Three I.V. injections of Mel B are given on days 1, 3 and 5, each con-

taining 3·6 mg./kg. body weight (maximum dose 200 mg.), and the course may be repeated after 3 weeks if the nervous system is severely affected. Toxic effects include vomiting, rashes and rarely hepatitis or encephalopathy.

Prophylaxis. Control of the tsetse fly is the most important measure in prevention. Those exposed to infection should be given pentamidine isethionate 3 mg. per kg. body weight in 3 ml. sterile distilled water by intramuscular injection every six months.

BACTERIAL INFECTIONS

LEPROSY (Hansen's disease)

This is a disease of low infectivity which is endemic in many parts of Asia, Central Africa, and South America. Infection with the acid-fast causative organism, Mycobacterium leprae, is acquired only by close contact over a prolonged period and the incubation period is therefore difficult to determine, though it may be several years.

Clinical Features. (1) Tuberculoid Leprosy. This is the benign variety of the disease in which small numbers of organisms stimulate a vigorous response by the tissues. The main reaction occurs in peripheral nerves: the patient complains of numbness, tingling, and loss of pain and temperature sense in the distal parts of the limbs and the affected nerves can be felt as hard thick cords. The great auricular nerve is very commonly affected. In addition, round, depigmented and anaesthetic areas appear on the skin. The disease usually runs a self-limiting course and the patient is non-infectious.

(2) Lepromatous Leprosy. This is the malignant variety of the disease: the patient's resistance to infection is low and granulomatous lesions teeming with M. leprae spread over the skin, particularly on the face and ears. As in the tuberculoid variety the earliest lesions are probably in the nerve fibrils, from which extension occurs into the skin and up the nerve trunks, but as there is very little inflammatory response nerve function is not disturbed until much later in the course of the disease. After a number of years of progressive ill-health death usually results from intercurrent infection.

Diagnosis is established by indentifying the characteristic acid-fast bacilli in scrapings from skin lesions but as bacilli are very scanty in the tuberculoid type, radial nerve biopsy may be necessary.

Treatment. The sulphones are specific therapy for leprosy, the active substance being 4–4′ diaminodiphenylsulphone (D.D.S.). This is given by mouth on two days each week, starting with 100 mg. each dose for the first month, 200 mg. the second month, 300 mg. the third month, and then continuing with 400 mg. per dose indefinitely. During sulphone therapy ferrous sulphate 200 mg. three times daily, intramuscular vitamin B_{12} 100 microgrammes twice weekly, with added yeast and Marmite, should be given to counteract the tendency to anaemia. Patients who develop severe toxic reactions to dapsone, such as hepatitis or haemolytic anaemia, or in whom the organisms become dapsone-resistant, may now be treated effectively with clofazimine (Lamprene) 100–200 mg. three times weekly.

Notification. Leprosy is a notifiable disease in Great Britain.

BACILLARY DYSENTERY

This is the result of infection with gram-negative bacilli of the genus Shigella, which cause acute inflammation and ulceration of the colon. The common pathogenic varieties of Shigella are Sh. dysenteriae (Shiga bacillus), Sh. flexneri and Sh. sonnei. The disease is spread by contamination of water with faeces from patients and carriers and although it is widespread throughout the world it is much more common in the tropics than elsewhere. Food may be infected by flies or by unsuspected carriers engaged in the transport or preparation of salads and other cold dishes. Severe bacillary dysentery in the tropics is usually due to Sh. dysenteriae or Sh. flexneri; in this country the milder disease due to Sh. sonnei is usually seen, mainly as small recurring outbreaks in residential institutions.

Clinical Features. The incubation period is up to one week. The disease starts abruptly and in its severest form (usually due to Sh. dysenteriae shiga) causes high fever, vomiting, and profuse diarrhoea with blood and mucus in the stools. There is rapid dehydration and the patient may collapse and die within a few hours. At the other end of the scale sonnei dysentery as seen in this country causes slight fever, colicky abdominal pains, vomiting, and diarrhoea, often without blood or mucus in the stools and with minimal constitutional upset. Complete recovery takes place within a week or so. In cases of intermediate severity symptoms may last for two or three weeks, but unlike amoebiasis this disease seldom if ever becomes chronic.

Acute *arthritis*, usually limited to one of the large joints of the limbs, sometimes develops within six months of infection with Sh. dysenteriae or Sh. flexneri. The joint pain and swelling may persist for some months.

Diagnosis. Microscopic examination of a specimen of mucus from the stool, mixed with a little saline on a slide and covered with a cover slip, shows a typical exudate with many pus cells, red blood cells and macrophages, and the organism may be isolated by culture on McConkey's medium.

Treatment. Strains of Shigella resistant to the sulphonamides are now common and the present drugs of choice are tetracycline 250–500 mg. 6-hourly or oral streptomycin 0·5 g. 6-hourly. Other drugs which may be given are ampicillin, polymyxin B, colomycin and furazolidine (Furoxone).

For severely ill patients complete rest and good nursing are of great importance and intravenous saline may be needed to combat dehydration and sodium depletion. For the first day or so only bland fluids should be given by mouth, in sufficient quantities to ensure a urinary output of at least two pints in 24 hours.

CHOLERA

This disease is due to infection with the 'comma vibrio' and is found particularly in India and the Far East. Epidemics occur from contamination of food or water supplies with faeces from patients or convalescent carriers; there are no chronic carriers. The severity varies very widely in different epidemics; in some the disease is relatively mild, while in others mortality rates of 75 per cent have been reported.

Clinical Features. After an incubation period of two to six days sudden diarrhoea begins and within an hour or so mucus-flecked fluid uncoloured by faecal material may be pouring from the patient, who is also vomiting, complaining of cramps and in acute circulatory collapse. Oliguria or anuria inevitably follow and death may occur within 48 hours. In milder cases complete recovery occurs within two or three weeks.

Diagnosis is established by culturing the vibrio from the stools.

Treatment. The most urgent measure is fluid and electrolyte replacement. In view of the circulatory collapse it is usually necessary to cut down on a vein to set up an intravenous infusion and two pints of normal glucose saline should be run in quickly, followed by a pint of alkaline hypotonic saline (6·0 g. sodium chloride and 18·0 g. sodium bicarbonate per litre) within the first two hours. But if there are severe cramps, little thirst and a good urinary output (indicating a predominant salt deficiency) the first pint should be hypertonic saline (16 g. sodium chloride per litre). It may be necessary to continue intravenous therapy for 48 hours. The amount of fluid given in all must obviously depend on the clinical state of the patient, but at least one third of it should be alkaline hypotonic saline. In view of the risk of pulmonary oedema the patient must be carefully watched for warning symptoms and signs such as cough, dyspnoea, basal râles, or rising jugular venous pressure.

A course of tetracyline, furazolidine or chloramphenicol, which inhibit most strains of the vibrio, should also be given.

Prophylaxis. Vaccination is effective for up to six months. Two doses of 0·5 ml. and 1 ml. are given at an interval of one week. Further booster doses of 1 ml. are necessary every six months for those who remain in endemic areas.

PLAGUE

Plague is endemic in the Far East, India, Central Africa, and parts of South America. The causative gram-negative bacillus, Pasteurella pestis, is transmitted by fleas from rats and other rodents to man.

Clinical Features. (1) **Bubonic plague** is by far the most common type. After an incubation period of two to four days there is sudden fever and grave constitutional upset, often with delirium. Enlarged and tender lymph nodes (buboes) appear after two or three days, usually in the groins but occasionally in the neck or axillae.

(2) **Septicaemic** and (3) **Pneumonic** plague are both rare; they are characterised by fever and profound toxaemia, with cough and signs of broncho-pneumonia in the latter variety, but buboes do not form. The mortality rate varies in different epidemics and may be as high as 80 per cent. Recovery from septicaemic or pneumonic plague is rare.

Diagnosis is established by isolating the organism from the blood or from material aspirated from a bubo.

Treatment. Combined therapy with the following drugs probably gives the best results, though even in treated cases the mortality rate may not fall below 20 per cent:

   (1) Streptomycin 0·5 g. intramuscularly every four hours until the temperature is normal, and then 1 g. daily until a total of 15 g. has been given, and

   (2) Chloramphenicol *or* tetracycline 0·5 g. every six hours for a week or 10 days.

Control of Outbreaks. Patients must be strictly isolated, all excreta being disinfected with care and fomites burnt. Attendants should wear protective overalls, rubber gloves, and plastic face-masks and their clothes should be treated with Malathion. Contacts must be vaccinated, either with Haffkine's heat-killed vaccine two 3 ml. doses at an interval of 10 days, or a single dose of the more efficient living avirulent vaccine. This gives protection for six months. In addition, contacts should take sulphadiazine 1 g. three times daily until a week after the last exposure and must be instructed to drink plenty of fluids during this time. Equally important is the energetic prosecution of campaigns against the rat and flea population of the district.

RELAPSING FEVER (Famine fever)

The causative organisms, spirochaetes of the genus Borrelia, are transmitted by lice and ticks. The disease is found in southern Europe, South America, the Middle East, Africa, and India.

Clinical Features. The incubation period is usually about a week, but varies from a day or so to a fortnight. The onset is remarkably sudden, with giddiness, headache, fever and rigor, pains in the back and limbs and sometimes vomiting. There is continuous high fever for several days and the patient soon becomes gravely ill, restless, and often delirious, with enlargement of the liver and spleen, sometimes purpura, and occasionally in severe cases, jaundice. On the fifth or sixth day the temperature drops to normal and there is a sudden dramatic clinical improvement, but after a week or so the first of a small series of relapses occurs, each febrile bout tending fortunately to be less severe than the last. The mortality rate is very variable in different epidemics, but may be as high as 30 per cent.

Diagnosis is established by identifying the spirochaete in the blood during the bouts of fever.

Treatment. Either tetracycline by mouth, 0·5 g. six-hourly, or benzyl penicillin by injection, 500,000 units six-hourly, should be given for four days. In addition, if the patient is not jaundiced he should be given a single intravenous injection of neoarsphenamine 0·45 g.

YAWS

This disease, due to the Treponema pertenue, is non-venereal but is spread by direct contact from patient to patient. The highest incidence is among children over the age of eighteen months.

Clinical Features. The first sign is a papular skin rash, which eventually ulcerates. Hyperkeratosis of the soles of the feet is common and there may be lymphadenopathy and lesions in the bones and periosteum. The disease usually runs a very chronic course over many years.

Diagnosis is established by identifying the Treponema pertenue. The Wassermann reaction is also positive.

Treatment. Oxytetracycline 0·5 g. six-hourly for five days is usually very effective. A second course should be given if the W.R. is still positive after three or six months.

SCHISTOSOMIASIS (Bilharzia)

This disease is due to infestation with trematodes (flukes) of the genus Schistosoma. Three species of Schistosoma are pathogenic to man: *S. haematobium* is found in Central and North Africa, especially in Egypt; *S. mansoni* is fairly widespread throughout Africa, in the West Indies and along the east coast of South America; *S. japonicum* is found in the Far East. The habitat of the adult worm is the vascular system, *S. haematobium* being found in the portal vein and its branches and in the vesical, uterine, and haemorrhoidal veins, while *S. mansoni* inhabits chiefly the portal and mesenteric veins. *S. haematobium* produces terminally spined eggs, which are found mainly in the urine; *S. mansoni* produces laterally spined eggs found mainly in the faeces. The irritation caused by these spined eggs is the initial cause of the symptoms.

Life Cycle. If the egg reaches water it hatches into a free-swimming larva which enters the intermediate host, a fresh-water snail. In the snail the larva forms into a sporocyst, which gives off a number of daughter cysts and these in turn produce enormous numbers of bifid-tailed cercariae which escape into the surrounding water. These cercariae have an independent life of about 48 hours, during which time they may gain access to human host by penetrating the unbroken skin or buccal mucosa. They pass via the bloodstream and lungs to the liver, where they develop within about two months into adult male and female worms. Thereafter the females start producing the spined eggs.

Clinical Features. After an incubation period of about three months, *S. haematobium* infestation causes haematuria, frequency, and dysuria, and though the illness is usually mild the symptoms are intractable. *S. mansoni* infestation has a shorter incubation period of about two months, followed by cough, headache, malaise, fever and rigors, abdominal pain, and enlargement of the liver and spleen. The general symptoms are usually followed by diarrhoea, with blood and mucus in the stools, due to the ulcerative and polypoid lesions in the colon. Urticarial and other skin rashes are often found and eosinophilia is common. Cirrhosis of the liver with ascites is a late complication of this variety of the disease. *S. japonicum* causes lesions very similar to those of *S. mansoni.* but there is frequently involvement of the central nervous system, causing cranial nerve palsies, hemiplegia, fits, or coma.

Diagnosis is established by identifying the eggs in the urine or faeces.

Treatment. Patients with no neurological symptoms should be given oral niradazole (Ambilhar) 25 mg./kg. body weight in divided doses daily for 7–10 days. It may cause E.C.G. changes or hallucinations, tremor and convulsions and may colour the urine red. Patients with cerebral symptoms and those who fail to respond to niradazole should be given intravenous sodium antimony tartrate, which is a more effective but also a more toxic drug. Injections are given on alternate days, starting with 30 mg., 60 mg., 90 mg. and then 120 mg. for nine injections. Great care must be taken to ensure that none of this preparation is injected outside the vein, as it is intensely irritant, and the injection should be given very slowly to the fasting patient. As it is a cardiac depressant it may cause hypotension and the patient should lie down for an hour after each injection.

TYPHUS FEVER

There are several varieties of typhus due to closely related rickettsiae. The most important is epidemic or louse-borne typhus, due to *R. prowazeki.* Other varieties are murine typhus, which is transmitted chiefly by fleas; Rocky Mountain fever, 'fievre boutonneuse' (prevalent along the Mediterranean coast), and Queensland or 'Q' fever, transmitted chiefly by ticks; and tsutsugamushi fever and scrub typhus, transmitted chiefly by mites.

EPIDEMIC LOUSE-BORNE TYPHUS has been one of the scourges of armies since prehistoric times and an aftermath of civil disasters which lead to overcrowding and destitution. Lice become infected by sucking blood from a patient with typhus and transmit the rickettsiae to other people in their faeces, which are rubbed into scratches and other lesions in the skin.

Clinical Features. The incubation is usually twelve days, with a range of five to fourteen days. There is usually a gradual onset with headache, shivering, backache, general malaise, and tenderness of the eyeballs, but by about the third day the patient is more seriously ill and has a flushed face, injection of the conjunctivae and tachycardia out of proportion to the fever. Epistaxis is common. About this time the temperature gradually rises towards its maximum (which is usually between 102–105° F.) and remains at this level with only slight morning remissions throughout the rest of the illness. The rash appears on the abdomen on the fifth day and spreads to the chest and shoulders; the limbs are sometimes involved too, but never the face. It takes many forms, but there are usually macules of varying sizes, a subcuticular mottling and sometimes petechial elements. As the rash develops the patient sinks into a stuporose and often delirious state from which he is difficult to rouse. By the second week the spleen is often palpable and the urine is scanty and contains albumen and casts. In patients who recover the temperature settles by lysis during the third week. The clinical severity and mortality rate of typhus vary widely in different epidemics, but in general most patients do recover.

Diagnosis is confirmed by the *Weil-Felix reaction*, which demonstrates a high agglutinin titre in the serum against B. proteus OX 19.

MURINE TYPHUS (and the other varieties of endemic rickettsial infection mentioned above) differ from epidemic louse-borne typhus in being primarily diseases of rodents and other small animals, from which infection is transmitted to man by fleas, ticks, and mites. The clinical illness is very similar to that of the epidemic disease, though usually much milder.

Diagnosis. The Weil-Felix reaction demonstrates agglutinins against B. proteus OX 19 in flea-borne murine typhus (as in epidemic typhus); against B. proteus OXK and only slightly OX 19 in mite-borne typhus; and against OXK, OX 19, and OX 2 in varying degrees in tick-borne typhus.

Treatment. Tetracycline 0·75 g. should be given six-hourly for forty-eight hours and then 0·5 g. six-hourly until the temperature has been normal for two days. Intravenous glucose-saline may be required to combat dehydration; intramuscular Chlorpromazine 50–100 mg. or morphine 15mg. may be needed to control delirium.

Control of Outbreaks. The important measures are (1) Delousing of patients on admission with D.D.T., their clothes being disinfested or burned. (2) Delousing of the population. This may be done by spraying dicophane dusting powder (which contains 10 per cent D.D.T.) into all apertures in the clothing, which must not be changed for 10 days thereafter. (3) Vaccination of doctors, nurses, and others specially exposed to infection with the Cox type yolk-sac vaccine, two doses of 1 ml. being given at an interval of two weeks followed by booster doses of 1 ml. every four months. Protective clothing must be worn while dealing with infested patients.

FURTHER READING

Hargreaves, W. H. and Morrison, R. J. G. *The Practice of Tropical Medicine*, Staples Press, London, 1965.

Manson-Bahr, Sir Philip H. (Editor) *Manson's Tropical Diseases*, 16th edition. Cassell, London, 1966.

CHAPTER EIGHTEEN

WORMS

1. NEMATODES (Round worms)

THREADWORMS (*Enterobius vermicularis*)

Threadworms are extremely common, particularly in childhood. They are about $\frac{1}{2}$–1 cm. long and look as their name implies, like threads of cotton. There are both male and female forms which inhabit the large bowel and rectum, being most numerous in the caecum. They may reach the anus where they cause considerable irritation.

Pairing of the worms occurs in the intestine and the eggs are passed out in the stools. These eggs may contaminate the fingers of the patient particularly if anal irritation is a feature. The eggs are then swallowed either in contaminated food or directly from sucking the fingers. The eggs then hatch and a new generation of worms develops in the intestine.

Clinical Features. Many patients may be unaware of threadworm infestation until the worms are noticed in the stools. The most common symptom is anal irritation and this may keep the child awake at night with the result that he is fretful next day.

The relationship between threadworms and acute appendicitis is still debated, but it seems probable that threadworms very rarely cause appendicular inflammation. The *diagnosis* is confirmed by finding the worm in the stools or the ova by means of perianal swabs.

Treatment. *Viprynium embenate* given either in tablet form or as a suspension as a single dose of 5·0 mg. base/kg. body weight and repeated in one week is satisfactory. It is low in side effects but colours the stools red.

Alternatively 'Pripsen', a preparation containing *piperazine* and standardised senna, is equally good. The dose for patients of six years and over is 10 g. of Pripsen granules (containing 4·0 g. of piperazine phosphate) as a single dose. Piperazine paralyses the worm which is then cleared out by the action of the senna.

Other treatment consists of general cleanliness with careful washing of the hands before meals. Anal itching may be reduced by an anti-histamine or hydrocortisone cream.

If attacks of infestation are recurrent it usually means that other members of the family are infected and it is then best to treat the whole family.

ASCARIS LUMBRICOIDES

Infection by ascaris lumbricoides is acquired by swallowing the fertilised egg. In the upper small intestine the egg develops into the larval form which penetrates the intestinal wall and enters the venous system and is then swept back to the heart and passes into the lungs where it may cause a pneumonitis. The larva is then coughed up in the sputum and swallowed and in the intestine develops into the adult worm. The adult ascaris is about 6–10 inches long and is white or yellow, resembling the common earth-worm. There are males and females.

Clinical Features. Frequently there are no symptoms and the diagnosis is made by finding a worm in the stools. Occasionally the worms in the intestine give rise to intestinal colic or biliary obstruction. If the infection is heavy, the larval form may give rise to a pneumonitis or to an urticaria, which is associated with eosinophilia in the blood.

Treatment. *Piperazine* as the phosphate is satisfactory. The dose for a young child is 3·0 g. and for an older child or adult is 4·0 g. of piperazine. Only a single dose is required. The drug acts by paralysing the muscle of the worm which is then passed alive per rectum. Alternatively *bephenium hydroxynaphthoate* (Alcopar) in a single dose of 5·0 g. for adults or 2·5 g. for children is also satisfactory.

HOOK-WORMS (*Ankylostoma duodenale* and *Necator americanus*)

Hook-worm infestation is extremely common, but is confined to tropical and subtropical countries. The adult worms are about 1·0 cm. long and inhabit the duodenum and jejunum. The eggs are passed out in the faeces; if they fall on moist warm soil they develop into the larval form which penetrates the intact skin of the next human victim. The larvae then pass back to the heart and then to the lungs. They penetrate the alveoli, and passing up the trachea re-enter the intestinal tract where they develop into mature worms.

Clinical Features. The adult worms are responsible for considerable ill-health by causing chronic bleeding from the duodenum. The patient suffers from anaemia, diarrhoea, and finally cachexia and even death may occur. The larval form may lead to areas of pneumonia with an associated eosinophilia in the blood. The point of penetration of the larvae through the skin is often inflamed and is known as the 'ground itch'. It must, however, be realised that very many people harbour hook worms and suffer little if any ill health.

Treatment. *Bephenium hydroxynaphthoate* is the drug of choice. For A. duodenale 5·0 g. is given as a single dose. For N. americanus 5·0 g. is given three successive days. Side effects include nausea and diarrhoea but are minimal. If anaemia is severe it should be treated with iron.

TRICHINOSIS

The adult form of this minute round worm (*Trichinella spiralis*) lives in the intestine of the pig; embryo worms find their way into the animal's bloodstream and develop in the muscles into small cysts about ½ mm. long.

If inadequately cooked pork from such a pig is eaten, an adult worm develops in the human intestine, and in time its embryos are disseminated in the bloodstream throughout the body.

Clinical Features. Small localised outbreaks occur from the eating of pork from an infected animal; pork sausage-meat, either fried too hastily or actually eaten raw, has a bad reputation in this connection. There is often nausea and vomiting lasting a day or two immediately after the ingestion of infected meat. About a week later (when the embryos are passing into the muscles and other tissues) there is fever, muscular pains, and tenderness, and frequently oedema of the eyelids and 'splinter haemorrhages' under the nails. The urine contains protein. The cysts can be found in the muscle on biopsy. The blood always shows a great excess of eosinophil cells This stage usually subsides slowly over several weeks, and the larvae in the muscles finally become calcified. Occasionally death occurs.

Treatment is purely symptomatic. In the stage of invasion the symptoms can best be controlled by prednisolone.

2. CESTODES (Tapeworms)

In order to complete their life cycle these parasites have to inhabit the bodies of two separate and unwilling 'hosts'. The adult tapeworm lives in the intestine of the main host, its ova passing out in the faeces. If the ova are ingested by a suitable 'intermediate host', the larval forms of the worm hatch out, gain access to the bloodstream and are distributed through the muscles of the body. If the intermediate is eaten by a main host, the cysts in the muscles develop into adult tape worms in the intestine of the latter.

Man acts as a main host for three worms. *Taenia saginata*, the common beef tapeworm, *Taenia solium*, the less common pork tapeworm, and *Diphyllobothrium latum*, the fish tapeworm. *T. saginata* and *T. solium* are the only tapeworms likely to be found in this country and infection is acquired by eating respectively imperfectly cooked beef or pork containing the larval forms. These tapeworms are white, flat, ribbon-like structures, about 1 cm. wide and many yards long, subdivided into a large number of segments, some of which break off from time to time and appear in the faeces. The head, which is no more than a pinhead in size, is firmly attached to the duodenum or upper part of the jejunum.

Clinical Features. There may be some abdominal discomfort or diarrhoea, or occasionally abnormal hunger. Frequently, however, the patient has no symptoms until he notices segments of worm in his stools. A white cell count sometimes shows an eosinophilia. Diagnosis is established by the identification of segments or ova of the tapeworm in the faeces.

Treatment. Most tapeworm infestations in Britain are due to *T. saginata*. This is best treated with *niclosamide*, which kills the worm. No preliminary starvation is necessary. Four tablets (0·5 g. each) are chewed and swallowed and the following day the dose is repeated. The treatment is nearly always successful.

With T. solium, niclosamide may cause disintegration of the worm with subsequent cysticercosis. The patient should, therefore, be put on a fluid diet for two days and be given a saline purge the night before treatment. He is then given *extract of male fern*. The dose is 8 ml. for an adult. It has an unpleasant taste and may be diluted in a suitably flavoured draught or given by duodenal tube. Capsules are not satisfactory as the head may be high up in the intestine and the anthelmintic may not be liberated at that level. One hour later a saline purge is given and the stools searched for the head of the worm. If it is not passed, the worm will grow again.

CYSTICERCOSIS

Cysticercosis is due to infestation of man by the cystic larval form of a cestode, usually taenia solium. Infection occurs either by eating food contaminated with the eggs of *T. solium* or sometimes patients who have an adult tapeworm in the lower intestine regurgitate food and thus allow the eggs to reach the upper intestine where they develop into the larval form. These larvae then penetrate the intestinal wall and are carried in the blood stream all over the body. Common sites for cysts to develop are the subcutaneous tissues, muscles, brain, eye, lungs, and heart. In this country the disease is seen mainly in those who have spent many years in India; it is rare.

Clinical Features. Cysticercosis may produce no symptoms, as the live cysts produce little in the way of a tissue reaction. When the cysts die, however, there may be considerable inflammatory reaction. Cysts in the brain are particularly troublesome and may cause epileptic fits. The dead cysts may become calcified and will then be visible radiologically.

Treatment. There is no treatment for cysticercosis except surgical removal of the cysts and control of the epilepsy by anticonvulsants. It is important that a patient who has an infestation of the bowel with *t. solium* should be treated efficiently; mepacrine should be avoided as this is particularly liable to produce vomiting, thus leading to the escape of larval forms from the upper intestine which penetrate the intestine and lead to systemic cystericosis.

HYDATID DISEASE

Hydatid disease is due to infestation by the cystic stage of *taenia echinococcus*. The worm is only about half a centimeter in length. It lives in the intestine of the dog. The ova are swallowed by the intermediate host, usually sheep, cattle, horses, or rarely man. The larvae then penetrate the intestinal wall and settle down in various organs and develop into the cystic form. Hydatid disease is rare in this country and is found more commonly in Australia, Iceland, South America, and the Middle East.

Clinical Features. Hydatid cysts are found most commonly in the liver and lungs. In the liver, hydatid cysts may reach a considerable size without causing symptoms. Sometimes the patient complains of a dragging pain in the abdomen. Pressure on the bile ducts may produce jaundice.

An hydatid cyst in the lungs may produce no symptoms. As it enlarges cough and sometimes haemoptysis occur. If it ruptures into a bronchus, the contents are coughed up and secondary infection develops in the cyst. Long-standing cysts may become calcified.

In hydatid disease the blood may show an eosinophilia, but this is by no means consistent. Casoni's test, which consists of the intradermal injection of fluid from an hydatid cyst, is positive in about 80 per cent of patients with the disease. False positions are, however, common.

Treatment. The treatment of hydatid cysts is either by removal of the whole cyst or by marsupialisation of the cyst which is then allowed to heal by granulation. Aspiration of the cyst is dangerous as it may lead to dissemination of daughter cysts.

FURTHER READING

Blacklock, D. B. and Southwell, T. *Guide to Human Parasitology*, 8th edition, Lewis, London, 1966.

CHAPTER NINETEEN

DISEASES OF THE SKIN

ECZEMA

There is some confusion about the meaning of the words 'eczema' and 'dermatitis'. It is perhaps best to regard dermatitis as any type of inflammation of the skin and eczema as a variety of dermatitis characterised by a red, weeping eruption usually associated with itching. Some dermatologists, however, make no such distinction and use the two words synonymously.

Some substances cause an eczematous reaction when applied to the skin of normal people; others do so only when applied to the skin of people who are specially sensitive. Less often eczema results from the eating of particular foods. Infantile eczema (*atopic eczema*) occurs in babies who have inherited an abnormal tendency to develop hypersensitivity to foreign proteins and these children frequently go on to suffer from hay fever, asthma, and persistent patches of eczema in the flexures of the limbs (*Besnier's prurigo*).

Contact eczema (or contact dermatitis) is extremely common. The substances which may cause eczema when applied to the skin are very numerous but may be classified into the following groups:

(1) *Chemical.* Drugs are important members of this group. Almost any drug may cause eczema on the skin of a sensitive individual, but penicillin and streptomycin are the worst offenders, and nurses, doctors, and students should be particularly careful when giving injections of these substances not to allow any of the solution to come in contact with their hands. Nickel (on suspender and brassière clips), lipstick, nail-varnish, and hair-dyes are common causes of contact eczema, and so are the dyes in furs and other articles of clothing. Soaps, bleaching-agents, and detergents constitute another big group.

(2) *Substances of Plant Origin.* In this country the plants which most often cause eczema are primulas and chrysanthemums.

(3) *Micro-organisms.* Infections of the skin such as impetigo and ringworm may be complicated by an eczematous reaction.

The **diagnosis** of contact eczema is usually suggested by the history of contact and the site and distribution of the lesions and may be confirmed by a *patch test*, in which the suspected substance is applied to an area of normal skin, covered with a square of cellophane or jaconet and left for 24 to 48 hours. A positive result is the development within three or four days of an eczematous reaction in the area of skin covered.

Treatment. The most important point is the removal of the cause, if this is known. Thus avoidance of contact with the offending drug, dye, plant, or whatever it may be, or change of work for patients with occupational eczema, is an obvious and usually effective remedy. For local symptomatic treatment hydrocortisone ointment has been replaced by more easily absorbed corticosteroids such as triamcinolone acetinide, fluorocinolone acetinide or betamethasone valerate. In addition the lesions may be occluded with a polythene sheet, but only a small area of skin should be covered at a time; complications include secondary infection, haemorrhage into the skin and local striae, particularly in areas such as the thighs where striae normally occur. It is often wise to combine the local corticosteroid with an antibiotic (as in the proprietary preparations Adcortyl A with Graneodin, Synalar N and Betnovate N cream).

DRUG ERUPTIONS

Drug eruptions are very common and may mimic the rashes of many other diseases, particularly measles and scarlet fever. There must be few drugs which never cause rashes; the barbiturates, especially phenobarbitone, and the sulphonamides are among those which do so most frequently. Streptomycin is another common offender. The other anti-tuberculous drugs, para-amino-salicylic acid (P.A.S.) and isoniazid, also cause rashes but less often. Thiouracil and phenylbutazone are other drugs worthy of special mention in this connection.

Iodides (usually taken in the form of potassium iodide in a cough mixture) occasionally cause remarkable large, fungating ulcerative lesions. The heavy metals *gold* and less often *arsenic* may cause a very severe generalised exfoliative dermatitis which is sometimes fatal. Nowadays *penicillin* rashes are among the commonest and most important. In a sensitised subject an injection of penicillin may cause an urticarial rash, angioneurotic oedema, or rarely death within a few minutes from anaphylactic shock. This last complication occurs particularly in allergic subjects with a history of infantile eczema, hay fever, and asthma; any such person who is known to have had a rash or any reaction following previous treatment with penicillin should on no account be given any more.

Treatment. In mild cases withdrawal of the drug is all that is needed. For relief of irritation an anti-histamine preparation should be given: promethazine hydrochloride 25 mg. or mepyramine maleate 100 mg. twice or three times daily are the most powerful of these but cause more drowsiness than chlorpheniramine maleate 4 mg. two or three times daily. Promethazine 50 mg. or chlorpheniramine 10 mg. may be given intramuscularly if the need is urgent. More severe cases should be treated with cortisone or an analogue, for example prednisolone 30–40 mg. daily; the dosage is gradually tailed off over a period of two to three weeks. Dermatitis due to heavy metals should be treated with dimercaprol (B.A.L.) intramuscularly 3 mg. per kilogram body-weight every six hours for three days.

For anaphylactic shock following injection of a drug give an immediate injection of adrenaline 1:1,000, 0·5 ml. subcutaneously, after which it may be necessary for an intravenous infusion of saline containing nor-adrenaline or aminophylline to be set up. It is a very good rule never to give any drug by injection without having a solution of adrenaline ready for use if needed.

INFECTIONS OF THE SKIN

Infection with coagulase positive staphylococci is responsible for furunculosis, sycosis barbae (folliculitis of the beard area), carbuncles, axillary hidradenitis, pemphigus neonatorum, and impetigo contagiosa. Only the last of these will be described here.

IMPETIGO CONTAGIOSA

This is an infection of the superficial layers of the skin and it occurs mainly in dirty, neglected, and debilitated children, sometimes as a complication of scabies or pediculosis. As the name implies it is very infectious and it is spread either by direct contact or by the use of contaminated towels or clothes.

Clinical Features. The first lesion is a pink macule up to half an inch in diameter, but within a few hours this becomes converted into a superficial vesicle, then a pustule which soon ruptures with the formation of a typical bright yellow crust. The face is the usual site. There is rarely any fever or constitutional disturbance.

Treatment. Antibiotics have revolutionised the treatment of this disease, which can now usually be cleared up within a day or two. At the present time a cream containing a mixture of bacitracin and neomycin is probably the most effective remedy. It is important to search for and treat any associated lesion, such as scabies or pediculosis capitis; the latter is particularly likely to be found in girls with long hair. The patient must of course be kept away from other children and must have his own towel and pillowcase, which should subsequently be sterilised by boiling.

FISSURED IMPETIGO (Intertrigo)

Fissures occur in natural folds in the skin, for example behind the ears and in the webs of the toes, in association with impetigo and also in other conditions such as chronic eczema. They tend to heal up after a week or two, but frequently recur. Daily painting with 1 or 2 per cent silver nitrate in spirit of nitrous ether is an old-fashioned but effective treatment. A cream or lotion containing hydrocortisone and neomycin is sometimes more effective.

RINGWORM

This is a group of common fungus infections of the skin which affect mainly the scalp, the groin, and the feet.

TINEA CAPITIS (Ringworm of the scalp)

The infection is seen mainly in children under ten, particularly boys, and never persists beyond adolescence. The scalp shows a number of rounded or oval patches which are covered with fine greyish-white scales and from which most of the hairs have fallen out. The ringworm fungus fluoresces a bright green colour under Wood's light, and this examination is therefore helpful in diagnosis. The fungus can also be identified microscopically in stumps of hair removed from one of the patches.

Treatment. Griseofulvin 250 mg. four times daily for a month or longer is now the treatment of choice. It may cause headache and urticaria and should be used with caution in patients sensitive to penicillin.

TINEA CRURIS

This infection occurs mainly in young adults, particularly men, and may be acquired by direct contact or from infected clothing or articles such as lavatory seats. It causes a red, slightly raised patch extending from the crutch for two or three inches down the inner aspect of each thigh. There is sometimes itching in the affected area. The infection is seen mainly in hot weather and is more common therefore in the tropics.

Treatment. Whitfield's ointment is usually very effective, but relapses in subsequent spells of hot weather are common. Griseofulvin may also prove effective.

TINEA PEDIS (Athlete's foot)

This infection occurs in two forms, one causing vesicles and subsequent desquamation on the sole of the foot, and the other causing fissuring and maceration of the skin in the clefts between the toes. Like tinea cruris, with which it may be associated, this infection is seen mainly in young adults and is acquired from the floors of public baths and changing-rooms.

Treatment. Whitfield's ointment, Castellani's paint, and undecylenic acid ointment are three among a number of effective remedies. Relapse is common, however, and to try to prevent it careful attention to the hygiene of the feet is important. They should be washed daily, carefully dried and powdered and the socks should be changed every day.

PARASITIC DISEASES

SCABIES

The animal causing scabies is a mite (*Sarcoptes scabei hominis*). It has four pairs of legs and the female, which causes the trouble, is about 0·3 mm. long, being therefore just visible to the naked eye. The male is smaller. The female makes a burrow up to a centimeter in length in the epidermis and lays about 30 to 40 eggs in it. Each egg hatches out in four to eight days into a larval form which leaves the burrow and eventually matures into the adult form.

Infection is mainly acquired by sleeping with an infected person. It may therefore be a venereal infection, or children may acquire it from their parents or from each other. Less often infected blankets, bedding, or clothes may transmit the infection.

Clinical Features. The burrow is the characteristic lesion of scabies and appears as a fine, often zig-zag, hair-like line in the epidermis, greyish or whitish in colour and 0·5–1 cm. in length. At the far end a tiny pinhead vesicle may be seen. These burrows occur mainly in the webs and sides of the fingers, the ulnar sides of the hands, the anterior axillary folds, the lower abdomen and penis and the lower part of the buttocks. They cause intense itching, particularly when the patient is warm in bed. As a result of scratching secondary infection is common and there may be an extensive papular and pustular eruption.

Diagnosis is usually easy from the history of intense itching and the discovery of typical burrows and may be confirmed by identifying the female acarus or its eggs in a microscopical preparation of scrapings from a burrow.

Treatment. This starts with a hot bath, the patient being instructed to scrub with a nail-brush and soap all areas where there are burrows. After drying himself the patient is painted from head to foot with a 25 per cent emulsion of benzyl benzoate (applicatio benzylis benzoatis, B.P.C.), sparing only the head and neck, which are never affected by scabies. After the solution has dried another coat of it is applied. Next morning the lotion is applied again and allowed to dry before the patient dresses. That night another hot bath is taken to wash off the remains of the benzyl benzoate and a complete change of clothing and bed linen is made. Gloves and other articles which are difficult to disinfest should be laid aside for three weeks, at the end of which time all acari they contain will have died. Residual itching after benzyl benzoate treatment is quite common: it is important to treat this with calamine lotion and reassurance as further benzyl benzoate or sulphur ointment will make it worse. It need hardly be said that all contacts with the patient, particularly those within his own family circle, should be treated at the same time to avoid reinfection.

PEDICULOSIS

Lice are blood-sucking parasites which mainly infest hairy parts of the body. The female produces several hundred eggs, each of which is attached to a hair and is commonly known as a nit. A larva is hatched out from the egg in six to nine days and develops into a mature louse in one to two weeks.

Pediculosis Capitis (Infestation with head lice)

The louse concerned is the *Pediculus humanus capitis*, which is about 3 mm. long and 1 mm. broad. It infests the scalp, the nits being attached mainly to hairs at the back and sides of the head. Since the louse deposits the eggs on hairs close to the scalp and since they have hatched out by the time the hair has grown an inch or so, the search for nits should be concentrated on hair close to the head. The diagnosis depends usually on the discovery of nits, since the lice themselves are few in number and difficult to find. Nits are greyish-white, shiny, oval, opalescent structures firmly attached to the hairs.

Infection may be acquired by direct transmission from person to person or by wearing infected headgear; and since the lice flourish particularly in long hair which is seldom washed, infestation occurs mainly in women and girls living under poor hygienic conditions. Patients recently infected usually complain of irritation of the scalp, but those who have had head lice for a long time often seem to suffer no inconvenience at all. When there has been much scratching septic lesions of the scalp are a common complication.

Treatment. The scalp and hair are soaked at bedtime in 2 per cent D.D.T. emulsion, then enclosed in a cap and washed with soap and water next morning. At the same time all headgear must be sterilised in the autoclave or by boiling. Nits which have been killed by the above treatment are removed by combing with a fine-toothed comb; they come away more readily if 2 per cent acetic acid is first applied to the hair and scalp. Mother and daughters should be treated at the same time to eliminate sources of reinfection.

Pediculosis Corporis (Infestation with body lice)

Pediculus humanus corporis is similar to the head louse but slightly bigger. It normally lives in the clothes and deposits its eggs in the seams and folds of woollen undergarments.

Clinical Features. Infestation causes a variable amount of itching; scratch marks are seen mainly around the shoulders, buttocks, and the fronts of the thighs and there may be a widespread eruption from secondary bacterial infection in these situations. Tramps and vagrants after lifelong infestation may develop a generalised pigmentation of the skin like that seen in Addison's disease (*'vagabond's pigmentation'*). The diagnosis is established by finding the louse or its ova in the seams of the patient's underclothes.

Treatment. Underclothes must be washed and ironed and bedding and other clothing autoclaved. It is sufficient for the patient to take a hot bath before putting on clean clothes.

In addition to their direct effects, infestation with head and body lice is important in the spread of typhus (p. 526) and relapsing fever (p. 524).

'Pediculosis' Pubis (Infestation with 'crab' lice)

This louse is not in fact of the species pediculus, its scientific name being *Phthirus pubis*. Its life history is similar to that of the pediculi, but it is smaller (about 2 mm. by 1·5 mm.) and does not spread typhus or any other disease.

Clinical Features. It infests particularly the pubic region, though in very hairy men the whole of the trunk, the thighs, and the upper arms may be involved. On close inspection the adult lice can be seen, lying flat on the skin and holding on to a hair at each side; the nits are very similar to those of pediculus humanus and are closely attached to the body hairs. Infection is acquired mainly by sexual intercourse and occurs usually therefore in young adults.

Treatment. Lethane is applied to the affected areas of the body and not washed off for a week. Underclothes should be disinfected by washing and ironing.

URTICARIA

In susceptible subjects local urticaria may follow trauma, stings, or insect bites. Generalised urticaria may be due to sensitivity to certain foods, particularly shellfish and strawberries, or to drugs, notably penicillin, or to parenteral serum or blood. In other patients the condition is associated with worm infestation; and in many the cause is never found.

Clinical Features. The typical lesion is an extremely itchy wheal surrounded by a zone of erythema. The wheals may be of any size and shape and may cover the greater part of the body. There may be associated swelling (*angioneurotic oedema*) in the subcutaneous tissue and mucous membranes, particularly in the mouth and throat. Papular urticaria without much wheal formation is common in children.

Treatment. Quick relief can usually be obtained by giving 0·5 ml. 1:1,000 adrenaline hydrochloride subcutaneously. An intramuscular antihistamine, such as promethazine hydrochloride 50 mg., may also be given. If there is laryngeal obstruction which is not quickly relieved by these measures emergency tracheotomy must be performed. Anti-histamines are given by mouth for more sustained effect; promethazine hydrochloride 25 mg. or mepyramine maleate 100 mg. are the most powerful of these but often cause troublesome drowsiness. Chlorpheniramine maleate 4 mg. has a slightly weaker anti-histamine effect but causes less sedation. The tablets are given two or three times daily. Ephedrine 30 mg. three times daily is worth trying if the symptoms persist. Cortisone suppresses the lesions, but its administration is rarely justified in this condition. The best local application is calamine lotion containing 2 per cent phenol.

ACNE VULGARIS

Acne is a complication of seborrhoea (or excessive sebaceous secretion). The essential lesion is the comedo, which is a sebaceous follicle whose mouth has been blocked with sebum mixed with epithelial debris, and these comedones frequently become pustular from infection of the retained sebaceous material. They are found on the face, chest, shoulders, and back. Their formation appears to be favoured by androgens and they appear therefore in the years following puberty and more often in boys than in girls. Adolescent acne tends to disappear spontaneously in early adult life, though when it is very severe it may persist and healing of the lesions may leave permanent scarring.

Treatment. Frequent washing with soap and water and regular squeezing out of the sebaceous plugs from the follicles are the important measures in mild cases. Plenty of fresh air and sunlight are usually beneficial and ultra-violet light in erythema doses may be given as an alternative. The best local application is a sulphur-containing preparation such as zinc sulphide lotion, B.P.C. Oral tetracycline 250 mg. twice daily for 2 months or longer may be of great benefit.

PSORIASIS

The cause of this common chronic skin disorder is unknown, though heredity is thought to play some part in its aetiology. In some patients the onset appears to be precipitated by an acute infection, by pregnancy, or by trauma.

Clinical Features. The typical lesion is a red spot or patch of varying size covered with a thick layer of scales, which can be scraped off with the finger-nail or curette, and which exhibits a characteristic silvery sheen. Further gentle scraping of the exposed red shiny surface causes bleeding; there is no exudation of serum. The lesions are most often seen on the knees and elbows, but practically the whole surface of the body may be involved. The scalp is a common site and there may be hyperkeratotic patches on the palms and soles. Affection of the nails causes them to be thickened, pitted, and striated. The condition usually persists for life, with occasional remissions and acute exacerbations.

Arthropathic psoriasis is seen only in middle-aged or elderly patients. In association with skin lesions as described above there is a characteristic destructive polyarthritis of the hands and feet, similar to rheumatoid arthritis (p. 336).

Treatment. The appearance of the lesions on exposed parts and the profuse scaling may cause great social embarrassment and it is important to stress to the patient and his relatives that the disorder is neither contagious nor infectious. He should also be encouraged to live an active normal life with as much fresh air and sunshine as possible, though a period of bed rest may be very beneficial during acute exacerbations. At such times a soothing local application such as 1 per cent ichthammol in lotio calaminae oleosa B.P.C. should be used, but in the chronic stage a stimulating preparation such as 4 per cent chrysarobin in petrolatum or 0·1 per cent dithranol ointment should be rubbed into the lesions twice daily. If the latter cause inflammation 3 per cent crude coal tar in a zinc and starch paste may be more suitable. Application of the newer absorbable corticosteroids and occlusion with polythene sheeting for several three-day periods (as for eczema, p. 534) nearly always clears the lesions temporarily, but must be used with caution. It is wise to treat only one palm-sized patch first, to use the ointment sparingly and to watch for signs of infection, haemorrhage or striae.

PITYRIASIS ROSEA

This is probably a virus infection and occasionally groups of three or four cases are seen in hostels and similar institutions. It produces one of the most characteristic rashes in dermatology. The first lesion (or *'herald patch'*) is an oval erythematous area about an inch across with a ring of tiny scales set a millimetre or so in from the edge of the patch, which is usually situated on the front of the chest. A few days later other similar but smaller oval patches appear, mainly on the trunk with their long axes in line with the ribs, though there may be a few on the upper arms and thighs. There may be slight itching but the general health is unimpaired and complete spontaneous recovery is the rule within about six to eight weeks. No treatment is necessary, but if irritation is troublesome calamine lotion containing $\frac{1}{2}$ to 1 per cent phenol may be used.

LICHEN PLANUS

The cause of lichen planus is unknown. The eruption is seen only in adults and although it usually clears up spontaneously in from three to nine months, relapses are common and in some patients the lesions may persist for years.

Clinical Features. The typical lesion is a small polygonal papule (little bigger than a pin's head) with a flat shiny surface of pink or violet hue. The papules may be limited to certain situations, such as the anterior aspect of the wrists and forearms, the genitalia, or the legs or they may be very profuse and widespread over most of the body, though the face and other exposed parts are rarely affected. Linear disposition of the lesions along scratch marks is common. In some of the patients bluish-white streaks or patches may be seen on the buccal mucosa. There is usually some irritation of the skin and sometimes this is intensely severe.

Treatment. Confinement to bed and sedation may be necessary in occasional very severe acute cases, but usually all that is necessary is an application such as calamine lotion with 2 per cent phenol to allay irritation. An anti-histamine tablet such as promethazine hydrochloride 25 mg. may help in this respect too. If itching continues hydrocortisone ointment may be tried. If the mouth, scalp, or genitalia are affected about a month's course of oral steroids may be given and is very effective.

ERYTHEMA MULTIFORME

This eruption consists of raised erythematous areas of irregular outline and varying size and shape; sometimes in addition there are vesicular, bullous, or nodular lesions. There may be associated ulcerative lesions on the buccal mucosa. Sometimes it appears as a cutaneous reaction to a focus of infection in the skin or elsewhere; sometimes it is a manifestation of acute rheumatism; sometimes it is a drug reaction; but usually the cause is never discovered. It is often preceded by herpes simplex.

Apart from slight fever there is little constitutional upset and spontaneous healing occurs within a couple of weeks, though recurrent attacks are common.

STEVENS-JOHNSON SYNDROME

This is a variety of erythema multiforme presenting acutely with fever, followed by the appearance of ulcers in the mouth and sometimes on the conjunctivae. Within a few days erythematous and bullous eruption spreads over the body, occurring particularly on the genitalia. The patient may be gravely ill for a week or two, but rapidly recovers when the temperature settles. Ophthalmic scarring, however, may lead to blindness. Prednisolone should be given.

LUPUS ERYTHEMATOSUS (see p. 330)

ROSACEA

This is a chronic hyperaemia of the face, particularly the cheeks and central part of the forehead, leading to permanent dilatation of capillaries and the formation of telangiectases. The patients are mostly anxious middle-aged women, many of whom also have vague digestive symptoms for which no definite cause can be found. The cosmetic disability is aggravated by the flushing associated with the menopause and with the taking of alcohol or hot spicy food. There may be associated papules and pustules and sometimes hyperplasia of the sebaceous glands. Oral tetracycline 250 mg. twice daily for 2 months and application of 3% sulphur in aqueous cream may be of benefit.

PEMPHIGUS

The cause of this very serious disease is unknown. Fortunately rare, it occurs equally in men and women and seldom appears before late middle-age. Before cortisone therapy it was nearly always fatal within two years.

Clinical Features. The essential lesion is a bulla which appears on normal skin with no surrounding erythema. Crops of these bullae appear on the skin and mucous membranes and soon rupture and become infected. Constitutional disturbance is severe.

Treatment. Cortisone or an equivalent must be given in high dosage, for example prednisolone 60 mg. daily. The dose is slowly reduced when fresh blisters cease to appear, but at least 15 mg. daily should be continued until the patient has been free of symptoms for three months when the drug may be further reduced in dosage and then stopped. With this treatment a fatal outcome is not so common.

DERMATITIS HERPETIFORMIS

This disease of unknown cause has a clinical similarity to pemphigus, since the lesions are predominantly vesicular or bullous and it tends to run a chronic or relapsing course. There are, however, important differences:

(1) The vesicles and bullae are set on an erythematous base and are often accompanied by urticarial and erythematous lesions.

(2) The blisters tend to appear in clusters, particularly on the buttocks and posterior aspect of the thorax.

(3) There are seldom lesions in the mouth.

(4) Constitutional upset is slight.

(5) Irritation of the skin is usually severe.

About 60% of these patients have a coeliac syndrome which responds to a gluten-free diet.

Treatment. Dapsone (diamino-diphenyl sulphone) is the drug of choice and so often successful that it is sometimes used as a diagnostic test in this condition. The dose is 100–300 mg. a day by mouth. Prednisolone and sulphapyridine are now less often used.

EXFOLIATIVE DERMATITIS

Exfoliative dermatitis is a syndrome in which there is a progressive desquamation involving the whole skin. It is characterised by the shedding of large amounts of the superficial layers of the skin, and is complicated by excessive heat loss and almost always by secondary infection. This may cause generalised lymphadenopathy. If of long standing the constant skin loss causes negative nitrogen balance and hypoproteinaemia, which may result in oedema. Special skin structures (sweat and sebaceous glands and hair follicles) may be destroyed, sometimes permanently. If healing occurs these structures may not regenerate, so that the patient is left hairless and unable to sweat. This may be a considerable hazard in hot climates, and result in heat stroke.

Many *causes* of exfoliative dermatitis are recognised, and the commoner are numerated below.

(1) Medicamentosa. Arsenic, gold, streptomycin, penicillin.

(2) Barbiturates. Usually appears after 8 to 10 days medication. Causes febrile erythroderma and stomatitis, going on to exfoliation.

(3) External applications. Penicillin, sulphonamides, chrysarobin, streptomycin.

(4) Untreated generalised eczema.

(5) Generalised psoriasis. Usually after chrysarobin has been applied.

(6) Generalised erythroderma. May complicate Hodgkin's disease, leukaemias, lymphosarcomas, and lipomelanic reticulosis.

(7) Mycosis fungoides and pityriasis rubra pilaris.

(8) Idiopathic group.

Treatment. Secondary infection should be treated appropriately, and the patient's body kept clean and warm. All other drugs should be withdrawn. If heavy metal poisoning is suspected a course of B.A.L. should be given (p. 558). Some cases respond well to local and systemic application of steroids, but with the exception of the iatrogenic group treatment often has to be continued for months or even years.

FURTHER READING

Ingram, J., *Clinical Dermatology*, Churchill, London, 1969.

CHAPTER TWENTY

VENEREAL DISEASES

The word venereal is derived from Venus, the goddess of love, and is applied to those diseases which are communicated by sexual intercourse. The important members of this group are syphilis, gonorrhoea and other causes of urethritis and vaginitis; rarer disorders include chancroid and lymphogranuloma venereum.

GONORRHOEA

The Neisseria gonorrhoea is a delicate organism which does not survive for long outside the body, and gonorrhoea is almost invariably acquired by coitus with an infected person. Recovery confers no immunity and it is therefore possible for the same individual to have repeated attacks of the disease. Young girls may acquire the disease from infected bed-linen and towels, but outbreaks of vulvo-vaginitis in children are in fact more often due to other organisms.

The Neisseria gonorrhoea is identified in smears of purulent exudates as a gram-negative kidney-shaped diplococcus which must be seen within the cytoplasm of polymorph leucocytes before the diagnosis can be made. It is rather difficult to grow in culture unless special media and increased carbon-dioxide tension are employed.

Clinical Features.

(1) **In Men.** Within about three to ten days of exposure to infection the first symptom is usually slight *scalding* on micturition, soon followed by a *purulent urethral discharge* and there may be tender swollen lymph nodes in the groin. If treatment is not given the infection tends to spread to the posterior urethra, as indicated by cloudiness in the second glass of voided urine. Infection of the *prostate* may follow and may cause acute retention of urine, while involvement of the *seminal vesicles* causes severe local pain and fever. Stricture in the posterior urethra is a late sequela. *Acute epididymitis*, indicated by severe pain, swelling, and tenderness which often spread to involve the testicle on the same side is a serious complication since it may be followed by sterility. With modern treatment spread beyond the anterior urethra is very rare.

(2) **In Women.** After a similar incubation period the disease usually presents with *painful, frequent micturition*, and *vaginal discharge*, though there may be no symptoms if the infection is confined to the cervix. Two-thirds of women infected do not seek medical advice, either through

fear or lack of presenting symptoms. Involvement of *Skene's* or *Bartholin's glands* may lead to large painful abscesses, though in fact Bartholin's abscess is much more often of streptococcal origin. If untreated the infection may spread to the uterus and Fallopian tubes, leading to the formation of a *pyosalpinx*; this presents with severe lower abdominal pain and fever and a tender adnexal mass can be felt on one or both sides on pelvic examination. It may be possible to demonstrate gonococci in cervical smears. Involvement of the tubes usually leads to permanent sterility.

Complications. Metastatic lesions due to transient bacteraemia are now very rare, but a purulent arthritis is occasionally seen. Gonorrhoeal rheumatism, however, is usually not due to bacteria in situ and may be in fact an associated Reiter's syndrome (p. 340). It may take the form of a flitting polyarthritis coming on a month or so after infection, or a single joint may be involved, particularly the knee, wrist or ankle. Associated tenosynovitis is common and iritis may occur.

Treatment. A single injection of procaine penicillin B.P., 1·2–2·4 g. (1,200,000–2,400,000 units), is usually adequate treatment for uncomplicated gonorrhoea. Women should receive the higher dose as they tend to respond less well. There are now strains of gonococci relatively resistant to penicillin; but most of the patients whose symptoms persist or relapse within a few days respond to procaine penicillin, fortified, B.P., 5 ml. (containing procaine penicillin 1·5 g. and benzylpenicillin 0·5 g.). A single injection of streptomycin 1 g. may be effective, but strains of gonococci completely resistant to it are increasing. Good results have also been obtained with oral demethylchlortetracyline in a single dose of 600–900 mg., erythromycin 500 mg. six-hourly for five days, or spiramycin 500 mg. six-hourly for two days, but the drugs are too expensive for routine use. It is important to remember that the treatment of gonorrhoea may suppress the appearance of a syphilitic lesion acquired at the same time and serological tests for the latter disease must always be made three and six months after the gonorrhoea has been treated.

SYPHILIS

As a result of improved treatment and the consequent reduced infectivity of patients with the disease, syphilis is much less common. It remains very important, however, because of the serious lesions which may appear in almost any organ of the body many years after the primary infection.

The causative organism, treponema pallidum, is a thin, actively motile spirochaete from 6–14 μm. in length, which can be recognised by its characteristic movements in preparations of the serous discharge from the early infectious lesions examined by the microscopic technique known as dark-ground illumination (D.G.I.). It cannot withstand drying and is transmitted only by direct contact.

Congenital syphilis is contracted by the foetus through the placenta in the later months of pregnancy; acquired syphilis is nearly always the result of sexual intercourse with an infected person, though occasionally extragenital infection may be acquired, for example by doctors or nurses, by handling syphilitic lesions. Congenital syphilis is fortunately extremely rare nowadays. It is a preventible disease, since if a woman with syphilis is given adequate treatment sufficiently early in pregnancy the child escapes infection. Routine serum tests should therefore be made on all women on their first attendance at ante-natal clinics.

Clinical Features. Congenital syphilis may cause intra-uterine death and result in *miscarriage* or *stillbirth*. or the child may be born apparently healthy only to develop various stigmata of the disease during childhood. Early manifestations are failure to gain weight in the first month or two of life and an infection in the nose ('*snuffles*') which interferes with the development of the nasal bones and leads eventually to the depressed bridge of the nose which is one of the most characteristic signs of the disease. A scaly yellow or copper-coloured *rash* is also common. Among the many lesions which may appear later in childhood are notches in the incisor teeth of the second dentition, which also tend to be widely spaced and to taper from the gum margin to the cutting edge (*Hutchinson's teeth*); scars known as *rhagades* radiating from the margins of the lips; and opacity of the cornea due to *interstitial keratitis* (I.K.). Aortic lesions are very rare in congenital syphilis, but juvenile forms of *tabes* and *general paresis* are occasionally seen.

Acquired syphilis passes through three stages, known as *primary* syphilis, *secondary* syphilis, and *tertiary* syphilis. The secondary stage occurs within a few months of primary infection, but many years may elapse before a tertiary lesion appears.

Primary syphilis is characterised by the appearance of a hard chancre (pronounced 'shanker') about a month after exposure to infection. In men the chancre usually occurs on the penis; in women it appears most often on the labia or cervix and in the latter situation readily escapes notice. Much more rarely the primary sore may be on the lip, tongue, tonsil, or nipple. The chancre is a hard, painless ulcer about 1 cm. in diameter, has a thin, serous discharge and is accompanied by painless enlargement of the regional lymph nodes. *Diagnosis* depends on identifying the treponema pallidum in the exudate with the use of the dark-ground microscope.

Secondary syphilis may cause some constitutional disturbance with *sore throat*, low *fever* and generalised *lymph-node enlargement*, but usually its manifestations are confined to the skin and the mucous membrane of the mouth. Various types of skin *rash* are seen, all having in common a symmetrical distribution over the body, absence of irritation, and a colour usually likened to raw ham. In the mouth painless, slimy, greyish patches known as '*snail-track ulcers*' are the typical lesions. Warty lesions known as *condylomata* may appear in the peri-anal and vulval regions. The cutaneous and mucosal lesions of the secondary stage are highly infective and the serum tests for antibody are invariably positive.

Tertiary Stage. A localised swelling known as a gumma may appear anywhere in the body many years after the primary infection; these lesions differ from those of primary and secondary syphilis in containing no spirochaetes and being therefore non-infective. In certain situations such as the liver, the lung, or the stomach, a gumma may be mistaken for a carcinoma; the distinction can be made by giving potassium iodide 1–2 g. which causes rapid disappearance of a gumma but has no effect on a carcinoma. The centre of a gumma often breaks down and leads to the formation of an ulcer with sharply punched-out margins.

Syphilitic *aortitis* is discussed on p. 143, and *neurosyphilis* on p. 283.

Treatment of Syphilis. Procaine penicillin injection B.P., 600 mg. (600,000 units), should be given daily for ten days. Alternatively itinerant or unco-operative patients may be given a single intramuscular injection of benzathine penicillin 2·4 g. (2·4 mega units) as this will maintain the necessary blood level (at least 0·03 units per ml.) for about two weeks. Patients sensitive to penicillin may be given tetracycline by mouth 750 mg. six-hourly for 10 to 15 days, though the long-term efficacy of this treatment has not yet been fully assessed. Patients with early infectious syphilis are kept under supervision for 2 years. Patients with late syphilis require two or more courses of treatment lasting 2–3 weeks each and may need prolonged follow-up. At each visit in addition to clinical examination and serum Wassermann and Kahn tests for syphilis antibody one of the tests using specific syphilitic antigen is performed, e.g. T.P.I. (Treponema Pallidum Immobilisation) or R.P.C.F.T. (Reiter Protein Complement Fixation Test). If there are clinical indications the C.S.F. is examined also.

An acute exacerbation of the lesions may occur within a day or so of starting treatment (the *Herxheimer reaction*) but this is never harmful in early syphilis and is over in a few hours. The Herxheimer reaction may have more serious effects in patients with syphilitic aortitis or gummata in special situations such as the larynx; penicillin therapy should be started under steroid cover in such patients.

NON-SPECIFIC URETHRITIS

Following the striking decline in the numbers of patients with gonorrhoea and syphilis, non-specific urethritis has become one of the most common conditions seen in V.D. departments. It may be due to known organisms such as virus (TRIC), mycoplasma organisms, mixed bacteria, Trichomonas vaginalis, Candida albicans, or at times to non-infective causes. It is seen mainly in young men.

After a variable incubation period which can probably be as long as two to three months, the patient develops scalding, frequency, and a purulent urethral discharge which contains no Neisseria gonorrhoea. In addition to urethral discharge some patients have conjunctivitis and acute arthritis affecting one or more of the large joints of the limbs, and the condition is then known as *Reiter's syndrome* (p. 340). The urethral discharge usually subsides fairly quickly, but the arthritis when present may persist for many months. A frequent local complication is subacute prostatitis.

Tetracycline 250 mg. six-hourly for five days should be given, but the response is often unsatisfactory.

SOFT SORE (Chancroid)

Chancroid is very rare in Britain, though it is occasionally seen in seaports. The causative organism is haemophilus ducreui (Ducrey's bacillus), a gram negative bacillus about 1–2 μm. in length.

Clinical Features. After an incubation period of two to fourteen days one or more small red papules appear on the genitalia or surrounding skin and within a few days develop into necrotic ulcers with undermined edges surrounded by an area of erythema and oedema. The inguinal lymph nodes enlarge and sometimes suppurate. The important distinction from syphilis is made by the shorter incubation period, the absence of induration in the lesions, the failure to demonstrate spirochaetes on dark-ground illumination and identification of Ducrey's bacillus in stained smears and on culture.

Treatment. A course of sulphadimidine or other sulphonamide is effective.

LYMPHOGRANULOMA INGUINALE

This is also very rare in Britain. It is a virus infection with an incubation period of up to three weeks.

Clinical Features. The initial lesion may be a small vesicle or ulcer on the genitalia, but more often the first evidence of the disease is enlargement of the inguinal lymph nodes. The swelling may become quite massive and eventually suppuration may occur with the discharge of yellow pus through multiple sinuses in the skin. There is often severe constitutional reaction with high fever. In women proctitis and subsequent rectal stricture may occur; sequelae in men include scarring and elephantiasis of the genitalia.

Diagnosis. A positive intradermal *Frei test* indicates that the patient now has or has had the disease.

Treatment. Some success may be achieved with either the sulphonamides or the tetracyclines, or the two drugs may be combined. Sulphonamides such as sulphadimidine should be given in doses of 3–4 g. daily for three to six weeks; tetracycline dosage is 500 mg. six-hourly for five days followed by 250 mg. six-hourly for three to six weeks or longer. Fluctuant buboes should be aspirated rather than incised.

FURTHER READING

Catterall, R.D., *A Short Textbook of Venereology*. E.U.P., 1965, 2nd edition 1972.

CHAPTER TWENTY-ONE

ABNORMAL REACTIONS TO DRUGS

INTRODUCTION

Drug reactions are becoming increasingly important as the range of substances used for diagnostic and therapeutic purposes is increased. The classification of these reactions is difficult for their underlying mechanism is often not fully understood.

(1) **Overdosage.** This term is self-explanatory. It must be realised, however, that patients vary in the amount of drug required to produce symptoms and signs of overdosage. Patients who develop evidence of overdosage with small doses are said to show *intolerance* to the drug.

(2) **Side Effects.** These effects although not therapeutically useful are inherent in the action of the drug. The constipation which complicates the use of ganglion blocking agents is a good example.

(3) **Secondary Effects.** These effects are not due to any action of the drug, but are a consequence of that action.

(4) **Idiosyncrasy.** This means that the subject reacts to the drug in some abnormal way.

(5) **Hypersensitivity Reactions.** These reactions imply that the patient is sensitive to the drug, usually from previous contact, and that the reaction is mediated by an antigen-antibody reaction.

(6) **Drug Interactions.**

In practice it is often very difficult to decide into which group a drug reaction falls, particularly to distinguish between idosyncrasy and hypersensitivity reactions.

The following is a description of a number of clinical syndromes which may occur as a result of taking drugs. The majority of these syndromes are hypersensitivity reactions.

ACUTE HYPERSENSITIVITY REACTION

This reaction occurs within a few minutes of administration of the drug. The main features are chest pain, dyspnoea, cyanosis, and a rapid fall in blood pressure. There is often, but not always, a history of previous exposure to the drug. This type of reaction is more common in those with a history of atopic disorders. It seems probable that these subjects are particularly liable to produce antibodies of the IgE class (see p. 320). These antibodies become attached to the surface of mast cells and when they combine with the appropriate antigen pharmacologically active substances such as histamine, bradykinin and 5-hydroxytryptamine are released from the cell.

Treatment begins with prophylaxis. It is important to ask the patient if he is sensitive to the drug about to be administered. If a reaction occurs adrenaline 0·5 ml. of 1:1,000 solution, must be given subcutaneously together with an anti-histamine (chlorpheniramine maleate 10·0 mg. I.V.).

DELAYED HYPERSENSITIVITY REACTION

The onset of symptoms with this type of reaction usually occurs from seven to fourteen days after the start of taking the drug. There is often a history of previous drug exposure. The common symptoms are *fever, skin rashes, joint pains*, and *lymphadenopathy*. The skin rashes although usually urticarial may occasionally be purpuric and sometimes even an exfoliative dermatitis occurs.

Among the drugs which produce these symptoms are the barbiturates, the sulphonamides, streptomycin, thiouracil, and particularly penicillin. Exfoliative dermatitis may follow the heavy metals, particularly gold or arsenic, as well as penicillin and the sulphonamides.

Treatment consists of stopping the drug. Usually this is sufficient. The disappearance of symptoms may be aided by an anti-histamine (promethazine hydrochloride 25 mg. twice daily or chlorpheniramine maleate 4 mg. three times daily). Prednisolone is occasionally required in severe cases. If the rash is troublesome the local application of calamine lotion reduces the itching.

BLOOD DYSCRASIAS

Blood dyscrasias are among the most important drug reactions. It would seem that many of them are hypersensitivity reactions and are due to combination of antigen, antibody and complement on the cell. Others are due to a direct effect on the blood cells or their precursors.

Agranulocytosis

This may occur with a number of drugs including amidopyrine, the sulphonamides, thiouracil, carbimazole, tridione, isoniazid, phenylbutazone, chloramphenicol, gold, and arsenic. In addition large doses of most cytotoxic drugs such as nitrogen mustard will produce agranulocytosis. With most drugs the agranulocytosis is reversible, provided the drug is not continued for too long, but with chloramphenicol recovery may not occur.

Clinical Features. There may be no symptoms and the depression in the granulocytes may be found by a routine blood count. Such patients are susceptible to infection and may present with general malaise, fever, and some infective process, usually a severe throat infection.

Treatment

(1) *Prophylaxis.* The patient should always be asked if he is susceptible to the drug before it is given. Certain drugs such as amidopyrine and

chloramphenicol should be avoided if possible. It is doubtful if routine blood counts on patients taking drugs which may cause agranulocytosis are much help as the fall in granulocytes may be sudden. The patient must, however, be told to report to the doctor if he becomes ill and in particular if he develops a sore throat; a blood count must then be performed.

(2) *Curative.* The drug must be stopped immediately. Procaine penicillin 600,000 units twice daily is given to prevent infection. If the white count does not improve within a few days, prednisolone 30 mg. daily should be given. The majority of patients will recover on this treatment. When granulopenia is due to heavy metals it should be treated with dimercaprol (p. 558).

Thrombocytopenia

Thrombocytopenia may occur as a result of drug administration. It has been described with sedormid, tridione, chloramphenicol, arsenic, gold, sulphonamides, and quinine. It may occur with excessive dosage of cytoxic drugs. Clinical features include purpura and bleeding from various sites.

Treatment. The drug should be stopped immediately. Prednisolone 30 mg. daily is the most effective treatment. It is doubtful whether blood transfusion is helpful and it should be reserved for those patients who require transfusion because of excessive blood loss. Fresh blood should be used, because transfused platelets are effective for only a few hours.

Aplastic Anaemia

Aplastic anaemia is not common following the taking of drugs. It may occur with benzol and its derivatives, with chloramphenicol and with a number of other drugs including gold and the sulphonamides. It may be associated with depression of other elements of the blood.

Treatment. The drug should be stopped. Repeated transfusion may be required. Prednisolone is not usually very helpful, but it is worth a trial in patients who are not recovering. If poisoning is due to heavy metals, dimercaprol should be used. Provided the drug is stopped quickly, recovery usually occurs. The exception is chloramphenicol, which rarely causes bone-marrow dyscrasias and usually only after repeated courses; if they occur, however, they are usually irreversible and ultimately prove fatal.

Haemolytic Anaemia

Drugs can occasionally cause haemolysis. It seems that a number of mechanisms may be responsible. Quinine has long been known to precipitate the acute haemolysis occurring in association with malaria and called *blackwater fever*. It is most likely that this is some kind of hypersensitivity reaction.

Potassium chlorate in large doses will produce haemolysis by a direct action on the cell; occasionally this occurs with quite a small dose of the drug and it can then be classed as an example of intolerance.

Finally in a small number of American negroes there appears to be some abnormality in one of the intracellular enzyme systems which is normally responsible for the integrity of the red cells. This results in acute haemolysis when such subjects take primaquine and is an example of true idiosyncrasy to a drug (p. 555).

Methaemoglobinaemia and Sulphaemoglobinaemia

These changes in the haemoglobin may occur with certain drugs, including phenacetin, potassium chlorate, and the sulphonamides. The patient appears cyanosed, but is not distressed or dyspnoeic. The diagnosis is confirmed by finding the absorption spectra of methaemoglobin or sulphaemoglobin in the blood. The only treatment usually required is to stop the offending drug. Methaemoglobinaemia can be temporarily reversed by giving methylene blue as a 1 per cent solution intravenously, the dose for an adult being 5 ml.

Megaloblastic Anaemia

Certain drugs including pyrimethamine and the anticonvulsants primidone and phenytoin may produce a megaloblastic anaemia which can be reversed by folic acid 10 mg. daily.

LIVER DAMAGE (see p. 89)

DRUG REACTIONS AND COLLAGEN DISEASES

Although some authors include a wide variety of syndromes under the term collagen diseases, this term should be confined to rheumatic fever, rheumatoid arthritis, disseminated lupus erythematosis, polyarteritis nodosa, dermatomyositis, and giant-cell arteritis. There has been considerable discussion whether drug reactions can cause these conditions. There is no doubt that a clinical picture similar to that of disseminated lupus erythematosis can be produced by hydralazine and by procaineamide, but it differs from the true disease in that recovery occurs when the drug is stopped. In addition, transient arteritis can occur in association with hypersensitivity reaction to a number of drugs, including penicillin and the sulphonamides. Whether such reactions play any part in the pathogenesis of true polyarteritis nodosa is more doubtful and it is unlikely that drug reactions are causally related to any of the other collagen diseases.

SERUM REACTIONS

Serum reactions can be divided into:
(a) Immediate reactions.
(b) Delayed reactions (serum sickness).

They are hypersensitivity reactions and are more common in those who have had serum before and in those with a history of allergic diseases such as asthma, hay fever, urticaria, or infantile eczema.

Immediate Serum Reactions

Clinical Features. Immediate serum reactions appear within a few minutes of injection and vary greatly in their severity. There may be merely swelling, with perhaps some local urticaria in the region of the injection. There may be a generalised rash without any other upset. In severe cases the patient complains of feeling unwell, with tightness in the chest and faintness, followed by collapse with cyanosis, a falling blood pressure and occasionally death.

Treatment. Mild reactions respond to the application of calamine lotion to the rash and an anti-histamine by mouth for a few days (chlorpheniramine maleate 4 mg. t.d.s. or promethazine 25 mg. b.d.). In severe cases subcutaneous adrenaline 0·5 ml. of 1 : 1,000 solution should be given immediately and may have to be repeated. This should be followed by an anti-histamine given by slow intravenous injection (chlorpheniramine maleate 10 mg. or promethazine hydrochloride 25 mg.). Rarely, hydrocortisone hemisuccinate 100 mg. intravenously will be required.

Delayed Serum Reaction (serum sickness)

This is due to a circulatory antigen, antibody to complement complex which causes transient damage to certain tissues.

Clinical Features. About a week to ten days after the patient has received serum he develops a rash, usually urticarial, pain and stiffness with some swelling in the joints, and usually a fever. Sometimes there is enlargement of the lymph nodes and a transient albuminuria. Rarely, a shock-like state develops with low blood pressure. This condition usually clears up in a few days.

Treatment. Local application of calamine lotion helps to relieve the itching. An anti-histamine such as chlorpheniramine maleate 4 mg. t.d.s. shortens the duration of the illness. In severe or resistant cases, prednisolone 20 mg. for a day or two and then tailed off will usually relieve the symptoms.

AVOIDANCE OF SERUM REACTIONS

When serum is given to a patient the following rules should be observed.

(1) The patient should be asked whether he has had serum before or whether he suffers from allergic diseases such as asthma, hay fever, eczema, or urticaria.

(2) If the answer to these questions is negative, 0·1 ml. of serum is injected subcutaneously. If there is no local or general reaction within half an hour, the full dose of serum is given intramuscularly.

(3) If the patient has a history of allergic disease or has had serum before, 0·1 ml. of serum diluted 1:10 is given subcutaneously; if there is no reaction within half an hour 0·1 ml. of serum is given subcutaneously; if after a further half an hour there is still no reaction, the full dose of serum is given intramuscularly.

(4) If the patient has a history of serum reactions or has a reaction to the test dose, he should be admitted to hospital. He is then given an anti-histamine followed by the serum in gradually increasing doses. It is usual to start with 0·1 ml. of a 1:100 dilution of serum and if this causes no reaction in half an hour the dose is doubled and so on until enough serum has been given. It is a very tedious process.

(5) Whenever serum is given it is essential that a syringe of fresh 1:1,000 adrenaline solution be at hand and also an anti-histamine suitable for I.V. injection (chlorpheniramine maleate 10 mg.). Whenever patients are given serum they must be observed for half an hour after the injection and must be warned of the possibility of a delayed serum reaction.

(6) Intravenous injections of serum should be avoided if possible. Where they are necessary, the same precautions should be adopted. Intravenous serum should not be given to those who have previously had serum or who have allergic disorders and in addition a test dose of 0·1 ml. of serum should also be given intramuscularly. As a general rule intravenous serum should be given only to patients in hospital.

(7) Following the administration of serum the patient should be actively immunised against the appropriate diseases. This should be delayed until at least one month after he has received the serum, as the circulating antibody from the serum may prevent the antigen from provoking active immunity.

GENETICALLY DETERMINED DRUG REACTIONS

Reactions to drugs may be due to specific hereditary enzymatic deficiency. About 10 per cent of American Negroes develop haemolytic anaemia when exposed to primaquine and other related drugs. It is now clear that these individuals lack the enzyme glucose-6-phosphate dehydrogenase and this deficiency is sex-linked. Precipitation of acute porphyria in genetically predisposed individuals by ingestion of barbiturates is well known. A dangerously prolonged response to the muscle relaxant succinylcholine may be due to a deficiency of the hereditary serum enzyme pseudocholinesterase. The height of the blood level of isonicotinic acid hydrazide which follows an oral dose depends on whether it is 'rapidly' or 'slowly' inactivated (acetylated). The gene for 'slow' inactivator is recessive and patients who are 'slow' inactivators, although they have a more rapid bacteriological response to isoniazid, are more likely to exhibit drug reactions than 'rapid' inactivators.

DRUG INTERACTION

The increasing use of drugs, particularly the prescribing of more than one drug at a time, has made drug interaction an important problem. Interaction may occur at several stages in the passage of drugs through the body:

(1) **In the gastro-intestinal tract** drugs may combine or their physical state may be altered so that absorption is modified. For example, iron combines with tetracycline decreasing its absorption and leading to lower blood levels of the antibiotic.

(2) **Competition for transport sites on the plasma proteins.** Many drugs are transported to their sites of action partially or almost totally bound to plasma proteins. When bound in this way they cannot produce their pharmacological effects and are not available to be metabolised or excreted. The activity of the drug depends on the unbound fraction.

When two drugs compete for a limited number of protein-binding sites there is a decrease in the bound fraction of each and an increase in the amount of free drug, with a corresponding enhancement of the pharmacological effect. The anticoagulant Warfarin, for example, is normally about 98% bound to plasma protein. If phenylbutazone is given concurrently competition for sites occurs and the bound fraction of Warfarin may drop to 96%; the amount of active Warfarin is therefore doubled and signs of overdosage may result.

(3) **Modification at sites of action.** The pharmacological action of a drug can be modified in several ways by the concurrent administration of another drug. For example:

    (a) Hypokalaemia produced by diuretics enhances the action of digitalis on the heart.

    (b) Tricyclic antidepressants reverse the effect of adrenergic blocking hypotensive agents, possibly by increasing the amount of noradrenaline at the adrenergic nerve endings.

    (c) The action of central nervous depressants such as barbiturates and alcohol is additive.

(4) **Enzyme induction.** Many drugs are metabolised by enzymes, usually in the liver. Certain drugs increase the activity of these enzymes so that drug breakdown is enhanced. For example, if a patient on an oral anticoagulent is given phenobarbitone the barbiturate increases the enzyme activity and the anticoagulant is metabolised more rapidly. An increased dose is therefore necessary to produce a satisfactory anticoagulant effect. Conversely, if the phenobarbitone is stopped enzyme activity decreases and signs of anticoagulant overdosage may appear.

(5) **Renal Excretion.** Competition for pathways in the kidney by two drugs given together may reduce the rate of excretion of both. Use is made of this phenomenon when probenecid is given with penicillin to reduce its excretion and so achieve a higher level of penicillin in the blood.

CHAPTER TWENTY-TWO

POISONING

The treatment of acute poisoning by substances taken by mouth divides itself into:

(a) Emptying and washing out the stomach.

(b) Specific treatment for the particular poison.

GASTRIC EMPTYING AND LAVAGE

In all patients who are conscious except those who have taken corrosive poisons, vomiting should be precipitated by making the patient drink a pint of warm water and then stimulating the pharynx with the fingers. This must be followed, except with corrosive poisons, by gastric lavage. A stomach tube of 1 cm. diameter is passed and 250 ml. of warm water is run into the stomach and then syphoned out. This should be repeated at least six times. If the nature of the poison is known, a suitable antidote may be left in the stomach (see below).

It is very important to avoid inhalation of gastric contents by the patient and during gastric lavage he should lie in the prone position with the head and shoulders lower than the rest of the body.

In the unconscious patient the risk of inhalation is increased. In these patients the help of an anaesthetist is advisable for gastric lavage which should be preceded by the passing of a cuffed endotracheal tube.

After four hours most poisons have left the stomach and so very little will be recovered by gastric lavage. Salicylates however cause pyloric spasm and gastric lavage is useful for up to 24 hours.

Finally, all vomit and the first return from gastric lavage should be kept and carefully labelled for further analysis.

TRICYCLIC ANTIDEPRESSIVES

This group includes imiprimine, nortriptyline and amitriptyline.

These drugs have become common agents in attempted suicide. The clinical picture is one of excitement followed by coma and sometimes convulsions. The pupils are dilated, the reflexes increased and the plantars extensor. In severe overdosage special features are hypotension, tachycardia and the occurrence of cardiac arrythmias. Frequently they may be combined with a phenothiazine or with a benzodiazepine compound such as chlordiazapoxide which produces a complicated clinical picture.

Treatment. There is no specific antidote and symptoms must be treated as they arise. Fits can be controlled by phenobarbitone. The cardiac arrythmias should be treated along the usual lines (see p. 115). Hypotension is difficult to treat and both vaso-constriction and cautious infusion with plasma volume expanders such as dextran have been used. Forced diuresis and dialysis are *not* effective.

ARSENICAL POISONING

Inorganic Arsenic, usually in the form of the oxide, acquired notoriety as a homicidal poison and is still sometimes taken with suicidal intent. Poisoning may also occur as a result of exposure to arsenical dusts which are produced in various industrial processes. It produces its toxic action by inhibiting the intracellular sulphydril enzymes which are essential to metabolism.

Acute Poisoning

Clinical Features. The main symptoms of acute poisoning by arsenic are burning in the throat, vomiting, abdominal pain, and diarrhoea. In severe cases circulatory collapse and death may follow.

Treatment. (1) The stomach should be emptied and then washed out with freshly prepared ferric hydroxide, which is made by adding 45 g. of ferric chloride to 15 g. of sodium carbonate (washing soda) in half a tumbler of water.

(2) *Dimercaprol* (B.A.L.) 300 mg. in oily solution is given I.M. six-hourly for two days and then decreased over the next few days. The action of dimercaprol is to offer SH groups with which the arsenic combines; it is thus unable to combine with the SH groups in intracellular enzymes.

Chronic Poisoning

The symptoms and signs of chronic arsenical poisoning are variable, but include:

    (1) Pigmentation of the skin which has a typical mottled ('rain-drop') appearance.
    (2) Polyneuritis.
    (3) Hyperkeratosis of the palms of hands and soles of the feet.
    (4) Chronic pharyngitis and perforation of the nasal septum.
    (5) Chronic diarrhoea.

Treatment. The patient should be removed from exposure to arsenic and given dimercaprol as for acute poisoning.

POISONING BY FERROUS COMPOUNDS

This form of poisoning has become common; it is usually due to children eating sugar-coated ferrous sulphate tablets in mistake for sweets.

Clinical Features, include vomiting with haematemesis, followed by collapse, pallor, and tachycardia. Collapse may occur after apparent recovery. Later acute hepatic necrosis may develop.

Treatment. (1) Vomiting should be induced.

(2) The stomach should then be washed out with 5 per cent sodium bicarbonate solution (one tablespoonful to one pint).

(3) The iron chelating agent desferrioxamine B mesylate is used to prevent further absorption of iron and to hasten excretion. Five grams in 100 ml. of water should be given orally. At the same time 2·0 g. are given intramuscularly twice daily.

In severe cases desferrioxamine can be given intravenously in 5 per cent glucose solution at a rate of 15 mg./kg. per hour to a maximum of 80 mg./kg. per 24 hours.

(4) The patient must be kept in bed and under observation for at least 48 hours after apparent recovery.

ANTICHOLINESTERASE POISONING

A number of these substances are used in medicine and also as insecticides. They also have a potential use in war, and are known as 'nerve gases'. They inhibit the enzyme cholinesterase either temporarily or for long periods, so that there is widespread overactivity of the parasympathetic nervous system and also neuromuscular block in voluntary muscle. Symptoms may include colicky abdominal pain, excess salivation, respiratory paralysis and the pupils are constricted.

Treatment. Atropine should be given in doses of 2·0 mg. intravenously or intramuscularly, and repeated as required. This will not however relieve neuromuscular block. Cholinesterase can be reactivated by pralidoxime 1·0 g. in 5 ml. of water I.V. or I.M., and repeated at four-hourly intervals as required. In severe cases some form of assisted ventilation may be necessary.

SALICYLATE POISONING

Poisoning by salicylates is common; it may be suicidal, or in children it may be accidental. The fatal dose in adults is in the region of 25 g. Doses of 2–4 g. have proved toxic in children. In addition, some subjects, particularly asthmatics, are sensitive to salicylates and death has occurred after as little of 0·3 g. of aspirin.

Clinical Features. In mild cases the main symptoms are nausea, vomiting, tinnitus and increased respirations. After larger doses there is mental confusion, the patient is flushed and sweating with a full pulse and over-breathing is very striking. In the early stages hyperventilation lowers the pCO_2 of the plasma and leads to a respiratory alkalosis; with increasing absorption of salicylate there is a metabolic acidosis with a fall in plasma bicarbonate. In children acidosis is common, whereas in adults a raised blood pH is more usual. In addition vomiting and sweating lead to dehydration and oliguria.

The urine gives a positive reaction to ferric chloride and may contain protein.

Treatment. (1) The stomach should be washed out with water. If the patient is in coma a cuffed intratracheal tube should be passed beforehand to avoid possible aspiration of vomited material into the lungs.

(2) In mild cases 5 per cent sodium bicarbonate solution should be given orally in doses of 2 g. four-hourly for 24 hours. Sodium bicarbonate, by making the urine alkaline, increases the rate of excretion of salicylate by the kidneys.

(3) In severe cases (plasma salicylate level of more than 30 mg./ 100 ml. in children and 50 mg./100 ml. in adults) treatment is aimed at correcting dehydration and producing a diuresis of alkaline urine and thus rapidly clearing salicylate from the body. Owing to the complex acid/base disorder which occurs in salicylate poisoning, it is important to estimate plasma pH, bicarbonate and pCO_2.

A central venous pressure line is also useful to guard against overloading the circulation and the bases of the lump should be examined regularly for signs of pulmonary oedema. In the first hour 500 ml. of $1 \cdot 2\%$ sodium bicarbonate (or $\frac{1}{6}$M sodium lactate) + 20 mg. of frusemide, followed by $1 \cdot 0$ litre of 5% dextrose + 20 mg. of frusemide are given intravenously. At the end of the hour the urinary flow should be greater than $3 \cdot 0$ ml./min. Subsequent rate of infusion will depend on central venous pressure and urinary volume. Every third bottle (500 ml.) of infusion fluid should contain 150mEq of sodium and every bottle of infusion fluid $10 \cdot 0$ mEq of potassium. Diuresis can be maintained either by adding mannitol (not more than 20 g./hour) to the infusion fluid or by further injections of frusemide intravenously. The urinary pH must be kept above $7 \cdot 5$.

If a diuresis is not produced by the end of the first hour there is probably impairment of renal function and dialysis will be required.

(4) 50 mg. of mephyton should be injected intravenously to prevent bleeding.

By this method a majority of adult patients with salicylate poisoning can be resuscitated. In a few patients with high plasmas salicylate levels (over 100 ml./100 ml.) and with renal or circulatory failure, haemodialysis will be required. Children are more sensitive to the toxic effects of salicylate.

CARBON MONOXIDE POISONING

Excluding road accidents, carbon monoxide is the commonest cause of accidental death in Great Britain; it is also used by the suicide. Poisoning may result from the escape of carbon monoxide from gas lights or gas fires, from car exhausts, from combustion stoves in a poorly ventilated room or from coal-mine explosions.

Carbon monoxide is odourless and lighter than air. It has a far greater affinity for haemoglobin than oxygen and forms a compound, carboxyhaemoglobin, which is bright-red colour. The carboxyhaemoglobin cannot carry oxygen and tissue anoxia results.

Clinical Features. Symptoms are minimal if less than 30 per cent of haemoglobin is combined with carbon monoxide and consist of nausea, lassitude, and headache. With higher concentrations the onset of symptoms is rapid. There is a transient increase in pulse rate and respiration followed by weakness, dimness of vision and finally coma, respiratory depression, and death.

The patient with carbon monoxide poisoning is often pale and cyanosed. The typical cherry red colour due to carboxyhaemoglobin is usually only seen at post mortem. The presence of this compound in the blood may be confirmed by its characteristic absorption spectrum.

Treatment. The patient must be removed from the poisoned atmosphere. Artificial respiration should be started immediately. If possible, pure oxygen should be given by the best available method. Cerebral oedema may develop in severe cases. The diagnosis is suggested by papilloedema and it should be treated by 500 ml. of 20% mannitol by infusion. Several days in bed are required after apparent recovery. Occasionally patients show evidence of permanent brain or cardiac damage after recovery.

CYANIDE POISONING

Hydrocyanic acid and potassium or sodium cyanide are very powerful poisons. They act by inhibiting a number of enzymes, the most important of which is cytochrome oxidase. They are used as pesticides and in metallurgy.

Clinical Features. The inhalation of hydrocyanic acid (which is a gas) results in death within a few minutes. After ingestion of cyanide salts, death may occur in anything from a few minutes up to several hours, depending on the dose. Generally speaking the absorption of about 1 mg. of cyanide is fatal.

Treatment. The aim of treatment in cyanide poisoning is to give substances which will combine with cyanide and prevent interference with enzyme systems. The following steps should be taken as rapidly as possible.

(1) Crush ampoules of amyl nitrite and allow the patient to inhale the vapour; this will form some methaemoglobin which combines with cyanide. This should be followed by sodium nitrite 0·3 g. in 10 ml. of water given I.V. over three minutes, to form more methaemoglobin.

(2) Sodium thiosulpate 50 ml. of 50 per cent solution should be given I.V. over ten minutes ; this also combines with cyanide.

(3) The stomach should be washed out with 5 per cent sodium thiosulphate.

(4) Oxygen and artificial respiration may be required.

If available 20 ml. of a 1·5% solution of cobalt edetate given intravenously over one minute is a specific remedy. It can be repeated if the response is adequate.

BARBITURATE POISONING

Barbiturate poisoning is the commonest type of poisoning in Great Britain and stands second to carbon monoxide as a cause of death. Chronic addiction to barbiturates also occurs.

Acute Poisoning

Barbiturates are usually taken in a deliberate suicidal attempt; occasionally by accident. Barbiturate and alcohol poisoning may be combined; these two drugs certainly have an additive effect, and it is believed by some that their actions are synergistic.

The speed of action and duration of effect depend on the type of barbiturate used.

Clinical Features. The symptoms of mild barbiturate overdosage are mental confusion with slurred speech, nystagmus, and unsteady gait. These are followed by deep sleep from which the patient can be roused though perhaps with difficulty. The corneal and pharyngeal reflexes remain and respiration is not markedly depressed. A bullous rash occurs in about 10% of patients with barbiturate overdosage.

In severe barbiturate overdosage there is deep coma, the patient cannot be roused and reflexes have disappeared. Finally death occurs from respiratory depression complicated by circulatory failure. The diagnosis can be confirmed by finding the drug in the urine, blood, or gastric contents.

The blood level of barbiturate is a poor guide as to prognosis as patients vary in their sensitivity to the drug.

Treatment. If the patient is conscious, no treatment will usually be required unless a large dose has just been taken, when it should be removed by gastric lavage.

In the unconscious patient management is:

(1) Ensure a clear airway, if the cough reflex is absent, an endotracheal tube should be introduced.

(2) Ensure adequate ventilation; in a cyanosed patient with respiratory depression some form of mechanical ventilation will be required.

(3) Gastric contents should be aspirated and the stomach washed out only if the drug has been taken within the previous four hours.

(4) Maintain hydration by giving 2·0 litres of intravenous fluid in 24 hours (N/5 dextrose saline).

(5) Treat intercurrent chest infections as they arise.

In severe intoxication however (absent reflexes—depressed respiration), an attempt should be made to increase the rate of barbiturate elimination. Renal excretion of phenobarbitone can be increased by producing a high flow rate of alkaline urine. This is not however effective with the short acting barbiturates which are largely broken down in the liver. For method see page 560).

The death rate from hospital admission with barbiturate poisoning is about 15 per cent.

Chronic Barbiturate Addiction

Chronic barbiturate addiction is by no means uncommon. Patients may indulge in bursts of intoxication or may take the drug regularly. Most addicts suffer from some form of psychological abnormality. If the drug is suddenly stopped a well-marked withdrawal syndrome occurs with weakness, nausea and vomiting, anxiety, and often convulsions.

MORPHINE POISONING

Acute morphine poisoning may result from overdosage during the therapeutic use of the drug or from a suicidal attempt. The lethal dose is variable, but has been given as between 60–240 mg., but it must be realised that repeated dosage quickly produces tolerance of the drug.

Clinical Features. The patient is comatose and cannot be wakened. The respiration rate is very slow. The skin is cyanosed and is cold and clammy. The pupils are pin-point in size. With severe poisoning the blood pressure may fall. Death results from respiratory depression.

Treatment. (1) If the drug has been taken by mouth, wash out the stomach with 1:2,000 potassium permanganate solution.

(2) Nalorphine is a specific antidote for morphine. The dose is 10 mg. intravenously repeated as required every 15 minutes until a total of 40 mg. has been given. The effects of nalorphine usually last for about two hours and if relapse occurs at this time the drug should be repeated. The aim of the treatment with nalorphine is to restore the respiratory rate to normal. Wakening the patient is not necessary. Nalorphine should not be given to morphine addicts as it may produce acute withdrawal symptoms.

(3) If there is severe respiratory depression with cyanosis, oxygen should be given and artificial respiration may be required.

(4) Occasionally respiratory stimulants such as nikethamide 4 ml. of a 25 per cent solution intravenously, or aminophylline 0·5 g. intravenously are useful in patients only partially relieved by nalorphine.

INSECT STINGS

Stings by bees, wasps, and other insects are very common. Usually except for some local pain and swelling which subsides in a few days, these stings cause little trouble. Rarely, a generalised reaction occurs which is occasionally fatal. This is seen particularly in those with a history of allergy.

Treatment consists in the local application of an anti-histamine cream. In the case of the bee, the sting is left behind and may be scraped out. If a severe general reaction occurs 0·5 ml. of 1·1,000 adrenalin is given subcutaneously and an anti-histamine is given intramuscularly (promethazine hydrochloride 50 mg. is satisfactory). In very severe cases hydrocortisone hemisuccinate 100 mg. should be given intravenously. Subjects who have had a severe reaction may be desensitised.

SNAKE BITES

The only poisonous snake in Great Britain is the adder. This snake is under 2 ft. in length, it is brownish in colour with zig-zag black markings on its back.

Clinical Features. There is considerable local swelling and discoloration in the region of the bite. General symptoms include dyspnoea, vomiting, weakness, and collapse. Death may occur, particularly in children.

The following recommendations for treatment are based on those given by T. C. Morton (1960), *Brit. med. J.*, II, 373, whose article should be consulted for further information.

(1) Young children should be removed to hospital if possible. In early cases 1–2 ml. of antivenin serum should be given into the bite. 8·0 ml. of serum should be given intramuscularly combined with hyaluronidase and preceded by an anti-histamine intravenously.

(2) Adults and children over ten years who have no symptoms for two hours after the bite require only rest and an anti-histamine.

(3) Adults with a severe reaction should be given 20 ml. of antivenin serum intramuscularly combined with hyaluronidase and preceded by an anti-histamine intravenously. Other measures in severe cases include hydrocortisone hemisuccinate 100 mg. intravenously. Serum sickness after antivenin is common. The doses given above refer to the Pasteur Institute's E. R. Serum.

LEAD POISONING

Lead poisoning may occur in a number of industries including lead smelting and lead burning, the manufacture of white and red lead and the making of accumulators. Children may also develop lead poisoning from sucking lead-containing paint. Poisoning is infinitely more probable when lead is absorbed through the lungs as dust or fumes rather than when taken by mouth. If lead is absorbed slowly it is stored in the bones. The development of the symptoms of lead poisoning depends not so much on the total amount of lead in the body, but on its rate of absorption or mobilisation from the bones.

Clinical Features

Lead Colic. Intestinal colic and constipation are the most common symptoms of lead poisoning. The pain is usually peri-umbilical and there are no abnormal signs in the abdomen.

Lead Neuropathy. In lead poisoning weakness develops in certain groups of muscles, usually the extensor muscles of the wrist and rarely of the foot. Sensory changes do not occur. The site of the lesion in lead 'neuropathy' is not certain, but is probably in the muscles.

Lead Encephalopathy. This manifestation of lead poisoning is rare. The patient complains of severe headaches and may suddenly develop epileptic fits.

Anaemia. A normocytic hypochromic anaemia occurs in lead poisoning, usually with punctate basophilia.

Gums. Patients with lead poisoning may show a bluish stippled line on the gum margin. It is only found in association with gingivitis and is due to the deposition of lead sulphide in the gums. The lead line may be found in patients without other manifestations of lead poisoning.

Other symptoms consist of weakness, loss of weight, joint pains, and a metallic taste in the mouth.

Generally speaking, a blood level of 80–100 microgrammes of lead per 100 ml. of blood or 200 microgrammes of lead per litre of urine are associated with symptoms of lead poisoning.

Treatment. Lead colic can be relieved by intravenous injections of 10 ml. of a 10 per cent solution of calcium gluconate. Lead can be cleared from the body by using a chelating agent. Certain of these substances form compounds with lead which are soluble and which are excreted by the kidneys. The agent of choice is calcium-disodium edathamil. The lead in the body displaces the calcium from this chelating agent and the resulting compound is excreted. The adult dose is 1 g. twice daily, given by slow intravenous infusion in saline, at intervals of twelve hours. Such treatment may be carried out for five days and then repeated if necessary. A high calcium diet should be given after treatment.

Prophylaxis. Prophylactic measures include:

(1) Avoidance of exposure to lead dust or fumes by ventilation, hygiene, and by wearing masks.

(2) Avoidance of absorption from the intestine by personal cleanliness, including washing of the hands, etc., before meals.

(3) Regular medical examination of those exposed to lead.

(4) A high calcium diet helps to prevent lead poisoning.

FOOD POISONING

Food poisoning may be due to bacteria or viruses, or their products, in the food, to poisonous substances or to allergy to something ingested.

BACTERIAL FOOD POISONING

(1) Staphylococcal

Some strains of staphylococci produce an entero-toxin which is fairly stable to heat and will resist boiling. The chief symptoms which start abruptly in from one to six hours, are nausea, vomiting, intestinal colic, and diarrhoea. The attack is short-lived and is all over within a few hours. It is not usually serious, but rarely there may be collapse with dehydration and deaths have occurred, particularly in young children and the aged.

Treatment. In most cases rest in bed with frequent sips of fluid and mist. kaolin and morphine (B.P.C.) 15 ml. four-hourly will control the symptoms. Rarely if there is collapse with severe dehydration and sodium chloride deficiency, intravenous fluids will be required.

(2) Salmonella

Certain of the salmonella group of organisms produce specific diseases such as typhoid and paratyphoid fevers. Others of the group, particularly S. typhi-murium, S. Newport, S. St. Paul, S. Thompson, and S. Dublin, produce an acute gastroenteritis which presents as a food poisoning.

Clinical Features. The onset is usually within forty-eight hours of eating infected food. The main symptoms are general malaise, headache, and fever combined with vomiting, intestinal colic, and diarrhoea. Occasionally there may be high fever with rigors, suggesting a septicaemia and the spleen may be palpable. The disease usually lasts several days.

The diagnosis is confirmed by culture of the pathogenic organism from the stools. This is important in indicating the most appropriate treatment and in helping to trace the source of infection.

Treatment. General measures include rest in bed and sips of fluid by mouth. If the diarrhoea has been severe, the oral fluids should consist of N/3 saline flavoured with fruit juice. Occasionally when vomiting is severe and prolonged, fluids and electrolytes must be given intravenously and this requires a daily estimation of the blood electrolytes and a full record of fluid balance. The diarrhoea and colic can be controlled by mist. kaolin and morphine 15 ml. four-hourly.

There is little evidence that antibiotic treatment modifies the course of Salmonella gastroenteritis.

(3) Virus

There is no doubt that certain outbreaks of gastroenteritis are due to a virus; they are usually mild and respond to symptomatic treatment.

MUSHROOM POISONING

Mushroom poisoning is usually due to *Amanita phalloides*. This mushroom has a yellow or olive yellow cap with white gills and there is a volva (cup) at the base of the stem.

Clinical Features. There is often a delay of several hours before the onset of symptoms. This is followed by severe abdominal colic with bloody diarrhoea and vomiting. Death may occur from shock or collapse. If the patient survives this stage, acute liver necrosis may develop and prove fatal.

Treatment. The stomach should be washed out. Atropine 1 mg. should be given intravenously and repeated as required. Fluid and electrolyte replacement will be necessary and this will have to be given intravenously. Antiphallinic serum should be given if available. It has been suggested that mashed rabbit stomach and brain should be given as these animals are resistant to mushroom poisoning. Otherwise, treatment is symptomatic.

ALLERGY TO FOOD

Some patients are hypersensitive to certain articles of food and may suffer from urticarial rashes, vomiting, diarrhoea, and even attacks of asthma. It is best for them to avoid such foods although desensitisation can be attempted.

Treatment. An attack due to allergy to food is treated as a sensitisation reaction (p. 553). If diarrhoea is a prominent symptom it can be relieved by a mixture containing morphine, such as mist. kaolin and morphine (N.F.) 15 ml. four-hourly.

FURTHER READING

Matthew, H., and Lawson, A. H. H. *Treatment of Common Acute Poisoning*, 2nd edition, Livingstone, 1970.

CHAPTER TWENTY-THREE

DISEASES DUE TO PHYSICAL AGENTS

DECOMPRESSION SICKNESS

Decompression sickness occurs when people who have been working at a high atmospheric pressure, such as workers in a caisson or diving bell, are suddenly decompressed. It may also occur in a subject who rises quickly to a height above 25,000 ft. In both circumstances, nitrogen rapidly comes out of solution both in the blood and in the tissues and forms bubbles. Oxygen and carbon dioxide also come out of solution, but rapidly diffuse away. These bubbles occur particularly in the nervous system and in adipose tissue, as nitrogen is soluble in fat.

Clinical Features. Within a few hours of decompression the patient complains of severe pain in the muscles and joints. This may be followed by evidence of involvement of the central nervous system, including vertigo, weakness of the limbs, and sphincter disturbances. Various skin rashes may develop.

Treatment. *Preventive.* Where possible workers should not be exposed to pressures greater than 18 lb. to the sq. in., for below this pressure sickness does not occur. If they work under higher pressures they should be slowly decompressed. *Curative.* If decompression sickness develops the subject should be recompressed again and then very slowly decompressed.

MOTION SICKNESS

Motion sickness may occur as a result of sea, land, or air travel. Although the exact mechanism is not known it would seem that repetitive stimulation of the vestibular apparatus plays a large part; it is not possible to produce sickness in animals who have had their vestibular apparatus removed, nor are deaf mutes seasick. Susceptibility to motion sickness varies, but is particularly common in migrainous subjects.

Clinical Features. The victim of motion sickness complains of feeling unwell with nausea, headache, and sometimes faintness. Finally symptoms are such as to require a rapid withdrawal from company and terminate in severe vomiting. The duration of the attack is variable and may last only a few hours, although susceptible subjects may be prostrate for several days.

Treatment. People susceptible to motion sickness should avoid undue movement. When at sea they should remain near the centre of the ship and if possible lie down with the eyes closed. In an aeroplane the head should be rested back on the head rest. Some food should be taken and if this is not possible, barley sugar should be sucked.

Certain drugs diminish the liability to sea-sickness. They are the hyoscine group and the anti-histamines. The most satisfactory drug is not decided, but there is a little evidence that hyoscine is better for short journeys and the anti-histamines for longer ones. The doses are:

Hyoscine, 0·5 mg.–1 mg. according to weight, taken 20 minutes before starting, is suitable for journeys lasting up to four hours. Side effects include dry mouth and paralysis of accommodation.

Cyclizine, 50 mg. three times daily or meclozine 50 mg. daily, are suitable for longer journeys.

Dimenhydrinate (dramamine) 25 mg. three times daily is also suitable, but rather liable to produce drowsiness.

These drugs can be used for children in reduced dosage.

DISORDERS DUE TO HEAT

A number of syndromes may result from exposure to heat, especially in those who have had no opportunity to become acclimatized.

Heat Stroke (Heat hyperpyrexia)

Heat stroke is due to a failure of the heat-controlling mechanism. It may occur merely as a result of exposure to heat or may complicate some pyrexial illness such as malaria. The symptoms are mental confusion, headaches, and inco-ordination proceeding to delirium, convulsions, and death. The body temperature is raised and may be 106° F. or higher. The skin is hot and dry, the sweating mechanism having failed.

Treatment. Heat stroke is a medical emergency and the body must be cooled as rapidly as possible until the rectal temperature is 102° F. This may be achieved by keeping the body surface moist by sponging or by sprays of water and encouraging evaporation by means of fans. The possibility of some complicating infection such as malaria must be remembered and appropriate treatment given.

Heat Exhaustion

Heat exhaustion may occur for a number of reasons and has to be subdivided on this basis:

(a) Salt Deficiency Heat Exhaustion

This is due to salt loss with inadequate replacement.

Clinical Features. The symptoms are those of salt deficiency, i.e. weakness, cramps, vomiting, and collapse with a low blood pressure. The plasma sodium and chloride levels are reduced and the urine may be low in chlorides.

Treatment is aimed at replacing the salt loss and this may be done by mouth, or by intravenous infusion if vomiting is troublesome.

(b) Anhidrotic Heat Exhaustion

Clinical Features. This form of heat exhaustion is usually associated with prickly heat. The symptoms are weakness and irritability and if exertion is attempted the patient may collapse. Examination shows that sweating is confined to localised areas, usually the face and axillae and sometimes the hands and feet. The condition may proceed to heat stroke.

Treatment is to remove the subject to a cooler environment.

In addition, heat exhaustion on effort may occur without clear evidence of either salt deficiency or anhidrosis.

Prickly Heat

Prickly heat is due to excessive sweating. It is a fine papular rash which sometimes becomes vesicular and usually gives a sensation of prickling (thus the name). It may become infected.

Treatment is removal to a cooler and less humid atmosphere.

Sunburn

Sunburn is due to the ultra-violet fraction of sunlight. It may be merely an erythema but if severe the erythema will be accompanied by some local oedema and sometimes headache and pyrexia.

Treatment. Sunburn may be prevented by graduated exposure to direct sunlight and by applying creams which exclude part of the ultra-violet end of the spectrum. If sunburn has occurred further exposure to sunlight should be avoided and some soothing lotion such as oily calamine applied.

DISORDERS DUE TO COLD

They may be either local or general. Local effects in temperate climates are commonly chilblains or Raynaud's phenomenon (p. 172). If cold is extreme, then the tissues of the extremities may freeze, and frostbite result. General effects result from the progressive cooling of the whole body, the syndrome of hypothermia.

Hypothermia

Old people may lose heat from their bodies faster than it can be generated, despite apparently adequate insulation with bedding or clothes, and so pass gradually into hypothermia. This occurs only when the external temperature is very cold.

Aggravating features are malnutrition, loss of mobility from arthritis or paralysis, urinary incontinence, and dementia.

Clinically, the patients become confused, then drowsy, and fall asleep, often in exposed positions. Unless rescued they pass into coma and ultimately die. On examination, their bodies are cold, and the rectal temperature low (usually 80–90° F.). Respiration is slow and shallow, the pulse very slow, and the blood pressure low. The E.C.G. is characteristic (p. 571). Treatment is by warming the body with relays of hot blankets,

E.C.G. in hypothermia, showing J waves from male, aged 80, rectal temperature 76°F., pulse rate 16/min.

correcting electrolyte abnormalities which may be present, and administering intravenous hydrocortisone (100 mg. i.v.) and an antibiotic. Prognosis depends upon how cold the body is on discovery, how old and how frail the patient is, and on co-incident disease. In general it is not good.

ALTITUDE SICKNESS

Altitude sickness is due to hypoxia occurring as a result of the decrease in the partial pressure of oxygen in the atmosphere at high altitudes. It may arise as a result of flying or mountain climbing. Up to 8,000 ft. no symptoms occur, but over 10,000 ft. symptoms may begin to appear. The susceptibility of people varies considerably, being less in the young and healthy and more marked in the elderly and those with respiratory or cardiac disease.

Some acclimatisation can occur to high altitudes. This is brought about by increased respiration, by increase in the pulmonary vascular diffusing surface and by polycythaemia.

Clinical Features

The earliest symptoms are some blunting of mental acuity with motor inco-ordination and slurred speech. These may be followed by headache and weakness. If the degree of hypoxia is increased there will be loss of consciousness and convulsions and finally death.

FURTHER READING

Hunter, D. *Diseases of Occupations*, 4th edition, E.U.P., 1969.

CHAPTER TWENTY-FOUR

THE STEROIDS

There are now a number of substances which in structure and actions are similar to cortisone and which are collectively known as the steroids. They all have the following actions to a greater or lesser extent.

(1) *Carbohydrate and protein metabolism*. The steroids cause breakdown of protein and the release of glucose, with increased resistance to the action of insulin. Occasionally patients receiving steroid hormones develop *diabetes mellitus*. Prolonged treatment with high doses of steroids causes withdrawal of bone matrix (osteoporosis, p. 172). This is associated with loss of calcium from the skeleton and a negative calcium balance.

(2) *Electrolyte balance*. This group of drugs leads to retention of sodium and water and loss of potassium through the kidneys. Oedema of the ankles and eventually hypertension may develop.

Potassium deficiency can be avoided in patients taking large doses of steroids over a long period by giving potassium as a slow release compound by mouth (see p. 396).

(3) *Effect on the inflammatory reaction*. The steroids suppress both the local and general response to infection. This may lead to a rapid spread of the infection without the usual symptoms and signs.

(4) *Effect on allergic reaction*. These drugs suppress both the allergic reaction and the formation of antibodies.

(5) *Peptic ulceration*. Corticosteroids may cause peptic ulcers or exacerbations of those already present. The reason for this is not known.

(6) *The eye*. Steroids may precipitate glaucoma in those prone to this condition. Prolonged use may also cause cataracts. Local steroids must be used with great care in infectious conditions of the eye as unless the infection is controlled it will spread with disastrous results.

(7) *Other effects*. Prolonged treatment with these drugs leads to an appearance similar to that found in Cushing's disease. In addition, mental disturbances may occur, particularly in people who have previously been unstable mentally; such a history is therefore an important contra-indication to treatment with corticosteroids.

(8) *Steroid therapy* which has persisted for six months or longer leads to atrophy of the adrenal cortex. This is a potentially dangerous situation, since the adrenals can no longer react to stress by boosting the secretion of cortical hormones and a state of collapse similar to an Addisonian crisis

may be induced by any acute infection, injury, or emotional shock. Such Addisonian shock may occur not only in patients still receiving long-term steroid therapy, but for up to two years after it has been discontinued. These patients must be warned that if they contract any acute illness or injury steroid therapy must be resumed immediately, or if they are still being treated the dose must be increased to two or three times its maintenance level until the acute episode is over.

Short courses of injections of ACTH every few months are sometimes given to patients on long-term corticosteroid therapy to stimulate and so prevent atrophy of the adrenal cortex. Sound in theory, this procedure has not yet been shown to be effective in practice.

Therapeutic Use

These drugs are used in the treatment of a number of diseases. They can be given locally or systemically. The more important diseases which can be treated are:

(1) *Collagen diseases.*	Rheumatoid arthritis. Rheumatic fever. Systemic lupus erythematosus. Polyarteritis nodosa. Giant-cell arteritis (temporal arteritis).
(2) *Allergic diseases.*	Asthma. Hay fever. Angioneurotic oedema. Eczema (applied locally). Serum sickness.
(3) *Blood diseases.*	Acute and chronic haemolytic anaemia. Idiopathic thrombocytopenic purpura. Acute leukaemia. Drug-induced bone-marrow depression.
(4) *Miscellaneous group.*	Nephrotic syndrome. Ulcerative colitis. Sarcoidosis.
(5) *Eye disease.*	Applied locally in various inflammatory diseases of the eye.
(6) *Replacement therapy.*	Addison's disease or after adrenalectomy.

The following preparations are available and are given with equivalent doses:

(1) Cortisone 100 mg. (4) Prednisone 20 mg.
(2) Hydrocortisone 80 mg. (5) Triamcinolone 16 mg.
(3) Prednisolone 20 mg. (6) Methyl prednisolone 16 mg.
(7) Dexamethasone 3·0 mg.

It is difficult to decide which is the best steroid to use. Except for replacement therapy, the steroid with the maximum therapeutic effect and the least salt-retaining properties would be the most satisfactory. It would appear that on these grounds dexamethasone is the best, but clinical experience is not very large with this drug. It is recommended, therefore, that prednisolone, with which there is a considerable amount of experience, should be used, but it is possible that it will be replaced by a better steroid in the future.

For replacement therapy, cortisone is usually the best, as a certain amount of salt retention is required in these circumstances.

Dosage

The correct dose of a steroid is the minimum amount of drug required to produce the desired effect, and it varies considerably. In general, if the dose does not exceed 10 mg. of prednisolone daily, side effects are much less common than with higher doses. For replacement therapy the dose usually is 50 mg. of cortisone; for other purposes it is usually necessary to start with 200–300 mg. of cortisone, though for maintenance of the effect as little as 25–50 mg. may be enough. Patients taking cortisone should be seen regularly and the following points noted:

(1) *General appearance*—any evidence of Cushing-like appearance.

(2) *Any dyspepsia suggestive of peptic ulcer.* If ulcer symptoms develop the steroid is usually stopped. If steroid therapy is vital it will have to be continued together with a full ulcer regime.

(3) *Blood pressure.*

(4) *Urine* must be tested for sugar.

(5) *Blood electrolytes* must be estimated in patients undergoing prolonged therapy with these drugs, particularly if there is evidence of renal damage. A close watch should be kept for undue potassium loss or sodium retention.

(6) *Any evidence of infection* (note that the symptoms may be masked). See under (8) on page 572.

(7) Enquire about backache, which might suggest the development of osteoporosis.

ANTIBIOTICS

Drug	Dose	Sensitive Organisms	Side Effects	Comments
Sulphonamides *Rapidly absorbed* Sulphadimidine Sulphadiazine Sulphafurazole Sulphamethizole	*Orally* 3 g. stat 1 g. 4 or 6 hourly 0·1 g. 4 or 6 hourly	Strep. pneumoniae Strep. pyogenes Meningococcus Gonococcus Shigellae E. coli.	Precipitation in the urinary tract. Nausea and vomiting. Rashes. Drug fever Agranulocytosis	High fluid intake required with rapidly absorbed sulphonamides except sulphamethizole. Sulphadiazine penetrates meninges very well.
Poorly absorbed Succinylsulphathiazole Phthalylsulphathiazole	4 g. stat. 3 g. 6 or 8 hourly			Poorly absorbed group used for intestinal infection and sterilising gut.
Long acting Sulphamethoxypyridazine Sulphamethoxydiazine	1 g. stat. 0·5 g. daily			High degree of protein binding leads to slow excretion and prolonged action.
Co-trimoxazole (Septrin–Bactrim) *Each tablet contains 80 mg. Trimethoprim and 400 mg. Sulphamethoxazole.*	tabs. 1–2 twice daily orally	Most pyogenic cocci and many Gram-negative organisms.		Most useful in bronchitis and urinary infections.
Nitrofurantoin	50–100 mg. t.d.s.	E. coli. B. Proteus.	Nausea (give after food) Neuritis Hyperpyrexia	Concentrated by the kidney and only used for renal infection.

Drug	Dose	Administration	Sensitive Organisms	Side Effects	Comments
Penicillin Benzylpenicillin	300 mg. (500,000 units) per injection 20,000 units	Intramuscularly Intrathecally	Strep. pyogenes Strep. pneumoniae Staph. aureus		Benzylpenicillin rapidly absorbed from injection site and excreted, must be given 6 hourly.
Procaine penicillin	600 mg. (600,000 units) per injection	Intramuscularly	Strep. viridans		Procaine penicillin more slowly mobilised 12 hourly injection satisfactory.
Benzathine penicillin	600,000 units	Intramuscularly	Meningococcus	Sensitisation reactions. Skin rashes and rarely collapse.	Benzathine penicillin slowly excreted. One injection adequate for sensitive organism.
			Gonococcus B anthracis Treponema pallida Actinomyces bovis		Very little to choose between them. Effective in all but severe infections provided organism is sensitive.
Oral penicillins Phenoxymethylpenicillin Phenethicillin	250 mg. q.i.d. 250 mg. q.i.d.	Oral			
Ampicillin	250 mg. q.i.d.	Oral	Similar to above with addition of Salmonellae Shigellae E. coli & H. influenzae		Useful in urinary and gut infection, and in chronic bronchitis.
Cloxacillin	500 mg. q.i.d. 250 mg. 4 hourly	Oral Intramuscular	Effective against resistant staphs.		Reserved for severe staph. infections.
Flucloxacillin	250 mg. q.i.d.	Oral			

Penicillin is the most generally useful antibiotic. A satisfactory treatment for infection by a sensitive organism is benzylpenicillin 300 mg. followed by either procaine penicillin 600 mg. 12 hours or phenoxymethylpenicillin 250 mg. q.i.d. In mild infections oral penicillin alone is adequate. In overwhelming infection or that by partially resistant organism larger doses must be given by injection. Penicillin does not cross the meningeal barrier in adequate concentrations and must be given intrathecally in meningitis. Hypersensitivity reactions are not uncommon and the patient must always be asked if he is sensitive to penicillin before treatment.

Drug	Dose	Administration	Sensitive Organisms	Side Effects	Comments
Tetracycline **Chlortetracycline** **Oxytetracycline**	250 mg. q.i.d.	oral	Broad Spectrum	1. Diarrhoea. 2. Gut superinfection with staphs. 3. Candida mouth infection. 4. Discoloration of growing teeth.	Particularly useful in recurrent bronchitis, urinary infections, lymphogranuloma brucellosis, typhus.
Demethylchlortetra-cycline	150 mg, q.i.d.	oral oral			Similar to above but longer action.

In spite of their wide antibacterial spectrum tetracycline must not be used indiscriminately because of side effects. Particular care is required in pregnancy and infancy, when they should be avoided if possible.

Drug	Dose	Administration	Sensitive Organisms	Side Effects	Comments
Chloramphenicol	500 mg. q.i.d. 3·0 g. daily	oral IV drip	Broad Spectrum including Salm typhii, H. influenzae and rickettsiae	Marrow aplasia rare but usually fatal.	H. influenzae meningitis Typhoid

Owing to side effects, chloramphenicol should only be used as indicated or in a severe infection resistant to other antibiotics.

Drug	Dose	Administration	Sensitive Organisms	Side Effects	Comments
Erythromycin	250 mg. q.i.d.	oral	Str. pneumoniae ,, pyogenes ,, viridans Staphs C. diphtheriae N. gonorrhoea H. influenzae and H. pertussis		Resistant staphs,, H. influenzae infection—Diphtheria. Useful in patient sensitive to penicillin.

Drug	Dose	Administration	Sensitive Organisms	Side Effects	Comments
Cephalorin	500 mg. q.i.d.	I.M.	Broad spectrum including penicillin resistant staphs, E. coli & proteus.	Possibly skin rashes	
Cephalexin	0·5–1·0 g. three times daily	oral	Broad spectrum		
Rifampicin	450–600 mg. daily	oral	Many gram + and some gram – organisms and M. tuberculosis.	Colours urine and sputum red. Disturbs hepatic function tests	Useful in tuberculosis.
Streptomycin	0·5 g. b.d.	I.M.	Myco tuberculosis, E. coli, H. influenzae, Shigellae; orally for gut infections	8th nerve damage: particularly in elderly and in renal failure,	Tuberculosis—Short courses in other infections by sensitive organisms.
	2·0–3·0 g. daily	oral			
Gentamycin	0·8–1·2 mg./kg. daily, divided into three doses	I.M.	Gram – organisms	8th nerve damage	Severe urinary infections and gram – septicaemias.
Colistin	50,000 units/kg./ 24 hours	I.M./ Locally	P. pyocyaneus	Rashes	Pyocyaneus infections.
Sodium fusidate	500 mg. three times daily	oral	Staphylococci		Used largely for resistant staphylococci.

INDEX

"a" wave, 97
Abortion, 40
Abortus fever, 509
Abreaction, 49
Achalasia of the cardia, 65
Acholuric jaundice, 471
Achondroplasia, 354
Acid/base disturbances, 397
Acidosis, 400, 401
  metabolic, 401
  respiratory, 400
Acne vulgaris, 539
Acrocyanosis, 173
Acromegaly, 436
Acrosclerosis, 334
Actinomycosis, 512
Acyanotic heart disease, 148
Addiction to drugs or alcohol, 20
Addisonian crisis, 451
Addison's anaemia, 469
Addison's disease, 450
Adenoviruses, 507
Adie's syndrome, 250
Adrenal function tests, 446
Adrenal gland, 446
  adenoma of, 447
  diseases of, 446
  insufficiency of, 450
Adrenal medulla, overaction of, 450
Adreno-cortical overaction, 447
Adreno-genital syndrome, 447
Aegophony, 190
Affective disorders, 13, 26
Agranulocytosis, 478
Air encephalography, 290
Air hunger, 186
Alastrim, 498
Alber's-Schonberg's disease, 353
Alcoholic cardiomyopathy, 146
Alcoholism, 20
Aldosteronism, primary, 449
Alimentary system, 61
  in hypercalcaemia, 346
  in renal failure, 377
  lesions causing anaemia, 471
Alkalosis, 400, 402
  metabolic, 402
  respiratory, 400
Allergy, and drug reactions, 550
  to food, 567
Altitude sickness, 571
Alveolar-capillary block, 183
Amentias, 14
Amoebiasis, 516
  hepatic, 518
Amoebic dysentery, 517
Amoebic colitis, 517
Amyloid disease, 432
  kidney in, 388
Amyotrophic lateral sclerosis, 294
Anaemia, 464
  aplastic, 478

caused by circulating haemolysins, 473
classification, 464
Cooley's, 472
definition, 464
drug induced, 552
haemolytic, 471
in lead poisoning, 565
in renal failure, 377
investigation, 465
iron deficiency, 466
macrocytic, 469
megaloblastic, 469
non-spherocytic, 473
pernicious, 469
sickle-cell, 472
sideroblastic, 468
Analgesic nephropathy, 388
Anaphylactic reactions, 326
Anaphylactoid purpura, 477
Anarthria, 257
Aneurysm, dissecting, 145
Angina pectoris, 155
  in aortic valve disease, 141
Angina of effort, 155
Angioneurotic oedema, 539
Ankylosing spondylitis, 339
Ankylostoma duodenale, 529
Anorexia nervosa, 41
Anosmia, 246
Anovulation, 455
Antibiotics, 575
Antibody production, disorders of, 323
Anticoagulants, in coronary artery disease, 160
  in pulmonary embolism, 168
Anti-depressants, 51
Anti-diuretic hormone, 357
  inappropriate secretion of, 421
Anti-excitement drugs, 52
Anti-nuclear factor, 330
Anxiety states, 9, 13, 26
Aorta, abdominal, 145
  coarctation of, 148
  syphilitic disease of, 143
Aortic aneurysm, 143
Aortic regurgitation, 142
Aortic stenosis, 140
Aortic valve disease, 140
Aphasia, 257
Apical systolic murmurs, innocent, 139
Aplastic anaemia, 478
Argyll-Robertson pupils, 251, 285, 286
Arrhenoblastoma, 447
Arrhythmias, 115
  in myocardial infarction, 160
Arterial disease, 170
  atheroma and, 424
Arterial occlusion, 172
Arterial pulse, 95
Arteriosclerotic parkinsonism, 299
Arthritis, in gout, 428
  in Reiter's syndrome, 340